Sport and Exercise Psychology Research

From Theory to Practice

Sport and Exercise Psychology Research

From Theory to Practice

Edited by

Markus Raab
Department of Performance Psychology, German Sport University
Cologne, Institute of Psychology, Cologne, Germany; School of Applied
Sciences, London South Bank University, London, United Kingdom

Paul Wylleman
Research Group Sport Psychology and Mental Support (SPMB),
Department of Movement and Sport Sciences, Faculty of Physical
Education and Physiotherapy and Faculty of Psychology and Educational
Sciences, Vrije Universiteit Brussel, Brussels, Belgium

Roland Seiler
Department II (Sport Psychology), Institute of Sport Science, University
of Bern, Bern, Switzerland

Anne-Marie Elbe
Department of Nutrition, Exercise and Sports, University of Copenhagen,
Copenhagen, Denmark

Antonis Hatzigeorgiadis
Department of Physical Education and Sport Science, University
of Thessaly, Trikala, Greece

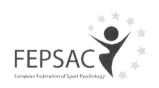

FEPSAC
European Federation of Sport Psychology

ELSEVIER

AMSTERDAM • BOSTON • HEIDELBERG • LONDON
NEW YORK • OXFORD • PARIS • SAN DIEGO
SAN FRANCISCO • SINGAPORE • SYDNEY • TOKYO
Academic Press is an imprint of Elsevier

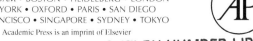

Academic Press is an imprint of Elsevier
125 London Wall, London EC2Y 5AS, United Kingdom
525 B Street, Suite 1800, San Diego, CA 92101-4495, United States
50 Hampshire Street, 5th Floor, Cambridge, MA 02139, United States
The Boulevard, Langford Lane, Kidlington, Oxford OX5 1GB, UK

Library of Congress Cataloging-in-Publication Data
A catalog record for this book is available from the Library of Congress

British Library Cataloguing-in-Publication Data
A catalogue record for this book is available from the British Library

ISBN: 978-0-12-803634-1

For information on all Academic Press publications
visit our website at https://www.elsevier.com/

Working together
to grow libraries in
developing countries

www.elsevier.com • www.bookaid.org

Publisher: Nikki Levy
Acquisition Editor: Nikki Levy
Editorial Project Manager: Barb Makinster
Production Project Manager: Jason Mitchell
Designer: Matthew Limbert

Typeset by Thomson Digital

Contents

Section I
Prerequisites of Sport and Exercise Psychology

6.   **Perspectives on Team Cognition and Team Sports**

Nathan McNeese, Nancy J. Cooke, Mike Fedele, and Rob Gray

Section II
Individual Differences in Sport and Exercise Psychology

7.   **Antecedents of Need Supportive and Controlling Interpersonal Styles From a Self-Determination Theory Perspective: A Review and Implications for Sport Psychology Research**

Doris Matosic, Nikos Ntoumanis, and Eleanor Quested

Section III
Perspectives From Sport Psychology

Section IV
Perspectives From Exercise Psychology

17. Empowering and Disempowering Coaching Climates: Conceptualization, Measurement Considerations, and Intervention Implications
Joan L. Duda and Paul R. Appleton

18. Escape From Cognitivism: Exercise as Hedonic Experience
Panteleimon Ekkekakis and Zachary Zenko

Contributors

Mark S. Allen, University of Wollongong, School of Psychology, Wollongong, Australia

Paul R. Appleton, School of Sport, Exercise and Rehabilitation Sciences, University of Birmingham, Birmingham, United Kingdom

Luis Calmeiro, Department of Sport and Exercise Sciences, Abertay University, School of Social and Health Sciences, Dundee, Scotland

Nancy J. Cooke, Human Systems Engineering, Arizona State University, Phoenix, AZ, United States

Margarida Gaspar de Matos, Department of Education, Social Sciences and Humanities, University of Lisbon, Faculty of Human Movement, Lisbon, Spain

Joan L. Duda, School of Sport, Exercise and Rehabilitation Sciences, University of Birmingham, Birmingham, United Kingdom

Panteleimon Ekkekakis, Department of Kinesiology, Iowa State University, Ames, IA, United States

Anne-Marie Elbe, Department of Nutrition, Exercise and Sports, University of Copenhagen, Copenhagen, Denmark

Kari Fasting, Department of Cultural and Social Studies, Norwegian School of Sport Science, Oslo, Norway

Mike Fedele, Human Systems Engineering, Arizona State University, Phoenix, AZ, United States

Cornelia Frank, Neurocognition and Action Research Group and Cognitive Interaction Technology Center of Excellence (CITEC), Bielefeld University, Germany

Evangelos Galanis, Department of Physical Education and Sport Science, University of Thessaly, Trikala, Greece

Ben Godde, Department of Psychology & Methods, Jacobs University, Bremen, Germany

Rob Gray, Human Systems Engineering, Arizona State University, Phoenix, AZ, United States

Lena Hübner, Institute of Human Movement Science and Health, Technische Universität Chemnitz, Chemnitz, Germany

Chris Harwood, School of Sport, Exercise and Health Sciences, Loughborough University, Loughborough, United Kingdom

Antonis Hatzigeorgiadis, Department of Physical Education and Sport Science, University of Thessaly, Trikala, Greece

André Klostermann, Department of Movement and Exercise Science, Institute of Sport Science, University of Bern, Bern, Switzerland

Sylvain Laborde, Department of Performance Psychology, German Sport University Cologne, Cologne, Germany; University of Caen, France

Sergio Lara-Bercial, School of Sport, Carnegie Faculty & International Council for Coaching Excellence, Leeds Beckett University, Leeds, United Kingdom

Clifford J. Mallett, School of Human Movement and Nutrition Sciences, The University of Queensland, Brisbane, Australia

Doris Matosic, School of Sport, Exercise, and Rehabilitation Sciences, University of Birmingham, Birmingham, United Kingdom

Nathan McNeese, Human Systems Engineering, Arizona State University, Phoenix, AZ, United States

Eleftheria Morela, Department of Physical Education and Sport Science, University of Thessaly, Trikala, Greece; Department of Nutrition, Exercise and Sports, University of Copenhagen, Copenhagen, Denmark

Claudia Niemann, Institute of Human Movement Science and Health, Technische Universität Chemnitz, Chemnitz, Germany

Nikos Ntoumanis, School of Psychology & Speech Pathology, Curtin University, Perth, Australia

Jeannine Ohlert, The German Research Centre for Elite Sport and Institute of Psychology, German Sport University, Cologne, Germany

Eleanor Quested, School of Psychology & Speech Pathology, Curtin University, Perth, Australia

Markus Raab, Department of Performance Psychology, German Sport University Cologne, Institute of Psychology, Cologne, Germany; School of Applied Sciences, London South Bank University, London, United Kingdom

Kirsten Kaya Roessler, Department of Psychology, Faculty of Health Sciences, University of Southern Denmark, Odense, Denmark

Nathalie Rosier, Faculty of Physical Education and Physiotherapy, Vrije Universiteit Brussel, Brussels, Belgium

Xavier Sanchez, Department of Medical and Sport Sciences, University of Cumbria, Lancaster, United Kingdom

Nele Schlapkohl, Department of Sport Science, Institute for Health, Nutrition and Sport, Europa University Flensburg, Flensburg, Germany

Roland Seiler, Department II (Sport Psychology), Institute of Sport Science, University of Bern, Bern, Switzerland

Alison L. Smith, Department for Health, University of Bath, Bath, United Kingdom

Natalia B. Stambulova, School of Health and Welfare, Halmstad University, Halmstad, Sweden

Yannis Theodorakis, Department of Physical Education and Sport Science, University of Thessaly, Trikala, Greece

Claudia Voelcker-Rehage, Institute of Human Movement Science and Health, Technische Universität Chemnitz, Chemnitz, Germany

Axel H. Winneke, Project Group Hearing, Speech and Audio Technology, Fraunhofer Institute for Digital Media Technology, Oldenburg, Germany

Paul Wylleman, Research Group Sport Psychology and Mental Support (SPMB), Department of Movement and Sport Sciences, Faculty of Physical Education and Physiotherapy and Faculty of Psychology and Educational Sciences, Vrije Universiteit Brussel, Brussels, Belgium

Zachary Zenko, Department of Kinesiology, Iowa State University, Ames, IA, United States

Christian Zepp, Department of Health and Social Psychology, Institute of Psychology, German Sport University, Cologne, Germany

Nikos Zourbanos, Department of Physical Education and Sport Science, University of Thessaly, Trikala, Greece

Preface

The scope of this book is to present a unique collective volume written by experts, with the aims of (1) providing a scientific guide for the sport and exercise psychology field and (2) providing a bridge from research to practice in our field.

WHAT IS IT ABOUT?

Sport and exercise psychology is a timely and interdisciplinary research field. This field has the benefit of incorporating experts with a wide range of expertise, ranging from basic research (eg, neurosciences and perceptual psychology) up to applied practice (interventions and injury prevention). This fascinating potential requires interdisciplinary perspectives since the research carried out in this field is continuously accumulating and expanding, as shown by recent international sport and exercise psychology conferences.

The nature of interdisciplinary research impels summarizing and synthesizing. While most research laboratories engage in a "'fast-forward' way of conducting empirical research and publishing, there are few attempts to summarize the current knowledge that is continuously acquired. Quite often significant contributions of young researchers remain unnoticed or underevaluated, due to the large volume of research output, and the quick and easy access to information via the Internet. By promoting the young researchers and giving them a forum to express their views, one can foresee the developments of the sport and exercise psychology field in the future. Moreover, by synthesizing the perspectives of these young researchers, one can add value and credibility to the field of sport and exercise psychology. The future of the field of sport and exercise psychology belongs to its current aspiring young researchers, and as such, it should be paved by synthesizing the "state of the art" of substantial contemporary scientific contributions in theoretical, empirical, and applied domains. This approach could produce a book that is not only a valid reference point to begin one's academic endeavors (eg, the student, the researcher), but also for the practitioner (eg, the athlete, the coach), and the specialist (eg, the sport psychologist, the sport science expert). Thus, new and innovative for the target group we have in mind this book can be used for basic and applied research and can be used for both sport psychology and exercise psychology. We invited past and present keynotes speakers as well as young award winners in our field nominated by the European Federation of Sport Psychology to suggest hot topics in their areas of research that pave the way to future development of sport psychology, which celebrated the 50th anniversary of the International Society of Sport Psychology in 2015 and will celebrate the 50th anniversary of the European Federation of Sport Psychology in 2019.

HOW IS THE BOOK STRUCTURED?

The book is structured in four sections and starts with a reflection of the past, present, and future of sport and exercise psychology by two past-presidents of the European Federation of Sport Psychology (Chapter 1).

Section I introduces basic processes involved in sport psychology–related topics such as, how to provide learning environments via instructions and feedback (Chapter 2), brain and behavior processes related to lifelong physical activity and fitness (Chapter 3), how perception and action interact (Chapter 4), how mental representations of movements develop (Chapter 5), and finally how we can access sport team dynamics (Chapter 6).

Section II focuses on individual behavior such as personal and contextual factors that promote healthy activity (Chapter 7), the effectiveness of self-talk (Chapter 8), personality-trait-like individual differences (Chapter 9), and acculturation through sport (Chapter 10). Section III focuses on perspectives from sport psychology such as the perspective of a scientific practitioner (Chapter 11), the perspective of career transitions (Chapter 12), a holistic perspective of athlete development (Chapter 13), the perspective from winning coaches (Chapter 14), the implications for sport psychologists in cases of sexual harassment and abuse (Chapter 15), and team diagnostics and interventions (Chapter 16). Section IV summarizes perspectives from exercise psychology such as how to promote adolescent physical activity (Chapter 17), exercise as a hedonic experience (Chapter 18), coaches' behavior as predictor of well-being in sport (Chapter 19), health promotion through health assets and active lifestyles (Chapter 20), and the relevance of emotional experience for health prevention and treatment (Chapter 21).

In sum 21 chapters provide a scientific guide to sport and exercise psychology from research to practice. This book is the culmination of the efforts of many people we would like to thank. First and foremost, we would like to thank the authors who put tremendous effort in completing this book that at the same time archives their impact to the field. For editorial management and coordination, we would like to thank Ms Markus, Cologne, who was very helpful in setting and monitoring deadlines and providing feedback on format. Finally, thanks to Nikki Levy and Barbara Makinster at Elsevier for rapid quality feedback and support for this book.

We hope that you will enjoy our road from research to practice that is simultaneously a tribute to our 50th anniversary celebration of FEPSAC the European Association of Sport Psychology in 2019.

Markus Raab, Paul Wylleman, Roland Seiler, Anne-Marie Elbe, and Antonis Hatzigeorgiadis Cologne, Dec. 2015

Chapter 1

European Perspective on Sport Psychology[a]

Paul Wylleman*, Roland Seiler**

*Research Group Sport Psychology and Mental Support (SPMB), Department of Movement and Sport Sciences, Faculty of Physical Education and Physiotherapy and Faculty of Psychology and Educational Sciences, Vrije Universiteit Brussel, Brussels, Belgium; **Department II (Sport Psychology), Institute of Sport Science, University of Bern, Bern, Switzerland

The 2015 FEPSAC European Congress of Sport Psychology held in Bern, Switzerland, was not only the 14th quadrennial congress of its kind, it also gathered the largest number of presenters in the history of FEPSAC, including 6 keynote lectures, 81 symposia, 38 workshops, and 8 special sessions and about 400 poster presentations (14th European Congress of Sport Psychology, 2015).

Situated within a broader perspective, the attractiveness and success of the 2015 congress can be considered the pinnacle of the development FEPSAC has experienced during the past decade. More particularly, FEPSAC's development has been characterized by, among others, the establishment of a biannual congress/conference schedule (ie, 2013 FEPSAC Conference in Paris, 2015 FEPSAC Congress in Bern, 2017 FEPSAC Conference in Nottingham, 2019 FEPSAC Congress in Münster), and by an increased international collaboration with major actors in the domains of psychology (eg, with the European Federation of Psychologists' Associations, EFPA) and sport sciences (eg, the European College of Sport Sciences, ECSS) in Europe. In this way, FEPSAC does not only provide for a growing number of researchers, applied sport psychologists, students, and others to gain and share knowledge and expertise, but also confirms its premiere position as leading organization representing the domain of sport psychology in Europe.

---

[a] This chapter is a substantially revised and updated version of the article of R. Seiler & P. Wylleman, "FEPSAC's role and position in the past and in the future of sport psychology in Europe," published 2009 in *Psychology of Sport and Exercise, 10*, 403–409.

Sport and Exercise Psychology Research. http://dx.doi.org/10.1016/B978-0-12-803634-1.00001-7

1

The current interest in, and the significance of, the domain of sport psychology[b] in Europe has, however, not always been so distinct nor always positive. In fact, it is important to remember that when the Fédération Européenne de Psychologie des Sports et des Activités Corporelles (FEPSAC) was founded in 1969, sport psychology was actually not "a desirable field" (Geron, 2003, p. 19). In order to understand sport psychology's huge—albeit slow—development in Europe during the past 25–30 years, this chapter will in first instance look back in order to trace the roots of European sport psychology and FEPSAC. We use historical documents and all publications from FEPSAC, as well as other reports on the history of sport psychology for a hermeneutical interpretation. After looking at the different developments that have shaped the past, a second part describes the challenges both FEPSAC and sport psychology in Europe are facing. Finally, this chapter concludes with some reflections on the possible future of the domain of sport psychology.

IDENTIFYING AND UNDERSTANDING THE HISTORICAL ROOTS

In this first section, the development of sport psychology in Europe is integrated in the context of the history of the continent with its enormous cultural and political variety, while also taking into account international developments.

Development of Sport Psychology in Europe Until World War II

Historical Roots of Sport Psychology in Europe

Many international sport psychology textbooks that include a section on the development of sport psychology agree in identifying the end of the 19th and the beginning of the 20th century as the onset of academic study in sport psychology. Interestingly, many authors locate the place of birth in North America where notably the names of Norman Triplett and Coleman Griffith are usually mentioned as key people, the latter often being considered to be the "founding father" of sport psychology (eg, Brewer & Van Raalte, 2002; Cox, Qi, & Liu, 1993; Weinberg & Gould, 2003).

This restricted view neglects that psychological questions concerning sport, physical activity, and physical education were treated widely in Europe, for example, in the tradition of Wilhelm Wundt in Leipzig, as well as in France, Italy,

---

[b] Based on the definition of the term "sport psychology" in European Federation of Sport Psychology (1995) Position Statement #1, and taking into account the terminology in various European languages and cultures, the term "sport psychology" is used to characterize psychologically based approaches to all sorts of sport, play, exercise, physical activity, or culture, including competitive and leisure sport, physical education, HEPA (health-enhancing physical activity), APA (adapted physical activity), and other areas. This does not ignore the definitional differentiation that has been initiated in the late 1980s mainly in the Anglo-Saxon world (Rejeski & Brawley, 1988).

and Hungary (Bäumler, 2002; Janssen, 2009; Kunath, 2003; Nitsch, Gabler, & Singer, 2000), resulting in a considerable number of publications between 1894 and 1900. These covered themes such as personality and character development, the relation between physical strain and mental performance in schools, pathological and psychohygenic effects of physical activity, and contributions on training and competition. However, all these contributions, though partially empirical and of high theoretical importance, were not based on experimental studies, and authors only occasionally worked in the field of sport and physical activity.

The term "sport psychology" (*psychologie du sport* in French) was seemingly first introduced in 1900 by Pierre de Coubertin, the founder of the Olympic Games of the modern era, in an essay where he distinguished combat sports from equilibrium sports (de Coubertin, 1900). The beginning of the 20th century was characterized by a further differentiation of sport, including the foundation of many international sport federations. The need increased for scientific treatment of evolving questions in sport psychology as well. This initiated a transition from a period of pioneering work to a period of institutionalization, resulting in the first international congress on sport psychology in 1913 in Lausanne, Switzerland (Comité International Olympique, 1913; see also Kunath, 2003). This conference was initiated and prepared well in advance by de Coubertin. In the same year, his essays in sport psychology were published (de Coubertin, 1913). Unfortunately, World War I interrupted this positive development.

Only 2 years after the end of World War I, in 1920, a psycho-technical laboratory was established by Robert Werner Schulte at the German High School for Physical Exercise (DHfL) in Berlin (Kunath, 2003; Nitsch et al., 2000), 5 years before Griffith founded his lab at the University of Illinois in 1925 (Brewer & Van Raalte, 2002). The research in Berlin covered a broad range of themes, including the effects of sport on personality and cognitive performance, as well as psychomotor peculiarities of different sports and skills, resulting in several books (Schulte, 1921, 1928; Nitsch et al., 2000).

In the Soviet Union, a similar development took place with the establishment by Rudik of a sport psychology laboratory in 1925 at the State Central Institute of Physical Culture in Moscow (Ryba, Stambulova, & Wrisberg, 2005). At the Lesgaft Institute for Physical Culture in the then Leningrad (now St. Petersburg), research in sport psychology was mainly conducted and published by Puni, who entered the institute as a student in 1929. He had conducted his first study on psycho-physiological effects of training in table tennis already in 1927 and was mainly interested in the psychology of performance (Ryba et al., 2005; Stambulova, Wrisberg, & Ryba, 2006).

Economic depression in the 1930s and the ideological agnosticism of the Nazi regime resulted in a rapid decline of sport psychology in Germany. The humanistic catastrophe of the persecution and genocide of the Jews and the destruction of major cities and areas during World War II almost completely stopped scientific research and exchange in sport psychology. Astonishingly enough the International Olympic Committee organized a scientific Congress at the occasion of the 50th anniversary of the Olympic movement during the war in 1944 in Lausanne. Almost 400 participants from 33 countries, many of them refugees in Switzerland, attended this congress on psychology and pedagogy of sport. On the sport psychology day, 16 papers were presented, and a proceedings book was published after the war in 1947 (Bureau International de Pédagogie Sportive et Institut Olympique de Lausanne, 1947). Maybe due to more vital problems in those years, this book hardly gained much attention.

Diversity of Theoretical Traditions and Cultures

An important aspect when looking at European sport psychology is the different psychological backgrounds. In different major language regions in Europe, such as French, German, Spanish, Russian, or English, diverse cultural and philosophical traditions had evolved. With this background, psychological concepts developed in a differentiated way, and since only few translations were available in the first half of the last century, exchange remained sparse.

One psychological tradition, the cultural–historical school, theoretically supports this observation. Established in the 1920s, and influenced strongly by the historical materialism of Marx and Engels, the cultural–historical school in Russian psychology (Rubinstein, 1958/1946) was represented among others by Vygotski, Lurija, and Leont'ew (Kölbl, 2006). This school claimed that psychological functions (1) are a result of the cultural and historical development of society, (2) are based on material foundations, and (3) evolve in the course of activity. The conceptions of a subjective internal representation of the external world and higher nervous functions were theoretical contrapositions against a simple reactive understanding of the human being, as suggested in behaviorism (Kölbl, 2006; Mintz, 1958).

Psychology in France was influenced by different contemporary trends. For example, Ribot established "scientific," that is, experimental, psychology in the tradition of Wundt in the last decennials of the 19th century (Nicolas & Murray, 2000). Others adopted the work of Merlau-Ponty's embodied phenomenology (1963/1942, 2012/1945), psychoanalytical approaches, or the traditions of Anglo-American psychology. Therefore, sport psychology in France developed with a variety of theoretical approaches and methods, still used for approaching the psychological problems emerging in the field of sport (Ripoll et al., n.d.).

Also in Germany, a variety of psychology schools developed. The so-called "traditional approach" of Wundt in Leipzig was diffused widely by many of his students, among whom Münsterberg who later assisted William James when he established his psychology laboratory in Harvard. However, Gestalt psychology also developed with many different views and schools (Berlin, Leipzig, Würzburg), with the field theory of Kurt Lewin becoming one of the most influential ones. The psychomotor coordination and motor control were important issues in many approaches in the time between the two World Wars and included interdisciplinary research questions and methods (Nitsch et al., 2000).

Another major aspect is the different understanding of the subject matter of sport psychology, that is, sport. The German tradition of Jahn in the 19th century promoted "Turnen" (gymnastics) as a nationalist program to promote the unification of the small states in what today is Germany (Ueberhorst, 1979). Turnen became a part of public schools' curriculum in Switzerland and Germany. In the French terminology, the "activité physique" (physical activity) plays a major role. The Soviet tradition used the term "fiziceskoj kul'tury" (physical culture) to indicate the integration of sport into the culture of developing the socialist personality. The English term "sport" originates in the Latin word "disportare" and means to distract or to amuse. When it was incorporated into continental European traditions and vocabularies, the meaning was in no way restricted to the element of competition, but rather complemented the traditional understanding of all kinds of physical exercise.

Development After World War II

Relaunch After the Destruction

World War II left behind a destroyed continent, including sport and scientific infrastructures and organizations, as well as huge economic difficulties (Nitsch et al., 2000). Right after the war, sport psychology in Europe suffered from a major contraction, but new attempts were made, starting with Puni who succeeded to launch a Department of Sport Psychology at the Lesgaft Institute of Physical Culture in Leningrad in 1946 and who obtained his second doctoral degree in 1952 with a thesis entitled "sport psychology" (Ryba et al., 2005). Research areas in this department included, among others, the role of imagery and self-talk in motor learning and tactical preparation as well as the psychological preparation for competitions, and resulted in a number of publications (Puni, 1961/1959).

In the same period, Rudik at the psychology department at the State Institute of Physical Culture in Moscow conducted a series of studies (Rudik, 1963/1958), and a conference was organized in Moscow in June 1958 (Rudik, 1958). The rivalry between Puni and Rudik seemed to both stimulate and hinder the development of Soviet sport psychology (Ryba et al., 2005).

In Germany, the first PhD theses in the field marked a new starting point of German sport psychology (Kohl, 1956; Möckelmann, 1952; Neumann, 1957). In the United States, the sport psychology laboratory at the University of Illinois was reestablished in Sep. 1950 (Kornspan, 2013).

Impact of Politics

The separation into, and the coexistence of, two political blocks in Europe may have had an important impact on the development of the field of sport psychology. Attempts to show superiority of the respective socioeconomical–political system resulted in an instrumentalization of Olympic sport. Especially the two German states, up until 1964 competing in a unified team at Olympic Games, invested in the development of top-level sport. While the use of sport psychology for the success of athletes was first established in the German Democratic Republic (GDR), the Federal Republic of Germany (FRG) also started to support sport science with the foundation of the Federal Institute of Sport Science in Cologne (Nitsch et al., 2000). Institutes of physical education and sport science were established at European universities.

With growing prosperity and leisure time, the importance of sport as a major societal and economic phenomenon increased in western European countries, whereas the socialist countries subordinated sport and physical activity to the goal of developing society and the socialist personality (Kunath & Müller, 1972). Despite an independent theoretical development of sport psychology in the eastern and western parts of Europe, contacts were established at an individual level, and during several national and international meetings and conferences (Kunath, 2003).

Foundation of FEPSAC

Sport psychology development in Europe was strongly boosted by the foundation of the International Society of Sport Psychology (ISSP) in Rome in 1965. Different explanations were put forward and can be found in the literature why, only 4 years after ISSP, the foundation of FEPSAC took place in 1969. These explanations contain: (1) a reaction after feeling threatened by North American sport psychology during the second World Congress in Washington, DC, in 1968, where no language except English was allowed (Kunath, 2003); (2) a reaction of the Warsaw Pact states after the protest notes of sport psychologists condemning the invasion of Czechoslovakia in 1968 (Apitzsch & Schilling, 2003); (3) a consequence of the low profile ISSP had in those years and President Antonelli's autocratic leadership style (Vanek, 1993); (4) as a socialist contraorganization against the capitalist ISSP (Morris, Hackfort, & Lidor, 2003).

The foundation of a European federation may instead be seen as an indispensable and logical step in order to respect the situation of two political and socioeconomical blocks, the variety of sport psychology traditions, and the cultural and language differences in European states, irrespective of what triggered the establishment of the federation.

The facts are as simple as this: the idea of a European Federation for Sports Psychology was born on December 4, 1968 at a sport psychology meeting held in Varna (Bulgaria), shortly after the second ISSP Congress. Preceded by intensive and emotional discussions, a decision was taken to prepare the foundation of a European Federation and to develop statutes and by-laws, and to meet again in 1 year's time in France. The factual association with the French name Fédération Européenne de Psychologie des Sports et des Activités Corporelles (FEPSAC) was founded at the first General Meeting held in Vittel (France) on June 4, 1969, on the occasion of the second European Congress on Sports Psychology (Kunath, 2003).

FEPSAC's Activities and Aims in the First 20 Years

Management of FEPSAC

Over the first two decades, the presidency of FEPSAC alternated between the two political blocks, with Guido Schilling (Switzerland, 1975–83) succeeding the first president Ema Geron (Bulgaria, 1969–74), followed by Paul Kunath (GDR, 1983–91) and Stuart Biddle (UK, 1991–99). The political blocks were fairly well balanced, with 11 Managing Council members from the socialist block and 14 from the western, capitalist block. The gender balance was worse: males only represented western sport psychology, whereas three female members represented socialist countries in the Managing Council until 1991. Ema Geron was the only woman to have served in the position of president during this period of time (Seiler, 1993a). European cultures and languages were quite equally represented in the first two decades, with Romance ($n = 5$), Slavic ($n = 8$), and Germanic ($n = 9$) languages complemented by other languages ($n = 3$) such as Hungarian, Finnish, or Turkish (Apitzsch & Schilling, 2003). The Managing Council meetings were held all over Europe, also representing a more or less balanced distribution between East and West.

Establish Scientific Exchange

In order to allow the scientific and personal exchange among European sport psychologists, FEPSAC established a tradition of European congresses at its foundation in 1969 in Vittel, France. The meeting in Varna, Bulgaria, in 1968, where the idea of FEPSAC was born, was declared to become, post hoc, the first European congress. Applied questions of psychological preparation were already an issue at this congress, contrasting the view of the "problem athlete" (Ogilvie & Tutko, 1966) by claiming that it is the competitive activity itself that poses problems.

After an initial period with a 3-year interval between congresses, a quadrennial frequency was maintained from 1975 onward. Seven congresses were organized until 1987, three in the eastern and four in the western part of the continent. This was diplomatically important in order to be able to continue the exchange on the content level, where common interests were found between the West and the East. Conference themes and keynote lectures covered a wide range of topics with different theoretical backgrounds and from different fields of sport, including psychological preparation, participation, differential sport psychology, and motor learning and control. Organizers were aware of the linguistic difficulties of congress participants: several congress languages were accepted, and multilingual proceeding books were published in most cases (Seiler, 2003b). Though somewhat easier for the presenters, the main disadvantage of this publication policy was that the texts were (and still are) not accessible for many due to language problems. In addition, many found the conferences difficult to attend because of travel restrictions in the socialist bloc.

Establish a Common Understanding and Theme

One of the first goals of FEPSAC was to establish a common terminology. While initiated as an ongoing project, the Scientific Committee made a start with the comparison of 63 sport psychological terms ranging from "activity" to "psychological tension." With the support of 28 representatives from 6 different countries and linguistic regions (Bulgaria, Czechoslovakia, Federal Republic of Germany, Hungary, Romania, Spain), a synthesis in French language was provided for the third European Congress 1972 in Cologne (Epuran, 1972). A manifesto was published in 1979 and released again in 1987, with the aim of obtaining a European understanding and definition of "sport psychology."

With a small print run, it did not reach—and was probably not aimed at attracting—the attention of a broader public. Influenced by Spielberger's research on stress and anxiety and the development of the State Trait Anxiety Inventory (Spielberger, Gorsuch, & Lushene, 1970), FEPSAC launched a European research project with the aim of collecting theoretical and empirical contributions on anxiety in sport. This project resulted in the first scientific FEPSAC publication (Apitzsch, 1983) and molded the 6th FEPSAC European Congress of Sport Psychology in Magglingen, Switzerland, in 1983.

Documentation of Status and Development

Annual reports were published from 1980 onward, based on a survey among the member countries and collecting important themes in research, education, or application across Europe, including theses and important publications, but also changes in the board of the respective national federations. The different traditions and the scientific development of sport psychology in Europe were documented in a brochure (Kunath, 1983), covering 11 European countries and made available at the 7th FEPSAC European Congress of Sport Psychology in Bad Blankenburg, German Democratic Republic, in 1987.

Strategic Orientation After 1989–91

When Germany was conveyed the honor to host the 8th FEPSAC European Congress of Sport Psychology in Cologne in 1991, nobody had expected the dramatic and rapid change in the political landscape of Europe from 1989. The fall of the Berlin Wall, and the perspective of pulling down the demarcation line between the two political and socioeconomic blocks, led politics in Germany to provide subsidies for scientific exchange and allowed the organizers of the Cologne Congress to invite a large number of colleagues from Central and Eastern European countries at heavily reduced costs. Despite the language difficulties—English and German were the two conference languages—mutual scientific exchange was fruitful and interesting, opening promising perspectives for the further development of sport psychology. On the other hand, the General Assembly no longer stuck to the unwritten rule to maintain a diplomatic balance between eastern and western Managing Council members, and elected a heavily western-dominated Managing Council, with only one member from the former Soviet bloc. Again, no woman was elected to the Managing Council between 1991 and 1995 (Apitzsch & Schilling, 2003).

In the following years, several factors influenced the further development of sport psychology, especially in the former socialist countries. The political will to demonstrate the superiority of the respective political and economic systems, for many years a strong argument for sport and sport science, was no longer a priority, resulting in reduced subsidies for the sport system. As a consequence, the number of institutions and positions decreased, and quite a few cutbacks occurred (Straub, Ermolaeva, & Rodionov, 1995). Economic difficulties in former socialist countries also affected the possibilities to conduct research and to travel to and participate in conferences during the 1990s. Especially in East Germany, many sport psychologists in university positions were dismissed because of their proximity to the former political system. Consequently, an enormous loss of knowledge and competence occurred (Nitsch et al., 2000). As an example of the stagnation, Janssen (2002) stated that the numbers of sport psychologists in the reunified Germany was 237 in 1991 and 238 10 years later in 2001. Contrary to this, in some western European countries, the development of academic sport psychology since 1990 had been considerable, notably in Greece and the United Kingdom.

Even if FEPSAC-responsible persons in this period may have had other visions, FEPSAC's activities since the European unification may, retrospectively speaking, be grouped in different strategic domains, namely fostering and facilitating mutual exchange and a common understanding and profile, supporting the young generation, working toward gender equality, and establishing sport psychology as a promising professional area.

Facilitating Contacts between Sport Psychologists Across Europe

One of the major platforms of any scientific organization to meet and exchange new ideas are regular congresses and conferences. With the aim to facilitate participation of sport psychologists from economically less privileged countries, namely the former socialist countries, FEPSAC chose venues for the European Congresses of Sport Psychology relatively central in Europe, namely Brussels, Prague, Copenhagen, and Halkidiki for the four conferences between 1995 and 2007. It was also a central aim to give colleagues from Europe, rather than just North America, for example, a platform by inviting them for keynote lectures, and respecting a linguistic and geographic representation for such selections (Seiler, 2003a). This also included a conscious decision not to opt primarily for world-famous names, even if those would probably have attracted more participants.

For a better information exchange among the member federations of FEPSAC in the 4-year intervals between the congresses, the FEPSAC Bulletin was established. This printed brochure, published twice a year from 1989, aimed at "improving the dissemination of news in the area of sport psychology in

Europe" (Apitzsch & Schilling, 2003, p. 12). The relatively low print run, the difficulties distributing copies in the member countries, and the high costs led the Managing Council to the decision to produce the Bulletin only electronically from 1999 and to stop it altogether when the FEPSAC Newsletter was made available in the newly established FEPSAC journal *Psychology of Sport and Exercise* in 2001.

The idea of a directory of European sport psychologists tried to support the momentum generated at the conference in Cologne in 1991 and aimed at facilitating the exchange among individual sport psychologists across Europe. In its totality, 296 entries, with detailed information about the individuals, were collected when the directory was published in 1993 (European Federation of Sport Psychology, 1993). However, since major problems occurred with data gathering in some countries, and information quickly lost correctness, the directory did not produce the expected sustainable effect. With the overwhelming success of the World Wide Web, a printed directory soon became obsolete.

Despite the efforts made by the Managing Council to encourage candidatures from Central and Eastern Europeans for the elections, a strong underrepresentation with only six representatives between 1991 and the current Managing Council (2015–19) remains. This made it difficult to maintain communication with these countries especially during the period when electronic communication was not so widespread as it is today. Two special meetings with leading sport psychologists from Central and Eastern Europe and a representative of the FEPSAC Managing Council were organized in Budapest in 1993 and in Prague in 1994 in order to record the challenges encountered by, as well as the needs and expectations of, sport psychologists from those countries (Seiler, 1993b). Consequently, Managing Council meetings have been held repeatedly in Central (but less in Eastern) European countries with the aim of promoting sport psychology and rending an educational service.

For a more frequent and intensified contact with the representatives of the member federations, a representatives' meeting was scheduled in the odd years between the General Assemblies and first held in 1993 in Jyväskylä, Finland (Apitzsch & Schilling, 2003). This allowed FEPSAC representatives from each member country, and not just those elected to the Managing Council, to meet and discuss issues of the day and to enhance communication.

A growing need emerged to forbear from the concept of national association as member. The statutes were adopted to allow international organizations and also institutions aligned with the aims of FEPSAC to become members, but also to accept more than one organization from one country. In addition, individual membership was established in the statutes in 2003.

Fostering a Common Understanding and Profile

A second issue was the establishment of themes pertinent to European sport psychology and making this information available to the academic and professional world. It was argued that many themes existed, with "probably as many similarities as differences between North American and European sport psychology" (Biddle, 1995, p. viii). A book on *European Perspectives on Exercise and Sport Psychology*, edited by Biddle (1995) included 15 chapters in English with 20 authors from 9 countries. A second FEPSAC textbook *Psychology for Physical Educators* was published 4 years later (Vanden Auweele, Bakker, Biddle, Durand, & Seiler, 1999), with a follow-up version, entitled *Psychology for Physical Educators—Students in Focus* in 2007, more focused on professional application (Liukkonen, Vanden Auweele, Vereijken, Alfermann, & Theodorakis, 2007). These publications gave European sport psychology a voice outside Europe.

Given the fact that in many of the European countries English was not yet a very widespread language in the early 1990s, the question of language was always an important one. The idea to establish a monograph series resulted from ideas and wishes in the first representatives' meeting in 1993 in Jyväskylä, Finland. Themes pertinent to European sport psychology could be made available in the form of small brochures at low cost, and people or institutions interested should be allowed to translate the content in languages other than English (Seiler, 2003b), and, more specifically, in Eastern European languages (Seiler, 1993b). Monograph # 1 on "Career transitions in competitive sports" was published in 1999 (Wylleman, Lavallee, & Alfermann, 1999), and Monograph # 2 on "Sport psychology in Europe" in 2003 (Apitzsch & Schilling, 2003). No further monographs have been issued since then.

The Managing Council of FEPSAC was also keen on increasing the profile and visibility of the organization by publishing position statements on relevant topics "with the aim to guide good practice for different target groups" and to be "based on scientific knowledge and represent the official opinion of FEPSAC" (Apitzsch & Schilling, 2003, p. 15). The nine statements published so far, starting in 1995, focused on the definition of sport psychology, children in sport, sport career transitions, gender and sport participation, sport career termination, sexual exploitation in sport, doping and substance abuse in competitive sport, quality of applied sport psychology services, and ethical principles (FEPSAC, 2015a).

While textbooks are important tools for increasing a common understanding among sport psychologists, high-quality peer-reviewed journals contribute more to the scientific profile. The lack of a European sport psychology platform led to the establishment of the European Yearbook of Sport Psychology (EYSP) in 1997. After only three issues, an opportunity was offered by Elsevier to FEPSAC to start a new official FEPSAC journal called *Psychology of Sport and Exercise* (PSE), a project successfully started in 2000 (Seiler, 2003b). Today, with six issues a year, PSE has become a major player in the field.

Encouraging Young Researchers in Sport Psychology

In accordance with the statutes, FEPSAC made efforts to encourage young colleagues to enter and remain in the field of sport psychology. Starting in 1991, a prize has been awarded during the Congress (Apitzsch & Schilling, 2003) for outstanding work in the field of sport psychology. Notwithstanding low numbers of participants when initiated, the FEPSAC Young Researchers Award has gained attention among the young researchers and has attained high standards.

With the financial support of the Erasmus program of the European Union, FEPSAC developed a European master's degree program in "Exercise and Sport Psychology," which opened in the academic year 1996–97 with 12 students and which has attracted over 200 persons since then (Vanden Auweele, 2003). An Intensive Course of 2 weeks, bringing together students and teachers from different countries, cultures, and scientific background, turned out to be an important element for the program, both scientifically and socially. An alumni network was established by those who have graduated from the program, resulting in the European Network of Young Specialists in Sport Psychology (ENYSSP). This network has become an active and innovative partner organization of FEPSAC in the field of sport psychology in Europe. Despite the termination of EU funding, there are ongoing efforts to continue the educational network across Europe and the program on new grounds and initiatives.

Working Toward Gender Equity in Sport Psychology

The first Managing Council in the unified Europe was a purely male committee. This did not reflect the fact that a majority of psychology students were (and still are) female. On the other hand, most of the national organisations had a strong underrepresentation of women in their Managing Council (Seiler, 1993a), and, on the other hand, a gender bias was also identified in the field of applied sport psychology in the United States (Roper, 2002), including various forms of gender discrimination experienced by female sport psychologists (Roper, 2008). In subsequent years, by encouraging the candidature of women, FEPSAC succeeded to steadily increase the number of women in the Managing Council up to four out of nine from 2011 to 2015. As a result of the elections in 2015, the Managing Council consists—for the first time in its history—of a majority of women (five out of nine) for the next term of office.

Establishing Sport Psychology as a Profession

Although sport psychology has struggled for acceptance as a scientific field for many years, the last 20 years have witnessed an upsurge in interest and activity in sport psychology as an applied professional field (Wylleman & Liukkonen, 2003). In light of the open European labor market, the debate on who should be a sport psychologist, the qualification and competences required, and further education became important issues. Credibility, transparency, and efficiency are important criteria for acceptance in the field of sport, and quality management approaches may help guarantee a high standard and distinguish it from less serious providers (Birrer & Seiler, 1999). The inclusion of formalized supervision has found a way into sport psychology (Stambulova, Johnson, & Linner, 2014), thus helping to increase the quality of the service provided.

The discussion about career development in applied sport psychology has not come to an end, and much remains yet to be done to ensure the development of the practitioners and the quality of the service delivery (Wylleman, Harwood, Elbe, Reints, & Caluwé, 2009). In 2003, the Forum of Applied Sport psychologists in Topsport (FAST) was initiated in order to unite and provide experienced sport psychologists working in top-level sport with a professional platform. While sharing their professional experiences, FAST established a body of knowledge that is now being disseminated to other colleagues also on a regional level (Wylleman et al., 2009). This may contribute to an increased quality in applied sport psychology services and, in the long run, better acceptance and improved job prospects for sport psychologists in Europe.

ACKNOWLEDGING THE CHALLENGES

In 2009, a view of FEPSAC's future was painted by way of delineating the challenges it may face through the processes of unification and diversity (Seiler & Wylleman, 2009). The development of FEPSAC has been, and still is, intrinsically linked to changes occurring in European society at large. Over the past 40 years, Europe has changed considerably; not only has it established a clear and well-defined economic and monetary zone, but it has also embraced many Central and Eastern European countries within the European Union (EU). While these changes not only represent a process of unification (eg, a unified labor market, and education system), they also reflect a process of increased diversity (eg, languages, cultural heritage, values, and norms). As these changes also have repercussions for the field of sport psychology in general, and for FEPSAC in particular, several of them will be addressed in this second part.

Challenges of Unification

As a European organization, FEPSAC has been able to play a vital role in establishing links and working relationships across supranational boundaries. In 2009, it was suggested that FEPSAC could broaden its aim from an organization representing sport psychology in Europe toward a European organization servicing groups and individuals interested and involved in sport psychology from within, as well as outside, the EU borders (eg, Norway, Russia, Switzerland, Israel). This challenge was met by FEPSAC as it strengthened its relationships with other continental sport psychology associations (eg, the International Society of Sport Psychology, ISSP; the Association of Applied Sport Psychology, AASP; the Asian-South Pacific Association of Sport Psychology, ASPASP; the North American Society for Psychology of Sport and Physical Activity, NASP-SPA), for example, by hosting a meeting of presidents of continental sport psychology associations and by organizing a roundtable with representatives of these associations (Wylleman et al., 2015). Especially this latter initiative allowed FEPSAC to consider how intercontinental initiatives could be initiated or encouraged (eg, organizing a symposium under the patronage of FEPSAC at each other's continental sport psychology congresses) as well as to discuss common issues (eg, organization of congresses/conferences, management of own journals, accreditation of members, ethical issues). Finally, with a steady influx of members of the European Network of Young Specialists in Sport Psychology (ENYSSP), the collaboration with FEPSAC has led to the formulation of joint initiatives (eg, in the area of the educational and vocational development of young sport psychologists).

As many of its group members provide similar services to its members, use similar tools (eg, electronic newsletter, website), and possibly look for "supraregional/supranational" criteria in the accreditation process of their applied sport psychologists, FEPSAC could invigorate the process of collaboration and exchange of ideas and information and support. It could also take the lead in the creation of interwoven networks around Europe working on shared projects locally (eg, provision of sport psychology support in traditional local sports), regionally (eg, workshops for parents of obese children), or around Europe (eg, guidelines on how to establish a private office as a sport psychology practitioner).

The process of unification within the EU has also led to a striving toward, among others, adding a European dimension to education, helping to develop quality assurance in higher education and elsewhere in education, encouraging lifelong learning, and the establishment of a European area of higher education (European Commission, 2007). Some of the ramifications on the educational process in the field of sport psychology include:

- the need to identify the educational paths (programs) in sport psychology currently provided across Europe, and to translate these paths quantitatively (in credits) as well as qualitatively (in terms of competencies);
- participating and/or establishing Pan-European networks so that students can participate (in an almost individualized way) in an array of (graduate or postgraduate) sport psychology programs;
- the need for a degree which is representative of a profile of competencies accepted by employers, and enabling people to join the labor market across Europe.

From the perspective of sport psychology in Europe, FEPSAC felt that there was a need to tackle challenges related to education and continued personal development. A three-way approach was followed. In first instance, there was a clear need to identify education in the field of sport psychology in Europe (Wylleman et al., 2009). While information on several sport psychology-related educational programs in Europe was available, a detailed overview (eg, organizing institute, content, duration, eligibility) of programs was lacking. Wylleman et al. suggested that FEPSAC, as the leading organization for sport psychology in Europe, should develop initiatives to enable guidelines for high-quality education, take the lead in analyzing sport psychology education programs throughout Europe, and develop or support initiatives in sport psychology education. In view of this, FEPSAC patronaged a study on sport psychology programs and courses and explored the possibility and objectives of a network of sport psychology educators in Europe (Hutter, van der Zande, Rosier, & Wylleman, in press). Findings showed that while education in sport psychology is available in most European countries, programs and courses vary widely (eg, level, size, applied focus). From the perspective of FEPSAC, the finding that educators in sport psychology from 30 European countries were also interested in exchanging information (eg, knowledge, staff, students, experiences, quality standards) and collaborating, was also important. This led in 2013 to the initiation of the FEPSAC-patronaged network for "Educators in Applied Sport psychologY" (EASY-network) (Hutter, 2014), which is aimed at providing educators with valuable information as well as a platform to share best practices.

While the EASY-network assists those interested in a career in sport psychology by providing an overview of not only sport psychology curricula, it was felt that education in sport psychology in Europe would also benefit from a more "hands-on" approach. After becoming an associated member of the European Federation of Psychology Associations (EFPA) in 2014, FEPSAC also considered the way in which the European Certificate in Psychology (Europsy) could provide the basis for a postgraduate sport psychology program. More particularly, initiatives have been taken to investigate to what extent the Specialist European Certificate, which builds on Europsy, could be used as a competence-building format leading up to a Specialist European Certificate in Sport Psychology. Besides the identification of competencies required in the field of sport psychology, it also led to the discussion of the role of, and the need for, interaction between all stakeholders, namely, academia, FEPSAC, and the labor market (eg, sport organizations, the health and fitness industry). By including this latter stakeholder, FEPSAC aims at identifying the expectations, requirements, and specificities of the labor market for sport psychology practitioners across Europe, as well as the setting and characteristics of professional career development in sport psychology and the financial remunerations of its practitioners.

Complementing education in sport psychology, a need was also identified for continued professional development (CPD) initiatives for (applied) sport psychologists. In 2012, FEPSAC patronaged the first edition of the international CPD program, "Psychological Excellence for Elite Performance" (PE4EP) (Hutter, 2012). Joining FEPSAC with two centers of excellence in elite sport and performance in Europe, namely the National Institute of Sport, Expertise and Performance (INSEP) and the Vrije Universiteit Brussel (VUB), the PE4EP program provides sport psychologists, elite coaches, and sport managers working in elite and Olympic sports a platform to develop their competencies and exchange professional experiences. Based upon a program combining presentations, workshops, group discussions, case studies, as well as individual and group exercises (eg, during the qualification round of Roland Garros), the topics of conflict and crisis management and of challenges in providing sport psychology in elite and Olympic sports, were already covered (FEPSAC, 2015b). Successful participation in the PE4EP program is rewarded with a joint postgraduate FEPSAC–INSEP–VUB certificate recognizing the academic and applied level of this CPD program. With these initiatives FEPSAC complemented already well-developed (or terminated) educational initiatives (eg, the European master's degree program in "Exercise and Sport Psychology," the European master's in "Sport and Exercise Psychology") and thus contributed to developments in the educational world in Europe, providing support to students, neophyte practitioners, as well as senior professionals.

A final aspect presented by this challenge of unification related to the structure of FEPSAC, in particular, to its legal status as a European society. As described earlier, the foundation of FEPSAC took place in 1969 by way of a simple "factual" organizational structure governed, from 1970 onward, by its statutes, its General Assembly, and its Managing Council. This factual functioning meant, for example, that the official address of FEPSAC was always linked to, and changed with its presidents (Emma Geron, Guido Schilling, Paul Kunath, Stuart Biddle, Glyn Roberts, Roland Seiler, and Paul Wylleman) and that the treasurers were personally responsible for opening and managing a bank account opened in name of FEPSAC. During the past 46 years, this system never faltered. In fact, it showed the clear commitment of, and confidence between its Managing Council members and its General Assembly.

However, as requirements with regard to financial transactions in Europe became more stringent, the factual status of FEPSAC was evaluated in 2011 as a possible threat to its continued existence as it did not allow anyone, for example, to open a bank account in name of FEPSAC or to apply for European grants. Specifically, as FEPSAC was no longer deemed to exist as a legal entity, the Managing Council initiated in 2012 a process to change its factual status into a legal status. After presenting a proposal during its 2013 informal members' meeting in Paris, the new statutes were unanimously accepted during its 2015 General Assembly in Bern. With the publication of its new statutes in the Belgian State Gazette, 2015 saw the birth of "FEPSAC 2.0," an international not-for-profit association (INPA) unified in line with European requirements. Given its newly acquired status, FEPSAC will now be able to fully focus on, among others, providing a platform for interest groups on specific topics (eg, via conferences, via dissemination, via special issues), providing offers for principal investigators of EU grants with FEPSAC as partner and responsible for specific milestones (eg, dissemination), applying as a coordinator for EU grants to foster research in specific areas, or to apply for organization grants to enhance organizational development of sport psychology in Europe and of FEPSAC.

Challenges of Diversification

FEPSAC is also coping with the challenges of a growing diversity within Europe. This is, for example, reflected in the development of regional rather than national societies representing the field of sport and exercise psychology (eg, Belgium, Spain), or in the growing (or reoccurring) interest of (applied) psychology societies for this specialized field (eg, the British Psychological Society). While these developments were already recognized by FEPSAC when it opened its group membership to all groups (aligned with the aims of FEPSAC) instead of limiting it to one (representative) national society (see the previous discussion), FEPSAC has taken initiatives aimed at supporting regional initiatives and collaboration among these (regional) groups.

It is important for FEPSAC to support the process of diversification of those involved in sport psychology in Europe. For example, there are indicators of a mounting diversity reflected in the increased involvement of women and youngsters in the field of sport and exercise psychology. FEPSAC as an organization has also taken up the need to respect a gender diversification in its Managing Council. Since it succeeded to steadily increase the number of women in the Managing Council since 2011, a majority of five women out of nine has been reached in the Managing Council elected in 2015, including the newly elected president Anne-Marie Elbe. This is seen as a strong signal toward gender equity and against any form of gender discrimination.

Taking into account the strong representation of female students entering higher education in the fields of education, health and welfare, and humanities and arts (European Commission, 2008), an increase in female sport psychologists may be anticipated during the next decade. The need for a survey of FEPSAC's individual members, as well as of the members of its group members, was thus already raised in 2009. This would allow FEPSAC to gain also more insight into the characteristics, requirements, and expectations toward its functioning as an organization for sport psychology and with regard to the provision of services to its members (eg, publications, congresses). FEPSAC should also continue to encourage female psychologists to enter the field of sport psychology and to assist them on their professional career path (Wylleman et al., 2009).

Furthermore, the participation rates of young students in the European master's degree program in Exercise and Sport Psychology, and the development of ENYSSP, are indicative of the fact that young people are looking toward sport psychology not only as a field of education, but also as an opportunity to develop a vocational career as a sport psychologist (Wylleman et al., 2009). Establishing collaboration with organizations that can have a role in employing sport psychologists is therefore an essential step FEPSAC has taken, for example, by liaising with European societies from the field of psychology (eg, the EFPA; the European Health Psychology Society, EHPS), as well as from the field of sport sciences and physical education (eg, the

European College of Sport Science, ECSS; the European Physical Education Association, EPEA).

An important challenge FEPSAC also faces is the diversity in the educational and vocational background of its members. It is therefore significant that as an associated member, FEPSAC also collaborates with the EFPA Task Force in Sport Psychology in order to define the minimum standards that European psychologists should meet in order to qualify for independent practice in the field of Sport Psychology, for example, by generating a proposal for the EuroPsy Specialist Certificate in Sport Psychology. However, FEPSAC also recognizes and takes fully into account the significant role of its members with an educational background in sport and exercise sciences and physical education. In order to formulate a proposal for certification criteria for members with this background, FEPSAC needs to continue and intensify its working relationship with ECSS as well as liaise with other organizations representing the field of sport and exercise sciences and physical education.

It is also interesting to note that this process has in fact also led to an increased communication or collaboration between FEPSAC and elite sport organizations in Europe. For example, through its patronaging of FAST, links have been made with the national Olympic Committees (NOCs) of Croatia, Cyprus, Greece, Iceland, Italy, Lithuania, the Netherlands, Norway, Portugal, and Switzerland (and even China and Brazil) as well as with several elite sport organizations (eg, INSEP; the Lawn and Tennis Association, LTA) around Europe. This collaboration has also led to elite sport organizations showing a strong interest in joining FEPSAC as a group member (ie, INSEP). It is clear that interaction with European NOCs (or its umbrella organization, the European Olympic Committees, EOCs) and elite sport organizations around Europe will enable FEPSAC to involve an important stakeholder as part of the process of accrediting applied sport psychologists and certifying professional development programs in elite sport psychology. A strong and sustained communication— for example, through FAST—with sport psychologists professionally involved in these NOCs and elite sport organizations will be essential in this.

Besides elite sport and health, sport, play, and physical activity are used in other areas of high societal importance. Examples are the potential of sport for the inclusion of people with mental or physical disabilities, for the integration in multicultural societies, to build up resilience and to overcome trauma, and in the work with underprivileged populations. Some of these topics were on the agenda at the FEPSAC Congress in 2015 in Bern (Schmid & Seiler, 2015) and will challenge sport psychology researchers in the future. Moreover, engagement in these evolving areas will also lead to a further diversification of the potential work fields for (applied) sport psychologists, provided that appropriate educational programs are offered.

In line with the gender representation in its Managing Council, FEPSAC is also confronted with the challenge of diversity in other ways. For example, by using specific awards FEPSAC is able to acknowledge the diversity of expertise present among its members (FEPSAC, 2015c). More particularly, by awarding the Young Researchers Award since the 8th FEPSAC European Congress of Sport Psychology in Cologne in 1991, FEPSAC is able to clearly identify and recognize the expertise of young and upcoming researchers in comparison to the more well-established researchers. In this way, young researchers are not "drawn" but actually stand out in the large sport psychology research community. Many of the 18 laureates have, since receiving this award, developed a strong career in sport psychology, be it as researcher, academic, and/or applied consultant. In a second example, FEPSAC has been able to recognize the diversity among its members with regard to the way in which they have supported sport psychology in general and FEPSAC in particular. With the "Ema Geron Award," installed by the Managing Council in 2011 in honor of FEPSAC's first president, FEPSAC recognizes the significance of a person or organization who, at the local, regional, and/or national level, has provided an exceptional contribution to the development of the domain of sport psychology. Since 2011, four sport psychologists have been awarded this honor. In a similar way, FEPSAC decided in 2007 also to recognize statutory honorary membership in order to acknowledge the significant contribution of an individual (or exceptionally to a group) member to the attainment of the goals and the advancement of FEPSAC and/or for rendering outstanding service to sport and exercise psychology in Europe. So far, four statutory honorary memberships have been awarded by the Managing Council.

In another example, FEPSAC's official journal *Psychology of Sport and Exercise* has steadily confirmed the need to categorize, for example, by maintaining the categorization of its articles in two areas, namely, sport or exercise psychology, or by exploring specific topics in the domain of sport psychology via special issues (eg, "Dual Career Development and Transitions," "The Development of Expertise and Excellence in Sport Psychology," "A Sport Psychology Perspective on Olympians and the Olympic Games").

A final, and perhaps poignant, example of diversification is linked to the organization of the FEPSAC European Congress of Sport Psychology. Notwithstanding its success, it was deemed that its quadrennial and plurithematic nature did not allow for a timely and monothematic approach. In 2011 the Managing Council decided therefore to organize a FEPSAC European Sport Psychology Conference, which would intercede between the quadrennial FEPSAC European Congresses of Sport Psychology 2011 and 2015. Specifically, it would be focused on a sport psychology theme poignant to the local organizing host and would last for only 2 days. The first FEPSAC European Sport Psychology Conference, organized in 2013 in Paris on the theme of "Applied sport psychology in Europe," was a clear success. With three keynote speakers, seven sessions and a poster session, and almost 200 participants, FEPSAC responded to a clear need among a specific section of the sport psychology community. The second FEPSAC European Sport Psychology Conference will be hosted in

Nottingham, United Kingdom, in 2017, followed in 2019 by the 15th FEPSAC European Congress of Sport Psychology in Münster, Germany.

By translating diversification in terms of specialization, FEPSAC has been able to provide a more specific service to its members and the sport psychology community at large. This entails that FEPSAC needs to further develop the initiative to organize a survey to gather more information on its members (eg, educational background, vocational development, working conditions) so as to be able to delineate specific requirements among the sport psychology community.

CONCLUSIONS

Using a hermeneutical interpretation of historical documents (from FEPSAC and other sources) as well as the experiential knowledge of both authors (as researcher and educator in sport psychology, applied sport psychologist, and FEPSAC president and Managing Council member), this chapter presented not only an overview of the development of sport psychology in Europe and the role FEPSAC played during the past decades, but also sketched their situation in the present and some of their (future) challenges.

It is argued that sport psychology in Europe developed with great variety, due to different cultural, linguistic, and psychological traditions, and that unification and diversification are challenges FEPSAC is and will be facing as the leading sport psychology organization in Europe.

It is clear that FEPSAC needs to be aware of, and take into account, the different developments that have shaped its past and are determining its present. As an international organization, with the aim of developing sport psychology across all of Europe, FEPSAC will have to manage the influential factors and conditions for an optimal attainment of its organizational goals. This task has been, and will be in the future, much more of a political or diplomatic mission instead of a purely scientific one. It should be acknowledged that Managing Council members from all over Europe have been the indispensable prerequisites that have allowed FEPSAC since its inception to prosper within a changing European political landscape.

With the benefit of hindsight, it could therefore be said that FEPSAC has had a strong and positive impact on the development of sport psychology in Europe by way of (1) its congresses and conferences; (2) joining sport psychology associations and groups within Europe; (3) the promotion of scientific, educational, and professional work in sport psychology in Europe; (4) the patronage of a journal and the dissemination of publications; and (5) the coordination of sport psychology activities on education, research, practice, and business affairs throughout Europe.

Of course, the development of sport psychology is also driven by academia, and more specifically by current and future research. Therefore, this chapter provides a good overview of the current and future development of sport psychology in Europe. First and foremost, it is important to acknowledge that researchers are focusing on physical activity, exercise, health, and well-being. Different chapters provide insight into research linking physical activity and active lifestyles with health prevention and treatment throughout the age span (from preadolescents to older adults). As noted by Ekkekakis and Zenko (Chapter 18), this avenue of research has, if not limited to academic metrics, certainly the possibility to have a societal relevance and impact.

Second, strong lines of research into the development of athletes are continuously being developed. These include intrapersonal (eg, self-talk, quiet eye) as well as interpersonal (eg, team cognition, team functioning) topics. Significant to note is that the use of a holistic perspective has become a well-established part of research into athletes' development (eg, career transitions). This book confirms also the growing awareness for the need of research into the development and functioning of coaches, including the role of coaches' behaviors in training (eg, learning of a motor action) and as part of their coaching (eg, interpersonal styles, winning).

In third instance, the role of the sport psychologist/sport psychology consultant is also addressed. This is the case for research looking into the development of interventions (eg, role of clients' individual differences, harassment, and abuse in sport) as well as with regard to their multirole profile (eg, scientist, educator, practitioner).

Finally, a special note should be made for the way in which researchers are also focusing on studying the role sport can potentially play within broader societal processes (eg, promotion of integration and multiculturalism). Taking into the account the tremendous changes Europe has faced (and is facing) at the political, the socioeconomical level, and within the context of sport, it adds to sport psychology research that has the ability to improve the lives of people around Europe.

In conclusion, while the challenges for sport psychology and our continent will be different in the future, it is hoped that with this book, FEPSAC is able to provide its readers with more insight into how to possibly prepare for them. With this book, FEPSAC continues its strong tradition to provide its members and the sport psychology community at large with enduring and high-quality publications.

REFERENCES

14th European Congress of Sport Psychology (2015). *The 2015 FEPSAC Congress in Bern is history!* Available from http://www.fepsac2015.ch/

Apitzsch, E. (Ed.). (1983). *Anxiety in sport.* Magglingen: FEPSAC.

Apitzsch, E., & Schilling, G. (2003). Milestones in the history of FEPSAC. *Sport psychology in Europe. FEPSAC—an organisational platform and a scientific meeting point* (pp. 9–18). Biel: FEPSAC (FEPSAC Monograph 2).

Bäumler, G. (2002). Sportpsychologie zwischen 1884 und 1900/Die Generation der Pioniere [Sport psychology between 1884 and 1900/the generation of pioneers]. In G. Bäumler, J. Court, &

W. Hollmann (Eds.), *Sportmedizin und Sportwissenschaft. Historisch-systematische Facetten [Sport medicine and sport science. Historical and systematical facets]* (pp. 287–318). Sankt Augustin: Academia.

Biddle, S. J. H. (1995). Introduction. In S. J. H. Biddle (Ed.), *European perspectives on exercise and sport psychology* (pp. xi–xviii). Champaign, IL: Human Kinetics.

Birrer, D., & Seiler, R. (1999). Quality management in applied sport psychology: a project for the professionalisation of sport psychology services in Switzerland. *Proceedings of the tenth European Congress of Sport Psychology, Part 1.* In V. Hošek, P. Tillinger, & L. Bílek (Eds.), *Psychology of sport and exercise: Enhancing the quality of life* (pp. 110–112). Prague: Charles University, Faculty of Physical Education and Sport.

Brewer, B., & Van Raalte, J. L. (2002). Introduction to sport and exercise psychology. In J. L. Van Raalte, & B. W. Brewer (Eds.), *Exploring sport and exercise psychology* (pp. 3–9). Washington, DC: American Psychological Association.

Bureau International de Pédagogie Sportive et Institut Olympique de Lausanne. (1947). *Traveaux des congrès de psychologie et de pédagogie sportive, tenus du 16 au 20 juin 1944 à Lausanne à l'occasion du 50e anniversaire du rétablissement des Jeux olympiques [Proceedings of the congresses of sport psychology and sport pedagogy, 16 to 20 June 1944 in Lausanne at the occasion of the 50th anniversary of the re-establishment of the Olympic Games].* Lausanne: Librairie de l'Université F. Rouge.

Comité International Olympique. (1913). *Congrès international de psychologie et physiologie sportives [International congress of psychology and physiology of sport].* Lausanne: Imprimerie E. Toso.

Cox, R. H., Qiu, Y., & Liu, Z. (1993). Overview of sport psychology. In R. N. Singer, M. Murphey, & L. K. Tennant (Eds.), *Handbook of research on sport psychology* (pp. 3–31). New York: Macmillan.

de Coubertin, P. (1900). La psychologie du sport [Psychology of sport]. *Revue des Deux Mondes, 160,* 167–179. Available from http://gallica.bnf.fr/ark:/12148/bpt6k75397n/f170.image.

de Coubertin, P. (1913). *Essais de psychologie sportive [Essays in sport psychology].* Lausanne: Librairie Payot.

Epuran, M. (1972). *63 termes de psychologie du sport [63 sport psychological terms].* Köln: FEPSAC, Comité Scientifique.

European Commission. (2007). *Higher education in Europe.* European Commission. Available from http://ec.europa.eu/education/policies/educ/higher/higher_en.html

European Commission. (2008). *Key data on higher education in Europe* (2007 ed.). European Commission. Available from http://eacea.ec.europa.eu/ressources/eurydice/pdf/0_integral/088EN.pdf

European Federation of Sport Psychology (FEPSAC) (1993). *Directory of European sport psychologists.* Lund: Lunds universitet reprocentralen.

European Federation of Sport Psychology (FEPSAC). (1995). *FEPSAC Position statement # 1 definition of sport psychology.* Available from http://www.fepsac.com/activities/position_statements/

FEPSAC. (2015a). *Position statements.* Available from http://www.fepsac.com/activities/position_statements/

FEPSAC. (2015b). *Psychological Excellence for Elite Performance.* Available from http://www.fepsac.com/pe4ep/

FEPSAC. (2015c). *FEPSAC awards.* Available from http://www.fepsac.com/activities/fepsac_awards/

Geron, E. (2003). FEPSAC president from 1969–1974: Emma Geron (Bulgaria and Israel). In E. Apitzsch, & G. Schilling (Eds.), *Sport psychology in Europe. FEPSAC—an organisational platform and a scientific meeting point* (pp. 19). Biel: FEPSAC (FEPSAC Monograph 2).

Hutter, V. (2012). FEPSAC newsletter. *Psychology of Sport & Exercise, 13*, 518–519.

Hutter, V. (2014). FEPSAC newsletter. *Psychology of Sport & Exercise, 15*, 226.

Hutter, V., van der Zande, J., Rosier, N., & Wylleman, P. (in press). Education and training in the field of applied sport psychology in Europe. *International Journal of Sport and Exercise Psychology*

Janssen, J.-P. (2002). Sportpsychologie in Ost und West nach 1950 [Sport psychology in east and west after 1950]. In G. Bäumler, J. Court, & W. Hollmann (Eds.), *Sportmedizin und Sportwissenschaft. Historisch-systematische Facetten [Sport medicine and sport science. Historical and systematical facets]* (pp. 319–371). Sankt Augustin: Academia.

Janssen, J.-P. (2009). Geschichte der Sportpsychologie unter besonderer Berücksichtigung der Entwicklung in Deutschland [History of sport psychology with special emphasis on the development in Germany]. In W. Schlicht & B. Strauss (Hrsg.), *Grundlagen der Sportpsychologie* (Enzyklopädie der Psychologie, Themenbereich D, Serie V, Band 1, S. 33–105). Göttingen: Hogrefe.

Kohl, K. (1956). *Zum Problem der Sensumotorik. Psychologische Analysen zielgerichteter Handlungen aus dem Gebiet des Sports [The problem of sensory-motricity. Psychological analyses of goal-oriented actions from the field of sport]*. Frankfurt: Kramer.

Kölbl, C. (2006). *Die Psychologie der kulturhistorischen Schule. Vygotskij, Lurija, Leont'ev [The psychology of the cultural-historical school]*. Göttingen: Vandenhoeck & Ruprecht.

Kornspan, A. S. (2013). Alfred W. Hubbard and the sport psychology laboratory at the University of Illinois, 1950–1970. *The Sport Psychologist, 27*, 244–257.

Kunath, P. (Ed.). (1983). *Sportpsychologie in europäischen Ländern—Stand und Tendenzen 1983 [Sport psychology in European countries—status and tendencies 1983]*. Leipzig: DHfK/FEPSAC.

Kunath, P. (2003). Psychology and sport: a historical review. In E. Apitzsch, & G. Schilling (Eds.), *Sport psychology in Europe. FEPSAC—an organisational platform and a scientific meeting point* (pp. 20–26). Biel: FEPSAC (FEPSAC Monograph 2).

Kunath, P., & Müller, S. (1972). Gegenstand und Aufgaben der sportpsychologischen Arbeit in der Deutschen Demokratischen Republik [Subject matter and tasks in sport psychology work in the German Democratic Republik]. In P. Kunath (Ed.), *Beiträge zur Sportpsychologie [Contributions to sport psychology]* (pp. 11–27). (Vol. 1). Berlin: Sportverlag.

Liukkonen, J., Vanden Auweele, Y., Vereijken, B., Alfermann, D., & Theodorakis, Y. (Eds.). (2007). *Psychology for physical educators. Student in focus* (2nd ed.). Champaign, IL: Human Kinetics.

Mintz, A. (1958). Recent developments in psychology in the U.S.S.R. *Annual Review of Psychology, 9*, 453–504.

Möckelmann, H. (1952). *Leibeserziehung und jugendliche Entwicklung [Physical education and juvenile development]*. Schorndorf: Hofmann.

Morris, T., Hackfort, D., & Lidor, R. (2003). From hope to Pope: the first twenty years of ISSP. *International Journal of Sport and Exercise Psychology, 1*, 119–138.

Neumann, O. (1957). *Sport und Persönlichkeit. Versuch einer psychologischen Diagnostik und Deutung der Persönlichkeit des Sportlers [Sport and personality. Attempt of a psychological diagnosis and interpretation of the personality of the sportsman]*. München: Barth.

Nicolas, S., & Murray, D. J. (2000). Le fondateur de la psychologie 'scientifique' francaise: Théodule Ribot (1839–1916) [The founder of the 'scientific' French psychology: Théodule Ribot (1839–1916)]. *Psychologie et Histoire, 1*, 1–42. Available from http://psychologieethistoire.googlepages.com/NICOLAS1.HTM.

Nitsch, J. R., Gabler, H., & Singer, R. (2000). Sportpsychologie: ein Überblick [Sport psychology: an overview]. In H. Gabler, J. R. Nitsch, & R. Singer (Eds.), *Einführung in die Sportpsychologie.*

Teil 1: Grundthemen [Introduction into sport psychology: Part: 1 Fundamental themes] (pp. 11–42). Schorndorf: Hofmann.

Ogilvie, B. C., & Tutko, T. A. (1966). *Problem athletes and how to handle them.* London: Pelham Books.

Puni, A. Z. (1961). *Abriss der Sportpsychologie [Essays in the psychology of sport].* Berlin, GDR: Sportverlag (Original work published in Russian in 1959).

Rejeski, W. J., & Brawley, L. R. (1988). Defining the boundaries of sport psychology. *The Sport Psychologist, 2,* 231–242.

Ripoll, H., Bilard, J., Durand, M., Keller, J., Levêque, M., & Therme, P. (n.d.). *Psychologie du sport. Questions actuelles [Sport psychology. Contemporary questions].* Paris: Revue EPS.

Roper, E. A. (2002). Women working in the applied domain: examining gender bias in applied sport psychology. *Journal of Applied Sport Psychology, 14,* 53–66.

Roper, E. A. (2008). Women's career experiences in applied sport psychology. *Journal of Applied Sport Psychology, 20,* 408–424.

Rubinstein, S. L. (1958). *Grundlagen der Allgemeinen Psychologie [Foundations of general psychology].* Berlin: Volk und Wissen (Original work published in Russian in 1946).

Rudik, P. A. (1958). Vtoros Vsesoiuznoe soveschchanie po psikhologii sporta [Second All-Union conference on the psychology of sport]. *Voprosy Psychologii, 4,* 175–181.

Rudik, P. A. (1963). *Psychologie. Ein Lehrbuch für Turnlehrer, Sportlehrer und Trainer [Psychology. A textbook for physical educators and coaches].* Berlin, GDR: Volk und Wissen (Original work published in Russian in 1958).

Ryba, T. V., Stambulova, N. B., & Wrisberg, C. A. (2005). The Russian origins of sport psychology: a translation of an early work of A.C. Puni. *Journal of Applied Sport Psychology, 17,* 157–169.

Schmid, O., & Seiler, R. (Eds.), (2015). Sport psychology. Theories and applications for performance, health and humanity. *Proceedings of the 14th European Congress of Sport Psychology,* July 14–19, 2015. Bern, Switzerland.

Schulte, R. W. (1921). *Leib und Seele im Sport. Einführung in die Psychologie der Leibesübungen [Body and mind in sport. Introduction into the psychology of physical exercise].* Charlottenburg: Volkshochschulverlag.

Schulte, R. W. (1928). *Die Psychologie der Leibesübungen. Ein Überblick über ihr Gesamtgebiet [Psychology of physical exercise. An overview of the entire area].* Berlin: Weidmannsche Buchhandlung.

Seiler, R. (1993a). The situation of female sport psychologists in Europe. *FEPSAC Bulletin, 5*(1), 15–16.

Seiler, R. (1993b). Conference of representatives of East European countries. *FEPSAC Bulletin, 5*(2), 8–11.

Seiler, R. (2003a). FEPSAC congresses: Topics and conference proceedings. In E. Apitzsch, & G. Schilling (Eds.), *Sport psychology in Europe. FEPSAC—an organisational platform and a scientific meeting point* (pp. 28–36). Biel: FEPSAC (FEPSAC Monograph 2).

Seiler, R. (2003b). Sport psychology as a science: publications of FEPSAC. In E. Apitzsch, & G. Schilling (Eds.), *Sport psychology in Europe. FEPSAC—an organisational platform and a scientific meeting point* (pp. 65–73). Biel: FEPSAC (FEPSAC Monograph 2).

Seiler, R., & Wylleman, P. (2009). FEPSAC's role and position in the past and in the future of sport psychology in Europe. *Psychology of Sport and Exercise, 10,* 403–409.

Spielberger, C. D., Gorsuch, R. L., & Lushene, R. E. (1970). *Manual for the State-Trait Anxiety Inventory (self-evaluation questionnaire).* Palo Alto, CA: Consulting Psychologists Press.

Stambulova, N. B., Wrisberg, C. A., & Ryba, T. V. (2006). A tale of two traditions in applied sport psychology: the heyday of Soviet sport and wake-up calls for North America. *Journal of Applied Sport Psychology, 18,* 173–184.

Stambulova, N., Johnson, U., & Linner, L. (2014). Insights from Sweden: Halmstad applied sport psychology supervision model. In J. G. Cremades, & L. S. Tashman (Eds.), *Becoming a sport, exercise, and performance psychology professional: a global perspective* (pp. 276–284). New York: Psychology Press.

Straub, W. F., Ermolaeva, M. V., & Rodionov, A. V. (1995). Profiles and professional perspectives: ten leading former Soviet Union sport psychologists. *Journal of Applied Sport Psychology, 7,* 93–111.

Ueberhorst, H. (1979). Jahn's historical significance. *Canadian Journal of History of Sport & Physical Education, 10*(1), 7–14.

Vanden Auweele, Y. (2003). Sport psychology and education. The European masters in exercise and sport psychology. In E. Apitzsch, & G. Schilling (Eds.), *Sport psychology in Europe. FEPSAC—an organisational platform and a scientific meeting point* (pp. 38–48). Biel: FEPSAC (FEPSAC Monograph 2).

Vanden Auweele, Y., Bakker, F., Biddle, S., Durand, M., & Seiler, R. (Eds.). (1999). *Psychology for physical educators.* Champaign, IL: Human Kinetics.

Vanek, M. (1993). Reflections on the inception, development, and perspectives of ISSP's image and self-image. In S. Serpa, J. Alves, V. Ferreira, & A. Paula-Brito (Eds.), *Proceedings of the 8th World Congress of Sport Psychology* (pp. 154–158). Lisbon: ISSP.

Weinberg, R., & Gould, D. (2003). *Foundations of sport and exercise psychology* (3rd ed.). Champaign, IL: Human Kinetics.

Wylleman, P., & Liukkonen, J. (2003). Sport psychology as a profession: case studies from around Europe. In E. Apitzsch, & G. Schilling (Eds.), *Sport psychology in Europe. FEPSAC—an organisational platform and a scientific meeting point* (pp. 50–63). Biel: FEPSAC (FEPSAC Monograph 2).

Wylleman, P., Lavallee, D., & Alfermann, D. (Eds.), (1999). *Career transitions in competitive sports.* Biel: FEPSAC. (FEPSAC Monograph 1). Available from http://www.fepsac.com/index. php/activities/publications/fepsac_books/fepsac_monographs

Wylleman, P., Harwood, C. G., Elbe, A. -M., Reints, A., & de Caluwé, D. (2009). A perspective on education and professional development in applied sport psychology. *Psychology of Sport and Exercise, 10,* 435–446.

Wylleman, P., Si, G., Ste-Marie, D., Cremades, G., Rosnet, E., & Elbe, A.-M. (2015). Roundtable: An international perspective on the organisation of sport psychology (FEPSAC, ISSP, NASPSPA, AASP, IAAP). During the *14th FEPSAC European Congress of Sport Psychology.* Bern, Switzerland: FEPSAC. Available from https://cast.switch.ch/vod/clips/8bcahx8vg/streaming.html

Section I

Prerequisites of Sport and Exercise Psychology

Chapter 2

Importance of Instructions in Sport and Exercise Psychology

Nele Schlapkohl*, Markus Raab**,†

*Department of Sport Science, Institute for Health, Nutrition and Sport, Europa University Flensburg, Flensburg, Germany; **Department of Performance Psychology, German Sport University Cologne, Institute of Psychology, Cologne, Germany; †School of Applied Sciences, London South Bank University, London, United Kingdom

INTRODUCTION

The effects of instructions on motor performance have been investigated in different ways. For instance, Wulf (2008) examined how the instructed focus of attention (external on movement effects vs internal on movement effectors) influences learning, Williams, Ward, Knowles, & Smeeton (2002) looked at whether guided or unguided learning is more efficient, and Masters (2000) studied how implicit and explicit learning (instructions via analogies vs rule-based) affect performance. In addition, instructions vary in terms of type and function depending on the content and context being targeted. For instance, in terms of content, instructions contain functions beyond performance improvements, such as boosting learners' motivation or improving communication (coaching effectiveness; Hänsel, 2002). In terms of context, coaches in competitive sports operate in a different learning situation from leisure-time coaches or physical education instructors. Competitive athletes handle instructions in a different way from novices or pupils.

Our main assumption is that instructions are a fundamental tool that is applied as part of the learning process and are an important facet of efforts to change behavior, but we do not know much about the effectiveness of different instructions discussed in sport and exercise psychology. It is interesting to note that even instructions accepted as an influential learning method have not yet found their way into encyclopedias of sport and exercise psychology (Eklund & Tenenbaum, 2004). In the following text we focus on four context domains: We look at competitive sports (competitive athletes), what content improves performance (motor learning with novices and in physical education), and how instructions can change behavior, such as in health-related studies through

Sport and Exercise Psychology Research. http://dx.doi.org/10.1016/B978-0-12-803634-1.00002-9
29

peer-to-peer instruction (two domains: schools and pupils' health, and functionally illiterate adults and their health).

Understanding the role of instructions during learning processes requires first looking into different kinds of motor learning, namely, implicit and explicit motor learning, and their respective instructions. Motor learning is central to many domains, including sports, but the terminology is not uniform enough to allow experience to be effectively shared or knowledge to be translated into practice (Kleynen et al., 2014). Implicit and explicit learning methods reveal differences between conscious and nonconscious attributes of the motor learning process, with implicit motor learning targeting more nonconscious attributes and explicit motor learning the more conscious attributes (Kleynen et al., 2014). Implicit and explicit instructions during a particular learning process vary. One method of instruction for implicit learning is the use of analogies. For explicit learning, instructions consist of a detailed description with step-by-step rules.

A recent metaanalysis looked at eight multiexperiment studies with 33 independent effects that compared analogy and rule-based instructions. The results showed that the analogy instructions had a more positive effect on motor learning (Tielemann, 2008). However, this advantage was identified only in novices and not in experts or school pupils. Furthermore, there is limited evidence of how specific instructions modulate movement patterns, as often only movement outcomes were measured, such as the points made in a table tennis relay or the number of holed golf putts (Tielemann, 2008).

In the past, studies of analogy and rule-based instructions have mainly been limited to novices and to a few sports such as table tennis, basketball, gymnastics, and skiing (see Tielemann, 2008, for an overview). The only sport analyzed extensively is table tennis (Koedijker, Oudejans, & Beek, 2007; Liao & Masters, 2001; Masters, Poolton, Maxwell, & Raab, 2008; Poolton, Masters, & Maxwell, 2006). Given that analogy instructions seem to have a more positive effect on motor learning (measured by movement outcome in novices) than rule-based instructions, several hypotheses have been put forward to explain the underlying mechanisms. It has been assumed that analogy learning leads to less declarative knowledge about the movement pattern than explicit learning. Additionally, explicit instructions depend on working memory for the retrieval of conscious, declarative knowledge. Cognitive capacity is limited, so it is possible that explicit learning causes cognitive overload (Masters & Maxwell, 2008; Maxwell, Masters, & Eves, 2003; Masters et al., 2008). Furthermore, the theory of reinvestment (Masters & Maxwell, 2008) suggests that motor processes can be disrupted if individuals consciously use declarative knowledge to control a movement in stressful situations. In sum, there is growing empirical evidence and attempts to explain the causes of effects of different instructions, but a recent review by Kleynen et al. (2014) suggested that current knowledge is far too limited to confirm the accuracy of the instructions and to explore the feasibility of the strategies identified in research, everyday practice, and education.

In this chapter we focus on instructions in different settings and directed toward people of different expertise. We aim to present an overview of studies in (1) motor learning with competitive athletes and novices, (2) physical education, and (3) health. In several studies we explored the question of whether implicit and explicit instructions have beneficial effects on performance and movement patterns. The findings extend the literature by accentuating the role of implicit learning for novices and school pupils and in health-related areas and that of explicit learning for experts.

MOTOR LEARNING WITH COMPETITIVE ATHLETES AND NOVICES

Most findings in research underline the role of implicit learning for novices. For example, Liao and Masters (2001) studied novices in an acquisition and a transfer phase. The authors found that an implicit group and an analogy group demonstrated less explicit knowledge and greater stability in movement execution in the transfer test than an explicit group. Poolton et al. (2006) used analogy and rule-based instructions in an acquisition phase. After the acquisition phase, they compared the instructions' effectiveness during a decision task of high or low complexity. The results showed no significant differences in hitting performance during the acquisition phase. However, during the high-complexity decision task, the hitting performance of the analogy group remained constant, whereas that of the corresponding rule-based group deteriorated.

In another study, Koedijker et al. (2007) examined performance under pressure with analogy instructions and rule-based instructions in an internally focused group and an externally focused group. They found that the accumulation of a large number of explicit rules was detrimental to performance under pressure. The authors argued that the amount of excess explicit verbal knowledge determined the robustness of hitting performance. One explanation of Koedijker et al.'s findings refers to cognitive load. To test the hypothesis that explicit learning leads to a higher cognitive load, Masters et al. (2008) analyzed the performance of an analogy and a rule-based group in a table tennis experiment with high- and low-complexity decision tasks. The analogy instructions were found to have the most positive impact in the high-complexity situation, in which cognitive overload was most likely diminishing the performance effects of the explicit instruction group.

Competitive Athletes

Implicit learning was found to be advantageous only for novices and not for experts (Schlapkohl, Hohmann, & Raab, 2012). To illustrate this from our own research, we tested whether previous findings could be generalized to higher levels of expertise. We investigated the effects of rule-based (explicit) and analogy (implicit) instructions on the performance of experts (for more information, see

Schlapkohl et al., 2012). Fifteen table tennis players were randomly assigned to two groups (analogy vs rule-based). All participants were junior national players in the German Table Tennis Association and attended a table tennis boarding school in Düsseldorf, Germany. A pretest/posttest/retention test design was used (Koedijker et al., 2007). Over the course of 4 weeks, an analogy and a rule-based group had to improve their wrist position during the topspin forehand. The delayed retention test followed after 12 weeks. For the tests, participants returned three types of passes (undercut, counter hit, or topspin forehand) that these expert players would be likely to encounter in training and play, in five different conditions (three technique and two decision blocks). Participants were expected to perform 10 topspin forehand hits in each block. The instructions differed depending on the group and the passes. For example, for the undercut, participants were given the analogy to pass like a discus thrower (Try to move the arm as if throwing a discus). For the counter hit, the participants should "Try to move the arm as if you were a soldier greeting a general." And for the topspin forehand, they should "Try to move the arm as if you were running your hand over a fitness ball." The explicit group got five rule-based instructions for each type of pass. For example, for the undercut (discus in the analogy instructions), they were given the following instructions:

1. Put your right foot behind you so that your feet are positioned slightly diagonal to the baseline.
2. Stretch your arm during the backward movement so that your bat is at the height of your right knee.
3. Try to move your bat with an explosive forearm and wrist movement to your forehead.
4. Try to hit the ball near the highest point of the trajectory.
5. Focus on an active trunk rotation to support the shift of your weight from the right to the left foot.

The results showed that the rule-based group reported a greater number of rules than participants in the analogy group. In terms of hitting performance, the results showed in both the technique and the decision blocks that participants in the rule-based group achieved better hitting performance. In terms of the movement pattern, analogy instructions produced a significantly smaller angle than rule-based instructions. The different kinds of movement patterns for the three analogies (soldier, stroke, and discus) also represent three different stroke directions, indicating that the choice of a specific analogy can have important consequences for the movement pattern (Fig. 2.1). This example (and many more studies—see the next section for novices, also Liao & Masters, 2001; Poolton et al., 2006) shows that rule-based instructions lead to more verbal knowledge. In terms of hitting performance, rule-based instructions lead to better performance than analogy instructions. This contrasts with previous findings with novices (Liao & Master, 2001; Poolton et al., 2006). Experts acquired many rules but the accumulation did not overload their working memory or

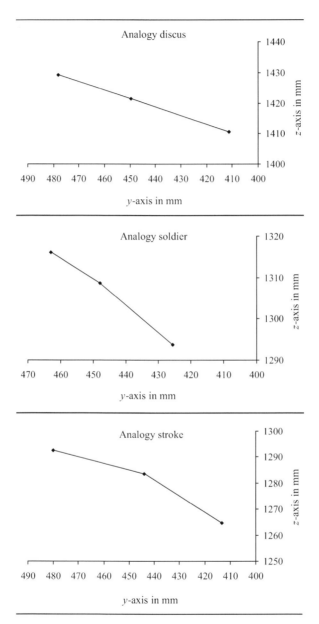

FIGURE 2.1   Analogy instructions: hitting movement when instructed with three different analogies.

influence their hitting performance. On the other hand, a single analogy did not improve experts' hitting performance. In line with our assumption, the results show that movement patterns differed significantly depending on the instruction or analogy given.

Novices

In our own research (Schlapkohl et al., 2012), we relied on the previous arguments and extended research integrating outcome and kinematic variables, using the type of instructions (analogy vs rule-based) in different acquisition and transfer conditions. Novices learned the table tennis topspin forehand with rule-based instructions or analogy instructions (Study 1) and therefore received decision training right from the acquisition phase (Study 2; for more information, see Schlapkohl et al., 2012). In Study 1, 56 novices in an analogy, a rule-based, and a control group were taught the table tennis topspin forehand. The experiment was separated into an acquisition phase, consisting of six blocks with 50 shots each, and a test phase, consisting of a retention test, a transfer test, and a decision test (with 50 shots each; see Liao & Masters, 2001; Poolton et al., 2006). For example, the analogy group got the "hypotenuse instruction" of Liao and Masters (2001, p. 310) "[Try] to pretend to draw a right-angled triangle with the bat." In contrast, the rule-based group read five detailed instructions:

1. Put your right foot behind you so that your feet are positioned slightly diagonal to the baseline.
2. Stretch your arm during the backward movement so that your bat is at the height of your hip.
3. Try to move your bat with an explosive forearm and wrist movement to your forehead.
4. Try to hit the ball in an upward movement before it reaches the highest point of the trajectory.
5. Focus on an active trunk rotation to support the shift of your weight from the right to the left foot. (German Table Tennis Association, 2001).

As in many other studies, the results revealed that with rule-based instructions novices could verbalize a significantly larger number of rules (Liao & Masters, 2001). Furthermore, the results showed that analogy instructions led to an optimized hitting bat-to-table angle and therefore better hitting performance than rule-based instructions, including under decision and transfer conditions. This result contrasts with the findings of Poolton et al. (2006), who found a decrease in the decision test in the rule-based group and stable performance in the analogy group.

In Study 2 (Schlapkohl et al., 2012), we extended Study 1 by adding a decision condition to the acquisition phase (Raab, Masters, & Maxwell, 2005). Sixty novices alternated practicing three blocks with instructions for the topspin forehand and three blocks with just a decision task. The instructions related not only to the execution of a topspin forehand ("how" instructions), but also to "what" to do. According to Masters and Maxwell (2008), when people try to solve a secondary task cognitively, their motor processes can be disrupted. To date, no differences have been found between analogy and rule-based instructions in an acquisition phase where a high cognitive load is implemented. The results of Raab et al. (2005) indicate that analogy instructions (with less declarative knowledge) even produced significantly better hitting performance in the acquisition phase with "how" and "what" decisions, stressing again the possible cognitive overload explanation previously mentioned. Furthermore, under transfer and decision conditions the novices showed an optimized bat-to-table angle and better hitting performance with analogies than with rule-based instructions. The interaction in the acquisition phase demonstrated the effectiveness of analogy instructions. Even if technical and tactical decision training are combined very early on in training, rule-based instructions could disrupt motor processes. Coaches and teachers need to be aware that too many rules and too much declarative knowledge disrupt the mechanics of the movement. Therefore, the simplicity of instructions during movement performance could be essential for athletes and their coaches if these studies can be replicated and generalized to other sports and performances.

PHYSICAL EDUCATION

In a study with 800 metaanalyses, Hattie (2008) identified what makes good tuition. In summary, he emphasized that the teacher plays a central role of the learning outcome (teacher clarity). That is, the pupils must understand what the teacher wants from them. The culture of correct feedback on the subject of the tuition should also be mentioned at this point (Hattie, 2008). Klingen (2005) reported that teachers were increasingly complaining that their pupils were unwilling to put in the necessary effort or did not have sufficient stamina to learn and practice, and sometimes even gave up or dodged demands after just a short time. How is it possible to instruct pupils with clarity and instill in them a sense of pleasure in playing sports? According to Achtergarde (2008), one approach is to increase autonomy, since regularity in sport assumes a certain level of autonomy (Ntoumanis and Matosik, Chapter 7; Ekkekakis and Zenko, Chapter 18). By allowing pupils to act independently and giving them the feeling that they are in control of their own sports activities, it is possible to generate stable patterns of behavior in relation to sports (Fuchs, 1997). Strauss (2008) emphasized this by saying: "Children and young people will only learn to view sport as part of their lives in general, including outside school, if we are able to teach them to act independently" (p. 8).

Analysis of sport psychology in school or in physical education is a new field (Makopoulou, Ntoumanis, Griffiths, & Li, 2014). To illustrate, from our own investigations we compared different instructions in physical education (with the focus on track and field athletics; Schlapkohl, Müller, Brogmus, Zink, & Blohm, 2011). The study examined which form of instructions was more effective at improving the motor performance of 44 school pupils. Differences in exercise variability, motivation, and sex were also analyzed. A 3-week, group-specific learning phase covering the disciplines of sprinting, ball throwing, and long jumping took place between the pre- and posttests (see instructions in Schlapkohl et al., 2011, Tables 2 and 3), and a retention test took place after 12 weeks. Analogy instructions for the discipline of sprinting included, for example, "Imagine that you are briefly in a puddle, but try not to get wet feet!" and "Try that as if you are cutting the air with your hands!" The rule-based group got five detailed rules.

From previous research we know that analogy instructions for novices in early learning are beneficial, but what are the results in pupils taking part in physical education classes? We found that after a 12-week break only analogy instructions led to significantly improved sprinting times and throwing distances. The group given analogy instructions also showed improved performance in the movement variability analysis. In terms of motivation, it is clear that analogy instructions are significantly more motivating. They have a particularly marked motivating effect on the work behavior of boys. These results suggest that we need further studies to analyze instruction differences in the school setting to have a broader understanding of this area.

HEALTH

A widespread aim of health projects is to get people to shape their daily diets and exercise regimes with self-determination, responsibility, and a sense of enjoyment (Johannsen & Schlapkohl, 2015). But the question of how to implement this in the long term often remains unanswered (Ekkekakis and Zenko, Chapter 18). Measures such as sanctions, training, "health days," or instructions by experts are not always successful. A new approach to giving instructions is the peer education approach (see also *Trendsport*, Bund, 2005), which involves training so-called lay disseminators as facilitators who instruct target groups from their own environment (Johannsen & Schlapkohl, 2015). The German Federal Centre for Health Education (BZgA) defines peer education in the area of health as "the teaching and sharing of information, values and patterns of behavior that promote health by members of the same age or status groups" (German Federal Centre for Health Education, 2003, p. 176). According to Backes, Schönbach, and Büscher (2002), the peer education approach impressively implements the theoretical principles of health promotion. It incorporates aspects such as promoting networks, self-organization, and empowerment (Heitmann & Schwaner-Heitmann, 2012). At the school level, for example, older pupils (leaders) will instruct younger pupils (participants) in working groups (eg, cooking, dancing, or football) or will act as exercise and play leaders in the playground.

An alternative approach focuses on examining the nutrition and physical activity skills of the leaders giving the instructions. Does the instructor's role bring about an implicit learning effect and motivation to exercise? Do the participants also learn from the pupils, and are they motivated by this? The target groups of this approach are pupils, people from an immigrant background and refugees, and functionally illiterate adults. Functionally illiterate adults are people whose reading, writing, and mathematical skills are inadequate to meet the demands of society despite having been to school. According to the Level One Study 2011, there are 7.5 million such people in Germany (Laschke et al., 2008; Groeneveld, Grünhagen-Monetti, Klinger, & Wilhelmi, 2011). In two cross-border, interdisciplinary, and interinstitutional projects at Europa University Flensburg and University College South Denmark, presented later in this chapter, researchers aimed first to take a very broad project approach with heterogeneous target groups and second to look at the successful transfer of instruction processes in practice (Laschke et al., 2008).

School and Health

The previously described project is an example of a school intervention. In it, 28 older pupils organized a health day (Feel Fit) and led individual activities on the subjects of nutrition and physical activity. Fifty-five primary school pupils took part in the action day, with teachers attending in a purely supporting role. The analysis examined what influence peer-to-peer instruction had on the pupils' learning skills and if there was an implicit effect on the pupils giving the instruction (leaders). The evaluation used a mixed-methods design to analyze the subprojects through quantitative and qualitative surveys. For the qualitative analysis, episodic interviews with teachers, focus group interviews with pupils, and analytical evaluations of target templates were carried out. The quantitative analysis involved a pre-, post-, and retention-test design with a questionnaire. The results indicated that in some cases participants' learning skills showed significant improvement in terms of cognitive knowledge about physical activity and its application in everyday life (German Federal Centre for Health Education, 2002). As the principal investigators of the study had assumed, the participating pupils' cognitive knowledge of physical activity improved as a result of the action day. However, the intervention did not change the participants' exercise behavior in their everyday lives. The action day was presumably too short to achieve this effect; an action week would be more worthwhile to test in future studies.

It was also found that the participants were far more motivated as previously to exercise as a result of the instructions given by the older pupils. There is significant evidence to support the assumption that facilitators' learning skills implicitly improve in all skills areas (knowledge of physical activity, application in everyday life, motivation to exercise; German Federal Centre for Health Education, 2002). Pupils who formulate and pass on their knowledge, give instruction, and lead exercises show a particular increase in their cognitive knowledge of physical activity, their motivation to exercise, and their long-term application of this knowledge in everyday life as well as improvements in their social behavior. Most of the results of the BZgA study can be applied to the school situation (German Federal Centre for Health Education, 2002). Learning skills were boosted as a result of the facilitators' subconscious learning situation (Backes et al., 2002; German Federal Centre for Health Education, 2002). The interviews produced comments such as: "When pupils explain something to other pupils, it is always on the same level. And when a teacher explains something to a pupil, there is always a gap. ... So when you have pupils explaining something on the same level, a lot more sticks. ... When pupils are motivated and given responsibility, they start to feel that they are a part of the whole. ... That's nice to see from the point of view of personality development" (teacher, personal communication).

Functionally Illiterate Adults and Health

This project is still ongoing, so no scientific analyses have been published as yet. The aim of the project is to teach functionally illiterate adults about nutrition and physical activity (Food & Move Literacy program; Johannsen & Schlapkohl, 2015). First, materials at an appropriate level for adults were created for the project. Second, functionally illiterate adults took over the role of instructor and helped other illiterate adults improve their nutritional and physical activity skills (peer-to-peer instruction). Over the course of five multiday workshops at eight adult education centers, students and lecturers developed a series of new practical and application-related methods along with teaching and learning materials for adult education. All teaching and learning materials developed as part of the INTERREG 4A project are being tested and further developed in an intervention phase in participating adult education center courses (the EU INTEEREG 4A project fosters intercultural activities between adjacent regions in border areas and is supported by the European Regional Development Fund). Following this, trained illiterate adults will instruct other illiterate adults and present the use of the materials in "train-the-trainer" courses.

CONCLUSIONS

The aim of this chapter was to present an overview of studies on instructions in competitive sports, sports played by novices, physical education, and health. In the various studies we explored the question of whether implicit and explicit instructions have different effects on performance and movement patterns. We aimed to extend the literature by accentuating the role of implicit learning for novices and pupils and in the area of health, as well as that of explicit learning for experts.

In conclusion, for experts in real game situations, movement performance must be accurate in order to provide short movement times. In table tennis, this allows players to return to a ready position earlier and thus gives them more time to attend to and process relevant information sources. With regard to our results, we advise coaches to train expert athletes using the explicit approach, that is, with rule-based instructions, for a fast and long-term learning process. Novices and pupils should be instructed implicitly, for example, with analogies, which are simple and efficient to use. In practice, this means that coaches and teachers should be aware that minor changes in specific instructions yield major changes in movements, which in turn can make a difference in the quality of competitive performance.

Additionally, we would suggest that teachers give pupils and functionally illiterate adults more responsibility and representative participation. Peer-to-peer instruction increases not only people's motivation to exercise but their knowledge of physical activity, as well. Implicit learning effects can also be observed among the leaders giving the instructions, leading to long-term consolidation in their everyday lives and improvements in their social behavior. As the results of the two case studies show, peer-to-peer learning/instruction as an innovative approach has met with strong interest on the part of stakeholders within various education systems. With this learning effect, both pupils and functionally illiterate adults take on the role of facilitator and have to come to grips with and formulate content. The effects they obtain from this are extremely important. In addition, the target group's sense of responsibility is reinforced and individual respect is conveyed.

This peer education approach can be transferred to both heterogeneous school and nonschool target groups and situations and to a wide range of themes and curricula (Heitmann & Schwaner-Heitmann, 2012). In future research, it would be interesting to extend the results to different environments and applications (eg, migrants and refugees), tasks (eg, motor learning during recess), methods of measuring (eg, neurophysiological measures), or institutions (eg, in adult education centers and physical education).

REFERENCES

Achtergarde, F. (2008). *Working independently in physical education. A book of sports methods.* Aachen, Germany: Meyer & Meyer.

Backes, H., Schönbach, K., & Büscher, I. (2002). Peer education. *A practical manual. Basic information, training concepts, methods, evaluation. Results of the model project commissioned by the Federal Centre for Health Education.* Meckenheim, Germany: Warlich.

Bund, A. (2005). How do young people learn "their" sport? Observations in the leisure sports environment. *Bewegungserziehung, 59,* 16–20.

Eklund, R. C., & Tenenbaum, G. (Eds.). (2004). *Encyclopedia of sport and exercise psychology.* Thousand Oaks, CA: SAGE.

Fuchs, R. (1997). *Psychology and physical exercise. Principles for theory-guided interventions.* Göttingen, Germany: Hogrefe.

German Federal Centre for Health Education. (2002). *Peer education—A practical manual.* Meckenheim, Germany: Warlich.

German Federal Centre for Health Education. (2003). *Key concepts of health promotion. Glossary on concepts, strategies and methods in health promotion.* Werbach-Gamburg, Germany: Verlag für Gesundheitsförderung.

German Table Tennis Association (Ed.). (2001). *Table tennis curriculum 2000 Stroke technique and footwork.* Frankfurt, Germany: German Table Tennis Association.

Groeneveld, M., Grünhagen-Monetti, M., Klinger, M., & Wilhelmi, I. (2011). Food literacy in the literacy course. *Making reading and writing appetising. Literacy and education.* Cologne, Germany: Bungarten.

Hänsel, F. (2002). Instructional psychology of motor learning. *Frankfurt am Main.* Germany: Lang.

Hattie, J. (2008). *Visible learning: A synthesis of over 800 meta-analyses relating to achievement.* New York, NY: Routledge.

Heitmann, H., & Schwaner-Heitmann, B. (2012). Pupils learn by teaching. Training pupils as working group leaders—concept and tools of the trade. *Pädagogik, 6,* 20–23.

Johannsen, U., & Schlapkohl, N. (2015). Intercultural expertise in supporting nutrition and physical activity. A research project with practical implementation. *Nutrition Survey International, 3,* 44–51.

Kleynen, M., Braun, S. M., Bleijlevens, M. H., Lexis, M. A., Rasquin, S. M., Halfens, J., ... Master, R. S. W. (2014). Using a Delphi technique to seek consensus regarding definitions, descriptions and classification of terms related to implicit and explicit forms of motor learning. *PloS One, 9,* 1–11.

Klingen, P. (2005). Motivating pupils—Promoting self-guidance. In *Sportunterricht schorndorf* (Vol. 54). Germany: Hofmann.

Koedijker, J. M., Oudejans, R. R. D., & Beek, P. J. (2007). Explicit rules and direction of attention in learning and performing the table tennis forehand. *International Journal of Sport Psychology, 38,* 227–244.

Laschke, M., Grundwald, S., Laes, B., Lehmkuhl-Wiese, M., Wolf, C., & Hausmann, C. (2008). *Project management. Manual for adult education establishments.* Hannover, Germany: Adult and Further Education Agency.

Liao, C. M., & Masters, R. S. W. (2001). Analogy learning: a means to implicit motor learning. *Journal of Sports Sciences, 19,* 307–319.

Makopoulou, K., Ntoumanis, N., Griffiths, M., & Li, F. X. (2014). In search for meaning, relevance, and importance in physical education. In K. Armour (Ed.), *Pedagogical cases in physical education and youth sport* (pp. 156–170). London, England: Routledge.

Masters, R. S. W. (2000). Theoretical aspects of implicit learning in sports. *International Journal of Sport Psychology, 31,* 530–541.

Masters, R., & Maxwell, J. (2008). The theory of reinvestment. *International Review of Sport and Exercise Psychology, 1,* 160–183.

Masters, R. S. W., Poolton, J. M., Maxwell, J. P., & Raab, M. (2008). Implicit motor learning and complex decision making in time-constrained environments. *Journal of Motor Behavior, 40,* 71–79.

Maxwell, J. P., Masters, R. S. W., & Eves, F. F. (2003). The role of working memory in motor learning and performance. *Consciousness and Cognition, 12,* 376–402.

Poolton, J. M., Masters, R. S. W., & Maxwell, J. P. (2006). The influence of analogy learning on decision making in table tennis: evidence from behavioural data. *Psychology of Sport & Exercise, 7,* 677–688.

Raab, M., Masters, R. S. W., & Maxwell, J. P. (2005). Improving the "how" and "what" decisions of elite table tennis players. *Human Movement Science, 24*, 89–99.

Schlapkohl, N., Hohmann, T., & Raab, M. (2012). Effects of instructions on performance outcome and movement patterns for novices and experts in table tennis. *International Journal of Sport Psychology, 6*, 522–541.

Schlapkohl, N., Müller, B., Brogmus, N., Zink, K., & Blohm, E. (2011). What forms of instruction improve motor skills and motivation in physical education? Initial results of an empirical research series. In N. Schlapkohl, & J. Schwier (Eds.), *School sports in Flensburg* (pp. 47–74). Flensburg, Germany: University Press Flensburg.

Strauss, B. (2008). Independent work in physical education—foreword. In F. Achtergarde (Ed.), *Independent work in physical education* (pp. 8). Aachen, Germany: Meyer & Meyer.

Tielemann, N. (2008). Modifying motor learning processes through instruction. *Effectiveness of analogies and movement rules.* Leipzig, Germany: Leipziger.

Williams, A. M., Ward, P., Knowles, J. M., & Smeeton, N. J. (2002). Perceptual skill in a real-world task: training, instruction and transfer in tennis. *Journal of Experimental Psychology, 8*, 259–270.

Wulf, G. (2008). Attentional focus effects in balance acrobats. *Research Quarterly for Exercise and Sport, 79*, 319–325.

Chapter 3

Benefits of Physical Activity and Fitness for Lifelong Cognitive and Motor Development— Brain and Behavior

Claudia Voelcker-Rehage*, Claudia Niemann*, Lena Hübner*, Ben Godde†, Axel H. Winneke‡

*Institute of Human Movement Science and Health, Technische Universität Chemnitz, Chemnitz, Germany; †Department of Psychology & Methods, Jacobs University, Bremen, Germany; ‡Project Group Hearing, Speech and Audio Technology, Fraunhofer Institute for Digital Media Technology, Oldenburg, Germany

In recent years, the influence of exercise and physical activity not only on physiological health and psychological well-being, but also on cognitive performance as well as on brain structure and function, has come into focus (eg, Etnier, Nowell, Landers, & Sibley, 2006; Hillman, Erickson & Kramer, 2008). In addition, studies examining the effects of exercise and physical activity on motor performance and motor learning processes (Roig, Skriver, Lundbye-Jensen, Kiens, & Nielsen, 2012) represent promising areas of research, especially for older adults and rehabilitation after stroke (Singh & Staines, 2015). The inclusion of brain research methods such as electroencephalography (EEG) or functional and structural magnetic resonance imaging (MRI) provide valuable information on how exercise and physical activity affect brain structure and function and which possible mechanisms might underlie their relationship with cognition/motor performance.

One line of research focuses on the immediate effects of acute bouts of exercise. Studies that fall into this category can be further divided into approaches measuring cognitive or motor performance during or directly after exercising. These studies are often complemented by EEG measurements to investigate underlying neurophysiological mechanisms. Another line of research investigates chronic effects of physical activity. Investigations in this field examine either the association between an individual's overall physical fitness level with, or

Sport and Exercise Psychology Research. http://dx.doi.org/10.1016/B978-0-12-803634-1.00003-0

43

the effect of a (long-term) exercise intervention on cognitive or motor performance. Only long-term intervention studies are assumed to lead to structural changes in the organism (eg, increased vascularization or growth of synaptic connections). For structural changes to occur, however, physiological changes must precede. Such physiological changes, which take place while the organism adapts to the physical demands of an activity, may already positively impact specific cognitive processes directly after an acute bout of exercise. The investigated age ranges vary between studies and the underlying mechanisms are still not completely understood.

Physical activity incorporates bodily movements produced by skeletal muscles including a variety of unspecified activities in daily life domains (eg, work, household). In contrast, structured *exercise* is characterized as physical activity that is planned, repetitive, and done with the purpose to improve physical fitness level. *Physical fitness level* (or: *fitness level*) in turn refers to the actual status of someone's physical fitness, often measured by defining the maximal rate of oxygen consumption (VO_2 max) or the participant's energy expenditure by use of physical activity questionnaires.

EFFECTS OF ACUTE BOUTS OF EXERCISE

Effects of Acute Bouts of Exercise on Cognitive Performance

The relationship between acute exercise and cognition has been investigated with various physical intervention methods, sample characteristics, cognitive assessments, and timepoints of measurement (McMorris, Sproule, Turner, & Hale, 2011). There is evidence that performance on complex cognitive tasks that tap into the executive control system, that is, those cognitive functions that are related to attentional control, working memory, and cognitive flexibility, suffers when performed *during* aerobic exercise (Pontifex & Hillman, 2007). These deficits, however, dissipate and even reverse when exercise is terminated, that is, cognitive performance *following* exercise improves on average (for a review, cf. Chang et al., 2012).

Most studies on acute exercise effects have been performed with young adults. A meta-analysis by McMorris, Sproule, Turner, and Hale (2011) reveals significantly faster response times in tasks of executive functions following moderate intensity exercise. Only few studies investigated healthy older adults or children.

Key factors that add to the variation in findings on the exercise-cognition relationship are the intensity and duration of the exercise. A recent meta-analysis by McMorris and Hale (2012) supports the assumption of an inverted U-shaped relationship between arousal and performance, referring to the Yerkes–Dodson Law (Yerkes & Dodson, 1908). Accordingly, the most beneficial and robust results for acute exercise on cognitive performance (particularly executive control) are achieved at submaximal, moderate intensities with durations between 20 and 60 min (McMorris et al., 2011; Tomporowski, 2003). High-intensity exercise, on the contrary, seems to be most beneficial in highly fit subjects (Budde et al., 2012). Alves and colleagues (2014) revealed improved performance in an attention task, but not in a short-term memory task in healthy middle-aged adults (participants of a physical fitness program) after a high-intensity interval training (HIT) indicating specific effects of bouts of high-intensity exercise with respect to the cognitive task. We have shown that attention was improved after high-intensity exercise in young adults with a high participation rate in physical activity, whereas this was not the case in low active individuals. This finding indicates that a higher participation rate in physical activity might lead to neurobiological adaptations that facilitate effects of high-intensity exercise on cognitive processes (ie, attention) (Budde et al., 2012; for further specification of effects of high-intensity exercise, see section "Combination of acute and chronic exercise" in this chapter).

Further, exercise effects differ with regard to the timepoint of assessment following exercising. Post exercise effects on executive functioning are evident immediately after exercise and last up to 30 to 40 min after exercise cessation (eg, Pontifex, Hillman, Fernhall, Thompson, & Valentini, 2009), but seem to diminish after two hours (Hopkins, Davis, VanTieghem, Whalen, & Bucci, 2012).

The finding that brief, moderate-intensity exercise can improve cognitive function has important implications for various target groups. For example, for adolescents in a school setting positive effects of single bouts of exercise on cognitive performance support the argument that physical activity could help to improve scholastic performance (Budde, Voelcker-Rehage, Pietrabyk-Kendziorra, Ribeiro, & Tidow, 2008), particularly for adolescents considered low cognitive performers (Budde, Windisch, Kudielka, & Voelcker-Rehage, 2010b). In older adults it could increase daily functioning and quality of life. Within the work context these findings suggest that an active lunch break could potentially increase job performance in the second half of the workday.

Several studies applied neurophysiological methods, predominantly EEG, during or after an acute bout of exercise to better understand underlying brain processes. It has repeatedly been shown that acute bouts of exercise modulate event-related potentials (ERPs). For example, there is some indication that acute bouts of moderate-intensity exercise lead to increased P3 amplitudes and earlier peak latencies alongside behavioral benefits (Drollette et al., 2014; Kamijo, Nishihira, Higashiura, & Kuroiwa, 2007; Magnie et al., 2000; Nakamura, Nishimoto, Akamatu, Takahashi, & Maruyama, 1999; Scudder, Drollette, Pontifex, & Hillman, 2012). This enlargement of the P3 amplitude can be interpreted as an increase in attentional resources in the brain (Kamijo, 2009, for an overview). Own pilot data collected from younger adults immediately after cycling for 20 min at a moderate intensity (40–60% of individual VO_2 peak values) reveal earlier P3 peaks and a trend for increased P3 amplitudes as compared to a rest condition (Winneke, Hübner, Godde, & Voelcker-Rehage, 2016). Little is known about acute intervention effects on ERPs in older adults. Only one study reported earlier P3 latencies in older adults immediately following moderate exercise as compared to a rest condition (Kamijo, 2009), indicating that acute bouts of exercise might be able to counter age-related cognitive decline. In a recent study by Drollette et al. (2014) children (age 8–10 years) showed earlier P3 latencies in a Flanker task following moderate exercise, indicating a higher processing speed. Interestingly, children classified as low performers showed particular behavioral gains in the more difficult incongruent Flanker condition accompanied by P3 amplitude enlargements, suggesting a gain in selective attentional resource allocation (cf. Hillman, Buck, Themanson, Pontifex, & Castelli, 2009, for similar results).

Results regarding the effect of exercise on the N2 ERP component are scarce and mixed; results with older adults are lacking. Themanson and Hillman (2006) did not find effects of acute exercise on the N2. Pontifex and Hillman (2007) in young adults reported a reduction in N2 amplitude while exercising accompanied by reduced performance, whereas Drollette and colleagues (2014) in children reported a reduction in N2 amplitude after 20 min of exercise together with improvement in performance. This reduction was interpreted as an facilitation in repsonse conflict.

Crabbe and Dishman (2004) did a quantitative synthesis of EEG studies investigating oscillations in the alpha frequency band (~8–12 Hz) after acute exercise including participants ranging from young to older adults. The authors reported overall increased absolute alpha power directly after exercise. For example, in 9- to 10-year-old children, larger alpha activity was revealed in the precuneus after 15 min of moderate bike exercise (Schneider, Vogt, Frysch, Guardiera, & Strüder, 2009). This has been interpreted as a reflection of an overall state of physical relaxation, which might improve the ability to concentrate and result in better cognitive performance following an acute exercise bout. Further, decreased coherence in the lower alpha band (8–10 Hz) after acute exercise of moderate intensity as compared to rest condition was shown, which is regarded as indicator for reduced cognitive effort after acute exercise (Hogan et al., 2013). Furthermore, individual alpha peak frequency (iAPF) was increased after exhaustive exercise but not after less intense exercise in young healthy adults (Gutmann et al., 2015). The increase in iAPF is interpreted as a marker of arousal and attention and is associated with increased information-processing speed (Gutmann et al., 2015). In a study with older adults, the participants revealed a stronger decrease in alpha event-related desynchronization) during a Stroop task following 20 min of exercise at a moderate intensity (Chang, Chu, Wang, Song, & Wei, 2015). Alpha desynchronization was particularly pronounced in frontal brain regions and was interpreted as a neural marker of enhanced task performance. These findings are supported by studies using functional near-infrared spectroscopy (fNIRS), which revealed that acute exercise led to enhanced prefrontal activity after exercise in older adults (Hyodo et al., 2012; Tsujii, Komatsu, & Sakatani, 2013), reflecting improved task processing.

To sum up the electrophysiological findings, research indicates enhanced attentional capacity related to acute exercise as reflected in increased P3 amplitudes. Studies looking at EEG frequencies (alpha frequency in particular) indicate an increase in neural resources that can be devoted to the cognitive task at hand, representing enhanced attention and better cognitive task performance.

Effects of Acute Bouts of Exercise on Motor Performance and Motor Learning

Effects of acute exercise on motor performance and motor learning have been studied for decades.[a] However, conducted exercise protocols (eg, exercise intensity, termination criteria) and performed motor tasks (eg, gross or fine motor skills) or whether the focus was on performance or learning varied across studies.

When measuring effects of acute exercise on motor performance, the performance or adaptation of a motor task was measured directly after exercise (Thacker, Middleton, McIlroy, & Staines, 2014; Wegner, Koedijker, & Budde, 2014). Findings are very heterogeneous. Some findings partially supported a claim of an inverted U-shape relationship between exercise intensity and motor performance (eg, with the gross motor Bachman ladder task, Pack, Cotten, & Biasiotto, 1974). Others found improvements after intense exercise in a task requiring fine motor control in high-fit young subjects (eg, Fitts' reciprocal tapping task; Dickinson, Medhurst, & Whittingham, 1979). A recent meta-analysis of effects of acute exercise on sport-related skills like passing in soccer by McMorris, Hale, Corbett, Robertson, & Hodgson (2015) did not only disprove an inverted U-shape relationship, but also found no significant effect of moderate-intensity exercise on motor performance and a detrimental effect of intense exercise.

So far, all studies were performed with young adults, with few exceptions. Wegner, Koedijker, and Budde (2014) investigated the effects of moderate-intensity exercise on manual dexterity performance in children (flower trail) and found no effect of acute exercise on fine motor performance. An EEG study by Thacker et al. (2014) revealed that acute bouts of moderate exercise led to an earlier onset of the early readiness potential in young participants indicating a positive effect on movement preparation in a subsequent motor task (self-paced wrist extension). Effects on task performance were not reported.

When measuring the effects of acute exercise on motor learning, performance was mostly measured by use of delayed retention tests (Mang, Snow, Campbell, Ross, & Boyd, 2014; Roig et al., 2012; Skriver et al., 2014) as the motor memory needs time to be transformed in performance improvement (for a review, see Kantak & Winstein, 2012). Findings regarding the effects of acute exercise on motor learning are again inconsistent. Interestingly, contrary to studies analyzing exercise effects on cognitive or motor performance, these studies used bouts of exercise of high intensity as lactate is assumed to

---

[a] In early studies, acute bouts of exercise were named as physical fatigue (eg, Pack, Cotten, & Biasiotto, 1974).

be a mediating mechanism. Positive effects of a high-intensity acute exercise protocol have been found on learning an implicit motor sequence task in terms of higher temporal precision but not spatial accuracy (force tracking) (Mang et al., 2014) and on retention performance (24 h and 7 days after practice), but not immediately after exercise (Roig et al., 2012; Skriver et al., 2014) as compared to a resting control group. The latter finding reflects that motor memory needs time for consolidation to be transformed into better motor performance. Roig and colleagues (2012) did not only compare the amount of motor learning after an acute bout of exercise with the amount of learning after a rest condition, but also varied the order of acute exercise and motor task. Interestingly, both, the experimental group practicing the motor task before the acute exercise and the group practicing the motor task after intense exercise performed better in the retention test seven days after practice than a non-exercising control group, with the post-exercise group performing best (Roig et al., 2012). This finding points to the need to further investigate the best timepoint of a bout of acute exercise (before or after practicing the motor task) to facilitate consolidation of motor learning processes.

Very recent studies provided neural underpinnings for the positive impact of acute bouts of exercise on motor learning processes. They revealed that acute bouts of exercise facilitate neuroplasticity in the (primary) motor cortex (M1) induced by repetitive transcranial magnetic stimulation (rTMS, ie, a noninvasive brain stimulation technique; Singh & Staines, 2015, for a review). M1 is the most important source of ascending projections to the motor neurons and is crucial for the voluntary control of movements. This enhanced neuroplasticity might occur because acute exercise affects neurochemical processes that are in turn known to facilitate M1 excitability, like higher levels of the neurotransmitters dopamine, serotonin, norepinephrine, and lactate (Singh, Neva, & Staines, 2014). In accordance to that, Skriver and colleagues (2014) showed that the same neurochemical processes (plus increased levels of insulin-like growth factor [IGF-1], epinephrine and vascular endothelial growth factor [VEGF]) were involved in motor skill acquisition and retention. Nevertheless, more studies are needed to examine the effects of acute exercise on motor functions and, motor learning including physiological and neurochemical measures. The aim is to understand the exact mechanisms and to give recommendations about exercise intensity, duration, and timing of exercise and motor paradigms (McMorris et al., 2015).

LONG-TERM EXERCISE OR PHYSICAL ACTIVITY EFFECTS

Long-Term Exercise or Physical Activity Effects on Cognition

Meta-analyses and review articles (Colcombe & Kramer, 2003; Kramer, Erickson, & Colcombe, 2006; Voelcker-Rehage & Niemann, 2013) have shown that physical activity (cross-sectional data and intervention studies) is positively associated with cognitive functioning across the lifespan. Colcombe and

Kramer (2003) analyzed 18 intervention studies on the influence of physical activity on various cognitive tasks in adults 55 years of age and older. They found the largest benefit of physical activity on executive control functions. Independent of cognitive task, method of training, and sample characteristics, physical activity enhanced cognitive performance by 0.5 standard deviations. The effect of physical activity was influenced by the length, the extent, and the type of intervention. Not only effects on executive control, but also on perceptual speed (Colcombe & Kramer, 2003) and memory performance were repeatedly shown (Flöel et al., 2008; Hötting, Schauenburg, & Röder, 2012; Klusman et al., 2010). Positive effects of moderate physical activity on cognitive performance have been shown already after only eight to 12 weeks of exercise (Albinet, Boucard, Bouquet, & Audiffren, 2010; Fabre, Chamari, Mucci, Masse-Biron, & Prefaut, 2002) two to three times a week and even in seniors who have been rather inactive previously.

Most exercise paradigms utilized cardiovascular exercise, also referred to as aerobic or cardiorespiratory exercise, where highly automated movements like walking or cycling are performed. Fewer studies investigated other types of exercise, such as motor-coordinative or resistance exercise. Similar to cardiovascular fitness, resistance exercise (resistance training) affects metabolic and energetic processes and to some extent intramuscular coordination. Unlike metabolic exercise, motor-coordination training comprises exercises for bilateral fine and gross motor body coordination such as balance, eye-hand coordination, and leg-arm coordination, as well as spatial orientation and reaction to moving objects/persons (Voelcker-Rehage, Godde, & Staudinger, 2011). Coordination training induces less change in energy metabolism than cardiovascular and resistance exercise. Instead, coordinative movements require perceptual and higher-level cognitive processes, such as attention, that are essential for mapping sensation to action and ensuring anticipatory and adaptive aspects of coordination. Thus, changes induced by coordinative exercise are likely to be related to changes in information processing and cognitive tasks that demand, besides attention, the ability to handle visual and spatial information. By contrast, perceptual and higher-level cognitive processes are less relevant in highly automated movements like walking or cycling, as used in cardiovascular exercise. Recently, dancing has come into focus as an attractive leisure-time activity among older adults. Dancing is a multimodal type of physical activity that addresses cardiovascular as well as coordinative and cognitive demands, and it is difficult to disentangle effects of cardiovascular from other fitness effects in dancing studies. In this section, we will detail the differential effects of different types of exercise and fitness on brain and cognitive function.

Cardiovascular Exercise

As for acute effects of exercise, there is increasing evidence for fitness-related modulations of cognitive ERPs. Other studies investigated the chronic exercise-cognition relationship by use of MRI or on a behavioral level only.

Higher physical activity levels are associated with shorter P3 latencies and/ or larger amplitudes in children (Hillman et al., 2014) and both younger (Kamijo & Takeda, 2010) and older adults (Fong, Chi, Li, & Chang, 2014; for reviews, cf. Kamijo et al., 2007). A cross-sectional study revealed that the amplitude of the N1 ERP component was increased in older adults participating in light and moderate aerobic exercise, as compared to a sedentary control group (Chang, Huang, Chen, & Hung, 2013b). This finding indicates that the exercise group was able to engage more attentional resources for the early stimulus encoding processes. Recent data from our lab revealed a linear positive relationship between VO_2 peak values and both behavioral performance and P3 amplitude in a working memory task in young adults (Winneke et al., 2016). Also a study with elementary school children revealed faster response times as well as shorter P3 latencies and increased P3 amplitudes on a flanker task and thereby underline the positive effect of physical activity intervention programs on attentional processes in children (Hillman et al., 2014). Interestingly, benefits of physical exercise in children were not only reported for general cognitive tasks but also for specific aspects of arithmetic problem solving (Moore, Drollette, Scudder, Bharij, & Hillman, 2014).

Findings regarding the N2 ERP component in context of physical activity are less and mixed. In a sample of middle-aged adults we showed a positive association between cardiovascular fitness levels and attentional control as well as N2 amplitudes (Fig. 3.1; Winneke, Godde, Reuter, Vieluf & Voelcker-Rehage, 2012), indicating greater conflict monitoring capacity (Yeung, Botvinick, & Cohen, 2004; for similar N2 results, cf. Gajewski & Falkenstein, 2015). Others report N2 and P2 latency reductions indicating reduced processing speed after aerobic exercise interventions (Özkaya et al., 2005). Contrary, Themanson and Hillman (2006) reported that in young adults the fitness level was not associated with modulations of the N2, but high-fit adults showed marked reductions in the amplitude of

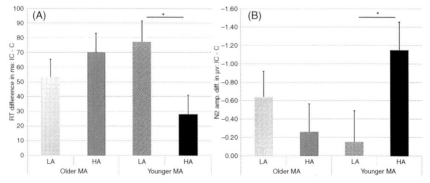

FIGURE 3.1   Interference induced by incongruent flanker (IC) quantified as (A) RT difference and (C) N2 amplitude difference at electrode Cz relative to congruent flanker (C) separated by age group and physical activity level *(LA = low active; HA = highly active).* * $p < 0.05$. *(Original figure appeared in Winneke et al., 2012.)*

the error-related negativity (ERN; cf. Themanson, Hillman, & Courton, 2006, for similar ERP results in older adults). Findings regarding the N2 and physical fitness in children and adolescents are also mixed with some studies reporting no association (Hillman et al., 2009), others reporting smaller N2 amplitudes in high-fit children yet better performance (Pontifex et al., 2011; Stroth et al., 2009).

Given the diversity of experimental designs and testing parameters together with the small number of studies, the effects of exercise interventions on ERP components, as markers of cognitive functioning and attentional control, require further investigation. Also, differences in maturity of brain development have to be considered particularly when comparing findings in children, young adults, and seniors.

The first functional MRI study on the exercise–cognition relationship was conducted by Colcombe and colleagues (2004) on older adults. Results indicated that after cardiovascular training, older adults applied cognitive resources more effectively and cognition was improved. Using a Flanker task, the data showed significantly higher levels of brain activation for physically active as compared to inactive older participants in prefrontal and parietal regions, and significantly lower activity in the anterior cingulate cortex (ACC). The same was true for older adults participating in a six-month aerobic exercise intervention (walking training) as compared to a stretching and toning control group (Colcombe et al., 2004). Higher prefrontal activation may contribute to better performance in a range of executive control functions, including attentional selection, working memory, task switching, and inhibitory control. Parietal structures that revealed higher activation in these studies are mainly associated with visuospatial processing, but also with language and tactile processing. Less activation in the ACC, on the contrary, indicates reduced response conflict.

Other studies confirmed the findings by Colcombe and colleagues (2004) (Holzschneider, Wolbers, Röder, Hötting, 2012; Prakash et al., 2011; Rosano et al., 2010). Interestingly, some studies revealed differential activation patterns. Following a 12-month aerobic exercise intervention, high-fit as compared to low-fit older adults revealed lower activation in the prefrontal cortex but higher activation in temporal regions during performance of incongruent Flanker trials (Voelcker-Rehage, Godde, & Staudinger, 2010, 2011). In the cognitive aging literature these contradictory findings are explained twofold: On the one hand, increasing task load is associated with increased recruitment (until a critical point is reached after which a decrease occurs) and training may serve to increase the engagement of task-relevant regions. On the other hand, increased efficiency in the processes linked to these regions might lead to reduced activations, that is, fewer neural resources required albeit maintaining or even improving performance. Moreover, higher activation in frontal brain areas, in older as compared to young adults, has often been interpreted as compensation for age-related changes (for review, see Reuter-Lorenz, & Lustig, 2005). Following this view, reduced activation after training might indicate a more youth-like or efficient brain and in turn less need for compensation. Thus, overactivation might be reduced in high-fit (Prakash et al., 2011) or trained older adults during less demanding, but also during challenging (Voelcker-Rehage et al., 2010, 2011) tasks. Both increased and decreased activation patterns may turn out to reflect physical activity-induced executive control improvement in older adults. Overall, cardiovascular activity seems to interact with brain activation during performance of executive control tasks, particularly, in frontal and parietal areas.

Research in children confirmed findings from research with older adults. In cross-sectional and longitudinal studies high-fit children (or after exercise intervention) revealed better executive control (Raine, Scudder, Saliba, Kramer, & Hillman, 2015; Chaddock et al., 2012a). Further, higher relational memory (Chaddock et al., 2010a) and learning benefits (Raine et al., 2013) were shown. These behavioral results from high-fit children were accompanied by more effective brain activation, as pronounced in either higher prefrontal cortex activity (Davis et al., 2011; Chaddock et al., 2012a, for the early task blocks) or reduced frontal activity (Chaddock et al., 2012a, for the later task blocks) and reduced parietal activity (Davis et al., 2011; Chaddock et al., 2012a, for the later task blocks), presumably reflecting a reduction of resources required to complete the task. Findings in children suggest that early cardiovascular fitness fosters executive control functioning and (less studied) memory performance and that this better performance may be related to functional and structural benefits, respectively.

In studies focusing on memory performance in adults, higher physical activity levels were paralleled by higher brain activation in the hippocampus and parahippocampal gyrus as well as in the frontal lobe during spatial learning or memory tasks in middle-aged (Holzschneider et al., 2012) and older adults (Smith et al., 2011). As both the frontal lobe and hippocampus are especially vulnerable to age-related functional changes (Grady, Springer, Hongwanishkul, McIntosh, & Winocur, 2006), one might assume that higher cardiovascular fitness or aerobic training contributes to better functioning of these regions. Depending on the sample and the type of task, cardiovascular activity may free up cognitive resources, to increase the engagement of task-relevant regions or to change performance strategies leading either to increased or reduced, but more efficient, activations in task-relevant areas.

Neural connectivity data bear the potential to reveal task-independent measures of brain function. Findings suggest that higher cognitive performance in high-fit older adults or following an extended aerobic intervention might be based on a higher functional connectivity within and between task-relevant brain regions at rest. Voss and colleagues (2010a; 2010b) demonstrated that higher functional connectivity of the so-called default mode network (DMN) was related to better executive control function. Whether other cognitive domains would also benefit from exercise-induced higher functional connectivity is currently not clear. Functional connectivity of the hippocampus with several other brain regions (Burdette et al., 2010) further seems to be enhanced through cardiovascular activity. This might positively influence memory function. To confirm this suggestion, additional research is required.

On the level of brain anatomy, Colcombe et al. (2003) again were the first to examine the association between brain volume and cardiovascular fitness in older adults. They found that age-related decline in brain volume in frontal, parietal, and temporal cortices was attenuated as a function of cardiovascular fitness (Colcombe et al., 2003). So far, brain regions that showed associations with cardiovascular fitness and/or training differ between studies. In older ages, a positive relationship has been found between cardiovascular training and frontal areas (eg, ACC) (Bugg & Head, 2011; Colcombe et al., 2003, 2006; Flöel et al., 2010; Gordon et al., 2008; Ruscheweyh et al., 2011; Weinstein et al., 2012), the temporal lobe (Colcombe et al., 2006; Gordon et al., 2008) or hippocampus (Erickson et al., 2009, 2011; Niemann, Godde, & Voelcker-Rehage, 2014b; Szabo et al., 2011), the parietal lobe (Benedict et al., 2013; Colcombe et al., 2003), and the basal ganglia (Verstynen et al., 2012). However, there were also studies that did not find any relationship between gray matter volume and cardiovascular activity parameter (Rosano et al., 2010; Smith et al., 2011). Also, in children higher levels of cardiovascular fitness or long-term exercise training have been related to larger volumes of the hippocampus (Chaddock et al., 2010a) and the basal ganglia (Chaddock et al., 2010b, 2012b, for an intervention analysis). Cognitive measurements were included in most of the studies and consistently revealed positive associations. However, cognitive domains differ substantially across studies: verbal skills in Gordon et al. (2008) and Benedict et al. (2013), episodic memory in Flöel et al. (2010) and Ruscheweyh et al. (2011), relational memory in Chaddock et al. (2010a), frequency of forgetting in Szabo et al. (2011), executive functions in Weinstein et al. (2012), Verstynen et al. (2012), Chaddock et al. (2010b and 2012a), and spatial memory in Weinstein et al. (2012) and Erickson et al. (2009 and 2011). So far, only one study examined the effect of cardiovascular exercise on brain parameters and cognitive functioning in middle-aged adults (Pereira et al., 2007), with a focus on the dentate gyrus. After a 3-month cardiovascular training, cerebral blood volume in the dentate gyrus of the hippocampus was enhanced and associated with improved cardiovascular fitness, suggesting better vascularization of this tissue. Furthermore, hippocampal blood volume was paralleled by better declarative memory performance of the participants (Pereira et al., 2007).

In comparison to gray matter volume, less research has been done on cardiovascular activity and white matter volume and integrity. Some research on white matter changes revealed a positive association with physical activity (Colcombe et al., 2003, 2006; Ho et al., 2011). However, the majority of studies did not find a relationship between white matter volume and physical activity (Erickson et al., 2010; Flöel et al., 2010; Gordon et al., 2008; Peters et al., 2009, for young adults; Ruscheweyh et al., 2011; Smith et al., 2011, for older adults). An association between white matter volume and cognitive performance has also not been established so far, although a positive association with information-processing speed is highly likely (Jacobs et al., 2011). First studies on white matter integrity in older adults suggested that high aerobic fitness may attenuate age-related decline in myelination of axons in portions of the corpus callosum (Johnson, Kim, Clasey, Bailey, & Gold, 2012), the cingulum (Marks, Katz, Styner, & Smith, 2011), and a frontoparietal brain network related to visuospatial functions, motor control, and coordination (Tseng et al., 2013). Similarly, increases in VO_2 max after a 12-month intervention period were related to increases of fractional anisotropy values in prefrontal and temporal regions (Voss et al., 2013b). However, also contradictory findings exist (Burzynska et al., 2014). In terms of white matter lesions and hyperintensities, more physical activity seems to be associated with less white matter hyperintensities in older adults without advanced diseases (for an exception in men, see Torres, Strack, Fernandez, Tumey & Hitchcock, 2015).

Resistance Training

Although some studies have reported conflicting findings on the role of resistance-exercise training in preventing cognitive decline with age, other studies have demonstrated a beneficial effect of such training on specific cognitive measures. A recent review of studies with healthy older adults revealed overall positive effects of resistance training on cognitive functions including information-processing speed, attention, memory formation, and specific types of executive function (Chang et al., 2012). In comparing resistance-exercise training with other types of exercise, such as flexibility, toning, relaxation, calisthenics, and even endurance exercises (Brown, Liu-Ambrose, Tate, & Lord, 2009; Cancela Carral & Ayan Perez, 2007; Özkaya et al., 2005), some studies showed that resistance training produced equivalent or even higher performance increases in specific cognitive functions. Further, resistance training seems to show clear dose-response effects. Intervention designs with loads of 60–80% 1RM (repetition maximum) with approximately seven movements in two sets separated by 2 min of rest at least twice per week for 2–12 months (usually 6 months), seem best suited to positively affect cognition.

The beneficial effects of resistance training were supported by functional MRI and ERP data indicating changes in (visual) processing strategies (Nagamatsu, Handy, Hsu, Voss, & Liu-Ambrose, 2012) and facilitation of early sensory processing and cognitive functioning in older individuals (Özkaya et al., 2005).

Motor-Coordination Training

Motor coordination measured after an exercise intervention or via motor fitness level is also positively associated with cognitive function. This has been shown for different age groups. In elementary school-aged children, motor fitness levels have been positively related to complex executive control tasks (Luz, Rodrigues, & Cordivil, 2015) and academic achievement (Lopes, Santos, Pereira, & Lopes, 2013). After 3 months (Koutsandréou, Niemann, Wegner, & Budde, 2016) or 6 months (Crova et al., 2014) of motor-demanding and cognitively challenging interventions, executive control performance of 9- to 10-year-old children was improved.

Drawing conclusions from intervention studies (in older adults) is difficult because not only the type of intervention differed (eg, multimodal exercise training including cardiovascular, strength, and motor fitness training, Vaughan et al., 2014; multimodal motor training including coordination, balance, strengthening, agility, and relaxation tasks, Forte et al., 2013; Voelcker-Rehage et al., 2011; flexibility and object manipulation training, Berryman et al., 2014; contemporary dance, Coubard et al., 2011; Kwok et al., 2011), but also cognitive dimensions included in the analyses vary as well as the intervention length (2–12 months). Even in studies using similar interventions and tasks, findings on cognition often could not be replicated (Forte et al., 2013; Klusmann et al., 2010; Vaughan et al., 2014). Nevertheless, positive effects of high motor coordination in older adults were reported on verbal fluency (Vaughan et al., 2014), measurements of fluid intelligence (Raven Standard Progressive Matrices, Kattenstroth, Kolankowska, Kalisch, & Dinse, 2010), information-processing speed (Okely, Booth, & Patterson, 2001; Vaughan et al., 2014; Voelcker-Rehage et al., 2011), Mini Mental State Examination (MMSE; a measure of cognitive impairment, Kwok et al., 2011), executive functions (Berryman et al., 2013; Forte et al., 2013; Okely et al., 2001; Vaughan et al., 2014; Voelcker-Rehage et al., 2011), and cognitive flexibility (Coubard et al., 2011). Some studies, however, failed to report positive effects. For example, Klusmann et al. (2010) could not replicate the findings for verbal fluency and executive control functions after 6 months of a similarly complex physical activity training, but found increases in episodic memory performance (cf. also, Hötting et al., 2012, for effects of a stretching and coordination training on episodic memory in middle-aged adults). There was also no positive influence of motor coordination found on problem solving and inhibition control (Coubard et al., 2011).

Studies on the effects of coordination trainings on neurophysiological measures are rare. An ERP study on task-switching revealed that P3 amplitudes were increased and reaction times were reduced in older adults with a history of regularly participating in Tai Chi as compared to sedentary older adults (Fong et al., 2014). Also, kindergarten children participating in an 8-week coordinative exercise program revealed faster response times as well as shorter P3 latencies and increased P3 amplitudes on a Flanker task at the end of the intervention relative to the beginning (Chang, Tsai, Chen, & Hung, 2013a). We conducted an MRI study on the effects of coordination training and were able to show that motor fitness was related to more efficient cognitive processing, indicated by less cortical activation in brain regions involved in cognitive control, that is, the superior and middle frontal cortex. In addition, motor fitness was related to higher activation of the right inferior frontal–posterior parietal network indicative of improved processing and integration of visuospatial information (Voelcker-Rehage et al., 2010). We further revealed that after a 12-month coordination training (60 min, 3 times per week) brain activation levels during a Flanker task increased particularly in the right inferior frontal gyrus and the superior parietal cortex, which form part of the so-called visuospatial attention network, as well as in the thalamus and caudate body (Voelcker-Rehage et al., 2011). These latter subcortical structures are important for process automation without conscious control. This fits well with other findings showing that high-fit older adults needed less dorsolateral prefrontal (cognitive) resources for movement control than low-fit participants (Godde & Voelcker-Rehage, 2010).

Furthermore, structural brain data indicate that older adults with higher levels of motor fitness or older adults participating in a 12-month coordination training program, revealed larger volumes of the hippocampus (Niemann et al., 2014b; c.f. Fig. 3.2). High motor fitness level as well as motor-coordination training seem to be beneficial to diminish age-related hippocampal volume shrinkage or even to increase hippocampal volume in older adults. Similarly, volume of the basal ganglia (caudate, putamen, and globus pallidus) also benefited from motor fitness and/or coordination training (Niemann, Godde, Staudinger, & Voelcker-Rehage, 2014a). Moreover, basal ganglia volume moderated the relationship between higher motor fitness levels and executive control performance. That is, in participants with low basal ganglia volume, motor fitness was positively correlated with executive control performance. This relationship became negligible when basal ganglia volume was larger. This finding indicates that motor fitness might prevent older adults from showing reduced executive control functioning when basal ganglia volume is low (or vice versa, that there is no additional benefit of motor fitness when basal ganglia size exceeds a certain volume).

To sum up, current research indicates that not only cardiovascular demands contribute to cognitive benefits in older adults, since interventions without any cardiovascular impact also revealed positive effects on the behavioral and neurophysiological level. Therefore, a coordination training including a

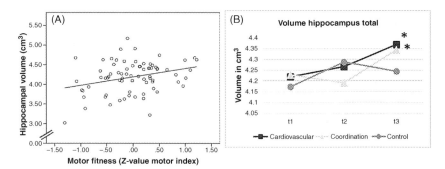

FIGURE 3.2 Cross-sectional and interventional findings of associations of coordinative activity with hippocampal volume of both hemisphere (in cm^3) in healthy older adults aged 62–79 years: (A) Significant relationship of hippocampal volume and motor fitness levels ($r=$ .28); (B) Hippocampal volume at baseline (t1) after 6 (t2) and 12 (t3) months of coordination (and cardiovascular) training. * $= p < 0.05$. *(Figure adapted from Niemann et al., 2014b.)*

variety of complex movements (for a discussion, see also Voelcker-Rehage & Niemann, 2013) might be essential for cognitive benefits.

Dancing

A first prospective study, by Verghese and colleagues (2003), showed leisure dancing to be associated with a reduced risk of developing dementia. A few years later, however, a cross-sectional study did not confirm this result. Adults aged 80 years, who had engaged in many years of nonprofessional dancing activity, did not demonstrate better cognitive performance in the domains of memory and executive control in comparison to nondancers (Verghese, 2006). Similarly, a pilot study with 13 healthy, older women did not reveal improvements in cognitive performance measured by the MMSE, after a 12-week jazz dance intervention (Alpert et al., 2009). Recent studies, again, showed more positive results. Older adults, with long-term dancing experience, showed better cognitive performance in the domains of fluid intelligence and attention in comparison to age-matched inactive controls (Kattenstroth et al., 2010). Furthermore, the same research group observed increasing performance in an overall index of cognition (comprised of concentration, attention, and nonverbal learning) in older adults participating in a 6-month dancing intervention (Kattenstroth, Kalisch, Holt, Tegenthoff, & Dinse, 2013).

We performed a first neuroimaging study, in which we tested the association of long-term senior dance experience with cognitive performance and gray matter brain volume in older women aged 65–82 years (Niemann, Godde, & Voelcker-Rehage, under review). In this study, we compared nonprofessional senior dancers with a control group consisting of physically active participants without any dance experience. No differences with respect to dance experience were revealed in the four tested cognitive domains (executive control, perceptual speed, episodic memory, long-term memory). Small effects of dance experience were observed in frontal gray matter volume in the right medial frontal gyrus and the left middle frontal gyrus. Volume of the left middle frontal gyrus was positively related to executive control performance, and volume of the hippocampus was positively related to long-term memory performance across the whole sample. Thus, although positive associations of cardiovascular as well as motor-coordination activity on brain structure and function have been previously revealed, data on the effects of dancing activity on the brain are sparse and further research is needed.

Genetic and Physiological Factors to Influence the Acute and Chronic Exercise-Cognition Relationship

Few studies have investigated the link between lifestyle factors such as physical activity, cognitive performance, and genetics. Of particular interest in this context is the catechol-O-methyltransferase (COMT) polymorphisms. The COMT gene has been identified as a candidate gene associated with executive functions (Goldberg & Weinberger, 2004). Numerous human studies showed advantages of met/met allele carriers over val homozygotes in tasks of executive functioning. Stroth and coworkers (2010) revealed that in a sample of healthy adults (17–47 years of age), COMT val homozygotes improved their cognitive performance (Stroop task, dots-mixed task), after 17 weeks of running training, to a greater extent than met allele carriers. Similarly, investigating the effect of a 6-month multicomponent training program (cognitive, aerobic, and activities of daily living) in healthy older adults, Pieramico et al. (2012) revealed the greatest exercise benefits in COMT val/val and val/met allele carriers (and DRD3 ser9gly carriers). We revealed a positive influence of overall fitness, and an interactive effect of fitness and COMT polymorphisms on Flanker accuracy performance (Voelcker-Rehage, Jeltsch, Godde, Becker, & Staudinger, 2015). Val/val carriers revealed the highest positive correlation between fitness and cognition suggesting that particularly val/val allele carriers benefit from exercise by improved cognitive functioning, whereas met/met carriers already perform close to their optimal level.

Endocrinological changes (especially glucocorticoids, eg, cortisol) have also been established as a factor that facilitates the positive effects of acute and/or chronic exercise on cognitive functioning (Lupien, Gillin, & Hauger, 1999; Budde et al., 2010a). Also neurotransmitter (eg, dopamine) and neurotrophic growth factors (eg, brain derived neurotrophic factors, BDNF) are assumed to play a key role in the exercise-cognition relationship. Dopamine has been shown to be affected by exercise in both animals (Hattori, Naoi, & Nishino, 1994; He et al., 2012; Kim et al., 2011) and humans (Kraemer et al., 1999; McMorris et al., 2008; Ruscheweyh et al., 2011; Winter et al., 2007) after both acute and long-term physical activity interventions. The association between physical activity and dopamine concentrations is, however, still controversially discussed; some studies did not find an increase in dopamine levels during (Nybo, Nielsen, Blomstrand, Moller, & Secher, 2003) or after (Wang et al., 2000) exercise.

BDNF as a major growth factor of the brain promotes angiogenesis, neurogenesis, synaptogenesis, gliagenesis, as well as the formation of dendrites and neuron body growth and thus, has an indirect impact on brain structure and cognitive functioning (for a review, see Voss et al., 2013a). Animal research showed that cardiovascular activity seems to enhance the release of BDNF in the hippocampus (Cotman & Berchtold, 2002; Ding, Vaynman, Akhavan, Ying, & Gomez-Pinilla, 2006; Gomez-Pinilla, Vaynman, & Ying, 2008), cortex (Ding, Li, Luan, Ding, Lai, Rafols et al., 2004), and basal ganglia (Ding et al., 2004). In humans, acute and chronic exposure to physical activity was shown to result in increased peripheral levels of BDNF (for a review, see Huang, Larsen, Ried-Larsen, Moller, & Andersen, 2014). Increased BDNF levels in response to cardiovascular activity were accompanied by better memory (Winter et al., 2007; Ruscheweyh et al., 2011), inhibition control (Ferris, Williams, & Shen, 2007), and spatial performance (Erickson et al., 2010). Fitness status was assumed to play a role in BDNF release. For example, in cardiovascular fit young adults, acute BDNF release in response to an acute bout of cardiovascular activity was higher than in less fit adults (Zoladz et al., 2008). In sum, endocrinological and neurochemical growth factors, crucial for brain structure and cognitive performance, are age dependent, but seem to be modifiable by physical activity, which boost the release.

Effects of Physical Activity on Motor Performance and Motor Learning

As compared to cognitive skills, less is known about the relationship between a chronic engagement in physical activity and the performance in motor tasks. No study investigated the effects of chronic physical activity on motor learning processes in humans so far. Existing studies about physical activity and motor performance were conducted with older adults; results are mixed.

Research indicates that older physically fit persons show superior motor performance as compared to their sedentary counterparts for tasks requiring lower limbs, like standing balance, walking speed, or the ability to rise from a chair (Krampe, Smolders, & Doumas, 2014; Pahor et al., 2006). Other studies showed this positive relationship also for the upper limbs in simple motor reaction time tasks (Spirduso, 1980), tasks requiring fine motor control (Bakken et al., 2001) and manual aiming ability (Claudino, Mazo, & Santos, 2013). Data from our own lab supported a positive association between physical fitness and fine motor performance in older adults showing that high-fit older adults performed better in tasks requiring fine motor control (visuomotor force tracking and Purdue Pegboard test) (Hübner, Godde, & Voelcker-Rehage, in preparation) than their less fit counterparts. (cf. Adamo, Alexander, & Brown, 2009; Etnier & Landers, 1998; Krampe et al., 2014 for no effects on fine motor control of the upper limbs).

Up to now, the underlying mechanisms remain unclear to a large extent. Some authors speculated that higher motor and sensory functions, better muscular performance, and conservation of proprioception of the more fit older adults might be responsible for the superior motor performance (Claudino et al., 2013). Animal studies showed that aerobic exercise interventions induced changes in the motor cortex and other areas involved in motor function (cerebellum, basal ganglia, substantia nigra) expressed by enhanced oxidative metabolism (Mc-Closkey, Adamo, & Anderson, 2001; Vissing, Andersen, & Diemer, 1996), hippocampal neurogenesis and synaptic plasticity (van Praag, Shubert, Zhao, & Gage, 2005). These findings indicate that regular exercise does not only modulate brain areas involved in cognitive processing, but also brain regions being active during motor performance. Again, more research is needed to be able to derive well-founded exercise recommendations to improve motor performance or motor learning processes. Findings could have great impact for certain target groups, for example, for rehabilitation of stroke patients.

COMBINATION OF ACUTE AND CHRONIC EXERCISE

Few studies investigated the interplay between the effects of acute and chronic exercise on cognitive functioning. Such a relationship is assumed because physiological changes, which take place while the organism adapts to the demands of an acute bout of exercise, may lead to structural changes in the long run. So far, these studies indicate that individual improvements in physical fitness lead to larger cognitive benefits through acute bouts of exercise (Hopkins et al., 2012). For example, Zervas, Danis and Klissouras (1991) investigated in an acute-chronic-mixed design the performance in a visual discrimination task in preadolescent children. Twenty-five minutes of treadmill running improved cognitive performance and was the highest after 6 months of aerobic training. The fitness effect seems to be especially prominent in highly complex cognitive tasks (Weingarten, 1973). However, so far, intervention lengths were limited (7 and 12 weeks) in studies, only children or young adults have been investigated, and study designs were not well controlled (Gutin, 1966; Weingarten, 1973). We assume that acute exercise effects sum up across an exercise intervention period and lead to pre- to posttest (chronic) changes in cognition and (neuro-) physiological markers.

Roig, Nordbrandt, Geertsen and Nielsen (2013) conclude in their review that fitness level does not interact with acute exercise in tasks requiring short-term memory. In contrast, in tasks requiring long-term memory, acute exercise seems to have a better effect in individuals with an average fitness level as with a low fitness level. Chang et al. (2012) in their review found benefits of high and low fit (but not moderately fit) participants on cognition directly after exercise.

Findings regarding exercise intensity effects are, however, ambiguous as some studies revealed higher cognitive benefits for high-fit or high-active participants in comparison to their less-fit or inactive counterparts (Budde et al., 2012; Pesce, Cereatti, Forte, Crova, & Casella, 2011) and others did not show any differential effects regarding fitness levels (Magnie et al., 2000; Themanson & Hillman, 2006).

To sum up, these results underline the importance to assess physical fitness status and a history of physical activity history (ie, sport participation in the last 12 months) in studies examining effects of acute exercise to control for the interplay of acute and chronic exercise effects.

OUTLOOK

In this chapter we provided an overview about different research facets of the exercise-cognition interaction. It turns out that certain research questions so far have been thoroughly investigated only in certain target groups (eg, chronic exercise effects mainly in older adults and acute exercise effects in younger adults). Further, research methods and paradigms differ immensely between studies. Systematic approaches that bring together the different research areas, methods and results are still missing. Especially the interaction of acute and chronic exercise effects on cognition need to be examined in greater depths, because, as we outlined in this chapter, existing findings seem to be ambiguous. Moreover, studies are needed to investigate whether effects of acute and chronic exercise on behavior and neurophysiological processes are the same in children, as well as younger and older adults. For example, it is unknown whether the exercise effects vary as a function of cognitive processes to a different degree in younger and older adults. Besides younger adults, adolescents, and older adults over the age of 65, another age group that is particularly interesting is that of middle adulthood, spanning the ages 35–65 years. In light of age-related cognitive changes, measures to prevent or to slow down the decline are important to take before first signs of deficits appear. Therefore, the optimal time to take preventive steps is probably the childhood and middle adulthood. As we have shown, physical exercise is a potential mean to modulate cognitive function. A few studies exist that look at the cognition-exercise relationship in middle-aged adults but more research is required to increase our understanding. In the same line of argumentation, more longitudinal studies and long-term follow-up measurements are desirable to further expand our knowledge of how the relationship develops over time. Also, research investigating the relationship between chronic physical activity or acute bouts of exercise and motor performance and motor learning in different age groups is needed. In this field of research, studies measuring neurophysiological processes are missing. Furthermore, only very lab-oriented motor tasks were used so far. Studies testing tasks that are more closely related to daily activities of older adults need to be conducted to better estimate the impact of physical activity and acute exercise on daily functioning and living.

GLOSSARY

Electroencephalography (EEG)

EEG measures the summed synchronous electrical activity of a large number of neurons via electrodes placed on the scalp. The EEG methodology has an excellent temporal resolution and allows for the online measurement of cognitive processing. EEG data are analyzed with two main approaches: continuous EEG data and event-related potentials.

Continuous EEG data that are not time-locked to certain events can be regarded as the linear sum of various oscillatory components. Decomposing the data by, for example, a Fourier transformation reveals typical oscillations in different frequency bands that can be associated with certain cognitive or brain states. *Alpha* oscillations ($\sim$8–13 Hz) are associated with a relaxed brain state without active processing of external or internal stimuli. The dominant EEG peak frequency within the individual alpha frequency band is the individual alpha peak frequency (iAPF). The term *event-related desynchronization (ERD)* describes decreases in brain oscillations as a consequence on an external event or stimulus. *Beta* oscillations (~14–30 Hz) are associated with motor behavior and changes in corticospinal output. Other typical oscillations can be observed in the theta (~4–8 Hz) or gamma (>30 Hz) frequency range. The phase consistency of oscillations between pairs of electrodes in each frequency band is called *coherence* and can be interpreted as functional interaction of corresponding brain areas. The power within a certain frequency band is a measure of the strength of the respective oscillations.

Event-related potentials (ERP) are short-lasting positive or negative voltage-changes that are synchronized with certain internal or external events such as stimuli, tasks, or responses. ERPs consist of typical components that are associated with perceptual, cognitive, or motor processes. The following components are of importance in the context of this chapter:

The *P1* and *N1* are the first positive and negative deflections in the ERP peaking around 50–100 ms and 100–150 ms after stimulus onset, respectively. They are associated with early sensory processing but can be modulated by attention. The second positive deflection (*P2*), reaching its peak about 150–200 ms after stimulus onset, reflects sensitivity to specific stimulus features and its occurrence probability. The second negative deflection in the ERP, the *N2*, reaches its maximum amplitude around 200–300 ms after stimulus onset and reflects endogenous cognitive components associated with novelty detection (N2a), executive control (N2b), and classification (N2c). A positive deflection peaking about 300–500 ms after stimulus onset is the *P3*. This component is related to the evaluation and classification of incoming information. *Latency* of the P3 is an index of the timing of respective cognitive processes; *amplitude* has been suggested to indicate processing intensity of the cognitive task at hand.

Other important components are the *readiness potential* (RP) and the *error-related negativity* (ERN or Ne). The RP, also called Bereitschaftspotential (BP), is a negative deflection starting about 1–2 s before the execution of a movement. The RP is further divided into the early and late RP (or early and late BP), reflecting different motor preparation processes. The ERN can be observed about 100 ms following an error was committed in various tasks even without the participant being aware of committing the error.

Structural and Functional Brain Imaging

Magnetic resonance imaging (MRI) is a brain-imaging technique that makes use of the magnetic properties of the atomic nucleus (nuclear magnetic resonance) and has an excellent spatial resolution. It is used for visualizing detailed pictures of the brain structure and to measure the volume of gray (*GM*) or white (*WM*) matter. While neuronal cell bodies, dendrites, and synapses occur as *GM* in the MR image, *WM* refers to the axons of neurons, being responsible for the transfer of information. *Myelin* is a fatty layer surrounding the axons of neurons that enables fast information processing between neurons, and is responsible for the white coloring. *WM integrity* represents a measure of the quality of the WM microstructure, for example, assessed by *fractional anisotropy* (value that refers to the coherence of the orientation of water diffusion).

With increasing age, the volume of the WM decreases and its microstructure and integrity changes leading to axon fiber splitting or swelling. These lesions are called *white matter hyperintensities (WMH)* and are associated with age-related slowing of cognitive, motor, and sensory processes as information transfer is less efficient.

Functional magnetic resonance tomography (fMRI) is a variant of MRI that reveals local brain function by measuring changes of the BOLD (blood oxygenation level dependent)-Signal, which is dependent on the oxygen saturation of the blood. The *default mode network (DMN)* is a network of interacting brain regions that is active when a person is not focused on the outside world, measurable with the fMRI technique.

Functional near-infrared spectroscopy (fNIRS) is another brain-imaging technique that makes use of changes in brain oxygenation during activation. Based on the different light absorption spectra of oxyhemoglobin (oxygenated form of hemoglobin) and deoxyhemoglobin (deoxygenated form of hemoglobin) for near-infrared light that is able to penetrate the skull and brain, activation in specific brain area can be visualized. *Transcranial magnetic stimulation (TMS),* also a noninvasive technique, applies a magnetic field near the sculp. Short electrical impulses are send to brain areas of interest (for example, the primary motor cortex), leading to changes in membrane function. TMS can be used to excite or to inhibit certain brain functions. *Repetitive transcranial magnetic stimulation (rTMS)* is one TMS technique, in which pulses are applied a repetitious manner.

Measuring Executive Functions

Executive functions are a key dimension of cognition and are comprised by components such as selective attention, response inhibition, and working memory. Different tests have been well established to examine individual executive functions:

The *flanker task* (Eriksen & Eriksen, 1974) requires (spatial) selective attention and executive control. In this task, irrelevant stimuli have to be inhibited in order to respond to a relevant target stimulus.

The *Stroop task* (Stroop, 1938) requires selective attention and inhibition control. The participant has to name the color of the ink (eg, blue, red, green) that the name of a color (*"blue," "red," "green"*) is printed in. If ink and color name do not match, reaction times increase because of this interference.

REFERENCES

Adamo, D. E., Alexander, N. B., & Brown, S. H. (2009). The influence of age and physical activity on upper limb proprioceptive ability. *Journal of Aging and Physical Activity, 17*(3), 272–293.

Albinet, C. T., Boucard, G., Bouquet, C. A., & Audiffren, M. (2010). Increased heart rate variability and executive performance after aerobic training in the elderly. *European Journal of Applied Physiology, 109*(4), 617–624.

Alpert, P. T., Miller, S. K., Wallmann, H., Havey, R., Cross, C., Chevalia, T., … Kodandapari, K. (2009). The effect of modified jazz dance on balance, cognition, and mood in older adults. *Journal of the American Academy of Nurse Practitioners, 21*(2), 108–115.

Alves, C. R., Tessaro, V. H., Teixeira, L. A., Murakava, K., Roschel, H., Gualano, B., & Takito, M. Y. (2014). Influence of acute high-intensity aerobic interval exercise bout on selective attention and short-term memory tasks. *Perceptual & Motor Skills, 118*(1), 63–72.

Bakken, R. C., Carey, J. R., Di Fabio, R. P., Erlandson, T. J., Hake, J. L., & Intihar, T. W. (2001). Effect of aerobic exercise on tracking performance in elderly people: a pilot study. *Physical Therapy, 81*(12), 1870–1879.

Benedict, C., Brooks, S. J., Kullberg, J., Nordenskjold, R., Burgos, J., Le Greves, M., … Schioth, H. B. (2013). Association between physical activity and brain health in older adults. *Neurobiology of Aging, 34*(1), 83–90.

Berryman, N., Bherer, L., Nadeau, S., Lauziere, S., Lehr, L., Bobeuf, F., … Bosquet, L. (2013). Executive functions, physical fitness and mobility in well-functioning older adults. *Experimental Gerontology, 48*(12), 1402–1409.

Berryman, N., Bherer, L., Nadeau, S., Lauziere, S., Lehr, L., Bobeuf, F., & Bosquet, L. (2014). Multiple roads lead to Rome: combined high-intensity aerobic and strength training vs. gross motor activities leads to equivalent improvement in executive functions in a cohort of healthy older adults. *Age (Dordrecht, Netherlands), 36*(5), 9710–9714.

Brown, A. K., Liu-Ambrose, T., Tate, R., & Lord, S. R. (2009). The effect of group-based exercise on cognitive performance and mood in seniors residing in intermediate care and self-care retirement facilities: a randomised controlled trial. *British Journal of Sports Medicine, 43*(8), 608–614.

Budde, H., Voelcker-Rehage, C., Pietrabyk-Kendziorra, S., Ribeiro, P., & Tidow, G. (2008). Acute coordinative exercise improves attentional performance in adolescents. *Neuroscience Letters, 441*(2), 219–223.

Budde, H., Voelcker-Rehage, C., Pietrassyk-Kendziorra, S., Machado, S., Ribeiro, P., & Arafat, A. M. (2010a). Steroid hormones in the saliva of adolescents after different exercise intensities and their influence on working memory in a school setting. *Psychoneuroendocrinology, 35*, 382–391.

Budde, H., Windisch, C., Kudielka, B. M., & Voelcker-Rehage, C. (2010b). Saliva cortisol in school children after acute physical exercise. *Neuroscience Letters, 483*, 16–19.

Budde, H., Brunelli, A., Machado, S., Velasques, B., Ribeiro, P., Arias-Carrion, O., & Voelcker-Rehage, C. (2012). Intermittent maximal exercise improves attentional performance only in physically active students. *Archives of Medical Research, 43*(2), 125–131.

Bugg, J. M., & Head, D. (2011). Exercise moderates age-related atrophy of the medial temporal lobe. *Neurobiology of Aging, 32*(3), 506–514.

Burdette, J. H., Laurienti, P. J., Espeland, M. A., Morgan, A., Telesford, Q., Vechlekar, C. D., … Rejeski, W. J. (2010). Using network science to evaluate exercise-associated brain changes in older adults. *Frontiers in Aging Neuroscience, 2*, 23.

Burzynska, A. Z., Chaddock-Heyman, L., Voss, M. W., Wong, C. N., Gothe, N. P., Olson, E. A., … Kramer, A. F. (2014). Physical activity and cardiorespiratory fitness are beneficial for white matter in low-fit older adults. *PLoS One, 9*(9), e107413.

Cancela Carral, J. M., & Ayan Perez, C. (2007). Effects of high-intensity combined training on women over 65. *Gerontology, 53*(6), 340–346.

Chaddock, L., Erickson, K. I., Prakash, R. S., Kim, J. S., Voss, M. W., Vanpatter, M., … Kramer, A. F. (2010a). A neuroimaging investigation of the association between aerobic fitness, hippocampal volume, and memory performance in preadolescent children. *Brain Research, 1358*, 172–183.

Chaddock, L., Erickson, K. I., Prakash, R. S., VanPatter, M., Voss, M. W., Pontifex, M. B., … Kramer, A. F. (2010b). Basal ganglia volume is associated with aerobic fitness in preadolescent children. *Developmental Neuroscience, 32*(3), 249–256.

Chaddock, L., Erickson, K. I., Prakash, R. S., Voss, M. W., VanPatter, M., Pontifex, M. B., … Kramer, A. F. (2012a). A functional MRI investigation of the association between childhood aerobic fitness and neurocognitive control. *Biological Psychology, 89*(1), 260–268.

Chaddock, L., Hillman, C. H., Pontifex, M. B., Johnson, C. R., Raine, L. B., & Kramer, A. F. (2012b). Childhood aerobic fitness predicts cognitive performance one year later. *Journal of Sports Sciences, 30*(5), 421–430.

Chang, Y., Pan, C. Y., Chen, F. T., Tsai, C. L., & Huang, C. C. (2012). Effect of resistance-exercise training on cognitive function in healthy older adults: a review. *Journal of Aging and Physical Activity, 20*, 497–517.

Chang, Y., Tsai, Y., Chen, T., & Hung, T. (2013a). The impacts of coordinative exercise on executive function in kindergarten children: an ERP study. *Experimental Brain Research, 225*(2), 187–196.

Chang, Y., Huang, C., Chen, K., & Hung, T. (2013b). Physical activity and working memory in healthy older adults: an ERP study. *Psychophysiology, 50*(11), 1174–1182.

Chang, Y., Chu, C., Wang, C., Song, T., & Wei, G. (2015). Effect of acute exercise and cardiovascular fitness on cognitive function: an event-related cortical desynchronization study. *Psychophysiology, 52*(3), 342–351.

Claudino, R., Mazo, G. Z., & Santos, M. J. (2013). Age-related changes of grip force control in physically active adults. *Perceptual & Motor Skills, 116*(3), 859–871.

Colcombe, S., & Kramer, A. F. (2003). Fitness effects on the cognitive function of older adults: a meta-analytic study. *Psychological Science, 14*(2), 125–130.

Colcombe, S. J., Erickson, K. I., Raz, N., Webb, A. G., Cohen, N. J., McAuley, E., & Kramer, A. F. (2003). Aerobic fitness reduces brain tissue loss in aging humans. *The Journals of Gerontology. Series A, Biological Sciences and Medical Sciences, 58*(2), 176–180.

Colcombe, S. J., Kramer, A. F., Erickson, K. I., Scalf, P., McAuley, E., Cohen, N. J., … Elavsky, S. (2004). Cardiovascular fitness, cortical plasticity, and aging. *Proceedings of the National Academy of Sciences of the United States of America, 101*(9), (pp. 3316–3321).

Colcombe, S. J., Erickson, K. I., Scalf, P. E., Kim, J. S., Prakash, R., McAuley, E., … Kramer, A. F. (2006). Aerobic exercise training increases brain volume in aging humans. *The Journals of Gerontology. Series A, Biological Sciences and Medical Sciences, 61*(11), 1166–1170.

Cotman, C. W., & Berchtold, N. C. (2002). Exercise: a behavioral intervention to enhance brain health and plasticity. *Trends in Neurosciences, 25*(6), 295–301.

Coubard, O. A., Duretz, S., Lefebvre, V., Lapalus, P., & Ferrufino, L. (2011). Practice of contemporary dance improves cognitive flexibility in aging. *Frontiers in Aging Neuroscience, 3*, 13.

Crabbe, J. B., & Dishman, R. K. (2004). Brain electrocortical activity during and after exercise: a quantitative synthesis. *Psychophysiology, 41*(4), 563–574.

Crova, C., Struzzolino, I., Marchetti, R., Masci, I., Vannozzi, G., Forte, R., & Pesce, C. (2014). Cognitively challenging physical activity benefits executive function in overweight children. *Journal of Sports Sciences, 32*(3), 201–211.

Davis, C. L., Tomporowski, P. D., McDowell, J. E., Austin, B. P., Miller, P. H., Yanasak, N. E., ... Naglieri, J. A. (2011). Exercise improves executive function and achievement and alters brain activation in overweight children: a randomized, controlled trial. *Health Psychology: Official Journal of the Division of Health Psychology, American Psychological Association, 30*(1), 91–98.

Dickinson, J., Medhurst, C., & Whittingham, N. (1979). Warm-up and fatigue in skill acquisition and performance. *Journal of Motor Behavior, 11*(1), 81–86.

Ding, Y. H., Li, J., Luan, X., Ding, Y. H., Lai, Q., Rafols, J. A., ... Diaz, F. G. (2004). Exercise pre-conditioning reduces brain damage in ischemic rats that may be associated with regional angiogenesis and cellular overexpression of neurotrophin. *Neuroscience, 124*(3), 583–591.

Ding, Q., Vaynman, S., Akhavan, M., Ying, Z., & Gomez-Pinilla, F. (2006). Insulin-like growth factor I interfaces with brain-derived neurotrophic factor-mediated synaptic plasticity to modulate aspects of exercise-induced cognitive function. *Neuroscience, 140*(3), 823–833.

Drollette, E. S., Scudder, M. R., Raine, L. B., Moore, R. D., Saliba, B. J., Pontifex, M. B., & Hillman, C. H. (2014). Acute exercise facilitates brain function and cognition in children who need it most: an ERP study of individual differences in inhibitory control capacity. *Developmental Cognitive Neuroscience, 7*, 53–64.

Erickson, K. I., Prakash, R. S., Voss, M. W., Chaddock, L., Hu, L., Morris, K. S., ... Kramer, A. F. (2009). Aerobic fitness is associated with hippocampal volume in elderly humans. *Hippocampus, 19*(10), 1030–1039.

Erickson, K. I., Prakash, R. S., Voss, M. W., Chaddock, L., Heo, S., McLaren, M., ... Kramer, A. F. (2010). Brain-derived neurotrophic factor is associated with age-related decline in hippocampal volume. *The Journal of Neuroscience: The Official Journal of the Society for Neuroscience, 30*(15), 5368–5375.

Erickson, K. I., Voss, M. W., Prakash, R. S., Basak, C., Szabo, A., Chaddock, L., ... Kramer, A. F. (2011). Exercise training increases size of hippocampus and improves memory. *Proceedings of the National Academy of Sciences of the United States of America, 108*(7), 3017–3022.

Eriksen, B. A., & Eriksen, C. W. (1974). Effects of noise letters upon the identification of a target letter in a nonsearch task. *Perception & Psychophysics, 16*(1), 143–149.

Etnier, J. L., & Landers, D. M. (1998). Motor performance and motor learning as a function of age and fitness. *Research Quarterly for Exercise and Sport, 69*(2), 136–146.

Etnier, J. L., Nowell, P. M., Landers, D. M., & Sibley, B. A. (2006). A meta-regression to examine the relationship between aerobic fitness and cognitive performance. *Brain Research Reviews, 52*(1), 119–130.

Fabre, C., Chamari, K., Mucci, P., Masse-Biron, J., & Prefaut, C. (2002). Improvement of cognitive function by mental and/or individualized aerobic training in healthy elderly subjects. *International Journal of Sports Medicine, 23*(6), 415–421.

Ferris, L. T., Williams, J. S., & Shen, C. L. (2007). The effect of acute exercise on serum brain-derived neurotrophic factor levels and cognitive function. *Medicine and Science in Sports and Exercise, 39*(4), 728–734.

Flöel, A., Witte, A. V., Lohmann, H., Wersching, H., Ringelstein, E. B., Berger, K., & Knecht, S. (2008). Lifestyle and memory in the elderly. *Neuroepidemiology, 31*(1), 39–47.

Flöel, A., Ruscheweyh, R., Kruger, K., Willemer, C., Winter, B., Volker, K., ... Knecht, S. (2010). Physical activity and memory functions: are neurotrophins and cerebral gray matter volume the missing link? *Neuroimage, 49*(3), 2756–2763.

Fong, D., Chi, L., Li, F., & Chang, Y. (2014). The benefits of endurance exercise and tai chi chuan for the task-switching aspect of executive function in older adults: an ERP study. *Frontiers in Aging Neuroscience, 6*, 295.

Forte, R., Boreham, C. A., Leite, J. C., De Vito, G., Brennan, L., Gibney, E. R., & Pesce, C. (2013). Enhancing cognitive functioning in the elderly: multicomponent vs. resistance training. *Clinical Interventions in Aging*, *8*, 19–27.

Gajewski, P. D., & Falkenstein, M. (2015). Long-term habitual physical activity is associated with lower distractibility in a Stroop interference task in aging: behavioral and ERP evidence. *Brain and Cognition*, *98*, 87–101.

Godde, B., & Voelcker-Rehage, C. (2010). More automation and less cognitive control of imagined walking movements in high- versus low-fit older adults. *Frontiers in Aging Neuroscience*, *2*, 139.

Goldberg, T. E., & Weinberger, D. R. (2004). Genes and the parsing of cognitive processes. *Trends in Cognitive Sciences*, *8*(7), 325–335.

Gomez-Pinilla, F., Vaynman, S., & Ying, Z. (2008). Brain-derived neurotrophic factor functions as a metabotrophin to mediate the effects of exercise on cognition. *The European Journal of Neuroscience*, *28*(11), 2278–2287.

Gordon, B. A., Rykhlevskaia, E. I., Brumback, C. R., Lee, Y., Elavsky, S., Konopack, J. F., … Fabiani, M. (2008). Neuroanatomical correlates of aging, cardiopulmonary fitness level, and education. *Psychophysiology*, *45*(5), 825–838.

Grady, C., Springer, M., Hongwanishkul, D., McIntosh, A., & Winocur, G. (2006). Age-related changes in brain activity across the adult lifespan. *Journal of Cognitive Neuroscience*, *18*(2), 227–241.

Gutin, B. (1966). Effect of increase in physical fitness on mental ability following physical and mental stress. *Research Quarterly*, *37*(2), 211–220.

Gutmann, B., Mierau, A., Hülsdünker, T., Hildebrand, C., Przyklenk, A., Hollmann, W., & Strüder, H. K. (2015). Effects of physical exercise on individual resting state EEG alpha peak frequency. *Neural Plasticity*, *5*, 717312.

Hattori, S., Naoi, M., & Nishino, H. (1994). Striatal dopamine turnover during treadmill running in the rat: relation to the speed of running. *Brain Research Bulletin*, *35*(1), 41–49.

He, J., Carmichael, O., Fletcher, E., Singh, B., Iosif, A., Martinez, O., … DeCarli, C. (2012). Influence of functional connectivity and structural MRI measures on episodic memory. *Neurobiology of Aging*, *33*(11), 2612–2620.

Hillman, C. H., Erickson, K. I., & Kramer, A. F. (2008). Be smart, exercise your heart: exercise effects on brain and cognition. *Nature Reviews Neuroscience*, *9*(1), 58–65.

Hillman, C. H., Buck, S. M., Themanson, J. R., Pontifex, M. B., & Castelli, D. M. (2009). Aerobic fitness and cognitive development: event-related brain potential and task performance indices of executive control in preadolescent children. *Developmental Psychology*, *45*(1), 114–129.

Hillman, C. H., Pontifex, M. B., Castelli, D. M., Khan, N. A., Raine, L. B., Scudder, M. R., … Kamijo, K. (2014). Effects of the FITKids randomized controlled trial on executive control and brain function. *Pediatrics*, *134*(4), e1063–e1071.

Ho, A. J., Raji, C. A., Becker, J. T., Lopez, O. L., Kuller, L. H., Hua, X., … Toga, A. W. (2011). The effects of physical activity, education, and body mass index on the aging brain. *Human Brain Mapping*, *32*(9), 1371–1382.

Hogan, M., Kiefer, M., Kubesch, S., Collins, P., Kilmartin, L., & Brosnan, M. (2013). The interactive effects of physical fitness and acute aerobic exercise on electrophysiological coherence and cognitive performance in adolescents. *Experimental Brain Research*, *229*(1), 85–96.

Holzschneider, K., Wolbers, T., Röder, B., & Hötting, K. (2012). Cardiovascular fitness modulates brain activation associated with spatial learning. *Neuroimage*, *59*(3), 3003–3014.

Hopkins, M. E., Davis, F. C., VanTieghem, M. R., Whalen, P. J., & Bucci, D. J. (2012). Differential effects of acute and regular physical exercise on cognition and affect. *Neuroscience, 215*, 59–68.

Hötting, K., Schauenburg, G., & Röder, B. (2012). Long-term effects of physical exercise on verbal learning and memory in middle-aged adults: results of a one-year follow-up study. *Brain Sciences, 2*(3), 332–346.

Huang, T., Larsen, K. T., Ried-Larsen, M., Moller, N. C., & Andersen, L. B. (2014). The effects of physical activity and exercise on brain-derived neurotrophic factor in healthy humans: A review. *Scandinavian Journal of Medicine & Science in Sports, 24*(1), 1–10.

Hübner, L., Godde, B., & Voelcker-Rehage, C. (in preparation). Cardiovascular fitness level is associated with fine motor performance and EEG beta power in older adults.

Hyodo, K., Dan, I., Suwabe, K., Kyutoku, Y., Yamada, Y., Akahori, M., ... Soya, H. (2012). Acute moderate exercise enhances compensatory brain activation in older adults. *Neurobiology of Aging, 33*(11), 2621–2632.

Jacobs, H. I., Leritz, E. C., Williams, V. J., Van Boxtel, M. P., Elst, W. V., Jolles, J., ... Salat, D. H. (2011). Association between white matter microstructure, executive functions, and processing speed in older adults: The impact of vascular health. *Human Brain Mapping, 34*, 77–95.

Johnson, N. F., Kim, C., Clasey, J. L., Bailey, A., & Gold, B. T. (2012). Cardiorespiratory fitness is positively correlated with cerebral white matter integrity in healthy seniors. *Neuroimage, 59*(2), 1514–1523.

Kamijo, K. (2009). Effects of acute exercise on event-related brain potentials. In: W. Chodzko-Zajko, A. F. Kramer, L. W. Poon, W. Chodzko-Zajko, A. F. Kramer, & L. W. Poon (Eds.), *Enhancing cognitive functioning and brain plasticity* (pp. 111–132). Champaign, IL US: Human Kinetics.

Kamijo, K., & Takeda, Y. (2010). Regular physical activity improves executive function during task switching in young adults. *International Journal of Psychophysiology, 75*(3), 304–311.

Kamijo, K., Nishihira, Y., Higashiura, T., & Kuroiwa, K. (2007). The interactive effect of exercise intensity and task difficulty on human cognitive processing. *International Journal of Psychophysiology: Official Journal of the International Organization of Psychophysiology, 65*(2), 114–121.

Kantak, S. S., & Winstein, C. J. (2012). Learning–performance distinction and memory processes for motor skills: a focused review and perspective. *Behavioural Brain Research, 228*(1), 219–231.

Kattenstroth, J. C., Kolankowska, I., Kalisch, T., & Dinse, H. R. (2010). Superior sensory, motor, and cognitive performance in elderly individuals with multi-year dancing activities. *Frontiers in Aging Neuroscience, 2*, 31.

Kattenstroth, J. C., Kalisch, T., Holt, S., Tegenthoff, M., & Dinse, H. R. (2013). Six months of dance intervention enhances postural, sensorimotor, and cognitive performance in elderly without affecting cardio-respiratory functions. *Frontiers in Aging Neuroscience, 5*, 5.

Kim, H., Heo, H., Kim, D., Ko, I., Lee, S., Kim, S., ... Kim, J. (2011). Treadmill exercise and methylphenidate ameliorate symptoms of attention deficit/hyperactivity disorder through enhancing dopamine synthesis and brain-derived neurotrophic factor expression in spontaneous hypertensive rats. *Neuroscience Letters, 504*(1), 35–39.

Kirchner, W. K. (1958). Age differences in short-term retention of rapidly changing information. *Journal of Experimental Psychology, 55*(4), 352.

Klusmann, V., Evers, A., Schwarzer, R., Schlattmann, P., Reischies, F. M., Heuser, I., & Dimeo, F. C. (2010). Complex mental and physical activity in older women and cognitive performance:

a 6-month randomized controlled trial. *The Journals of Gerontology. Series A, Biological Sciences and Medical Sciences, 65*(6), 680–688.

Koutsandréou, F., Wegner, M., Niemann, C., & Budde, H. (2016). Effects of motor vs. cardiovascular exercise training on children's working memory. *Medicine and Science in Sports and Exercise*, doi: 10.1249/MSS.0000000000000869.

Kraemer, W. J., Volek, J. S., Clark, K. L., Gordon, S. E., Puhl, S. M., Koziris, L. P., … Sebastianelli, W. J. (1999). Influence of exercise training on physiological and performance changes with weight loss in men. *Medicine and Science in Sports and Exercise, 31*(9), 1320–1329.

Kramer, A. F., Erickson, K. I., & Colcombe, S. J. (2006). Exercise, cognition, and the aging brain. *Journal of Applied Physiology (Bethesda Md.: 1985), 101*(4), 1237–1242.

Krampe, R. T., Smolders, C., & Doumas, M. (2014). Leisure sports and postural control: can a black belt protect your balance from aging? *Psychology and aging, 29*(1), 95.

Kwok, T. C., Lam, K. C., Wong, P. S., Chau, W. W., Yuen, K. S., Ting, K. T., … Ho, F. K. (2011). Effectiveness of coordination exercise in improving cognitive function in older adults: a prospective study. *Clinical Interventions in Aging, 6*, 261–267.

Lopes, L., Santos, R., Pereira, B., & Lopes, V. P. (2013). Associations between gross motor coordination and academic achievement in elementary school children. *Human Movement Science, 32*(1), 9–20.

Lupien, S. J., Gillin, C. J., & Hauger, R. L. (1999). Working memory is more sensitive than declarative memory to the acute effects of corticosteroids: a dose-response study in humans. *Behavioral Neuroscience, 113*(3), 420–430.

Luz, C., Rodrigues, L. P., & Cordovil, R. (2015). The relationship between motor coordination and executive functions in 4th grade children. *European Journal of Developmental Psychology, 12*(2), 129–141.

Magnie, M. N., Bermon, S., Martin, F., Madany-Lounis, M., Suisse, G., Muhammad, W., & Dolisi, C. (2000). P300, N400, aerobic fitness, and maximal aerobic exercise. *Psychophysiology, 37*(3), 369–377.

Mang, C. S., Snow, N. J., Campbell, K. L., Ross, C. J., & Boyd, L. A. (2014). A single bout of high-intensity aerobic exercise facilitates response to paired associative stimulation and promotes sequence-specific implicit motor learning. *Journal of Applied Physiology (Bethesda, Md.: 1985), 117*(11), 1325–1336.

Marks, B. L., Katz, L. M., Styner, M., & Smith, J. K. (2011). Aerobic fitness and obesity: relationship to cerebral white matter integrity in the brain of active and sedentary older adults. *British Journal of Sports Medicine, 45*(15), 1208–1215.

McCloskey, D. P., Adamo, D. S., & Anderson, B. J. (2001). Exercise increases metabolic capacity in the motor cortex and striatum, but not in the hippocampus. *Brain Research, 891*(1), 168–175.

McMorris, T., & Hale, B. J. (2012). Differential effects of differing intensities of acute exercise on speed and accuracy of cognition: a meta-analytical investigation. *Brain and Cognition, 80*(3), 338–351.

McMorris, T., Collard, K., Corbett, J., Dicks, M., & Swain, J. P. (2008). A test of the catecholamines hypothesis for an acute exercise cognition interaction. *Pharmacology, Biochemistry and Behavior, 89*(1), 106–115.

McMorris, T., Sproule, J., Turner, A., & Hale, B. J. (2011). Acute, intermediate intensity exercise, and speed and accuracy in working memory tasks: a meta-analytical comparison of effects. *Physiology & Behavior, 102*(3–4), 421–428.

McMorris, T., Hale, B. J., Corbett, J., Robertson, K., & Hodgson, C. I. (2015). Does acute exercise affect the performance of whole-body, psychomotor skills in an inverted-U fashion? A meta-analytic investigation. *Physiology & Behavior, 141*, 180–189.

Moore, R. D., Drollette, E. S., Scudder, M. R., Bharij, A., & Hillman, C. H. (2014). The influence of cardiorespiratory fitness on strategic, behavioral, and electrophysiological indices of arithmetic cognition in preadolescent children. *Frontiers in Human Neuroscience, 8,* 258.

Nagamatsu, L. S., Handy, T. C., Hsu, C. L., Voss, M. W., & Liu-Ambrose, T. (2012). Resistance training promotes cognitive and functional brain plasticity in seniors with probable mild cognitive impairment. *Archives of Internal Medicine, 172*(8), 666–668.

Nakamura, Y., Nishimoto, K., Akamatu, M., Takahashi, M., & Maruyama, A. (1999). The effect of jogging on P300 event related potentials. *Electromyography and Clinical Neurophysiology, 39*(2), 71–74.

Niemann, C., Godde, B., Staudinger, U., & Voelcker-Rehage, C. (2014a). Exercise-induced changes in basal ganglia volume and cognition in older adults. *Neuroscience, 281,* 147–163.

Niemann, C., Godde, B., & Voelcker-Rehage, C. (2014b). Not only cardiovascular, but also coordinative exercise increases hippocampal volume in older adults. *Frontiers in Aging Neuroscience, 6,* 170.

Niemann, C., Godde, B., & Voelcker-Rehage, C. (in preparation). Senior dance experience, cognitive performance and brain volume in older women.

Nybo, L., Nielsen, B., Blomstrand, E., Moller, K., & Secher, N. (2003). Neurohumoral responses during prolonged exercise in humans. *Journal of Applied Physiology (Bethesda, Md.: 1985), 95*(3), 1125–1131.

Okely, A. D., Booth, M. L., & Patterson, J. W. (2001). Relationship of physical activity to fundamental movement skills among adolescents. *Medicine and Science in Sports and Exercise, 33*(11), 1899–1904.

Özkaya, G. Y., Aydin, H., Toraman, F. N., Kizilay, F., Özdemir, Ö., & Cetinkaya, V. (2005). Effect of strength and endurance training on cognition in older people. *Journal of Sports Science & Medicine, 4*(3), 300.

Pack, M. D., Cotten, D. J., & Biasiotto, J. (1974). Effect of four fatigue levels on performance and learning of a novel dynamic balance skill. *Journal of Motor Behavior, 6*(3), 191–197.

Pahor, M., Blair, S. N., Espeland, M., Fielding, R., Gill, T. M., Guralnik, J. M., et al. (2006). Effects of a physical activity intervention on measures of physical performance: results of the lifestyle interventions and independence for elders pilot (LIFE-P) study. *The Journals of Gerontology: Series A: Biological Sciences and Medical Sciences, 61,* 1157–1165.

Pereira, A. C., Huddleston, D. E., Brickman, A. M., Sosunov, A. A., Hen, R., McKhann, G. M., ... Small, S. A. (2007). An in vivo correlate of exercise-induced neurogenesis in the adult dentate gyrus. *Proceedings of the National Academy of Sciences of the United States of America, 104*(13), 5638–5643.

Pesce, C., Cereatti, L., Forte, R., Crova, C., & Casella, R. (2011). Acute and chronic exercise effects on attentional control in older road cyclists. *Gerontology, 57*(2), 121–128.

Peters, J., Dauvermann, M., Mette, C., Platen, P., Franke, J., Hinrichs, T., & Daum, I. (2009). Voxel-based morphometry reveals an association between aerobic capacity and grey matter density in the right anterior insula. *Neuroscience, 163*(4), 1102–1108.

Pieramico, V., Esposito, R., Sensi, F., Cilli, F., Mantini, D., Mattei, P. A., ... Ferretti, A. (2012). Combination training in aging individuals modifies functional connectivity and cognition, and is potentially affected by dopamine-related genes. *PLoS One, 7*(8), e43901.

Pontifex, M. B., & Hillman, C. H. (2007). Neuroelectric and behavioral indices of interference control during acute cycling. *Clinical Neurophysiology, 118*(3), 570–580.

Pontifex, M., Hillman, C., Fernhall, B. O., Thompson, K., & Valentini, T. (2009). The effect of acute aerobic and resistance exercise on working memory. *Medicine Science in Sports Exercise, 41*(4), 927–934.

Pontifex, M. B., Raine, L. B., Johnson, C. R., Chaddock, L., Voss, M. W., Cohen, N.J., ... Hillman, C. H. (2011). Cardiorespiratory fitness and the flexible modulation of cognitive control in pre-adolescent children. *Journal of Cognitive Neuroscience, 23*(6), 1332–1345.

Prakash, R. S., Voss, M. W., Erickson, K. I., Lewis, J. M., Chaddock, L., Malkowski, E., ... Kramer, A. F. (2011). Cardiorespiratory fitness and attentional control in the aging brain. *Frontiers in Human Neuroscience, 4*, 229.

Raine, L. B., Lee, H. K., Saliba, B. J., Chaddock-Heyman, L., Hillman, C. H., & Kramer, A. F. (2013). The influence of childhood aerobic fitness on learning and memory. *PLoS One, 8*(9), e72666.

Raine, L. B., Scudder, M. R., Saliba, B. J., Kramer, A. F., & Hillman, C. (2015). Aerobic fitness and context processing in preadolescent children. *Journal of Physical Activity & Health*.

Reuter-Lorenz, P. A., & Lustig, C. (2005). Brain aging: reorganizing discoveries about the aging mind. *Current Opinion in Neurobiology, 15*(2), 245–251.

Roig, M., Skriver, K., Lundbye-Jensen, J., Kiens, B., & Nielsen, J. B. (2012). A single bout of exercise improves motor memory. *PLoS One, 7*(9), e44594.

Roig, M., Nordbrandt, S., Geertsen, S. S., & Nielsen, J. B. (2013). The effects of cardiovascular exercise on human memory: a review with meta-analysis. *Neuroscience & Biobehavioral Reviews, 37*(8), 1645–1666.

Rosano, C., Venkatraman, V. K., Guralnik, J., Newman, A. B., Glynn, N. W., Launer, L., ... Aizenstein, H. (2010). Psychomotor speed and functional brain MRI 2 years after completing a physical activity treatment. *The Journals of Gerontology. Series A, Biological Sciences and Medical Sciences, 65*(6), 639–647.

Ruscheweyh, R., Willemer, C., Kruger, K., Duning, T., Warnecke, T., Sommer, J., ... Flöel, A. (2011). Physical activity and memory functions: an interventional study. *Neurobiology of Aging, 32*(7), 1304–1319.

Schneider, S., Vogt, T., Frysch, J., Guardiera, P., & Strüder, H. K. (2009). School sport—a neurophysiological approach. *Neuroscience Letters, 467*(2), 131–134.

Scudder, M. R., Drollette, E. S., Pontifex, M. B., & Hillman, C. H. (2012). Neuroelectric indices of goal maintenance following a single bout of physical activity. *Biological Psychology, 89*(2), 528–531.

Singh, A. M., & Staines, W. R. (2015). The effects of acute aerobic exercise on the primary motor cortex. *Journal of Motor Behavior, 47*, 328–339 (ahead-of-print).

Singh, A. M., Neva, J. L., & Staines, W. R. (2014). Acute exercise enhances the response to paired associative stimulation-induced plasticity in the primary motor cortex. *Experimental Brain Research, 232*(11), 3675–3685.

Skriver, K., Roig, M., Lundbye-Jensen, J., Pingel, J., Helge, J. W., Kiens, B., & Nielsen, J. B. (2014). Acute exercise improves motor memory: exploring potential biomarkers. *Neurobiology of Learning and Memory, 116*, 46–58.

Smith, J. C., Nielson, K. A., Woodard, J. L., Seidenberg, M., Durgerian, S., Antuono, P., ... Rao, S. M. (2011). Interactive effects of physical activity and APOE-ε4 on BOLD semantic memory activation in healthy elders. *Neuroimage, 54*(1), 635–644.

Spirduso, W. W. (1980). Physical fitness, aging, and psychomotor speed: a review. *Journal of Gerontology, 35*(6), 850–865.

Stroop, J. R. (1938). Factors affecting speed in serial verbal reactions. *Psychological Monographs, 50*(5), 38.

Stroth, S., Kubesch, S., Dieterle, K., Ruchsow, M., Heim, R., & Kiefer, M. (2009). Physical fitness, but not acute exercise modulates event-related potential indices for executive control in healthy adolescents. *Brain Research, 1269*, 114–124.

Stroth, S., Reinhardt, R. K., Thöne, J., Hille, K., Schneider, M., Härtel, S., ... Spitzer, M. (2010). Impact of aerobic exercise training on cognitive functions and affect associated to the COMT polymorphism in young adults. *Neurobiology of Learning and Memory, 94*(3), 364–372.

Szabo, A. N., McAuley, E., Erickson, K. I., Voss, M. W., Prakash, R. S., Mailey, E. L., ... Kramer, A. F. (2011). Cardiorespiratory fitness, hippocampal volume, and frequency of forgetting in older adults. *Neuropsychology, 25*(5), 545–553.

Thacker, J. S., Middleton, L. E., McIlroy, W. E., & Staines, W. R. (2014). The influence of an acute bout of aerobic exercise on cortical contributions to motor preparation and execution. *Physiological Reports, 2*(10), e12178.

Themanson, J. R., & Hillman, C. H. (2006). Cardiorespiratory fitness and acute aerobic exercise effects on neuroelectric and behavioral measures of action monitoring. *Neuroscience, 141*(2), 757–767.

Themanson, J. R., Hillman, C. H., & Curtin, J. J. (2006). Age and physical activity influences on action monitoring during task switching. *Neurobiology of Aging, 27*(9), 1335–1345.

Tomporowski, P. D. (2003). Effects of acute bouts of exercise on cognition. *Acta Psychologica, 112*(3), 297–324.

Torres, E. R., Strack, E. F., Fernandez, C. E., Tumey, T. A., & Hitchcock, M. E. (2015). Physical activity and white matter hyperintensities: a systematic review of quantitative studies. *Preventive Medicine Reports, 2,* 319–325.

Tseng, B. Y., Gundapuneedi, T., Khan, M. A., Diaz-Arrastia, R., Levine, B. D., Lu, H., ... Zhang, R. (2013). White matter integrity in physically fit older adults. *Neuroimage, 82,* 510–516.

Tsujii, T., Komatsu, K., & Sakatani, K. (2013). Acute effects of physical exercise on prefrontal cortex activity in older adults: a functional near-infrared spectroscopy study. *Advances in Experimental Medicine and Biology, 765,* 293–298.

van Praag, H., Shubert, T., Zhao, C., & Gage, F. H. (2005). Exercise enhances learning and hippocampal neurogenesis in aged mice. *The Journal of Neuroscience: The Official Journal of the Society for Neuroscience, 25*(38), 8680–8685.

Vaughan, S., Wallis, M., Polit, D., Steele, M., Shum, D., & Morris, N. (2014). The effects of multimodal exercise on cognitive and physical functioning and brain-derived neurotrophic factor in older women: a randomised controlled trial. *Age and Ageing, 43*(5), 623–629.

Verghese, J. (2006). Cognitive and mobility profile of older social dancers. *Journal of the American Geriatrics Society, 54*(8), 1241–1244.

Verghese, J., Lipton, R. B., Katz, M. J., Hall, C. B., Derby, C. A., Kuslansky, G., ... Buschke, H. (2003). Leisure activities and the risk of dementia in the elderly. *The New England Journal of Medicine, 348*(25), 2508–2516.

Verstynen, T. D., Lynch, B., Miller, D. L., Voss, M. W., Prakash, R. S., Chaddock, L., ... Wojcicki, T. R. (2012). Caudate nucleus volume mediates the link between cardiorespiratory fitness and cognitive flexibility in older adults. *Journal of Aging Research,* 939285.

Vissing, J., Andersen, M., & Diemer, N. H. (1996). Exercise-induced changes in local cerebral glucose utilization in the rat. *Journal of Cerebral Blood Flow & Metabolism, 16*(4), 729–736.

Voelcker-Rehage, C., & Niemann, C. (2013). Structural and functional brain changes related to different types of physical activity across the life span. *Neuroscience and Biobehavioral Reviews, 37*(9 Pt B), 2268–2295.

Voelcker-Rehage, C., Godde, B., & Staudinger, U. M. (2010). Physical and motor fitness are both related to cognition in old age. *The European Journal of Neuroscience, 31*(1), 167–176.

Voelcker-Rehage, C., Godde, B., & Staudinger, U. M. (2011). Cardiovascular and coordination training differentially improve cognitive performance and neural processing in older adults. *Frontiers in Human Neuroscience, 5,* 26.

Voelcker-Rehage, C., Jeltsch, A., Godde, B., Becker, S., & Staudinger, U. M. (2015). COMT gene polymorphisms, cognitive performance, and physical fitness in older adults. *Psychology of Sport and Exercise, 20*, 20–28.

Voss, M. W., Erickson, K. I., Prakash, R. S., Chaddock, L., Malkowski, E., Alves, H., … Kramer, A. F. (2010a). Functional connectivity: a source of variance in the association between cardiorespiratory fitness and cognition? *Neuropsychologia, 48*(5), 1394–1406.

Voss, M. W., Prakash, R. S., Erickson, K. I., Basak, C., Chaddock, L., Kim, J. S., … Kramer, A. F. (2010b). Plasticity of brain networks in a randomized intervention trial of exercise training in older adults. *Frontiers in Aging Neuroscience, 2*, 32.

Voss, M. W., Vivar, C., Kramer, A. F., & van Praag, H. (2013a). Bridging animal and human models of exercise-induced brain plasticity. *Trends in Cognitive Sciences, 17*(10), 525–544.

Voss, M. W., Heo, S., Prakash, R. S., Erickson, K. I., Alves, H., Chaddock, L., … Kramer, A. F. (2013b). The influence of aerobic fitness on cerebral white matter integrity and cognitive function in older adults: results of a one-year exercise intervention. *Human Brain Mapping, 34*(11), 2972–2985.

Wang, G. J., Volkow, N. D., Fowler, J. S., Franceschi, D., Logan, J., Pappas, N. R., … Netusil, N. (2000). PET studies of the effects of aerobic exercise on human striatal dopamine release. *Journal of Nuclear Medicine: Official Publication, Society of Nuclear Medicine, 41*(8), 1352–1356.

Wegner, M., Koedijker, J. M., & Budde, H. (2014). The effect of acute exercise and psychosocial stress on fine motor skills and testosterone concentration in the saliva of high school students. *PLoS One, 9*(3), e92953.

Weingarten, G. (1973). Mental performance during physical exertion: the benefits of being physically fit. *International Journal of Sport Psychology, 4*, 16–26.

Weinstein, A. M., Voss, M. W., Prakash, R. S., Chaddock, L., Szabo, A., White, S. M., … Erickson, K. I. (2012). The association between aerobic fitness and executive function is mediated by prefrontal cortex volume. *Brain, Behavior, and Immunity, 26*(5), 811–819.

Winneke, A. H., Godde, B., Reuter, E.-M., Vieluf, S., & Voelcker-Rehage, C. (2012). The association between physical activity and attentional control in younger and older middle-aged adults: an ERP study. *The Journal of Gerontopsychology and Geriatric Psychiatry, 25*, 207–221.

Winneke, A. H., Hübner, L., Godde, B., & Voelcker-Rehage, C. (in preparation). Brief bout of exercise boosts neurophysiological marker of attentional control.

Winter, B., Breitenstein, C., Mooren, F. C., Voelker, K., Fobker, M., Lechtermann, A., … Knecht, S. (2007). High impact running improves learning. *Neurobiology of Learning and Memory, 87*(4), 597–609.

Yerkes, R. M., & Dodson, J. (1908). The relation of strength of stimulus to rapidity of habit-formation. *Journal of Comparative Neurology and Psychology, 18*, 459–482.

Yeung, N., Botvinick, M. M., & Cohen, J. D. (2004). The neural basis of error detection: conflict monitoring and the error-related negativity. *Psychological Review, 111*(4), 931–959.

Zervas, Y., Danis, A., & Klissouras, V. (1991). Influence of physical exertion on mental performance with reference to training. *Perceptual and Motor Skills, 72*(3 Pt 2), 1215–1221.

Zoladz, J., Pilc, A., Majerczak, J., Grandys, M., Zapart-Bukowska, J., & Duda, K. (2008). Endurance training increases plasma brain-derived neurotrophic factor concentration in young healthy men. *Journal of Physiology and Pharmacology, 59*(Suppl. 7), 119–132.

Chapter 4

Visual Perception and Motor Action: Issues in Current Quiet-Eye Research

André Klostermann

Department of Movement and Exercise Science, Institute of Sport Science, University of Bern, Bern, Switzerland

The coupling between motor control processes and visual perception has been extensively studied in the last decades. In this vein of research, it is often found that with increasing motor expertise, not only motor control but also visual-perceptual processes become optimized, as indicated by a more precise and stable, as well as more economical, performance. For example, Sailer, Flanagan, and Johansson (2005) investigated gaze behavior and eye–hand coordination while learning a novel visuomotor task. In the study, the participants had to (re) position a cursor at different targets displayed on a computer screen by using a control handle. The results showed that with increasing visuomotor expertise, the gaze increasingly supported the cursor movements by marking future cursor goals. The authors suggested that the planning and control of the hand movements are increasingly supported by oculomotor predictions of future states.

In sport science, peak performance is well established to be dependent not only on anatomic, physiologic, and psychological factors (Janelle & Hillman, 2003) but also on the level of perceptual expertise (Williams, Davids, & Williams, 1999). In this context, perceptual–cognitive skills describe the capability of athletes to identify task-relevant information in the environment and to integrate this with existing knowledge for the purpose of decision making or controlling the motor response (Broadbent, Causer, Williams, & Ford, 2014; Mann, Williams, Ward, & Janelle, 2007). Research within this domain has shown, among others that experts are better able to extract relevant information earlier, which, in turn, allows them to more accurately select and execute appropriate motor responses (Abernethy, Farrow, Gorman, & Mann, 2012). Not least, this advantage can be attributed to more efficient gaze strategies because experts optimize visual information processing by reducing the amount of fixations, while at the same time increasing their durations (Gegenfurtner, Lehtinen,

Sport and Exercise Psychology Research. http://dx.doi.org/10.1016/B978-0-12-803634-1.00004-2

& Säljö, 2011; Mann et al., 2007). As a consequence, the point of gaze can be stabilized at crucial cues in the environment for longer periods of time (for an overview, see Mann et al., 2007). A particular gaze strategy was observed by Joan Vickers (1992, 1996), who found very stable gaze patterns in expert golf and basketball players, especially in successful trials. Vickers (1996, 2007) labeled this gaze behavior the quiet eye (QE), which is characterized by relatively long last fixations on task-relevant targets or areas in the visual field before movement initiation.

The functionality of this gaze strategy has been shown for various sport tasks (for overviews, see Mann et al., 2007; Vickers, 2007). The findings thus far suggest that the QE is a strong empirical phenomenon that seems to persist under various constraints. However, as will be shown in this work, there are still several issues that need to be addressed toward untangling this gaze strategy. Therefore, after introducing the QE phenomenon in more detail, problems with recent gaze analysis processes will be worked out. In the third section, it will be argued that instead of further describing the phenomenon, it is necessary to develop empirical methods to address its mechanisms, as discussed in the fourth section. Thereafter, other empirical and theoretical aspects of the QE that merit further consideration in the future will be discussed, such as the relevance of its spatial anchoring. Finally, a summary of the chapter will be provided.

QUIET-EYE PHENOMENON

In her seminal work, Vickers (1996) investigated the gaze behavior in the free-throw shooting of elite basketball players who differed in their free-throw performances. In total, the gaze behavior of 8 expert and 8 near-expert free-throw shooters in 10 hits and 10 misses was analyzed. Vickers found that, compared with the near-expert shooters, the experts showed longer final fixation durations before initiating the final throwing movement; additionally, this duration was longer in hits than in misses. These extended fixation durations were characterized by earlier onsets (ie, the beginning) of the final fixation, but no differences were found in the offsets (ie, the ending). This particular gaze strategy was labeled the QE and defined as:

> *a final fixation or tracking gaze that is located on a specific location or object in the visuomotor workspace within 3° of visual angle (or less) for a minimum of 100 ms. The onset of the quiet eye occurs prior to the final movement, and the offset occurs naturally when the gaze deviates off the location or object by more than 3° of visual angle for a minimum of 100 ms.*

(Vickers, 2007, p. 11)

This definition has since been developed by adapting the fixation parameters to more biologically plausible limit values (eg, a fixation is detected if the point of gaze remains within 1.2 degrees of visual angle for at least 120 ms; Klostermann, Kredel, & Hossner, 2013b). In addition, researchers are increasingly paying attention to a priori established definitions of the critical movement phase, such as by applying previously established definitions (eg, throwing task: Klostermann, Kredel, & Hossner, 2014a; basketball free throw: Wilson, Vine, & Wood, 2009).

In the field of QE research, studies have been done not only on motor tasks that demand visual processing of stationary objects but also on QE effects in targeting sports that require tracking of moving objects. For example, Causer, Bennett, Holmes, Janelle, and Williams (2010) analyzed the gaze behavior of 24 elite and 24 subelite shooters in shotgun shooting, which is an externally paced task that requires one to act within short periods of time. In contrast to earlier QE investigations, this task constrains prospective aspects of the visuomotor control such that, in particular, fast detection of the target and sustained tracking of the target before trigger release are decisive for high performance. This very effect was empirically shown because the elite shooters initiated their last fixation about 35 ms earlier, on average, than the subelite shooters, and earlier QE onsets were found when comparing hits versus misses (difference of about 20 ms). Similarly, the elite shooters tracked the target on average about 7% of the average shooting time longer than the subelite shooters and also for hits when compared to misses on average about 5% longer relative tracking times were revealed.

Based on these empirical findings, in another line of research, the practice-oriented question arose on whether the QE gaze strategy can be implemented in motor skill training to accelerate the learning process. In a typical study, a classical golf-putting teaching protocol was compared with the same protocol but with additional gaze instructions intended to extend the final fixation duration (Vine & Wilson, 2010). By a majority, the results of these QE interventions were quite promising because not only was the gaze behavior altered in the intended direction, that is, toward increased QE durations in the experimental groups, but improved performance was also shown in post- and retention tests compared with the traditional training protocols (for an overview, see Vine, Moore, & Wilson, 2012). Meanwhile, positive QE training effects were found not only in several sport-specific tasks but also in a broader range of gross (eg, military marksmanship; Moore, Vine, Smith, Smith, & Wilson, 2014) and fine motor skills (eg, surgical knot tying; Causer, Vickers, Snelgrove, Arsenault, & Harvey, 2014), as well as in clinical populations (eg, throwing and catching in children with developmental coordination disorder; Miles, Wood, Vine, Vickers, & Wilson, 2015).

In sum, positive QE effects on motor performance and learning have been observed in more than 70 studies (Vickers, 2011). Thus, it seems fair to state that this phenomenon occurs more frequently than just by random chance. However, the mechanism behind the QE phenomenon is still not well understood until now. For example, some results have suggested that experts in particular profit from long QE durations. As previously mentioned, in the study by Vickers (1996), intraindividual performance effects were found only in the expert free-throw shooters, whereas the near-experts descriptively showed longer QE durations in misses than in hits. Similarly, in a golf-putting task, intra-individual correlations between radial error and QE measures were found only in the expert golf players, whereas no such relation was observed in the near-experts (Klostermann, Kredel, & Hossner, 2014b). These findings not only raise interesting questions regarding the purview of the QE but also challenge the theoretical explanations of the phenomenon. In the following, the focus will be shifted from a descriptive to an explanatory perspective. This shift will be taken in three steps: first, by discussing fundamental problems of the gaze registration methodology; second, by tackling issues regarding the alleged causal role of the QE on performance enhancement; and third, by focusing on potential QE mechanisms that have recently been discussed in the literature.

MEASURING THE QUIET EYE

In future QE research, the objectivity and reliability of gaze behavior analyses should be improved to fully capture human gaze behavior and to increase the studies' comparability. This methodological problem with the gaze registration is based on: (1) the rather low temporal resolution of conventional mobile eye-tracking systems and (2) the ambiguity of the data output obtained by such systems.

The first issue arises from the challenge of measuring the high-velocity movements of the oculomotor system. The human eye moves rapidly within milliseconds to different points in space. Depending on their amplitude, these saccadic eye movements can reach velocities of up to 600 degrees/s (Baloh, Konrad, Sills, & Honrubia, 1975) and can last no longer than 30 ms (Rayner, 1978). As a consequence of these high velocities, thorough analyses of the gaze behavior with conventional video-based eye-tracking systems are impossible because saccades will be missed as a function of their low resolution (30 Hz regularly; eg, Vickers, 1996). This, in turn, affects the analyses of the saccadic gaze behavior and, as a direct consequence, the calculation of slow eye movements and the final fixation duration. Such inaccuracies entail problems in many ways. Among others, they might complicate or even hinder researchers from doing replication studies because of the difficulty of comparing the rather inaccurate measurements. Furthermore, the comparability of different QE studies, in particular on different motor tasks, is severely aggravated. The possibility to directly compare studies would allow, for example, the structuring of databases and the carrying out of intrastudy data analyses. The latter could be used to facilitate research on the suggested relation between QE duration and task demands. Thus, the QE effects on different motor tasks could be directly compared without need for further data collection.

The second issue originates from the type of data output generated by conventional eye-tracking systems, which usually provide the gaze data in the form of video footage. In this approach, a scene camera films in the direction that the head is aligned toward, and the current point of gaze of the participant is indicated by an overlaid fixation cross. The resulting data have to be analyzed frame-by-frame, meaning that for each video frame, blinded raters manually map the position of the fixation cross to predefined areas of interest in the video and then count, for example, the number of frames in which the cross remains within one area of interest. Obviously, this procedure has severe drawbacks. First, the spatial accuracy of the analyses is rather low because the rater-based frame-by-frame mappings represent, in most cases, rough guesses instead of objective measures. Second, such analyses are very time consuming so that only small samples can be drawn, questioning the generalizability of the data and, in addition, only small sample sizes are taken, questioning the reliability of the data (Kredel, Klostermann, & Hossner, 2015).

To overcome these shortcomings, a precise and high-frequency eye-tracking method that allows for both automated gaze data analyses and an algorithmic calculation of gaze point positions is required. Kredel et al. (2015) introduced such improved method, consisting of a mobile eye-tracking system (EyeSeeCam, 220 Hz) integrated into a three-dimensional motion capture device (Vicon). This method not only allows gaze registration with satisfactory temporal resolution but also simultaneous capture of the translational and rotational motion of the eyes and the head, respectively. Thus, a vector-based three-dimensional representation of the gaze point can be calculated; in turn, within the Vicon workspace, the position and velocity of this gaze point can be read into fixation and saccade detection algorithms, respectively. Consequently, the positional data for each gaze point can also be mapped onto areas of interest by applying respective methods (eg, on the basis of the nearest-neighbor approach; for an overview, see Holmqvist et al., 2011). Accordingly, the analyses of large eye movement data sets become possible, providing precise and reliable information about the gaze behavior of the participant.

Thus, by applying such integrated eye-tracking system, the methodological problems in gaze analyses outlined previously can be solved. However, at present, this approach can be applied only in a laboratory setting, which, in turn, comes with drawbacks in external validity. Consequently, researchers should keep in mind the focus of their study. If the researcher is interested in studying mechanisms, this methodological approach is mandatory. However, if achieving a high ecological validity is the priority, the methodological restrictions in field research have to be accepted. Nonetheless, in this mutual trade-off, two further possible expedients exist. The first is to create conditions of high external validity, such as in field research, and to link these to a high internal validity, which is possible only in the laboratory (Heuer, 1988). The second is to come up with further technological improvements in integrated eye-tracking devices, such as local positioning systems that can also be applied outside of the laboratory (Kredel et al., 2015). Nonetheless, researchers always have to ensure that the effect that occurs under these circumstances is replicated as it appears in the real world, that is, as performance-enhancing long QE durations. In the best case, researchers manage to replicate similar effects to those reported in earlier, more ecologically valid studies (Klostermann et al., 2013b).

STUDYING THE QUIET EYE

Such technology as previously described allows for investigating a series of research questions that hone in on a theoretical foundation of the QE phenomenon. In this regard, a trendsetting experiment was done by Williams, Singer, and Frehlich (2002), who manipulated the level of complexity of a series of billiard shots (Experiment 1) and constrained the execution time (Experiment 2) to assess the effects of the manipulation on the billiard players' QE duration. The results indicated successful manipulation because, independent of performance and expertise with increasing complexity, the QE duration increased; in addition, the manipulation of the execution time was shown to affect the QE duration. However, the experimental design had a correlational character; thus because the QE and performance were measured as dependent factors, causality was only indicated but could not be inferred. To solve this problem, the QE characteristics have to be directly addressed to test its components as independent and, for example, motor performance as dependent variable. Such experimental paradigm was introduced by Klostermann et al. (2013b; Experiment 1), who directly manipulated the QE duration by controlling the movement and gaze behavior of the participants.

In these experiments, the participants have the task of hitting with a ball as accurately as possible virtual target disks presented on a life-size screen (Fig. 4.1a). The underhand throwing movement and the fixation duration at the target are experimentally manipulated such that: (1) the initiation of the movement is aligned to the appearance of the target and (2) the target appears at different instants of time (Fig. 4.1b). The participants structure their throwing movement according to five audio tones presented in each trial. The first three tones serve as the starting signals "Ready" and "Set"; the throwing movement

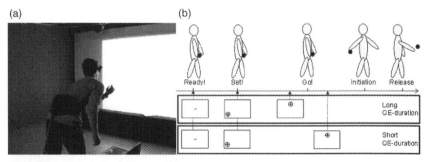

FIGURE 4.1 (a) Participant equipped with the integrated mobile eye-tracking system (Eye-SeeCam) throwing at the final target position. (b) Timeline of the experimental paradigm in two QE-duration conditions. For example, the target initially appeared in the lower left corner jumping later (Short QE-duration) or earlier (Long QE-duration) to the final positions at 6 o'clock.

has to start at the "Go" signal. On tone number four, the throwing hand has to be in the most backward position; on tone number five, the ball has to be released. The beginning of the forward swing before ball release is defined as the initiation of the final movement. At the same time, the jumping target disk has to be visually tracked. To this end, the target disk appears, first, in one of the four screen corners, and this moment is kept constant (at the second tone). However, the instant of time at which the target disk jumps into its final position, where it has to be hit, is manipulated. When the instructions are perfectly followed, the timing differences result in different final fixation onsets (early vs late) and, in turn, in the opportunity to exploit time intervals of different lengths for the final fixation. Consequently, different QE durations can be expected as a function of the experimental manipulations.

Applying this paradigm, Klostermann et al. (2013b; Experiment 1) investigated whether QE effects can be replicated, thereby questioning, because of the experimental approach, whether long QE durations actually cause high motor performance or occur only as a by-product. Consequently, the onset of the final fixation on the target was manipulated such that the participants had to hit the target as precisely as possible under either short (the target could be fixated starting at 400 ms before movement initiation) or long (the target could be fixated starting at 800 ms before movement initiation) QE-duration conditions. Two main findings were obtained. First, the gaze results corroborated the manipulation because the participants actually had significantly shorter QE durations ($M = 549.9$ ms, $SD = 208.2$ ms) in the short, compared with the long, QE duration condition ($M = 817.7$ ms, $SD = 376.1$ ms). Second, as a function of the varying QE duration conditions, the radial error of the ball impact point to the center of the target was significantly higher in the short ($M = 122.8$ mm, $SD = 21.3$ mm) than in the long QE duration condition ($M = 114.2$ mm, $SD = 15.1$ mm). Consequently, it was shown that long QE durations are not a by-product but a cause of high performance. In addition, because this rather artificial laboratory task could also reveal QE effects, the door was opened to experimentally tackle on an explanatory level research questions regarding the mechanisms of the QE.

MECHANISMS OF THE QUIET EYE

As early as in the first studies, QE results have been discussed in terms of possible mechanisms that might explain the tight link between perception and motor performance. Based on the observed interindividual and intraindividual differences in basketball free-throw shots as a function of the QE onset but not of the QE offset, Vickers (1996) argued that a long final fixation duration before movement initiation is required to adequately set the shot parameters, such as force and timing, as well as the coordination of the limbs. In other words, Vickers (1996) suggested that the visual information processed during the QE period optimizes the preparameterization of the respective movement. This suggestion builds on the cognitive understanding of human motor control, in particular, on the idea that the motor system draws on centrally stored motor programs for the control of a class of actions. According to Schmidt (1975), a motor program must be adapted to situational conditions by setting appropriate program parameters to achieve specific task goals.

However, surprisingly few studies have investigated this hypothesized mechanism, and only recently have research activities increased. In those studies, this hypothesis of optimized movement parameterization was tested by manipulating the demands of the motor task investigated. The idea here is that different task demands should evoke different information processing demands. This relation was previously shown in the classical experiment by Henry and Rogers (1960), who found longer preprogramming times (assessed by increased reaction times) with increasing task complexity. Drawing on the parameterization hypothesis, therefore, task demand manipulations should affect the QE because increasing processing demands require longer QE durations. The previously mentioned experiment by Williams et al. (2002) was the first to test this relation. In particular, the effects of task demand manipulations on the QE duration suggest a correlation between information-processing load and QE duration, elucidating the relevance of the QE in information processing over movement parameterization (Horn, Okumura, Alexander, Gardin, & Silvester, 2012; Mann, Coombes, Mousseau, & Janelle, 2011).

Drawing on the information-processing approach outlined earlier and assuming a segmentation of this process (Schmidt, 1982; stimulus identification, response selection, and response programming), the results of Williams et al. (2002) essentially relate to the stage of response programming (the more complex the task, the longer the QE duration). Hence, if indeed the QE optimizes movement parameterization, as suggested by Vickers (1996) and Williams et al. (2002), it seems reasonable to predict that the remaining stages of stimulus identification and response selection also profit from long final fixation durations. These predictions were tested by applying the paradigm on experimental manipulation of the QE duration introduced earlier. More precisely, in addition to QE manipulation, either (1) the availability of visual information about the target position over the QE interval (Klostermann et al., 2014a; Experiment 2) or (2) the predictability of the target position before the target onset (Klostermann et al., 2013b; Experiment 2) were experimentally manipulated. Drawing on the findings by Williams et al. (2002), it was expected that for the remaining processing stages as well, the functionality of long QE durations should vary as a function of task demands.

In the first study, in addition to the two QE conditions (short vs long), the visual information-processing duration was manipulated (immediate vs delayed) (Fig. 4.2; top). After the presentation of a fixation cross, peripheral flicker cues appeared at the prospective target position, evoking saccades to the respective position either earlier or later in relation to the timing of the movement phases. In the following, the target disk was presented exactly at this position either immediately or delayed. Thus, over QE durations of different lengths, positional target information could be processed either continuously or in part. Again, the

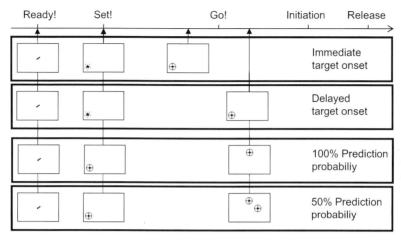

FIGURE 4.2   Top: timeline of Experiment 1 for the delayed versus immediate target onset conditions in the long QE duration condition. For example; the flicker cue evokes an earlier final fixation at the bottom left corner and the target is presented at the flickered position either immediate or delayed. Bottom: timeline of Experiment 2 for the 100% prediction probability versus the 50% prediction probability conditions in the short QE duration condition. For example, the target appears at the bottom left corner and jumps earlier either at the 12 o'clock or 3 o'clock position.

gaze results confirmed the intended QE manipulation because, independent of the target onset, QE durations of different lengths were found. Consequently, the visual information-processing duration over the QE period was successfully manipulated, ranging from 200 ms (short QE/delayed target onset), to over 400 ms (short QE/immediate target onset and long QE/delayed target), to 800 ms (long QE/immediate target onset). Furthermore, the findings elucidate a relation between visual information-processing duration and the QE because, despite the same QE durations, the throwing performance deteriorated when the visual information-processing duration was experimentally shortened; in addition, longer stabilizations of the oculomotor system alone did not affect performance. In other words, the performance-enhancing effects of long QE durations depend on the presence of respective visual information and the necessity to process this information (Klostermann et al., 2014a; Experiment 2).

The second study manipulated the prediction probability of the final target position such that the target appeared either always at the same position or at two different positions (100% vs 50% prediction probability) (Fig. 4.2; bottom). These two prediction conditions were also tested in short versus long QE duration conditions. The results again confirmed the intended QE manipulation because the QE duration was found to differ only as a function of the QE duration manipulation but not of the prediction manipulation. In addition, the performance results showed that longer QE durations positively affected throwing performance only in the condition with increased demands. In contrast, in the conditions with 100% prediction probability, no performance difference was found for long versus short QE durations. Again, these results elucidate the functional role of long QE durations in information processing. The participants could make use of long QE durations only in those trials that demanded the processing of positional information for response programming because preprogramming, such as in the 100% prediction conditions, was not possible. In the 50% prediction conditions, with the QE durations being too short, the time was not sufficient to optimally specify the motor response (Klostermann et al., 2013b; Experiment 2). Thus, the QE interval seems to be exploited for the optimization of information processing such that a minimum QE duration is needed to complete the processes. As long as these processes cannot be finalized, shorter QE durations harm the processes of movement parameterization and, in turn, deteriorate motor performance.

EXPLAINING THE QUIET EYE

Thus far, the empirical evidence suggests a tight link between the QE and information processing such that long durations seem to optimize movement parameterization. However, experimentally, this functionality has been shown only for the phase of movement preparation (ie, open-loop motor control) because task-demand effects have been found either at the QE onset (Williams et al., 2002) or in motor performance as a function of an experimentally manipulated QE onset (Klostermann et al., 2013b; Klostermann, 2014). In fact, Vickers (2009) explicitly suggested that the QE optimizes only these processes, thereby questioning the relevance of the late QE phase and the functionality of the QE in online motor control processes (p. 286).

Nevertheless, there is ample evidence that the late QE phase might also matter. Among the first to show this dependency were Oudejans, van de Langenberg, and Hutter (2002), who analyzed the throwing performance of basketball players in the basketball jump shot. As a function of the players' movement phases, the vision was occluded either early or late in the throwing movement by using Plato liquid crystal goggles. The results showed that the loss of either early or late visual information deteriorated performance as a function of the players' shooting style. Those players that used a low-style technique, in which the hands and the ball are finally stabilized in front of the face, showed performance drops when early visual information was restricted. In contrast, the exact opposite was observed in those players who shot with a high-style technique, in which the hands and the ball are finally stabilized above the head (de Oliveira, Oudejans, & Beek, 2008). More recently, Vine, Lee, Moore, and Wilson (2013) and Klostermann et al. (2014b) extended this finding by showing the relevance of the late QE in golf-putting tasks. In a shoot-out competition, Vine et al. (2013) observed decrements in late QE components in missed trials compared with the preceding successful trials. In addition, Klostermann et al. (2014b) found that, intraindividually, only the QE offset correlated with high putting accuracy, indicating that the later the offset, the smaller the radial error.

Although these studies imply the relevance of the QE for online control processes, as previously discussed for the QE onset and the resulting long QE durations in movement preparation, they lack experimental control because only correlations, but no causalities, could be presented. Consequently, in future experimental studies, attention has to be directed to this issue. For example, within the throwing paradigm introduced earlier, experimental manipulations of the QE offset seem to be indicated. Moreover, it seems advisable to again manipulate the processing demands in the late QE phase in order to assess QE efficiency aspects in the late QE phase as well. This could be done, for example, by applying a dual-task paradigm, as introduced by Khan, Lawrence, Buckholz, and Franks (2006). Drawing on the suggestion that the QE generally enhances information processing, the functionality of a late QE offset should be more pronounced in dual-task trials than in trials without dual-task demands.

Moreover, questions not only on offline versus online processes of movement parameterization but also on the relevance of spatial anchoring in the context of the QE phenomenon need to be investigated. Studies addressing this issue have been done by Rienhoff, Baker, Fischer, Strauss, and Schorer (2012), and by Klostermann, Koedijker, and Hossner (2013a). By using a moving window paradigm in a dart-throwing task, Rienhoff et al. (2012) showed relations between the QE position and throwing precision only in those conditions with occlusion of the foveal visual field but not with occlusion of the peripheral visual field. On one hand, this result suggests a certain relevance of spatial anchoring; on the other hand, it also seems to contradict the relevance of the QE in information processing. However, because the foveal occlusion was perfectly related to the center of the dart disc, it also seems plausible that the participants were still able to sufficiently extract positional information (Klostermann et al., 2014a; Experiment 1).

A relevance of the QE anchoring, however, was also found by Klostermann et al. (2013a), who showed in a precision throwing task a relation between the QE location and the intended effect of the throwing movement. The participants had to throw balls either as precisely as possible into a box or in such a way that the balls rolled into a goal located behind the box. Thus, spatial manipulations of the task goal had to be solved with the same throwing movement. The results showed that the manipulation of the task goals resulted in spatially aligned shifts in the anchoring of the QE such that, in the box condition, the participants focused on the front edge of the box hole, whereas in the goal condition, the anchoring was spatially shifted in the same direction (Fig. 4.3).

Taking together the results of Rienhoff et al. (2012) and Klostermann et al. (2014a), one can conclude that a possible relation seems to exist between the anchoring and the efficiency of the QE. However, more work is needed to investigate the actual relevance of the QE location. Again, an experimental approach should be favored so that predictions on the QE efficiency as a function of different functional QE locations can be tested. In this respect, one would, for instance, expect to find performance-enhancing effects of experimentally

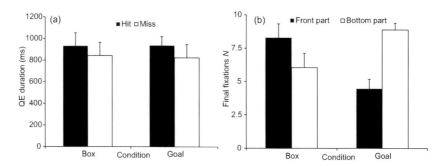

FIGURE 4.3   (a) QE duration (M and S.E.) as a function of condition (box vs goal) and throwing success (hit vs miss). (b) QE duration (M and S.E.) as a function of condition (box vs goal) and location (bottom part vs front part).

controlled, relatively late QE offsets when the participants focus the golf ball in a golf-putting task; in contrast, this functionality should disappear when the participants are instructed to finally fixate less functional cues, such as the left foot.

Finally, perhaps the most exciting challenge in QE research at present is to find an explanation for the QE expertise effect. This is of particular interest because the prolongation of the QE duration in experts, which has been shown in numerous studies and for a broad range of motor tasks (for an overview, see Vickers, 2007), is counterintuitive rather than self-explanatory. In general, research in motor learning shows that with increasing experience, humans tend to economize their behavior such that, among others, movements are executed with less interference and with the impression of an automatic execution (Fitts & Posner, 1967; Schneider & Shiffrin, 1977). When transferring this rationale to the QE phenomenon, one would expect to find similar learning effects, especially when drawing on the optimized movement parameterization hypothesis: As a function of the reduced effort in expert performance, a reduced information processing load has to be assumed such that, as a consequence, shorter— but definitely not longer—QE durations should result from acquired expertise. Similarly, the suggested facilitation of an optimal control strategy introduced by Vine et al. (2012) seems to be trapped in the same problem because with increasing motor experience, attention should be less and less needed for motor execution and thus could instead be devoted to other tasks (Beilock, Carr, MacMahon, & Starkes, 2002). This ambiguity indicates that there is probably more behind the QE phenomenon than the current cognitive explanations suggest. This implies that, besides further empirical activity, an intensification of theoretical work seems to be indispensable. In this regard, the first conceptual drafts have been suggested, such as the idea of psychomotor quieting (Vine et al., 2012) or of a general inhibition mechanism (Klostermann, 2014). However, without doubt, more work is needed to obtain a complete understanding of the mechanisms underlying the QE phenomenon.

CONCLUSIONS

The QE was discussed as a specific performance-enhancing gaze strategy that has attracted distinct attention in sport science research over the last years. A range of studies was presented, highlighting the strong relation between long QE durations and high motor performance at an intraindividual as well as an interindividual level. In addition, the success of QE training protocols in fostering motor learning was shown. Drawing on this strong empirical base, it was worked out that, first and foremost, future research should focus on the fundamental question on the explanatory mechanisms behind the QE effect in motor control and learning. In this respect, several requirements were highlighted, in particular regarding the application of high-resolution eye-tracking systems that allow for objective and automated gaze analyses and the necessity of experimental designs that allow for testing the alleged causal role of the QE in motor performance. In the final sections, the optimized movement parameterization hypothesis for the QE phenomenon was introduced, and three studies confirming this theoretical approach were presented. Finally, several shortcomings and future research questions were discussed to stress the imperative of more empirical and, in particular, theoretical work to further our understanding of the mechanism behind the QE.

REFERENCES

Abernethy, B., Farrow, D., Gorman, A. D., & Mann, D. L. (2012). Anticipatory behaviour and expert performance. In: N. J. Hodges, & A. M. Williams (Eds.), *Skill acquisition in sport: research, theory and practice* (pp. 287–305). London: Routledge.

Baloh, R. W., Konrad, H. R., Sills, A. W., & Honrubia, V. (1975). The saccade velocity test. *Neurology, 25*, 1071–1076.

Beilock, S. L., Carr, T. H., MacMahon, C., & Starkes, J. L. (2002). When paying attention becomes counter-productive: impact of divided versus skill-focused attention on novice and experienced performance of sensorimotor skills. *Journal of Experimental Psychology, 8*, 6–16.

Broadbent, D. P., Causer, J., Williams, A. M., & Ford, P. R. (2014). Perceptual-cognitive training and its transfer to expert performance in the field: future research directions. *European Journal of Sport Science, 24*, 1–10.

Causer, J., Bennett, S. J., Holmes, P. S., Janelle, C. M., & Williams, A. M. (2010). Quiet eye duration and gun motion in elite shotgun shooting. *Medicine and Science in Sports and Exercise, 42*, 1599–1608.

Causer, J., Vickers, J. N., Snelgrove, R., Arsenault, G., & Harvey, A. (2014). Performing under pressure: quiet eye training improves surgical knot-tying performance. *Surgery, 156*, 1089–1096.

de Oliveira, R. F., Oudejans, R. R. D., & Beek, P. J. (2008). Gaze behavior in basketball shooting: further evidence for online visual control. *Research Quarterly of Exercise and Sports, 79*, 399–404.

Fitts, P. M., & Posner, M. I. (1967). *Human performance*. Oxford: Brooks and Cole.

Gegenfurtner, A., Lehtinen, E., & Säljö, R. (2011). Expertise differences in the comprehension of visualisation: a meta-analysis of eye-tracking research in professional domains. *Educational Psychological Review, 23*, 523–552.

Henry, F. M., & Rogers, D. E. (1960). Increased response latency for complicated movements and a "memory drum" theory of neuromotor reaction. *Research Quarterly, 31*, 448–458.

Heuer, H. (1988). The laboratory and the world outside. In: O. G. Meijer, & K. Roth (Eds.), *Complex movement behaviour: "the" motor-action controversy* (pp. 405–417). Amsterdam: North-Holland.

Holmqvist, K., Nyström, M., Andersson, R., Dewhurst, R., Jarodzka, H., & van de Weijer, J. (2011). *Eye tracking. A comprehensive guide to methods and measures.* Oxford: University Press.

Horn, R. H., Okumura, M. S., Alexander, M. G. F., Gardin, F. A., & Silvester, C. T. (2012). Quiet eye duration is responsive to variability of practice and to the axis of target changes. *Research Quarterly for Exercise and Sport, 83*, 204–211.

Janelle, C. M., & Hillman, C. H. (2003). *Expert performance in sports: Advances in research on sport expertise.* Champaign, IL: Human Kinetics.

Khan, M. A., Lawrence, G., Buckolz, E., & Franks, I. M. (2006). Programming strategies in simple and choice reaction time rapid aiming tasks. *Quarterly Journal of Experimental Psychology, 59*, 524–542.

Klostermann, A. (2014). Finale fixationen, sportmotorische Leistung und eine Inhibitionshy-pothese: mechanismen des "quiet eye". *Sportwissenschaft, 44*, 49–59.

Klostermann, A., Koedijker, J., & Hossner, E. -J. (2013a). Zielinstruktionen, räumliche quiet-eye-verankerung und bewegungsparametrisierung: hinweise auf einen wirkmechanismus. *Zeitschrift für Sportpsychologie, 20*, 59–64.

Klostermann, A., Kredel, R., & Hossner, E. -J. (2013b). The "quiet eye" and motor performance: task demands matter! *Journal of Experimental Psychology, 39*, 1270–1278.

Klostermann, A., Kredel, R., & Hossner, E. -J. (2014a). The quiet eye without a target: the primacy of visual information processing. *Journal of Experimental Psychology, 40*, 2167–2178.

Klostermann, A., Kredel, R., & Hossner, E. -J. (2014b). On the interaction of attentional focus and gaze: the quiet eye inhibits focus-related performance decrements. *Journal of Sport & Exercise Psychology, 36*, 392–400.

Kredel, R., Klostermann, A., & Hossner, E. -J. (2015). Automated vector-based gaze analysis for perception-action coupling diagnostics. In: T. Heinen (Ed.), *Advances in visual perception research* (pp. 45–59). Hauppauge, NY: Nova Science Publisher.

Mann, D. T. Y., Coombes, S. A., Mousseau, M. B., & Janelle, C. M. (2011). Quiet Eye and the bere-itschaftspotential: visuomotor antecedents to expert motor performance. *Cognitive Processing, 12*, 223–234.

Mann, D. T. Y., Williams, A. M., Ward, P., & Janelle, C. (2007). Perceptual-cognitive expertise in sport: a meta-analysis. *Journal of Sport & Exercise Psychology, 29*, 457–478.

Miles, C. A. L., Wood, G., Vine, S. J., Vickers, J. N., & Wilson, M. R. (2015). Quiet eye training facilitates visuomotor coordination in children with developmental coordination disorder. *Research in developmental disabilities, 40*, 31–41.

Moore, L. J., Vine, S. J., Smith, A., Smith, S. J., & Wilson, M. R. (2014). Quiet eye training improves small arms military marksmanship. *Military Psychology, 25*, 355–365.

Oudejans, R. R. D., van de Langenberg, R. W., & Hutter, R. I. (2002). Aiming at a far target under different viewing conditions: visual control in basketball jump shooting. *Human Movement Science, 21*, 457–480.

Rayner, K. (1978). Eye movements in reading and information processing. *Psychological Bulletin, 85*, 618–660.

Rienhoff, R., Baker, J., Fischer, L., Strauß, B., & Schorer, J. (2012). Field of vision influences sensory-motor control of skilled and less-skilled dart players. *Journal of Sports Science and Medicine, 11*, 542–550.

Sailer, U., Flanagan, J. R., & Johansson, R. S. (2005). Eye-hand coordination during learning of a novel visuomotor task. *Journal of Neuroscience, 25*, 8833–8842.

Schmidt, R. A. (1975). A schema theory of discrete motor skill learning. *Psychological Review, 82*, 225–260.

Schmidt, R. A. (1982). *Motor control and learning: A behavioral emphasis* (1st ed.). Champaign, IL: Human Kinetics.

Schneider, W., & Shiffrin, R. M. (1977). Controlled and automatic human information processing: I. Detection, search, and attention. *Psychological Bulletin, 84*, 1–66.

Vickers, J. N. (1992). Gaze control in putting. *Perception, 21*, 117–132.

Vickers, J. N. (1996). Visual control when aiming at a far target. *Journal of Experimental Psychology, 22*, 342–354.

Vickers, J. N. (2007). *Perception, cognition, and decision training. The quiet eye in action.* Champaign, IL: Human Kinetics.

Vickers, J. N. (2009). Recent advances in coupling perception and action: the quiet eye as a bi-directional link between the gaze, focus of attention and action. In: M. Raab, J. Johnson, & H. Heekeren (Eds.), *Progress in brain research 174: mind and motion: the bidirectional link between thought and action* (pp. 279–288). The Netherlands: Elsevier.

Vickers, J. N. (2011). Mind over muscle: the role of gaze control, spatial cognition, and the quiet eye in motor expertise. *Cognitive Processing, 12*, 219–222.

Vine, S. J., Lee, D., Moore, L. J., & Wilson, M. R. (2013). Quiet eye and choking: online control breaks down at the point of performance failure. *Medicine and Science in Sports and Exercise, 45*, 1988–1994.

Vine, S. J., Moore, L. J., & Wilson, M. R. (2012). Quiet eye training: the acquisition, refinement and resilient performance of targeting skills. *European Journal of Sport Science, 14*, 235–242.

Vine, S. J., & Wilson, M. R. (2010). Quiet eye training: effects on learning and performance under pressure. *Journal of Applied Sport Psychology, 22*, 361–376.

Williams, A. M., Davids, K., & Williams, J. G. (1999). *Visual perception and action in sport.* London: E & FN Spon.

Williams, A. M., Singer, R. N., & Frehlich, S. G. (2002). Quiet eye duration, expertise, and task complexity in near and far aiming tasks. *Journal of Motor Behavior, 34*, 197–207.

Wilson, M. R., Vine, S. J., & Wood, G. (2009). The influence of anxiety on visual attentional control in basketball free throw shooting. *Journal of Sport & Exercise Psychology, 31*, 152–168.

Chapter 5

Learning a Motor Action "From Within": Insights Into Perceptual-Cognitive Changes With Mental and Physical Practice

Cornelia Frank

Neurocognition and Action Research Group and Cognitive Interaction Technology Center of Excellence (CITEC), Bielefeld University, Germany

A human's repertoire of motor actions changes throughout the lifespan. Individuals continuously learn and relearn to perform goal-directed motor actions in various settings such as their everyday life, their sports, or during their rehabilitation. Consider, for instance, the child who learns to take his first steps, the athlete who learns the appropriate technique for sprinting in track and field, or the injured elderly woman who relearns how to properly walk after several weeks of immobilization. How does the human motor action system (re)learn to adequately solve a motor task in any given situation such that it serves to achieve an intended effect within the environment?

The two most common means to (re)learn a motor action are through physical practice (ie, repeatedly executing a motor action) and mental practice (ie, repeatedly imagining the execution of a motor action). Motor imagery denotes imagining oneself performing a particular motor action without actually executing it at the same time (Jeannerod, 1994, 1997; Jeannerod & Decety, 1995; for a discussion on its conceptualization, see Morris, Spittle, & Watt, 2005). Thus, whereas actual or physical practice implies overtly rehearsing a motor action, mental practice in the sense of motor imagery training can be understood as the covert rehearsal of a motor action by way of motor imagery (as opposed to other forms of mental practice such as self-talk, for instance; for classification, see, eg, Driskell, Copper, & Moran, 1994; Morris et al., 2005).

Sport and Exercise Psychology Research. http://dx.doi.org/10.1016/B978-0-12-803634-1.00005-4

Accordingly, the term "mental practice" is used as a synonym for the repeated use of motor imagery (ie, motor imagery training; see also Schack, Essig, Frank, & Koester, 2014) throughout this chapter.

Using a variety of different empirical approaches to motor learning as it is induced by mental and physical practice, both practice types have been shown to contribute to the learning of a motor action (Seidler & Meehan, 2013). The two most commonly used indicators of motor learning are changes in motor performance and changes in brain activation (ie, behavioral and neural changes); research directly addressing the role of mental representations[a] (ie, cognitive changes) has remained scarce.

Traditionally, researchers have agreed that persisting changes in motor performance are a valid indicator of motor learning (Schmidt & Lee, 2011) when (1) changes in motor performance occur and persist over time (ie, retention) or when (2) changes in motor performance of a particular task lead to changes on a related task (ie, transfer; for details on the performance–learning distinction, see, eg, Kantak & Winstein, 2012). Similarly, researchers investigating the influence of mental practice on the motor action system and drawing comparisons between mental and physical practice traditionally have focused on overt variables, that is, behavioral changes or changes in motor performance as a variable to measure the degree of learning (Corbin, 1967a, 1967b; for reviews and metaanalyses, see Driskell et al., 1994; Feltz & Landers, 1983; Feltz, Landers, & Becker, 1988; Grouios, 1992; Hinshaw, 1991; Richardson, 1967a, 1967b).

Metaanalyses have shown that mental practice is more effective than no practice, but less effective than physical practice (Driskell et al., 1994; Feltz & Landers, 1983; Feltz et al., 1988). For instance, Driskell et al. (1994) conducted a metaanalysis on the effects of mental practice in comparison to irrelevant practice and physical practice. The authors reported small to moderate effect sizes from their analysis of 35 studies, with an overall average effect size of $d = 0.53$ for mental practice. In contrast, moderate to strong effect sizes were reported for physical practice, with an average of $d = 0.78$.[b] From their metaanalysis, the authors concluded that mental practice is not as effective as physical practice, but that it can have a positive effect on performance. Furthermore, combined mental and physical practice has been suggested to be as effective as physical practice or even superior to physical practice only (Corbin, 1967a; Gomes et al., 2014; Hall, Buckolz, & Fishburne, 1992; McBride & Rothstein, 1979). To date, mental practice is considered a potentially effective means to improve performance and, in this sense, to promote learning.

More recently, researchers have become interested in examining the covert variables that are associated with permanent improvements in motor

---

[a] Mental representation and cognitive representation are being used interchangeably in this chapter (for details on mental representations of human motor action and action control, see theoretical background in this chapter; for a more detailed discussion, see, eg, Land, Volchenkov, Bläsing, & Schack, 2013).

[b] Effect sizes reported throughout this chapter refer to Cohen's d (Cohen, 1992).

performance, and thus motor learning as induced by either mental or physical practice. From a neuroscientific view, motor learning has been studied by looking at changes in the brain, both in its anatomy and its physiology. The adaptation of the brain (ie, neural changes) as a result of physical practice has received a great deal of attention (Wadden, Borich, & Boyd, 2012). Research has provided insights into central changes within the motor action system and prompted conclusions regarding the neural aspects of learning a motor action and the neural plasticity of the brain (for a recent metaanalysis, see Hardwick, Rottschy, Miall, & Eickhoff, 2013; for reviews, see also, eg, Dayan & Cohen, 2011; Doyon & Benali, 2005; Doyon & Ungerleider, 2002; Halsband & Lange, 2006; Kelly & Garavan, 2005; Ungerleider, Doyon, & Karni, 2002).

Likewise, motor imagery and mental practice have been studied by investigating adaptations within the human brain. In the realm of the principle of functional equivalence (Finke, 1979; Jeannerod, 1994, 1995; Johnson, 1980) and the simulation theory (Jeannerod, 2001, 2004, 2006), the study of action representation from a neurophysiological point of view has received tremendous research interest (for overviews, see, eg, Decety, 2002; Guillot, Di Rienzo, & Collet, 2014). According to Jeannerod (2001), both actual and simulated (eg, imagined) actions are considered actions, as each involves a covert stage of action (ie, a simulation stage; s-stage). In other words, "actual" actions imply a covert and an overt stage of action, whereas "simulated" actions imply a covert stage of action only. To this extent, all of the different types of s-stages to some degree involve the activation of the motor action system. Along these lines, mental practice is thought to be effective because it is functionally equivalent to (ie, adheres to the same principles as) physical practice, and as such activates and induces changes within the motor action system.

Although considerable research attention has been directed to the different stages of action, such as the imagery and the execution of an action (Decety, 1996, 2002; Jeannerod & Frak, 1999), it has only been within the last two decades that advances have been made regarding the changes in the brain during the learning of a motor action, examining the effects of mental practice on brain activation, in comparison to both no practice and physical practice (Allami et al., 2014; Avanzino et al., 2015; Jackson, Lafleur, Malouin, Richards, & Doyon, 2003; Pascual-Leone et al., 1995; Zhang et al., 2012, 2014). From neurophysiological studies investigating learning as induced by mental practice and/or physical practice, both mental and physical practice have been found to lead to significant changes in brain activation during skill acquisition. For instance, employing positron emission tomography, Jackson et al. (2003) investigated cerebral functional changes in the brain induced by mentally practicing foot movements and compared these changes to those induced by physically practicing foot movements (Lafleur et al., 2002). Similar to the findings reported by Lafleur et al. (2002), the results showed mental practice to be associated with functional cerebral reorganization. More recently, Zhang et al. (2014) examined changes in functional connectivity in a resting state as a result of mental practice, using functional magnetic resonance imaging. The authors reported alterations in cognitive and sensory resting state networks in various brain systems after learning by way of motor imagery (ie, mental practice), but no alterations in connectivity were found in the control condition (ie, no practice). From this, the authors concluded that modulation of resting-state functional connectivity as induced by mental practice may be associated with functional reorganization in the brain.

Neurophysiological studies such as those previously exemplified give evidence on functional changes in brain activation as a result of physical and mental practice, providing valuable insights into the learning of a motor action by either mental or physical practice. What is not clear from studies focusing on changes in neural representations, however, is what these changes mean in cognitive terms with regard to changes in one's mental representation. Functional changes on a neural level, as described in the studies presented earlier, as a result of mental and physical practice suggest that functional changes on a cognitive level (ie, concept formation in one's mental representation) may take place during the imagery and the execution of an action. Research investigating perceptual–cognitive changes associated with permanent improvements in motor performance, which could provide a closer look at both mental and physical practice, is lacking.

In sum, from findings elucidating behavioral or neural changes associated with motor learning as induced by mental and physical practice, it is not clear what these behavioral and neural changes mean on a cognitive representational level. As such, they do not allow for specific conclusions regarding the cognitive representation of a particular motor action in long-term memory and its development over the course of learning. Given these limitations, it seems crucial to go beyond either behavioral or neural changes and to highlight the role of mental representation itself, if the aim is to thoroughly understand the complexity of the adapting motor action system during learning. In other words, both behavioral and neural variables have been employed mainly to measure the degree of learning within the motor action system and to draw conclusions with respect to underlying representations of an action (Hodges & Williams, 2012; Rose & Christina, 2006). Learning thus has usually been inferred from and empirically studied by either changes in motor performance or changes in the brain. At the same time, conclusions about underlying representations have been drawn based on these changes, inheriting the assumption of an isomorphic relationship between the two. If representations are the basis of action organization, however, the mental representation itself in the organization and during the learning of a motor action might prove to be a valuable indicator of motor learning. Accordingly, having a closer look at the functional role of representations may shed further light on motor learning as induced by mental and physical practice.

The aim of the present chapter is to introduce and discuss recent evidence on perceptual–cognitive changes that occur throughout the process of learning a motor action by way of mental and physical practice in early skill acquisition. For this purpose, recent work on cognitive changes (ie, changes in mental representation) and perceptual changes (ie, changes in "quiet eye") as induced by mental and physical practice is presented, addressing the following questions: How does the mental representation change during the learning of a motor action? Do mental and physical practice differ in their influence on the mental representation of a motor action throughout the learning process? How does the quiet eye change during the learning of a motor action? Do these changes relate to representation development?

Accordingly, the present chapter entails an introduction to the theoretical background, a review of the current state of research, and an overview of recent insights into perceptual–cognitive changes as induced by physical and mental practice: Following a short introduction to motor learning perspectives in general, perceptual–cognitive approaches to complex action are sketched. Second, details on methods to investigate mental representation of complex actions are given. Third, after having sketched the current state of research investigating the representation of complex action over the course of learning, three recent learning experiments are described that systematically examined the influence of physical and mental practice on mental representation and gaze behavior in complex action. Finally, the chapter ends with concluding remarks on the relevance of this perspective for motor learning, motor imagery, and quiet-eye research.

PERSPECTIVES ON MOTOR LEARNING

According to Bernstein (1967), motor control and learning are centered around finding suitable solutions to a particular motor problem. In this sense, the process of learning a motor action reflects more and more elaborate problem solving. In general, researchers agree on the changing nature of the learning process from unskilled to skilled action (Anderson, 1982, 1995; Fitts, 1964; Fitts & Posner, 1967; Gentile, 1972; Masters & Poolton, 2012; Meinel & Schnabel, 1987): During early motor learning, the agent must solve an entirely unfamiliar motor task, attempting to find an appropriate solution for a specific motor problem [eg, cognitive stage: Fitts & Posner, 1967; *Entwicklung der Grobkoordination* (development of rough coordination): Meinel & Schnabel, 1987], whereas during later learning, the motor action that serves to solve the motor problem at hand is being refined based on prior experience [eg, associative stage and autonomous stage: Fitts & Posner, 1967; *Entwicklung und Stabilisierung der Feinkoordination* (development and stabilization of precise coordination): Meinel & Schnabel, 1987].

Research on motor learning has a long-standing tradition (Adams, 1987; Summers, 2004), during which researchers in the field have been trying to determine what mechanisms underlie motor control and learning. Although a number of theories on motor learning exist to date, the specific mechanisms of learning a motor action are still a matter of debate (for an overview, see, eg, Hodges & Williams, 2012; Magill, 2011; Schmidt & Lee, 2011). In general, two main approaches to the basic mechanisms of motor learning can be distinguished: central (ie, cognitive) and peripheral (ie, ecological) approaches, also known as the motor approach and the action approach to motor control and learning (Meijer & Roth, 1991). In addition to these two camps reflecting two distinct positions, perceptual–cognitive approaches on motor learning have evolved (details on each of the approaches follow).

A fundamental assumption of central or cognitive approaches to motor learning is the idea that movements are internally represented (eg, motor program: Keele, 1968; schema: Schmidt, 1975). In other words, central approaches to motor learning provide cognitive, memory-based explanations, assuming some form of representation that changes over the course of learning (Adams, 1971; Anderson, 1982; Fitts & Posner, 1967; Schmidt, 1975). Whereas skilled motor action is thought to rely on well-developed representations (or motor programs or schemas, respectively), motor learning, according to central approaches, is a consequence of the permanent refinement of representations, resulting in more appropriate representations and movement parameter specifications, guiding movement execution in an increasingly reliable manner.

Peripheral or ecological approaches represent a more recent view on motor learning, thereby challenging the traditional cognitive view. From a peripheral point of view, motor control and learning are approached by focusing on the reciprocal relation between the person and the environment. Originating from the theory of direct perception (Gibson, 1977, 1979), ecological approaches assume a direct relationship between perception and action (ie, perception–action coupling), thereby dissociating from representational accounts (Michaels & Beek, 1995). Motor action, in this sense, resides in the direct relation of the person and the environment (Turvey, 1991; Turvey & Kugler, 1984). Accordingly, practice results in the setting up of direct perception–action relations. Thus, motor learning reflects the growth and refinement of the perception–action coupling that guides the realization of affordances (ie, motor action). In other words, motor learning is considered as the establishment of laws for an elaborate coupling of perception and action (Newell, 1991; Schmidt & Fitzpatrick, 1996).

More recently, perceptual–cognitive approaches have received growing research interest in the area of motor control and learning (eg, theory of anticipative behavioral control: Hoffmann, 1993; theory of event coding: Hommel, Müsseler, Aschersleben, & Prinz, 2001; simulation theory: Jeannerod, 2001). Dating back to the original idea of a bidirectional link between an action and its effects (ie, ideomotor theory: Herbart, 1825; James, 1890; for an overview, see Koch, Keller, & Prinz, 2004; Shin, Proctor, & Capaldi, 2010), perceptual–cognitive approaches emphasize the role that the effects of an action play during the selection, planning, and execution of an action. The basic idea of perceptual–cognitive approaches is that motor actions are guided by way of representations holding information about the perceptual effects of motor actions. In this sense, actions are primarily guided by cognitively represented effects. Specifically, motor actions serve the individual to cause changes within the environment (ie, perceptual effects), and these perceptual effects, in turn, serve as an essential control variable to guide future motor action. Thus, perceptual–cognitive approaches to motor action assume a close functional relationship between motor action and the corresponding cognitively represented perceptual effects (Mechsner, 2004; Nattkemper & Ziessler, 2004). Whereas skilled action is thought to rely on well-developed effect representations, motor learning is a result of the constitution and development of effect representations. Accordingly, practice leads to more detailed effect representations, which more efficiently guide and control our actions.

Perceptual–Cognitive Perspective: Cognitive Action Architecture Approach

One such perceptual–cognitive approach, arising in the tradition of Bernstein (1967) and situated at the interface of cognitive psychology and movement science, is the cognitive action architecture approach (CAA-A; Schack, 2002, 2004). Against the background of ideomotor theory (James, 1890), assuming a bidirectional link between actions and action effects, and the common coding theory (Prinz, 1997), postulating that actions are coded commonly in terms of their effects, the CAA-A centers around the hierarchical organization of motor actions, with a particular focus on action effects, their cognitive representation, and their relation to the functional structure of motor actions.

According to the CAA-A (Schack, 2002, 2004), motor actions are organized in a stratified manner, with two main systems (ie, the mental system and the sensorimotor system) contributing to the construction of motor action (Fig. 5.1). Each of the two systems encompasses two levels of action organization. Specifically, from the higher to the lower levels in the hierarchy, the mental system comprises the level of mental control (ie, level IV) and the level of mental representation (ie, level III), and the sensorimotor system is composed of the level of sensorimotor representation (ie, level II) and the level of sensorimotor control (ie, level I). Thus, the motor action system is thought to operate on four different levels: two levels with regulatory functions (ie, the level of mental control and the level of sensorimotor control) serving as control entities, and two levels with representational functions (ie, the level of mental representation and the level of sensorimotor representation) serving as reference entities. Whereas the sensorimotor system, being the "sub" part (ie, the lower part) of both systems within the hierarchy, is concerned with the direct transformation of intentions into actions, that is, the transformation of the intent to move into actual movement, the mental system, being the "super" part (ie, the higher part) within the

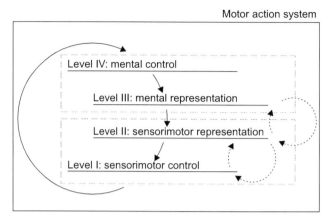

FIGURE 5.1   The levels of action organization within the motor action system during early stages of motor learning. *(Adapted from Schack (2002), p. 59; reprinted from Frank (2014), with permission.)*

hierarchy, is concerned with the indirect transformation, that is, the transformation of the intent to move into real movement (mediated via plans, strategies, etc.; Goschke, 1996). When a motor action is being performed, all four levels of the system are involved, with each level contributing in its specific manner (for an overview of and more details on the CAA-A, see also Schack, 2004; Schack, Bläsing, Hughes, Flash, & Schilling, 2014).

Basic Action Concepts and Mental Representation of Complex Action

The realization of a movement necessitates the involvement of each level, with each level fulfilling distinct functions, but the role that mental representations play within the organization of actions is of particular importance (Schack, 2002, 2004). Action organization and thus the controllability of the motor action system are thought to be closely tied to mental representations of actions (Land et al., 2013). Well-developed mental representations form the basis of well-organized actions and as such ensure that actions can be controlled within the motor action system (Bläsing, 2010; Schack & Mechsner, 2006). Specifically, the level of mental representation serves as a cognitive reference system for subsequent action control, mediated via basic action concepts (BACs): On this level, the intended effect is transferred into a model of the motor action to be executed, by delivering reference values for action execution (Schack, 2002, 2004).

Analogous to the idea that objects are being represented by way of object concepts in long-term memory (Ach, 1921; Hoffmann, 1986, 1993; Rosch, 1978), actions have been suggested to be represented by way of action concepts (Schack, 2002, 2004). According to the CAA-A, the BACs represent cognitive compilations or chunks with regard to the realization of an action goal. Specifically, these compilations are thought to be composed of body pos-tures and movement elements together with their sensory consequences relating to an action goal. To illustrate, "grip check" as a BAC of the golf putt is a cogni-tive chunk serving a particular action goal (ie, to ensure an optimal grip during the preparation of the putting movement before initiation of the backswing). As such, it is composed of the corresponding body posture (eg, standing upright, hips flexed) and movement elements (eg, take grip, move fingers) together with their sensory consequences (eg, feel fingers touching each other and the surface of club; eg, on the tennis serve, see Schack & Mechsner, 2006).

Structuring and Dimensioning of Mental Representations

Mental representations of actions, according to the CAA-A, are considered rep-resentational frameworks composed of BACs (Schack, 2002, 2004; for more details, see Schack, 2012). The structuring of the mental representation is de-fined by the relations between the BACs. The relations between the BACs, in turn, are feature based. That is, each proximity or distance between the concepts of a given set is determined by corresponding features (ie, type, number, and relevance of features), both functional and sensory ones that are closely inter-connected. This feature binding is referred to as the dimensioning of the mental representation; the present chapter, however, focuses on mental representation structure, namely, the relations between and the groupings of BACs, and its change over time.

Learning of a Complex Motor Action and Mental Representation Development

Whereas the organization of skilled motor action is thought to be based on a well-developed mental representation, with automatized processes taking place primarily within the sensorimotor system (for more details, see Schack, 2002), no such well-developed representation is available during the organization of a motor action that is new to an individual. Instead, representations develop dur-ing the learning process (Schack, 2002, 2003; Schack & Ritter, 2013). In other words, for intelligent and thus stable motor action, a cognitive reference on the level of mental representation is essential. However, such a cognitive reference is lacking in the beginning of the learning process, being no more (if at all) than a simple, unrefined version of a reference estimated based on prior experience with a similar motor action.

During the process of motor learning, this cognitive reference is thought to develop from a simple and general representation to a more elaborate and refined version. Specifically, during early stages of skill acquisition [cognitive stage: Fitts & Posner, 1967; *Entwicklung der Grobkoordination* (development of rough coordination): Meinel & Schnabel, 1987], the motor action system is being challenged, with all levels of action organization being in charge. Accord-ing to Schack (2002), the direct interaction of the person with the environment with regard to a particular motor task allows lower sensorimotor patterns and higher conceptual structures to evolve (Fig. 5.1) and as such helps stabilize the perceptual–cognitive system within the human motor action system during early stages of motor learning.

Motor learning, from this point of view, is considered the change and functional development of representational networks of complex action in long-term memory and thus reflects the adaptation of the structuring and dimensioning of mental representations (Schack, 2002, 2003, 2004). Similarly, mental practice effects are thought to be reflected in terms of order formation in memory. Thus, motor learning, according to the CAA-A, reflects an adaptation on the level of mental representation such that the relations and the groupings of action concepts (ie, mental representation structure) are modified over the course of the learning process.

Assessing Mental Representations

The study of mental representations of complex actions has been approached by a variety of different methods such as verbal protocol analysis, sorting and categorization tasks, or recognition and recall tasks (for a methodological overview, see Hodges, Huys, & Starkes, 2007). In the realm of the CAA-A (Schack, 2002, 2004), the structural dimensional analysis of mental representations (SDA-M; Schack, 2012) has been developed as a means to provide psychometric data on the structure and dimension of mental representations of complex movements in long-term memory. With the help of SDA-M, it is possible to measure both the distance and the grouping of BACs (ie, the structuring) as well as the binding of features to BACs (ie, the dimensioning) within the representation of a complex action (for details, see Schack, 2012).

The SDA-M consists of several steps (Schack, 2002, 2004): In a first step, a split procedure delivers a distance scaling between the BACs of a suitably predetermined set. In a second step, a hierarchical cluster analysis is used to outline the structure of the given set of BACs. In a third step, a factor analysis reveals the dimensions in this structured set of BACs, and in a last step, the cluster solutions are tested for invariance within and between groups (for details, see Schack, 2012). In the following paragraphs, each of the steps is presented in more detail.

Before testing for mental representations via SDA-M, a set of BACs for the action of interest is determined. For instance, for the purpose of the line of studies presented in the following, BACs of golf putting were utilized (Frank, Land, & Schack, 2013). To specify the BACs of the golf putt, several steps were taken: With the help of standard textbooks (Pelz & Frank, 2000) and the biomechanical analysis of the golf putt, the movement and movement phases were described in detail in a first step. From this, the parts of the movement considered most relevant resulted in a preliminary set of 27 meaningful body postures. Next, the 27 body postures were further rated and verified by golf experts ($n = 5$). In a last step, a final set of 16 BACs were selected based on the experts' ratings. With this procedure, 16 BACs for the putt were identified (for details, see Table 5.1).

As a first step of the SDA-M, a splitting task delivers a distance scaling between the BACs of the predetermined set of concepts. This task is performed in front of a computer with the screen displaying the BACs (ie, two at a time) of the action to be investigated. While one selected BAC is permanently displayed on the screen (anchor concept; eg, "grip check"), the remaining BACs are presented successively in randomized order. Participants are asked to decide, one after another, whether a given BAC is related to the anchor concept during movement execution (eg, first decision: "grip check" vs "accelerate club," second decision: "grip check" vs "look to the hole," etc.). Once a given list of BACs is finished (eg, each of the BACs has been compared to the anchor concept "grip check"), another BAC serves as an anchor concept and the procedure continues, until each BAC has been compared to the remaining BACs of the set. Second, a hierarchical cluster analysis is used to outline the groupings of BACs and thus

TABLE 5.1 Basic Action Concepts of the Putt in Golf

No.	Basic action concept	Movement phase
1	Shoulders parallel to target line	Preparation
2	Align club face square to target line	
3	Grip check	
4	Look to the hole	
5	Rotate shoulders away from the ball	Backswing
6	Keep arms–shoulder triangle	
7	Smooth transition	
8	Rotate shoulders toward the ball	Forward swing
9	Accelerate club	
10	Impact with the ball	Impact
11	Club face square to target line at impact	
12	Follow-through	
13	Rotate shoulders through the ball	
14	Decelerate club	Attenuation
15	Direct clubhead to planned position	
16	Look to the outcome	

the structuring of mental representation for individuals or groups (ie, individual dendrograms or mean group dendrograms). For cluster analyses, an alpha level is chosen (eg, $\alpha = 0.05$), resulting in a critical value (eg, $d_{crit} = 3.41$). Links between BACs above this critical value are considered statistically irrelevant. In other words, BACs linked above this line are treated as being not related, whereas BACs linked below this line result in a cluster and therefore are treated as being statistically related. As a third step, a factor analysis can be used to determine the dimensioning within the structured set of BACs (for more details, see Schack, 2012). In a final step, cluster solutions are tested for invariance within and between individuals or groups. In addition, the degree of similarity between two cluster solutions can be determined with an analysis of similarity based on adjusted Rand indices. Specifically, analyses of invariance serve to compare cluster solutions. Two cluster solutions are considered variant, that is, significantly different, for $\lambda < 0.68$, while two cluster solutions are invariant for $\lambda \geq 0.68$. In addition, the adjusted Rand index (Rand, 1971; Santos & Embrechts, 2009) can be used to examine the similarity between a given cluster solution and a reference. The adjusted Rand index (ARI) serves as an index of similarity on a scale from -1 to 1. On this scale, the value "-1" indicates that two cluster solutions are different and the value "1" indicates that two cluster solutions are the same. Indices between these extremes rank similarity between two cluster solutions. Typically, well-structured mental representations of expert performers serve as a reference.

Cross-Sectional Research Investigating Representations Across Skill Levels

The body of research on the functional role of mental representation in motor action has been conducted mainly in the field of expertise, thereby drawing comparisons across skill levels (for a review, see, as well, Hodges et al., 2007). For instance, Allard and Burnett (1985) found basketball experts classified problems relating to their sport according to functional principles, whereas novices did so by adhering not to functional but to superficial features. Specifically, expert players classified pictures representing various aspects of the game into distinct and discriminating meaningful categories (eg, offensive and defensive fundamentals), whereas novices classified pictures by way of obvious characteristics such as number of players (eg, individual and team). Moreover, French and Thomas (1987) were among the first to show that skill-related knowledge differs according to skill level. Specifically, expert basketball players differed not only in their superior performance (eg, shooting skill) from their novice counterparts, but also in their basketball-specific knowledge (eg, position of the players). In addressing differences in problem representations between elite and nonelite athletes, Huber (1997) found that more features defined the central concepts of elite athletes, and the interrelations between the concepts were more numerous compared to nonelite athletes. Furthermore, the organization of movement-related knowledge has been systematically investigated. McPherson and coworkers addressed problem representations and condition–action–goal linkages across skill levels by analyzing verbal reports. Experts' problem representations were found to differ from those of novices. For instance, the authors reported more elaborate conceptual networks of declarative and procedural knowledge (ie, condition–action–goal linkages) in both skills and tactics (McPherson, 1993; for an overview, see McPherson & Vickers, 2004; French & McPherson, 2004).

In the realm of the CAA-A, Schack and Mechsner (2006) were the first to investigate the structuring and dimensioning of mental representations across skill levels using the SDA-M. By examining representational networks of the tennis serve in experts and nonexperts, the authors elicited distinct differences in mental representations across skill levels. Specifically, skilled individuals held functionally structured representations of the tennis serve (ie, reflecting well the three movement phases preactivation, strike, and final swing), whereas unskilled individuals did not have such structured representations available. Such differences in mental representations across skill level have been shown to generalize to various motor skills in a variety of sports such as dance (Bläsing, 2010) and volleyball (Velentzas, Heinen, Tenenbaum, & Schack, 2010) and have as well been reported in the area of manual action (Braun et al., 2007) and gait (Schega, Bertram, Foelsch, Hamacher, & Hamacher, 2014; Stöckel et al., 2015).

Research investigating the structure of mental representation of complex action can be condensed into three main findings (Schack & Mechsner, 2006): (1) the mental representation of skilled individuals can be characterized by a distinct structure, with the representation reflecting order formation of BACs; (2) the structure of a skilled individual's mental representation is functional in the sense that the formation of BACs corresponds to the biomechanical and functional task demands; and (3) mental representation structures are similar across skilled individuals. In contrast, mental representation structures of unskilled individuals differ remarkably, and their representations do not hold a distinct, functional structure. From this and other research, it appears that skilled action, but not unskilled action, is based on well-developed representations that help the individual control the motor action system during action execution. In this sense, elaborate representations allow for refined movement execution, resulting in appropriate actions and thus stable performance in a given situation.

Longitudinal Research Investigating Representations Over the Course of Learning

Whereas much attention has been directed toward differences between skilled and nonskilled individuals in their mental representations of complex action, less research has addressed questions relating to the development of an individual's mental representation during motor learning.

Physical Practice

With regard to physical practice, Körndle and coworkers (Körndle, 1983; Zimmer & Körndle, 1988) were among the first to show that cognitive units of action-related knowledge evolve during motor learning and are being integrated into hierarchies during this process. For instance, Körndle (1983) compared individuals who learned a pedaling task quickly (ie, fast learners) to those who learned the task slowly (ie, slow learners) and showed that fast learners differed from slow learners during the learning process, both in their pedaling performance (ie, as measured by way of effective forces and velocity) and in their representations (ie, as measured by way of feature ratings and interviews). Specifically, fast learners were able to give precise statements (eg, keep upper body still; place whole foot on footboard), while slow learners gave no more than global statements (eg, keep balance; go rapidly) on the learning process after practice, indicating different degrees of hierarchy in their representation structures. Continuing this work, Lippens (1992) examined subjective theories during motor learning. Subjective theories as cognitions of the self and the world during rowing were investigated by way of a sorting task. The author reported distinct differences between fast and slow learners. Specifically, fast learners were better able to identify relevant knowledge (eg, sound of oar blade and water) and to quickly and more efficiently access their knowledge. In contrast, slow learners spent more time on their knowledge search and used more numerous terms in their descriptions, thereby getting lost in details more often. From this, the author concluded that representations of rowing become hierarchically integrated during learning. Similarly, Seiler (1995) researched the nature and change of representational frames during motor learning, thereby supporting the idea of hierarchical structuring of representations during motor learning (for related work, see also, eg, Blaser, Stucker, Körndle, & Narciss, 2000; Kromer, 2007; Wiemeyer, 1994; for an overview, see Schack, 2003). In research directly testing for changes in underlying representations of complex motor action during learning, action-related knowledge has been shown to change over the course of learning such that representations of complex action adapt and become hierarchically structured.

Mental Practice

With regard to mental practice, research on the development of mental representations during motor learning as induced by mental practice is scarce. A first step toward considering the influence of mental practice on both the (covert) level of representation and the (overt) level of performance was taken by Narciss (1993). Narciss examined the change of internal representations and biomechanical characteristics of the breaststroke in swimming over the course of practice. In this study, one group of students practiced physically, and another group of students practiced mentally in addition to physical practice. Both groups improved their breaststroke performance over time. Interestingly, the combined (mental and physical practice) group revealed a more developed internal representation in comparison to the physical-practice-only group after practice. Narciss did not further discuss this somewhat unexpected finding but concluded that it may prove fruitful to consider both the covert level of representation and the overt level of performance in future studies. Although the study reflects seminal work on the influence of mental practice on the mental representation of a complex action, the effects of mental and physical practice were not investigated systematically in this study.

In sum, compared to research addressing differences in experts' and novices' representations of complex action, much less research has been conducted that investigates the development of representations during motor learning. Moreover, apart from one study that directly addressed mental representation development with mental practice and physical practice during the learning of a motor action, studies systematically investigating the influence of mental practice on mental representation development, especially in comparison to physical and no practice, are lacking. However, if one aims to thoroughly understand the motor action system and to study motor learning by overt and covert types of practice (ie, physical and mental practice) "from within," it is essential to learn about the distinct contributions of each practice type to perceptual–cognitive adaptations within the motor action system.

RECENT INSIGHT INTO PERCEPTUAL-COGNITIVE CHANGES WITH PHYSICAL AND MENTAL PRACTICE

To systematically investigate the influence of mental and physical practice on the motor action system with a particular focus on the functional development of mental representations, motor learning was recently studied in a series of three learning experiments conducted in a laboratory setting. In a first step, the influence of physical practice on mental representation development during motor learning was investigated (Study 1; Frank et al., 2013). Specifically, this study aimed at answering the question of whether novices' mental representation structure of a complex action changes as a result of physical practice, and whether this change reflects a functional development in the direction of an expert structure. In a second step, the influence of both physical and mental practice on mental representation development during the learning of a motor action was examined (Study 2; Frank, Land, Popp, & Schack, 2014), aiming at both replicating findings from Study 1 and answering the question of whether novices' mental representation structure develops differently according to type of practice (ie, mental and physical practice). In a third step, the influence of physical and mental practice on both mental representation development and gaze behavior (ie, the quiet eye) during motor learning was studied. By doing so, the aim was to gain a more thorough picture of the perceptual–cognitive background of performance changes during the learning of a motor action.

For each of the studies, novices were invited to practice the golf putt for 3 consecutive days in a laboratory setting. Each of the learning studies consisted of a pretest and an acquisition phase of 3 days, followed by a posttest and a retention test after 3 days of no practice. The type of practice differed according to the specific purpose of each study.

In each of the studies, mental representation structures of the putt were assessed using SDA-M to learn about the change and development of mental representations of complex action over time. For this particular purpose, BACs of the putt have been identified (see Table 5.1). Each of the 16 BACs can be assigned to a particular movement phase from a functional and biomechanical perspective (Hossner, Schiebl, & Göhner, 2015): preparation (BACs 1–4), backswing (BACs 5–7), forward swing (BACs 8–11), and attenuation (BACs 12–16). The preparation phase consists of the performer setting up and aligning her/his body with the hole. The backswing phase consists of the start of the backswing and transition between back and forward swing. The forward swing phase relates to the acceleration of the clubhead as well as to the mechanical and functional qualities associated with clubhead–ball impact. Finally, the attenuation phase consists of the follow-through and evaluation of the outcome. In each of the studies, the change and development of mental representations of complex action were assessed (1) by comparing representation structures from pretest to posttest to retention test to learn if any changes had taken place and (2) by comparing representation structures to an expert structure for each time of measurement, to learn whether the change in structures reflected a functional development. In the following, each of the studies will be presented in more detail (for more details, see Frank, 2014).

Study 1: *Mental Representation and Physical Practice*

Building on the finding that mental representations of complex actions differ across skill levels, the study aimed to shed light on an individual's development of a mental representation of a complex action during motor learning (for details, see Frank et al., 2013). We explored whether the mental representation structure of a complex action changes over the course of practice, and if so, whether this change reflects a development toward a more elaborate and functional structure, such as that of an expert. Novice golfers were randomly assigned to either a putting practice group ($n = 12$) or a no-putting control group ($n = 12$). Each participant was tested before and after an acquisition phase of 3 days as well as after a 3-day retention interval. SDA-M was used to record the mental representation structures of the putt. Outcome performance of the practice group was measured using two-dimensional error scores of the putt (ie, putting accuracy and consistency). Findings revealed that to-gether with improvements in putting performance, mental representations of the putt were found to change with practice, developing toward more func-tional ones. Specifically, mental representation structures of the (physical) practice group changed from pretest to posttest to retention test and became more similar to a golf expert structure over the course of practice, reflecting distinct phases of the putting movement (ie, preparation, forward swing, and impact). In contrast, mental representation structures of the control group, who neither executed nor practiced the putt, did not change and remained dissimilar in comparison to an expert structure (Fig. 5.2). This study showed that, along with improvements in (overt) performance, the (covert) mental representation of a complex action functionally develops as a result of prac-tice, suggesting that motor skill acquisition is associated with functional ad-aptations of action-related knowledge in long-term memory.

Study 2: *Mental Representation and Mental Practice*

Drawing on the finding that novices' mental representations of complex action functionally adapt with practice, this study further addressed the development of an individual's mental representation according to type of practice (for de-tails, see Frank et al., 2014). Specifically, the aim was to learn if and how mental practice (ie, motor imagery training) adds to this adaptation process. Hence, the question investigated was whether the mental representation structure of a complex action changes as a result of either mental or physical practice as well as a combination of both, and if so, whether the changes reflect a development toward a more elaborate and functional structure.

For this purpose, novice golfers ($N = 52$) were assigned to either a mental practice group, a physical practice group, a mental–physical combined practice group, or a no-practice group. In other words, participants in the practice groups practiced the putt by either imagining it, executing it, or imagining and executing it. Again, the complex task to be practiced was the golf putt. Participants were tested prior to and after a practice phase, as well as after a 3-day retention inter-val. As in the study of Frank et al. (2013), both mental representation structures of the putt and outcome performance (putting accuracy and putting consistency) were assessed. Findings revealed significant performance improvements over the course of practice together with functional adaptations in mental representa-tion structure. In line with findings from Frank et al. (2013), mental represen-tations of the putt developed over the course of practice. Interestingly, mental practice, either solely or in combination with physical practice, led to even more elaborate representations compared to physical practice only. Specifically, men-tal representation structures of the groups practicing mentally became more similar to a functional structure, thereby reflecting well the functional phases of the putting movement, whereas those of the physical practice group revealed less development toward a functional structure (Fig. 5.3). Furthermore, putting

(a)

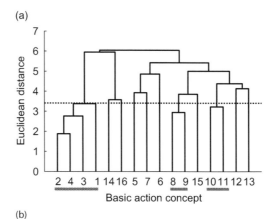

(b)

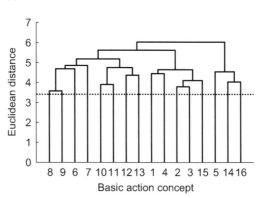

FIGURE 5.2 Mean group dendrograms of (a) the practice group ($n = 12$) and (b) the control/no-practice group ($n = 12$) for the golf putt at retention test. The numbers on the x axis relate to the basic action concept (BAC) number, and the numbers on the y axis display Euclidean distances. The lower the link between related BACs, the lower is the Euclidean distance. The horizontal dotted line marks d_{crit} for a given α level ($d_{crit} = 3.41$; $\alpha = 0.05$): Links between BACs above this line are considered unrelated; horizontal gray lines on the bottom mark clusters. BACs: (1) shoulders parallel to target line, (2) align club face square to target line, (3) grip check, (4) look to the hole, (5) rotate shoulders away from the ball, (6) keep arms–shoulder triangle, (7) smooth transition, (8) rotate shoulders toward the ball, (9) accelerate club, (10) impact with the ball, (11) club face square to target line at impact, (12) follow-through, (13) rotate shoulders through the ball, (14) decelerate club, (15) direct clubhead to planned position, and (16) look to the outcome. *(Reprinted from Frank et al. (2013), with permission.)*

performance improved over the course of practice. Specifically, combined mental and physical practice was most effective ($d = 0.64$), followed by physical practice ($d = 0.54$), mental practice ($d = 0.28$), and no practice (ie, combined practice > physical practice > mental practice > no practice), reflecting the well-known pattern of magnitude of improvement according to type of practice (Driskell et al., 1994, for instance, reported moderate to strong effect sized

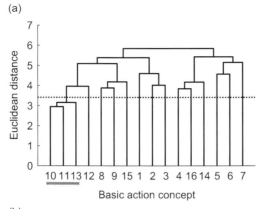

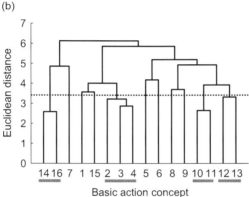

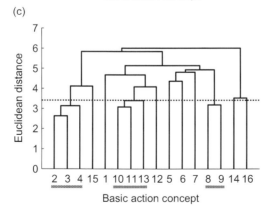

FIGURE 5.3   Mean group dendrograms of (a) the physical practice group (n = 13), (b) the mental practice group (n = 13), and (c) the combined mental and physical practice group (n = 13) for the golf putt at retention test. The numbers on the x axis relate to the basic action concept (BAC) number, and the numbers on the y axis display Euclidean distances. The lower the link between related BACs, the lower is the Euclidean distance. The horizontal dotted line marks d_{crit} for a given α level (d_{crit} = 3.41; α = 0.05): Links between BACs above this line are considered not related; horizontal ▶

for physical practice, $d = 0.78$, and small to moderate effect sizes for mental practice, $d = 0.53$). Statistically, combined practice proved more effective than mental practice only and no practice with respect to performance.

This study replicated the finding by Frank et al. (2013) that the mental representation of a complex action develops with practice. More importantly, however, this study shows that the mental representations of participants incorporating mental practice into their practice regime were more functional in structure than the representations of participants not incorporating mental practice. Notably, these (covert) adaptations did not seem to transfer one-to-one to the (overt) motor output. From these findings, mental practice seems to promote the cognitive adaptation process during motor learning, leading to more elaborate representations than physical practice only.

This finding suggests that mental practice effects may not primarily become evident in terms of overt performance during early skill acquisition. Driskell et al. (1994), having a closer look at mental practice effects relative to level of expertise (ie, novice vs experienced individuals) in their metaanalysis, found mental practice to be more beneficial for cognitive tasks in comparison to motor tasks in novices, whereas experienced individuals profited both in cognitive and motor tasks (between-task comparison). In the same vein, the findings reported previously point toward the idea that mental practice particularly promotes the cognitive level of action organization in novices practicing a motor action (within-task comparison). This suggests that mental practice particularly affects the perceptual–cognitive level at an early stage of motor learning and might not necessarily or only minimally have to be reflected in overt outcome performance. However, future research is needed to test this proposition and to further investigate the causal role of representations and their relation to performance changes as reported previously.

Study 3: *Mental Representation, Gaze Behavior, and Physical and Mental Practice*

The aim of the third study was to further examine the perceptual–cognitive background of performance changes that occur within the motor action system as a result of mental and physical practice, thereby providing insights into mental representations and gaze behavior in complex action (Frank, Land, & Schack, 2016). Accordingly, we investigated whether mental representation

◄ **FIGURE 5.3** gray lines on the bottom mark clusters. BACs: (1) shoulders parallel to target line, (2) align club face square to target line, (3) grip check, (4) look to the hole, (5) rotate shoulders away from the ball, (6) keep arms–shoulder triangle, (7) smooth transition, (8) rotate shoulders toward the ball, (9) accelerate club, (10) impact with the ball, (11) club face square to target line at impact, (12) follow-through, (13) rotate shoulders through the ball, (14) decelerate club, (15) direct clubhead to planned position, and (16) look to the outcome. *(Reprinted from Frank et al. (2014), with permission.)*

structures and the quiet eye (Vickers, 1992, 1996, 2009; Klostermann, Chapter 4) change with both physical practice and combined mental and physical practice in early skill acquisition, and if so whether the changes reflect a functional development (ie, structuring of mental representations together with prolongation of the quiet eye).

Based on their baseline performance, novices ($N = 45$) were assigned to one of three groups: combined mental and physical practice, physical practice, and no practice. Participants in the practice groups again trained on a golf putting task over the course of 3 days either by repeatedly executing and imagining or by solely executing it. Dependent variables (ie, putting performance, mental representation structure of the putt, and the quiet eye prior to putting) were measured prior to and post practice as well as after a retention interval. The quiet eye was measured using a mobile eye-tracking system. Combined mental and physical practice led to the most developed representation structures of the putt, whereas physical practice alone was associated with fewer changes in mental representation structure. As an extension, combined practice led to the most elaborate gaze behavior prior to the execution of the putt. Specifically, final fixations prior to the onset of the putting movement (ie, the quiet eye) during retention were longest for the group practicing mentally in addition to physical practice, followed by the physical practice and the no-practice control group. Statistically, quiet-eye durations prove to be longer after combined practice in comparison to no practice. Interestingly, better developed representation structures were related to longer quiet-eye durations after learning. Putting performance improved similarly in both practice groups over the course of practice.

Thus, although similar improvements in motor performance were evident, changes on a perceptual–cognitive level (ie, mental representation structure and gaze behavior) differed among the groups. A combination of mental and physical practice was associated with a significant development in representation structure and a significant prolongation of the quiet eye, whereas physical practice without mental practice was associated with only small changes in representation structures and quiet-eye durations. This indicates that the combination of mental and physical practice particularly promotes the covert perceptual–cognitive adaptation process within the motor action system in early skill acquisition. However, similar to previous findings, these (covert) perceptual–cognitive adaptations did not become evident on (overt) motor output.

With regard to the quiet eye, findings from the study reported previously extend research on differences in quiet-eye behavior between skilled and unskilled individuals by providing insight into quiet-eye changes over the course of practice. To the best of our knowledge, it is the first study to show that quiet-eye duration becomes longer in novices practicing a complex movement and that it develops along with mental representations. Mental representation structures and quiet-eye durations related to one another after learning, indicating that more elaborate information processing during movement preparation, as expressed by longer quiet-eye durations, is based on more elaborate underlying mental representations in long-term memory. This further supports the notion that the quiet eye is rooted in the cognitive domain (Gonzalez et al., 2015; Klostermann, Kredel, & Hossner, 2014; Williams, Singer, & Frehlich, 2002), reflecting critical action-related information processing that is based on the representation available.

Altogether, this body of work clearly demonstrates that motor learning by mental and physical practice is associated with perceptual–cognitive adaptations within the motor action system and with functional changes in mental representation structures of complex action in particular. Importantly, findings indicate that mental practice (ie, repeated motor imagery) and physical practice (ie, repeated motor execution) differ in their influence on the different levels of action organization (Frank et al., 2014). As stated earlier, the principle of functional equivalence (Finke, 1979; Jeannerod, 1994, 1995; Johnson, 1980) and the simulation theory (Jeannerod, 2001, 2006) propose that imagining and executing an action are functionally equivalent, with both states of action to some degree involving the activation of the motor action system. Although much research has investigated the functional equivalence between different stages of action (such as the imagery and the execution of an action; eg, Decety, 1996, 2002; Jeannerod & Frak, 1999), research addressing the (similar or differential) influence that each of the states of action has on the motor action system during learning has remained scarce (for related discussions, see, eg, Guillot, Moschberger, & Collet, 2013; Munzert, Lorey, & Zentgraf, 2009; Wakefield, Smith, Moran, & Holmes, 2013). In other words, the unique potential of mental practice and physical practice to induce changes on different levels within the motor action system during learning remains to be explored in a systematic manner. As a first step forward, the studies previously reported provide initial evidence on a differential influence of mental and physical practice with regard to different levels of action organization. In particular, findings revealed more functional representation structures and longer quiet-eye durations after learning for the groups practicing by way of motor imagery (either solely or in combination with motor execution). This is indicative of mental practice operating primarily on higher levels within the motor action system during early skill acquisition (for a more detailed discussion, see Frank, 2014; Frank et al., 2014). However, future research is needed to further disentangle the differential influence of imagery and execution with regard to particular levels of action organization.

In sum, the studies reported previously provided insights into cognitive changes (in terms of representation) as well as perceptual changes (in terms of the quiet eye) during learning. These findings complement existing evidence on behavioral and neural changes as induced by mental and physical practice (Allami et al., 2014; Driskell et al., 1994) and as such might contribute to a better understanding of the adapting motor action system during learning.

SUMMARY

Both physical practice (ie, repeatedly executing a motor action) and mental practice (ie, repeatedly imagining the execution of a motor action) have been shown to lead to performance improvements, and in this sense, to promote motor learning. However, motor learning as induced by mental and physical practice has rarely been studied with a specific focus on the perceptual–cognitive changes occurring in the motor action system that is the development of an individual's representation of a complex action and related gaze behavior (ie, the quiet eye) in particular.

Accordingly, the goal of the chapter was to introduce and discuss recent evidence on perceptual–cognitive changes that occur throughout the process of learning a motor action by way of mental and physical practice in early skill acquisition. After an introduction of the theoretical and methodological background, the chapter turned to research focusing on mental representation of complex action and its changes over the course of learning. By presenting recent work on the learning of a motor action by way of physical and mental practice, it was possible to shed light on the perceptual–cognitive background of performance changes (ie, changes in mental representation and the quiet eye) that occur during the learning of a motor action, both in general and according to practice type (ie, mental and physical practice).

Specifically, mental representations and gaze behavior (ie, the quiet eye) in complex action have been shown to develop over the course of learning. In this sense, the learning of a motor action is associated with functional order formation in long-term memory as well as longer action-related information processing prior to the onset of the motor action. Furthermore, this development seems to depend on practice type: The findings presented in the present chapter indicate that mental practice and physical practice differentially influence the motor action system, and that mental practice particularly promotes perceptual–cognitive adaptations during early skill acquisition. However, future research is needed to disentangle the influence of repeated imagery versus execution of a motor action on the different levels of action organization and on subsequent performance of a motor action.

Overall, these results complement behavioral and neural evidence in the field of motor cognition and learning and at the same time underline the importance of advancing knowledge of motor learning from a perceptual–cognitive point of view in future work.

CONCLUSIONS

Several conclusions can be drawn from the research presented in this chapter. First, it is important to consider not only motor but also perceptual and cognitive adaptations that (co)occur over the course of learning a motor action. That is, besides considering learning "from the outside" in terms of permanent changes in motor performance, learning "from within" as induced by mental and physical practice can be studied in terms of order formation in memory as reflected by a functional development in representation structure toward that of an expert.

Second, such perceptual–cognitive approaches as presented in the chapter allow for advancing research in the area of motor imagery and mental practice. By directly examining the representation of the action to be imagined and its changes over time, it becomes possible to further explore the similarities and differences of mental practice and physical practice with regard to the overall motor action system, studying not only behavioral and neural adaptations, but also perceptual–cognitive adaptations that occur within the motor action system as a result of the repeated use of motor imagery. Third, with regard to quiet-eye research, employing a longitudinal design made it possible to demonstrate that the quiet eye becomes longer in novices practicing a motor action, and that quiet-eye durations relate to the degree of development in underlying representation structures. This perspective opens up a perceptual-cognitive explanation of the quiet-eye phenomenon. Furthermore, from the findings presented in this chapter, it seems valuable to bridge quiet eye and motor imagery research to study action-related information processes as they apply to the imagery of complex action in the future.

Overall, advancing research on action representation from a perceptual–cognitive point of view seems to be a promising approach to motor cognition, as it reflects a valuable complement to behavioral approaches (focusing on motor variables such as outcome performance or kinematics) and neurophysiological approaches (focusing on neurocognitive/neuromuscular variables such as brain activity/muscular activity). By building bridges between approaches and disciplines, it becomes possible to approximate changes that occur within the motor action system over time in their entirety (Moran, Guillot, MacIntyre, & Collet, 2012; Munzert & Zentgraf, 2009). Future research, therefore, should further aim at integrating different approaches across different disciplines to reach a better understanding of the complex phenomenon of learning a motor action, the perceptual, cognitive and motor aspects thereof, and the similarities and differences in the learning by way of executing or imagining a motor action.

ACKNOWLEDGMENT

This research/work was supported by the Cluster of Excellence Cognitive Interaction Technology "CITEC'(EXC277)" at Bielefeld University, which is funded by the German Research Foundation (DFG).

REFERENCES

Ach, N. (1921). *Untersuchungen zur psychologie und philosophie. Über die begriffsbildung. Eine experimentelle untersuchung [Investigations on psychology and philosophy. On concept formation. An experimental investigation].* Bamberg, Germany: C. C. Buchners.

Adams, J. A. (1971). A closed-loop theory of motor learning. *Journal of Motor Behavior, 3,* 111–150.

Adams, J. A. (1987). Historical review and appraisal of research on the learning, retention, and transfer of human motor skills. *Psychological Bulletin, 101,* 41–74.

Allami, N., Brovelli, A., Hamzaoui, E. M., Regragui, F., Paulignan, Y., & Boussaoud, D. (2014). Neurophysiological correlates of visuo-motor learning through mental and physical practice. *Neuropsychologia, 55,* 6–14.

Allard, F., & Burnett, N. (1985). Skill in sport. *Canadian Journal of Psychology, 39*, 294–312.

Anderson, J. R. (1982). Acquisition of cognitive skill. *Psychological Review, 89*, 369–406.

Anderson, J. R. (1995). *Learning and memory.* New York, NY: Wiley.

Avanzino, L., Gueugneau, N., Bisio, A., Ruggeri, P., Papaxanthis, C., & Bove, M. (2015). Motor cortical plasticity induced by motor learning through mental practice. *Frontiers in Behavioral Neuroscience, 9*, 105.

Bernstein, N. A. (1967). *The co-ordination and regulation of movements.* Oxford, England: Pergamon Press.

Blaser, P., Stucke, K., Körndle, H., & Narciss, S. (2000). *Auswirkungen eines leistungstrainings im brustschwimmen auf den zusammenhang von bewegungsrepräsentation und bewegungsausführung [Effects of practicing breast-stroke swimming on the relation of movement representation and movement execution].* Cologne, Germany: Strauss.

Bläsing, B. (2010). The dancer's memory: expertise and cognitive structures in dance. In: B. Bläsing, M. Puttke, & T. Schack (Eds.), *The neurocognition of dance* (pp. 75–98). London, England: Psychology Press.

Braun, S. M., Beurskens, A. J. H. M., Schack, T., Marcellis, R. G., Oti, K. C., Schols, J. M., & Wade, D. T. (2007). Is it possible to use the SDA-M to investigate representations of motor actions in stroke patients? *Clinical Rehabilitation, 21*, 822–832.

Cohen, J. (1992). A power primer. *Psychological Bulletin, 112*, 155–159.

Corbin, C. (1967a). The effects of covert rehearsal on the development of a complex motor skill. *The Journal of General Psychology, 76*, 143–150.

Corbin, C. (1967b). Effects of mental practice on skill development after controlled practice. *Research Quarterly, 38*, 534–538.

Dayan, E., & Cohen, L. G. (2011). Neuroplasticity subserving motor skill learning. *Neuron, 72*, 443–454.

Decety, J. (1996). Do imagined and executed actions share the same neural substrate? *Cognitive Brain Research, 3*, 87–93.

Decety, J. (2002). Is there such a thing as functional equivalence between imagined, observed and executed action? In: A. N. Meltzoff, & W. Prinz (Eds.), *The imitative mind: Development, evolution, and brain bases* (pp. 291–310). Cambridge, England: Cambridge University Press.

Doyon, J., & Benali, H. (2005). Reorganization and plasticity in the adult brain during learning of motor skills. *Current Opinion in Neurobiology, 15*, 161–167.

Doyon, J., & Ungerleider, L. G. (2002). Functional anatomy of motor skill learning. In: L. R. Squire, & D. L. Schacter (Eds.), *Neuropsychology of memory* (pp. 225–238). New York, NY: Guilford.

Driskell, J., Copper, C., & Moran, A. (1994). Does mental practice enhance performance? *Journal of Applied Psychology, 79*, 481–492.

Feltz, D., & Landers, D. (1983). The effects of mental practice on motor skill learning and performance: a meta-analysis. *Journal of Sport Psychology, 5*, 25–57.

Feltz, D. L., Landers, D. M., & Becker, B. J. (1988). A revised meta-analysis of the mental practice literature on motor skill learning. In: National Research Council (Ed.), *Enhancing human performance, part III: Improving motor performance.* Washington, DC: National Academy Press.

Finke, R. A. (1979). The functional equivalence of mental images and errors of movement. *Cognitive Psychology, 11*, 235–264.

Fitts, P. M. (1964). Perceptual-motor skill learning. In: A. W. Melton (Ed.), *Categories of human learning* (pp. 243–255). New York, NY: Academic Press.

Fitts, P. M., & Posner, M. I. (1967). *Human performance.* Belmont, CA: Brooks/Cole.

Frank, C. (2014). *Mental representation and learning in complex action: A perceptual-cognitive view on mental and physical practice.* Doctoral dissertation, Bielefeld University, Bielefeld, Germany.

Frank, C., Land, W. M., & Schack, T. (2013). Mental representation and learning: the influence of practice on the development of mental representation structure in complex action. *Psychology of Sport and Exercise, 14*, 353–361.

Frank, C., Land, W. M., Popp, C., & Schack, T. (2014). Mental representation and mental practice: experimental investigation on the functional links between motor memory and motor imagery. *PLoS One, 9*, e95175.

Frank, C., Land, W. M., & Schack, T. (2016). Perceptual-cognitive changes during motor learning: the influence of mental and physical practice on mental representation, gaze behavior, and performance of a complex action. *Frontiers in Psychology, 6*, 1981.

French, K. E., & McPherson, S. L. (2004). Development of expertise in sport. In: M. R. Weiss (Ed.), *Developmental sport and exercise psychology: a lifespan perspective* (pp. 403–423). Morgantown, WV: Fitness Information Technology.

French, K. E., & Thomas, J. R. (1987). The relation of knowledge development to children's basketball performance. *Journal of Sport Psychology, 9*, 15–32.

Gentile, A. M. (1972). A working model of skill acquisition with application to teaching. *Quest, 17*, 3–23.

Gibson, J. J. (1977). The theory of affordances. In: R. Shaw, & J. Bransford (Eds.), *Perceiving, acting, and knowing: toward an ecological psychology* (pp. 67–82). Hillsdale, NJ: Erlbaum.

Gibson, J. J. (1979). *The ecological approach to visual perception.* Boston, MA: Houghton Mifflin.

Gomes, T. V. B., Ugrinowitsch, H., Marinho, N., Shea, J. B., Raisbeck, L. D., & Benda, R. N. (2014). Effects of mental practice in novice learners in a serial positioning skill acquisition. *Perceptual and Motor Skills, 119*, 1–18.

Gonzalez, C. C., Causer, J., Miall, R. C., Grey, M. J., Humphreys, G., & Williams, A. M. (2015). Identifying the causal mechanisms of the quiet eye. *European Journal of Sport Science, 10*, 1–11.

Goschke, T. (1996). Wille und kognition: zur funktionalen architektur der intentionalen handlungssteuerung [Volition and cognition: on the functional architecture of intentional action control]. In: H. Heckhausen, & J. Kuhl (Eds.), *Motivation, volition, handlung [Motivation, volition, action]* (pp. 583–663). Göttingen, Germany: Hogrefe.

Grouios, G. (1992). Mental practice: a review. *Journal of Sport Behavior, 15*, 42–59.

Guillot, A., Moschberger, K., & Collet, C. (2013). Coupling movement with imagery as a new perspective for motor imagery practice. *Behavioral and Brain Functions, 9*, 8.

Guillot, A., Di Rienzo, F., & Collet, C. (2014). The neurofunctional architecture of motor imagery. In: T. D. Papageorgiou, G. I. Christopoulos, & S. M. Smirnakis (Eds.), *Advanced brain neuroimaging topics in health and disease: methods and applications* (pp. 421–443). Rijeka, Croatia: InTech.

Hall, C., Buckolz, E., & Fishburne, G. (1992). Imagery and the acquisition of motor skills. *Canadian Journal of Sport Sciences, 17*, 19–27.

Halsband, U., & Lange, R. K. (2006). Motor learning in man: a review of functional and clinical studies. *Journal of Physiology, 99*, 414–424.

Hardwick, R. M., Rottschy, C., Miall, R. C., & Eickhoff, S. B. (2013). A quantitative meta-analysis and review of motor learning in the human brain. *NeuroImage, 67*, 283–297.

Herbart, J. F. (1825). *Psychologie als wissenschaft [Psychology as science].* Königsberg, Germany: Verfasser.

Hinshaw, K. (1991). The effects of mental practice on motor skill performance: critical evaluation and meta-analysis. *Imagination, Cognition and Personality, 11*, 3–35.

Hodges, N. J., & Williams, A. M. (2012). *Skill acquisition in sport. Research, theory and practice.* London, England: Routledge.

Hodges, N. J., Huys, R., & Starkes, J. L. (2007). Methodological review and evaluation of research in expert performance in sport. In: G. Tenenbaum, & R. C. Eklund (Eds.), *Handbook of sport psychology* (pp. 161–183). Hoboken, NJ: Wiley.

Hoffmann, J. (1986). *Die welt der begriffe [The world of concepts]*. Berlin, Germany: Verlag der Wissenschaften.

Hoffmann, J. (1993). *Vorhersage und erkenntnis [Prediction and understanding]*. Göttingen, Germany: Hogrefe.

Hommel, B., Müsseler, J., Aschersleben, G., & Prinz, W. (2001). The theory of event coding (TEC): a framework for perception and action planning. *Behavioral and Brain Sciences, 24*, 849–937.

Hossner, E.-J., Schiebl, F., & Göhner, U. (2015). A functional approach to movement analysis and error identification in sports and physical education. *Frontiers in Psychology, 6,* 1339.

Huber, J. (1997). Differences in problem representation and procedural knowledge between elite and nonelite springboard divers. *The Sport Psychologist, 11*, 142–159.

Jackson, P. L., Lafleur, M. F., Malouin, F., Richards, C. L., & Doyon, J. (2003). Functional cerebral reorganization following motor sequence learning through mental practice with motor imagery. *NeuroImage, 20*, 1171–1180.

James, W. (1890). *The principles of psychology*. New York, NY: Holt.

Jeannerod, M. (1994). The representing brain: neural correlates of motor intention and imagery. *Behavioral and Brain Sciences, 17*, 187–245.

Jeannerod, M. (1995). Mental imagery in the motor context. *Neuropsychologia, 33*, 1419–1432.

Jeannerod, M. (1997). *The cognitive neuroscience of action*. Oxford, England: Blackwell.

Jeannerod, M. (2001). Neural simulation of action: a unifying mechanism for motor cognition. *NeuroImage, 14*, S103–S109.

Jeannerod, M. (2004). Actions from within. *International Journal of Sport and Exercise Psychology, 2*, 376–402.

Jeannerod, M. (2006). *Motor cognition: what actions tell the self*. Oxford, England: Oxford University Press.

Jeannerod, M., & Decety, J. (1995). Mental motor imagery: a window into the representational stages of action. *Current Opinion in Neurobiology, 5*, 727–732.

Jeannerod, M., & Frak, V. (1999). Mental imaging of motor activity in humans. *Current Opinion in Neurobiology, 9*, 735–739.

Johnson, P. (1980). The functional equivalence of imagery and movement. *Quarterly Journal of Experimental Psychology A, 34*, 349–365.

Kantak, S. S., & Winstein, C. J. (2012). Learning–performance distinction and memory processes for motor skills: a focused review and perspective. *Behavioral Brain Research, 228*, 219–231.

Keele, S. W. (1968). Movement control in skilled motor performance. *Psychological Bulletin, 70*, 387–403.

Kelly, A. M., & Garavan, H. (2005). Human functional neuroimaging of brain changes associated with practice. *Cerebral Cortex, 15*, 1089–1102.

Klostermann, A., Kredel, R., & Hossner, E. -J. (2014). The quiet eye without a target: the primacy of visual information processing. *Journal of Experimental Psychology, 40*, 2167–2178.

Koch, I., Keller, P. E., & Prinz, W. (2004). The ideomotor approach to action control: implications for skilled performance. *International Journal of Sport and Exercise Psychology, 2*, 362–375.

Körndle, H. (1983). *Zur kognitiven steuerung des bewegungslernens [On the cognitive control of motor learning]*. Doctoral dissertation, University of Oldenburg, Oldenburg, Germany.

Kromer, M. (2007). *Veränderungen von gedächtnisrepräsentationen im motorischen lernprozess: theoretische überlegungen und eine pilotstudie zum konzept impliziter bewegungsrepräsenta-tion* [*Changes of memory representations during motor learning: Theoretical reflections and a pilot study on the concept of implicit movement representations*]. Doctoral dissertation, German Sport University Cologne, Cologne, Germany.

Lafleur, M. F., Jackson, P. L., Malouin, F., Richards, C. L., Evans, A. C., & Doyon, J. (2002). Motor learning produces parallel dynamic functional changes during the execution and imagination of sequential foot movements. *NeuroImage, 16,* 142–157.

Land, W. M., Volchenkov, D., Bläsing, B., & Schack, T. (2013). From action representation to action execution: exploring the links between cognitive and biomechanical levels of motor control. *Frontiers in Computational Neuroscience, 7,* 127.

Lippens, V. (1992). *Die innensicht beim motorischen lernen. Untersuchungen zur veränderung der subjektiven theorien bei lern- und optimierungsprozessen am beispiel des ruderns [The inner view on motor learning. Investigations on the change of subjective theories during learning and optimization processes using the example of rowing].* Cologne, Germany: Strauss.

Magill, R. A. (2011). *Motor learning and control: Concepts and applications.* New York, NY: McGraw-Hill.

Masters, R. S. W., & Poolton, J. M. (2012). Advances in implicit motor learning. In: A. M. Williams, & N. J. Hodges (Eds.), *Skill acquisition in sport: Research, theory, and practice* (2nd ed., pp. 59–75). London, England: Routledge.

McBride, E. R., & Rothstein, A. L. (1979). Mental and physical practice and the learning and retention of open and closed skills. *Perceptual and Motor Skills, 49,* 359–365.

McPherson, S. L. (1993). Knowledge representation and decision-making in sport. In: J. Starkes, & F. Allard (Eds.), *Cognitive issues in motor expertise* (pp. 159–188). Amsterdam, The Netherlands: Elsevier.

McPherson, S. L., & Vickers, J. N. (2004). Cognitive control in motor expertise. *International Journal of Sport and Exercise Psychology, 2,* 274–300.

Mechsner, F. (2004). Perceptual-cognitive control of bimanual coordination. *International Journal of Sport and Exercise Psychology, 2,* 210–238.

Meijer, O., & Roth, K. (1991). *Complex movement behaviour: "The" motor-action controversy.* Amsterdam, The Netherlands: North-Holland.

Meinel, K., & Schnabel, G. (1987). *Bewegungslehre, sportmotorik [Kinesiology, movement science].* Berlin, Germany: Volk und Wissen.

Michaels, C. F., & Beek, P. J. (1995). The state of ecological psychology. *Ecological Psychology, 7,* 259–278.

Moran, A., Guillot, A., MacIntyre, T., & Collet, C. (2012). Re-imagining motor imagery: building bridges between cognitive neuroscience and sport psychology. *British Journal of Psychology, 103,* 224–247.

Morris, T., Spittle, M., & Watt, A. (2005). *Imagery in sport.* Champaign, IL: Human Kinetics.

Munzert, J., & Zentgraf, K. (2009). Motor imagery and its implications for understanding the motor system. In: M. Raab, J. Johnson, & H. Heekeren (Eds.), *Progress in brain research (Vol. 174). Mind and motion: The bidirectional link between thought and action* (pp. 279–288). Amsterdam, The Netherlands: Elsevier.

Munzert, J., Lorey, B., & Zentgraf, K. (2009). Cognitive motor processes: the role of motor imagery in the study of motor representations. *Brain Research Reviews, 60,* 306–326.

Narciss, S. (1993). *Empirische untersuchungen zur kognitiven repräsentation bewegungsstruktureller merkmale. Ein wissenspsychologischer ansatz zur theoretischen fundierung des mentalen trainings [Empirical investigations on the cognitive representation of structural movement features. A knowledge-based psychological approach to the theoretical foundation of mental practice].* Doctoral dissertation, University of Heidelberg, Heidelberg, Germany.

Nattkemper, D., & Ziessler, M. (2004). Cognitive control of action: the role of action effects [Editorial]. *Psychological Research, 68*, 71–73.

Newell, K. M. (1991). Motor skill acquisition. *Annual Review of Psychology, 42*, 213–237.

Pascual-Leone, A., Dang, N., Cohen, L. G., Brasil-Neto, J. P., Cammarota, A., & Hallett, M. (1995). Modulation of muscle responses evoked by transcranial magnetic stimulation during the acquisition of new fine motor skills. *Journal of Neurophysiology, 74*, 1037–1045.

Pelz, D., & Frank, J. A. (2000). *Dave Pelz's putting bible: The complete guide to mastering the green.* New York, NY: Doubleday.

Prinz, W. (1997). Perception and action planning. *European Journal of Cognitive Psychology, 9*, 129–154.

Rand, W. (1971). Objective criteria for the evaluation of clustering methods. *Journal of the American Statistical Association, 66*, 846–850.

Richardson, A. (1967a). Mental practice: a review and discussion, part I. *The Research Quarterly, 38*, 95–107.

Richardson, A. (1967b). Mental practice: a review and discussion, part II. *The Research Quarterly, 38*, 263–273.

Rosch, E. (1978). Principles of categorization. In: E. Rosch, & B. B. Lloyd (Eds.), *Cognition and categorization* (pp. 27–48). Hillsdale, NJ: Erlbaum.

Rose, D. J., & Christina, R. W. (2006). *A multilevel approach to the study of motor control and learning.* San Francisco, CA: Benjamin-Cummings.

Santos, J. M., & Embrechts, M. (2009). On the use of the adjusted rand index as a metric for evaluating supervised classification. In: C. Alippi, M. Polycarpou, C. Panayiotou, & G. Ellinas (Eds.), *Lecture notes in computer science (Vol. 5769). Artificial neural networks—ICANN 2009* (pp. 175–184). Berlin, Germany: Springer.

Schack, T. (2002). Zur kognitiven architektur von bewegungshandlungen—modelltheoretischer zugang und experimentelle untersuchungen [On the cognitive architecture of motor actions—theoretical approach and experimental investigations]. Habilitation dissertation, German Sport University Cologne, Cologne, Germany.

Schack, T. (2003). Kognition und emotion [Cognition and emotion]. In: H. Mechling, & J. Munzert (Eds.), *Handbuch bewegungswissenschaft bewegungslehre [Handbook of movement science kinesiology]* (pp. 313–330). Schorndorf, Germany: Hofmann.

Schack, T. (2004). The cognitive architecture of complex movement. *International Journal of Sport and Exercise Psychology, 2*, 403–438.

Schack, T. (2012). Measuring mental representations. In: G. Tenenbaum, R. C. Eklund, & A. Kamata (Eds.), *Measurement in sport and exercise psychology* (pp. 203–214). Champaign, IL: Human Kinetics.

Schack, T., & Mechsner, F. (2006). Representation of motor skills in human long-term memory. *Neuroscience Letters, 391*, 77–81.

Schack, T., & Ritter, H. (2013). Representation and learning in motor action. Bridges between experimental research and cognitive robotics. *New Ideas in Psychology, 31*, 258–269.

Schack, T., Bläsing, B., Hughes, C., Flash, T., & Schilling, M. (2014a). Elements and construction of motor control. In: A. G. Papaioannou, & D. Hackfort (Eds.), *Routledge companion to sport and exercise psychology* (pp. 308–323). London, England: Routledge.

Schack, T., Essig, K., Frank, C., & Koester, D. (2014b). Mental representation and motor imagery training. *Frontiers in Human Neuroscience, 8*, 328.

Schega, L., Bertram, D., Foelsch, C., Hamacher, C., & Hamacher, D. (2014). The influence of visual feedback on the mental representation of gait in patients with THR: a new approach for an experimental rehabilitation strategy. *Applied Psychophysiology and Biofeedback, 39*, 37–34.

Schmidt, R. A. (1975). A schema theory of discrete motor skill learning. *Psychological Review*, *82*, 225–260.

Schmidt, R. C., & Fitzpatrick, P. (1996). Dynamical perspective on motor learning. In: H. N. Zelaznik (Ed.), *Advances in motor learning and control* (pp. 195–223). Champaign, IL: Human Kinetics.

Schmidt, R. A., & Lee, T. D. (2011). *Motor control and learning: a behavioral emphasis*. Champaign, IL: Human Kinetics.

Seidler, R. D., & Meehan, S. K. (2013). Introduction to the special topic: a multidisciplinary approach to motor learning and sensorimotor adaptation [Editorial]. *Frontiers in Human Neuroscience*, *7*, 543.

Seiler, R. (1995). *Kognitive organisation von bewegungshandlungen. Empirische untersuchungen mit dem inversionsprinzip [Cognitive organization of motor actions. Empirical investigations on the principle of inversion]*. Sankt Augustin, Germany: Academia.

Shin, Y., Proctor, R., & Capaldi, E. (2010). A review of contemporary ideomotor theory. *Psychological Bulletin*, *136*, 943–974.

Stöckel, T., Jacksteit, R., Behrens, M., Skripitz, R., Bader, R., & Mau-Moeller, A. (2015). The mental representation of the human gait in young and older adults. *Frontiers in Psychology*, *6*, 943.

Summers, J. (2004). A historical perspective on skill acquisition. In: N. J. Hodges, & M. A. Williams (Eds.), *Skill acquisition in sport: Research, theory and practice* (pp. 1–26). London, England: Routledge.

Turvey, M. T. (1991). Action and perception from an ecological point of view. In: R. Daugs (Ed.), *Sportmotorisches lernen und techniktraining: internationales symposium [Motor learning and movement behavior]* (pp. 78–95). Schorndorf, Germany: Hofmann.

Turvey, M. T., & Kugler, P. N. (1984). An ecological approach to perception and action. In: H. T. A. Whiting (Ed.), *Human motor actions. Bernstein reassessed* (pp. 373–412). Amsterdam, The Netherlands: Elsevier.

Ungerleider, L. G., Doyon, J., & Karni, A. (2002). Imaging brain plasticity during motor skill learning. *Neurobiology of Learning and Memory*, *78*, 553–564.

Velentzas, K., Heinen, T., Tenenbaum, G., & Schack, T. (2010). Functional mental representation of volleyball routines in German youth female national players. *Journal of Applied Sport Psychology*, *22*, 474–485.

Vickers, J. N. (1992). Gaze control in putting. *Perception*, *21*, 117–132.

Vickers, J. N. (1996). Visual control when aiming at a far target. *Journal of Experimental Psychology*, *22*, 342–254.

Vickers, J. N. (2009). Advances in coupling perception and action: the quiet eye as a bidirectional link between gaze, attention, and action. In: M. Raab, J. G. Johnson, & H. R. Heekeren (Eds.), *Progress in brain research (Vol. 174). Mind and motion: The bidirectional link between thought and action* (pp. 279–288). Amsterdam, The Netherlands: Elsevier.

Wadden, K. P., Borich, M. R., & Boyd, L. A. (2012). Motor skill learning and its neurophysiology. In: N. J. Hodges, & A. M. Williams (Eds.), *Skill acquisition in sport* (pp. 247–265). London, England: Routledge.

Wakefield, C., Smith, D., Moran, A. P., & Holmes, P. (2013). Functional equivalence or behavioural matching: a critical reflection on 15 years of research using the PETTLEP model of motor imagery. *International Review of Sport and Exercise Psychology*, *6*, 105–121.

Wiemeyer, J. (1994). *Interne bewegungsrepräsentation. Grundlagen, probleme und perspektiven [Internal movement representation]*. Cologne, Germany: BPS.

Williams, A. M., Singer, R. N., & Frehlich, S. G. (2002). Quiet eye duration, expertise, and task complexity in near and far aiming tasks. *Journal of Motor Behavior*, *34*, 197–207.

Zhang, H., Xu, L., Zhang, R., Hui, M., Long, Z., Zhao, X., & Yao, L. (2012). Parallel alterations of functional connectivity during execution and imagination after motor imagery learning. *PLoS One*, 7, e36052.

Zhang, H., Long, Z., Ge, R., Xu, L., Jin, Z., Yao, L., & Liu, Y. (2014). Motor imagery learning modulates functional connectivity of multiple brain systems in resting state. *PLoS One*, 9, e85489.

Zimmer, A. C., & Körndle, H. (1988). A model for hierarchically ordered schemata in the control of skilled motor action. *Gestalt Theory*, 10, 85–102.

Chapter 6

Perspectives on Team Cognition and Team Sports

Nathan McNeese, Nancy J. Cooke, Mike Fedele, Rob Gray
Human Systems Engineering, Arizona State University, Phoenix, AZ, United States

INTRODUCTION: TEAMS, TEAM COGNITION, AND SPORTS

Sports are an important aspect of almost every culture and something with which most people identify. Sports have also helped to define what most people consider a team. Like sports, teams permeate society. A team is more than a collection of individuals. Dyer (1984; Salas, Cooke, & Rosen, 2008, p. 541) defines a team as a "social entity composed of members with high task interdependency and share valued common goals." This definition is fairly standard, though there have been a number of variations on the theme. Most notably, Salas, Dickinson, Converse, and Tannenbaum (1992, p. 4) define a team as "a distinguishable set of two or more people who interact dynamically, interdependently, and adaptively toward a common and valued goal/object/mission, who have each been assigned specific roles or functions to perform, and who have a limited life span of membership." Often, teams and groups are discussed interchangeably. Although teams and groups have many of the same characteristics, they are different. A team is a special type of group with members who have interdependent and heterogeneous roles and responsibilities (Cooke, Salas, Kiekel, & Bell, 2004). Each member on a team has a specific and different role on the team, with each role necessary to accomplish the task. Whereas for a group, members may have the same roles or their roles are never defined. Also, members of a group can work side-by-side without interacting. Interaction among team members is central to the definition of team.

There are many reasons that teams can be found in many different contexts including healthcare, emergency crisis management, and command and control. Possibly, the most impactful reason is that teams are effective and productive. Assuming that the team adequately works together, they are able to bring together many resources to approach problems in a more efficient manner than is a single individual.

Sport and Exercise Psychology Research. http://dx.doi.org/10.1016/B978-0-12-803634-1.00006-6

Yet, even though teams are used in many contexts, when asked to describe a team, many turn to the domain of sports. This is because sports teams are extremely popular, familiar, and abundant in society. Over the years, team sports have become incredibly popular due the growth of football (both North American and European), basketball, baseball, and hockey. These different sports are connected through the concept of *teamwork*.

Teamwork is critical to the success of sports teams. Team members must work together (the activity of sport) toward a common goal (overcoming the other team and winning the game). If a team fails to exhibit high levels of teamwork, then their performance will most likely suffer. Although it is easy to say that a team must exhibit good teamwork to function as an effective team, articulating the essential aspects of teamwork on the field is much more difficult.

Team sports are clearly dependent on the physical activities of individuals. However, there is significant cognitive processing required to execute those activities in a skilled manner and to coordinate those activities with those of teammates. Therefore, effective teamwork is dependent on types of activities: physical action and cognitive processing. These two activities are interrelated and must act in concert at *both* an individual and team level. Team sports consist of multiple layers of both individual and team physical and cognitive activities. Although team sports are bounded by teamwork, they are still inherently composed of individuals. Because of this, individuals must coordinate their own individual physical movement in concert with their cognition.

An example of the physical/cognitive interaction at an individual level in sports is demonstrated when an individual basketball team member is bouncing the basketball up and down. The team member must physically move his or her hand and arm to bounce the ball while cognitively processing where and how fast to bounce the ball. As the interaction of physical coordination and cognitive processing is occurring at an individual level, it is also occurring at a team level. The relationship and interaction of physical coordination and cognitive processing becomes even more complicated at the team level due to team-level situational variables. Now, the individual team member must continue to individually bounce the basketball, but also access the multiple aspects of teamwork. Cognitively, the player must now process what his/her teammates are doing and what the opponents are doing as well. This information is then processed and physical action may take place in response. Thus, at a team level, the basketball player is maintaining his or her individual actions, but also now reacting physically and cognitively to the team environment. The interaction between physical and cognitive activities at the team level or *team cognition* drives teamwork.

Team cognition is defined here as cognitive activity that occurs at a team level (Cooke, Gorman, Myers, & Duran, 2013). Team cognition is what allows a team member to pass a soccer ball to an open teammate who then scores. Team cognition is a rich research area that has been studied in many contexts and through multiple different research streams such as shared mental models

(Mohammed, Ferzandi, & Hamilton, 2010), situation awareness (Gorman, Cooke, & Winner, 2006), training (Salas & Cannon-Bowers, 2001), stress (Cannon-Bowers & Salas, 1998), and temporal limitations (Mohammed, Hamilton, & Lim, 2009). Over time, the overarching finding is that team cognition is critically linked to team performance (Salas et al., 2008).

Team cognition has historically been studied from two perspectives. The first perspective, *shared knowledge*, is the more common perspective for understanding team cognition. Traditionally, researchers who study team cognition as shared knowledge have viewed teams from an information-processing perspective in which there are inputs to the team, processes that occur on the team, and outputs (Hinsz, Tindale, & Vollrath, 1997). This perspective has tended to focus on the inputs of team cognition, often measured in terms of the knowledge of individual team members. Based on the way knowledge is measured, it is defined as being relatively static and not adapting to environmental change. The focus is on how knowledge compares across team members with knowledge similarity typically being the target for effective teamwork. This perspective has resulted in the construct of a shared mental model (Mohammed et al., 2010). Traditionally, shared mental models portray knowledge as being static and team cognition resulting from the sharing of individual knowledge.

Though this perspective of team cognition is valuable, there are conceptual and methodological gaps. More specifically, this perspective does not account for the cognitive processing that occurs at a team level. It also does not account for the dynamic nature of many environments (like team sports) that require concomitant dynamic cognition. The authors of this chapter prescribe to an *ecological* perspective of team cognition. Although, shared knowledge can be important for team effectiveness, our view is that the cognitive interaction (communication, coordination) that is taking place at the team level is even more critical. That cognition is dynamic, meaning that it is constantly changing and evolving in response to the environment in which it occurs. We feel that this perspective is particularly valuable for studying team cognition within the context of sports. Team sports are extremely dynamic and rely heavily on interactions among teammates, two features that are addressed within the ecological perspective to studying team cognition.

The theory of interactive team cognition (ITC), an ecological theory, holds that team cognition occurs at the team level through team member interactions and is dynamic. Furthermore, the theory states that the interaction that occurs during teamwork *is* team cognition. Aspects of team interaction, such as communication and coordination, are examples of team-level cognitive processing (Cooke et al., 2013). This means that team cognition can be studied by observing team communication and coordination. Methodologies of analyzing team communication and coordination have been developed, which facilitate the expansion of the concept of team cognition beyond teamwork or taskwork knowledge (as the shared knowledge perspective implies). ITC is a means to study team cognition that could be very valuable in the sports context. The theory will be reviewed in more detail later in the chapter, and specifically in the context of team sports.

In the remaining sections of this chapter, we review the shared knowledge perspective, paying particular attention to the construct of the shared mental model that exemplifies how team cognition has been studied. We will also explore and describe work that has focused on sports and the shared mental model construct. Next, we discuss the ecological perspective, highlighting the theory of ITC in depth. We then review literature focused on ecological dynamics found within the sport community. This is recent work that is not traditionally considered within the domain of team cognition, but that is consistent with ITC. Once the different perspectives have been fully reviewed, we then present a discussion on how these perspectives of team cognition relate to the sports context. In response, we suggest an integrative perspective. This is a perspective that takes aspects from both the shared knowledge and ITC perspectives and applies them to studying team cognition of team sports. Each perspective that we mention and outline in this paper has specific benefits to the sports context, so an integrative perspective might be what is necessary to understand team cognition within the team sports context.

INFORMATION PROCESSING PERSPECTIVES ON TEAM COGNITION: SHARED KNOWLEDGE AND SHARED MENTAL MODELS

Static Perspectives on Teamwork

Organizations and teams collaborate in a multitude of diverse scenarios. Members within teams provide inputs to the team in terms of specific behaviors and attitudes that, in turn, can have an effect on team performance. Inputs, processes, and outcomes evolve as teams collaborate over time (Kozlowski, Gully, Nason, & Smith, 1999). Traditionally, teamwork has been studied from this information-processing perspective. The input–process–output (I-P-O) model has been a common model for understanding how teams operate. The model involves assessing the mediating processes that describe why particular inputs impact team performance. Specifically, the model posits that teams take inputs from team members and the environment and process information that results in a team output (Ilgen, Hollenbeck, Johnson, & Jundt, 2005).

Under the umbrella of the I-P-O framework is the idea of a shared mental model (SMM). SMMs have become a major construct for explaining team processes. These combined mental blueprints between teammates provide team members with the opportunity to coordinate team actions without explicitly communicating information (Klimoski & Mohammed, 1994). SMMs are a popular way to express how teammates' knowledge is interrelated. Cooke, Salas, and Cannon-Bowers (2000) state that the definition of an SMM tends to vary across researchers, as some prefer to refer to the construct as "team knowledge."

Blickensderfer, Cannon-Bowers, and Salas (1999) discuss task and team knowledge as the two types of information teammates bring to a particular scenario. All teammates have separate perceptions of a situation, individual knowledge of the task, current surroundings, and knowledge of teammates that has built up over time. Shared mental models aid team situation awareness (SA) or the awareness of change in the environment by a team. Endsley (1995) posited a particular model of SA suggesting that workload, stress, system complexity, amount of automation, and aspects of design affect situation awareness. Specifically, the author suggests that the advancement and evolution of technology has possibly created problems for situation awareness as the human becomes increasingly disconnected from the environment by the technology. For instance, pilots and copilots need to be sharing information about their current states to achieve a coordinated, successful flight. Typically, lackluster performance occurs when situation awareness is faulty. Furthermore, team situation awareness has many components and is the culmination of multiple mental processes (Cooke, Stout, & Salas, 2001).

Transactive memory is another shared knowledge topic that researchers have used to describe why certain teams may be more efficient than others. Transactive memory structures are mental representations of specific individuals' knowledge capabilities known to teammates and are relevant due to their link to performance. Austin (2003) conducted a study involving the connection between transactive memory systems and performance in developed, persisting groups. Measured by knowledge stock and specialization, and transactive memory consensus and accuracy, a team's transactive memory structure was positively related to group goal performance, and internal and external group evaluations. Teams who trained together scored higher on performance measures than teams who trained separately.

Although these frameworks have been quite popular, their limitations have been discussed extensively. Marks, Mathieu, and Zaccaro (2001) argue that the I-P-O framework is not dynamic enough to capture the complex nature of teams. Further, the focus on the attainment of knowledge similarity or overlap belies that heterogeneous definition of team. These limitations of the shared knowledge perspective on team cognition remain consistent as team cognition is extended to the domain of sports.

Shared Mental Models and Sports

Examples of mental models can be seen in any individual or team sport. For instance, in basketball, when a team calls a specific offensive play, all players on the court are (hopefully) aware of their own personal roles and the sequence of interactions that is supposed to occur. The players' beliefs about how the team is supposed to operate will affect the outcome. Possibly, the play involves a point guard passing to a winger, and while that occurs, the center is supposed to go set a back screen for the opposing winger on the other side of the court. If the winger who was passed to expects the opposing winger to come off the back screen in a particular manner, and he/she violates that belief, an errant pass and turnover could occur. If everything happens in a fluid, expected sequence, there is a greater opportunity for success. However, the fascinating aspect of sports is that a wonderfully executed play can be shunned by a high performing defense, which draws from their own mental model.

The processes of anticipating and predicting the behaviors of one's teammates are vital to the overall coordination and performance of a team (Tannenbaum, Salas, & Cannon-Bowers, 1996). The idea of anticipation has been at the forefront of sports research, as teammates are constantly anticipating each other's actions to gain an edge on the opponent. Safeties in football are constantly reading the eyes of the quarterback to decide what area of the field they need to cover. The quarterback is, in turn, anticipating the movements of defensive players, and trying to deceive them with movements like fake hand-offs, look-offs, and pump fakes.

In dealing with sports, physical actions are vital because they determine the result of the contest. But the cognitive processes that lead to these actions must be addressed in order to comprehend these athletic endeavors. Research has found that differences between experts and novices in information processing appear to be in the anticipation of actual behaviors (Reimer, Park, & Hinsz, 2006). In particular, McPherson and Kernodle (2003) showed that tennis experts and beginners experience differences in problem-solving scenarios, which align with players' choices while actually playing. The participants were initially presented with a scheme of scenarios. Experts accessed information beyond what was represented in the schemes and developed a representation that included more strategic components. However, in real gameplay, over 80% of experts shot choices were considered strategic or tactical in the context of a given scenario according to the player's position, opponents' positions, and position of the ball. Fifty percent of the time beginners made shot choices with no strategic plan (McPherson & Kernodle, 2003).

There has been research dedicated to understanding shared mental models (SMM) in sports. Giske, Rodahl, and Høigaard (2015) conducted a study that involved expert hockey and handball athletes. The athletes were surveyed about whether their teams had or had not established shared goals, such as their overall offensive rush pattern. Furthermore, investigators wanted to understand the underlying processes of how these shared goals evolved. For instance, they questioned whether these teams participated in certain types of training to obtain an overall collective identity. There was also a measure in place to reveal whether or not the teams had established shared beliefs or expectations about the opponent they had to face on any given day. They found that teammates held an SMM and their pregame presumptions supported that SMM. Generally, it is common for sports teams to have an overarching philosophy, and for their practices and preparations to coincide with this overall strategy (Giske et al., 2015).

Attempting to elicit knowledge through interviews is a routine technique for researching team cognition in sports. Bourbousson, Poizat, Saury, and Sève (2012) used personal interviews to observe the types of shared knowledge that a basketball team evidenced. Their categories of sharedness consisted of moments of nonsharedness (1% of the game), partial sharedness (87% of the game), and complete sharedness (12% of the game). It is worth noting that these were individual interviews, and the responses to the questions were gathered and compared to all the other teammates' answers. This is a common aggregation method, however, it has limitations associated with aggregating data from individuals who have different roles and backgrounds.

Silva, Garganta, Araujo, Davids, and Aguiar (2013) discusses the shared knowledge approach and compares it to the ecological dynamic approach. The shared knowledge perspective suggests that team members are able to coordinate their actions because of a shared mental model that they have developed about a particular strategy. Researchers are skeptical about how this approach can explain how long it takes this mental model to come together. Also in a sports venue, the environment is quite dynamic. How could a shared model account for the constantly changing opponent and teammate behaviors? The ecological approach could possibly be a more useful framework to apply to the study of team cognition in sports. Supporters of the ecological perspective believe that an SMM could be important for understanding pregame operations, but is not sufficient for comprehending the in-game volatilities of an athletic competition (Silva et al., 2013).

Limitations

It is important to note the difference between the research areas of sports psychology and team cognition. Sports psychology is more closely related to clinical psychology in the sense that it deals with the interpersonal counseling of players. Also, it tends to focus on the individual rather than the team. Sports psychology is an important field, but research has not focused on understanding the team as whole. The study of team cognition as shared knowledge has assumed a collective approach, which involves studying the team at the level of the individuals within it, and aggregating those results to the team as a whole. This suggests that team knowledge is the sum of the individual's knowledge within the team, whereas others have suggested that team cognition goes beyond the sum of the parts (Cooke et al., 2013). This approach also assumes that team member knowledge should be similar, which is contrary to the view that a team is composed of team members with different roles, skills, and background knowledge. This collective methodology aligns with the shared knowledge perspective for which comparison of individual knowledge is the focus. Recently, other approaches have been proposed that consider the team as the unit of analysis, thereby avoiding the aggregation issue.

ECOLOGICAL PERSPECTIVES ON TEAM COGNITION: INTERACTIVE TEAM COGNITION

Interestingly, recent perspectives on team cognition have, in reaction to the static shared knowledge perspective, begun to characterize the construct more dynamically and ecologically. The theory of ITC (Cooke et al., 2013) exemplifies this perspective and may provide further insight on capturing the teamwork dynamics of sports teams.

ITC holds that team cognition is cognitive activity at the team level. This theory focuses on cognitive processing over cognitive structure or knowledge. When teams plan, decide, assess the situation, perceive, or solve problems as a unit of two or more individuals, they display cognitive activity at the team level (Cooke et al., 2013). Team coordination and communication are outward manifestations of this cognitive processing. Therefore, observations of communication and coordination provide a direct measure of team-level cognitive processing. It is acknowledged that this is a broader view of "cognition" than the view of cognition as knowledge. This approach is ecological in the sense that team interactions, which are central to the theory, are tightly coupled with events happening in the environment, including the behavior of other teammates.

To make this theory more concrete, consider the three-person Unmanned Aerial System (UAS) task in which ITC was developed (Cooke & Shope, 2004). In this task, there are three team members, each taking on quite different roles, with the team goal of taking as many good photos of designated ground targets as possible. The three roles include pilot or air vehicle operator, mission planner, and photographer or payload operator. When teams approach a designated target waypoint in the simulated environment, the mission planner must provide information about the upcoming target to the pilot. Then the pilot and photographer negotiate the position of the UAS and the camera settings (eg, the required zoom and focus will require a specific UAS altitude range). Once a good photo is taken, the photographer should let the other team members know that they can move on. These interactions have to happen to get a good photo and to maximize team effectiveness, the timing is important. This type of coordination has been likened to that of sports teams—specifically North American football (Pedersen & Cooke, 2006).

The ecological nature of the interactions is associated with the push and pull of information. Even without drawing on task-related knowledge, which ITC acknowledges as important, the actions of the pilot are directed by the information passed by the mission planner. The information that is outside of the head is pivotal in the team's actions. ITC considers the affordances of other teammates as central to teamwork.

There are three assumptions of ITC (Cooke et al., 2013, pp. 256–257):

1. Team cognition is an activity, not a property or a product;
2. Team cognition should be measured and studied at the team level; and
3. Team cognition is inextricably tied to context.

The first assumption is tied to the idea that team cognition can be defined apart from knowledge. In particular, cognitive processing is a team activity. The second assumption argues that team cognition should be studied at the team level, as opposed to measuring at the individual level, followed by aggregation. The third assumption acknowledges the importance of context or the environment.

The ITC theory was not only inspired by logical arguments about dynamics, context, and team-level measurement, but also by empirical data (Cooke et al., 2013). Although some data on degrees of shared knowledge do demonstrate correlations with team performance, in other cases there is little or no connection. In the UAS experiments, teams that demonstrated skill acquisition over a series of 40-min missions would show little or no changes in shared knowledge, but would demonstrate changes in interactions (ie, response to novel events, interactions, verbal process behaviors). Further, forgetting in teams was better predicted by quality of interactions prior to the retention interval rather than shared knowledge. In analyses of these same data, dynamical systems modeling has been applied to communication flow data (who is talking to whom) and other interaction data and different patterns have been associated with the flexibility or adaptability of the team (Gorman, Cooke, & Amazeen, 2010). Perturbations from the environment can also impact the dynamics, with some teams returning to their original interaction trajectories faster than others. These and other similar results suggest that interactions are at least as important as shared knowledge and in some cases, more important.

There are interesting implications that accompany ITC. First, the idea that interactions in the form of communication and coordination are directly observable means that team-level cognitive processing is directly observable, a phenomenon relegated to inference in individuals. Also, unlike shared knowledge approaches that require off-task knowledge elicitation, the measurement of communication and coordination can occur during the task and in a manner that is not disruptive. This unobtrusiveness is important so that the task performance of interest is not altered by the measure. Not only is the measurement unobtrusive, but to the extent that the processing and analysis of the data can occur in real time or near real time then monitoring the performance of the team can also occur in real time. ITC also suggests that interventions should be directed toward interactions, rather than knowledge.

What is the role of individual and shared knowledge in ITC? Knowledge is not discounted; in some tasks that are knowledge intensive (vs processing intensive) such as team-based scientific discovery, knowledge may be more important. But as knowledge takes a back seat to real-time processing of information in the environment, the interaction will be more predictive of team performance. Knowledge at a particular level (rules of the game, capabilities of teammates and other teams) is important as a prerequisite, as are shared goals and objectives.

What are the implications for ITC in sports teams? Interactions can extend beyond behavior or movements and to communications or cognitive coordination. Communication data can be explicitly or implicitly nonverbal. Gestures and hand signals can be analyzed and much information can be gained without extensive content analysis. Quantity and flow of communication have been important indicators of team cognition and performance. How can these data be collected unobtrusively on sports teams? Video analysis is one possibility, though that is necessarily after the fact. Voice-activated microphones and recorders are yet another possibility. There are yet other implications for ITC and sports teams. If data can be collected in real time, then team performance can be monitored in real time and feedback or other interventions could be administered that would impact team interactions. Further, opposing teamwork could be analyzed from this vantage point and interventions to get an understanding of how to apply perturbations to disrupt team interactions.

Overall, ITC provides a perspective on team cognition that addresses the criticisms of shared knowledge approaches that are individually oriented and focused on static knowledge.

Although ITC has not yet been applied to sports teams, there is recent research on ecological dynamics of sports teams that is closely aligned with the ITC perspective. First, the dynamics of teamwork are considered, which are important to a full understanding of teamwork in any domain, but central to sports teams. Second, in the ecological dynamics approach, teamwork is addressed at the team level by examining shared affordances and interactions among teammates. This attention to factors external to the individual addresses the criticism levied against shared knowledge approaches that aggregate measures taken at an individual level, purportedly losing the essence of teamwork. This new area of ecological dynamics in sports teams is discussed in the next section.

ECOLOGICAL DYNAMICS AND SPORTS

In the past decade, there has been growing interest in using an ecological approach to study team coordination in sports (reviewed in Araujo, Silva, & Davids, 2015). As discussed earlier, this approach shares several common principles with ITC. In particular, in the ecological approach, team coordination can only be understood within the context of the performance itself as it relies on shared attunement to perceptual information (Silva et al., 2013), rather than shared prior knowledge between teammates.

For example, consider the example of an athlete attempting to pass a ball to the teammate, while at the same time preventing an opponent from intercepting the ball. How does the player with ball know when to pass and how does the player receiving the ball know when to break for the ball? In the ecological approach, this coordination problem could be solved if both the passer and receiver based their actions on the higher-order perceptual variable τ_{Diff}, which gives the difference between the time of arrival of the defender at the pass landing point and time of arrival of the receiver at the same location. τ_{Diff} is optically specified by the ratio of the angular gap between each player and the landing location and the rate of change of this gap (Correia & Araujo, 2009). This variable is informative because it directly specifies whether there is an opportunity for a pass (ie, $\tau_{Diff} > 0$) or not (ie, $\tau_{Diff} < 0$). Coordination between players occurs in this case occurs because both players are attuned to τ_{Diff} (ie, are relying on it to control motor action) and thus would simultaneously detect when the environment affords the opportunity for a pass. On the surface because the perceptual information needed for the action is available to anyone with a functional visual system, it might be assumed that practice is less important for the development of team coordination in the ecological approach. However, it has been shown that practice is often required for actors to become attuned to such higher-order variables as novice performers often rely on simpler (and less effective) information sources (Smith, Flach, Dittman, & Stanard, 2001). Furthermore, these information sources must be scaled by the action capabilities of both performers (Fajen, 2007), which again would presumably occur during practice. For example, the τ_{Diff} value that affords passing also depends on the maximum running speed that can be achieved by the receiver and the maximum velocity at which the passer can accurately pass the ball. In summary, the keys to team coordination in the ecological approach are that: (1) both players are attuned to the same information sources and (2) both players' perceptions are effectively calibrated for the action capabilities of their teammates.

In terms of the specifics of the research, previous ecologically oriented research on team coordination has utilized both micro- and macrolevel methodologies. At a micro level, researchers have begun to identify candidate perceptual information sources that could be used for coordinated behavior. Again because the information sources only exist online, research in this area has involved the analysis of either real (via video) or simulated game play. An example of this type of research can be seen in the recent study examining team coordination in rugby (Correia, Araujo, Cummins, & Craig, 2012). In this study, a virtual reality simulation of three-on-three play in rugby was used to investigate how gaps between players are used as information to make passing decisions. The main findings were that the position and rate of opening of player gaps strongly influenced participants' behavior, with the nature of the effect being related to rugby expertise. On the one hand, when the gap directly in front of the participant carrying the ball had the fastest opening rate, participants ran with the ball in most cases. On the other hand, when an adjacent gap was opening at the fastest rate, participants would most likely pass the ball. Furthermore, the relationship between the chosen behavior and gap information was significantly stronger in more experienced professional players as compared to recreational or nonrugby players. Therefore, what on the surface could be thought of as behavior that involves a complex decision process (eg, should I run, pass short, or pass long) can be understood by examining the relationships between players' actions and the available perceptual information (ie, gaps). It will be interesting for future research to examine whether similar gaps in information influences the running behavior of teammates not carrying the ball, as would be predicted by the ecological approach.

At a macro level, some recent studies have sought to understand the nature of the coordinated behaviors that emerge from the interaction between teammates. These efforts have been greatly aided by the availability of GPS tracking information used now by many sports teams. The logic behind these efforts is that if, as suggested by both ITC and the ecological approach, team coordination is emergent, then there may be many metrics that can be used to capture this process that cannot be derived from using a bottom-up approach (ie, by looking the execution of "plays" and coaches' strategy).

For example, consider the emergent properties of team centroid and team stretch index. A team's centroid is defined as the mean lateral and longitudinal position coordinates of each player on a team, whereas the stretch index is defined as the average radial distance of all players of a team from the centroid. Centroid and stretch are emergent properties as they are characteristics that arise naturally from game play rather than being explicitly controlled (eg, coaches do not implement strategies to directly influence team centroid). Research examining these metrics has revealed some important relationships with team coordination and success. For example, in their study of small-sided soccer games, Frencken, Lemmink, Delleman, and Visscher (2011) found that the crossing of offensive and defensive centroids was a reliable indicator of a play that would end in a goal being scored. More recently, Clemente, Couceiro, Martins, Mendes, and Figueiredo (2013) have shown that centroid analyses can be used to detect instances when teams change the side/flank of their attack during a game.

For stretch index, it has been demonstrated that the magnitude of stretch is a reliable indicator of when a team is attacking (expanded index) or defending (contracted index) (Moura, Martins, Anido, Barros, & Cunha, 2012). This variable has also been used to calculate the effective playing space, defined as the area on the field that a team actually utilizes (as opposed to the total physical area) during a game. One could imagine making interesting links between this measure and differences in team strategy (eg, spreading the floor in basketball or a prevent defense in football). It will be important for this relatively new line of research to further relate these macrolevel measures of coordination to performance measures (eg, goals and wins) and to understand the relationship between the microlevel perceptual information and macrolevel outcomes.

In sum, the ecological approach to team coordination in sports is a rapidly developing research area that is highly commensurate with the ideas of ITC.

INTEGRATIVE PERSPECTIVE OF STUDYING TEAM COGNITION IN TEAM SPORTS

Overall, research focused on team cognition within the context of team sports has been minimal. Although we have highlighted some work specific to each team cognitive perspective, it is still minimal when compared to the amount of work that has been conducted in other research contexts. For example, a significant amount of work has focused on team cognition in the contexts of command and control, aviation, medical teams, and emergency crisis teams (Cooke et al., 2013; Mohammed et al., 2010). As a result, specific knowledge relating to team cognition and those contexts has been generated and interventions created for making teams in these domains more effective. There is a significant opportunity to study and apply team cognition in the sports context. This a exciting and critical gap to fill, as much can be learned about both team cognition at a high level and team cognition within the specific context of sport.

Sports provides a very unique context for many reasons. For example, members of sports teams must not only interact with each other, but must additionally account for their coach and the opposing team. Each of these contextual variables has the potential to impact team cognition in different ways compared to a nonsports team. The implications are that the team cognition community must understand *how* to study team cognition during team sports. Identifying and understanding *how* to study team cognition during sports means both identifying the most suitable team cognitive perspectives, as well as the specific methodologies that are most appropriate for the sports context. In this section, we discuss what perspective to use when studying team cognition and sports. Due to the unique aspects of the sports context, this might not be a case of one perspective being more appropriate than the other. Rather, an integration of both perspectives could be the most fruitful. This is an idea that we will further articulate within this section.

In the previous sections, we highlighted two different perspectives to studying team cognition: (1) *information processing/shared knowledge* and (2) *ecological*. When the two are compared, the information-processing approach exemplified in the shared knowledge perspective dominates the sports context. Typically, team cognition and sports research has focused on using the construct of a shared mental model to frame the discussion. For the most part, the ecological perspective has not been applied to team cognition during sports. The aforementioned literature on ecological dynamics and sports is not traditionally considered team cognition work. Rather, work is found within related communities and encompasses attributes aligned with the ecological perspective of team cognition. No research has yet employed the theory of ITC to the team sports context.

Simply, regardless of the perspective that is utilized, more work needs to be conducted in this area. Moving forward with this research stream, it is critical to evaluate what each perspective brings to the table. The goal of this chapter is not to say that one of these perspectives is better than the other. Both perspectives are extremely valuable and should continue to be used to study team cognition in a variety of settings. Rather, the goal here is to articulate how the perspectives align with the sports context and based on that alignment recommend *how* to conceptually understand the sports context in the best way. Although it would be optimal if it were as clear-cut as saying researchers should use the *X* perspective to study team cognition and sports, it is not that easy. As we have analyzed each perspective and its added benefits to the sports context, we have concluded that this is not a case of using the shared knowledge perspective *or* the ecological perspective. Rather, it is more that researchers should use the shared knowledge perspective *and* the ecological perspective. Both perspectives are beneficial to studying team cognition and sports and both should be applied to this specific context.

We recommend that the best perspective for studying team cognition and sports is an integrative perspective that mixes aspects of both the shared and ecological perspective. The perspectives are complementary to each other in that during dynamic communication and coordination (ecological perspective), knowledge (shared knowledge perspective) is constantly being shared among the team members. It is a mix of cognitive process and cognitive structure. The close relationship that communication, coordination, and knowledge all share within team cognition allow for aspects of both perspectives to be utilized in conjunction.

Sports is a context that is multifaceted, so it is important to employ a holistic perspective that accounts for the many variables that take place at both an individual/team level and are static/dynamic. A blending of the two perspectives allows team cognition researchers to study team cognition at multiple levels while accounting for the many domain-specific variables. The differences among the perspectives are actually their strengths when applied to the sports context. To better understand why we are suggesting that researchers utilize an integrative perspective, we explain team sports in a way that directly orients aspects of the existing perspectives to specific aspects of sport. Through this, it will become apparent that in order to fully understand team cognition during team sports, it is necessary to employ aspects of each approach.

Let us consider the team sports context. What is a sports team—who makes up that team? Well, it starts with individual players playing together to then make up a team. So, sports teams consist of both individuals and the overall team. As highlighted in the introduction, the roles of the individual and the overall team are critical to the success of the team. The interaction of the individual teammates with each other results in teamwork and team cognition. It is critical to consider that teamwork is built on both individual knowledge and team interaction. The individual knowledge that each team member brings to the team may or may not manifest itself in the team interactions. One could make an argument that individual knowledge builds the foundation of team cognition. This approach leads us back to the shared knowledge perspective. It is important to understand individuals' knowledge and how it is shared among the team because it directly impacts the team, and subsequently team cognition. Sports teams are dependent on individual performances within the overall team. These individual performances are directly linked to individual knowledge. As team cognition researchers, it is critical to understand that there is significant value in understanding individual players' knowledge and how that is shared within the team. This shared knowledge not only accounts for an overlap of individuals' knowledge but also creates new team knowledge through the team interactions.

The team interaction (among individuals) that creates new knowledge is team cognition. In addition to accounting for the individual knowledge and what it is shared (shared knowledge), researchers must also study the interactions that take place at a team level because these interactions account for the action of team cognition (ecological-ITC). Whereas the team is composed of individuals, team sports ultimately take place at a team level. The team is playing *together*. For this reason, team cognition should be studied at the team level. After all, it is referred to as *team* cognition, not *individually shared* cognition. The ecological perspective allows for the study of team cognition at the team level. This is critically important because the communication and coordination that occurs at the team level is ultimately what team cognition is (although individual knowledge scopes the interactions).

Both individuals and the team ultimately result in the team cognition that occurs during sports teamwork. For these reasons, it is critical that researchers attempt to study team cognition in a manner that will allow for an understanding of individual knowledge and how it is shared, as well as the interactions that take place at a team level. Both explicitly account for team cognition in sports teams.

Knowledge has been mentioned throughout our discussions on team cognition. In the sports context, it is important to consider what knowledge truly is. Knowledge in this context is both static and dynamic. For example, understanding that there are two goals within a soccer field and that when the ball goes into one, a goal is scored is static knowledge. This is knowledge that not is changing. Rules of sports are static knowledge. The overall understanding of how you play a sport is static knowledge. This knowledge is incredibly significant to a sports team. If an entire team understands the rules correctly, but one of their teammates does not, it might result in a penalty. Therefore, it is important to understand the role that static knowledge has within team cognition. Part of a team's cognition should be devoted to static knowledge, whereas part should be devoted to dynamic knowledge. The shared knowledge perspective is better at measuring and understanding static knowledge. Traditionally, there was the assumption that team cognition was static and not changing. Once each team member shared his or her knowledge, team cognition then developed and did not change.

Further, cognition is much broader than knowledge that is either static or dynamic. Team cognition includes not only knowledge, but the cognitive processing that takes place at a team level. Teams make decisions, plans, and solve problems as a unit and do so very quickly in the sports context. ITC focuses on the cognitive processing, but acknowledges that the knowledge is a critical prerequisite to that processing.

Now, after many years, we now know that team cognition is incredibly dynamic and changes based on situational knowledge of both the team and their environment. Sports are dynamic. Although it varies based on the sport, the field of play is often constantly changing. Players are constantly moving around and changing their physical actions in response to the many situations of the game. Due to this, knowledge of both teammates and the environmental landscape requires constant adaptation. Team cognition reacts to this adaptation through team-level cognitive processing.

The ecological perspective accounts for the cognitive processing within the team. More specifically because the ITC theory studies the team while they are interacting with each, it is most appropriate to capture the dynamic nature of both communication and coordination. Communication and coordination are dynamic activities of interaction, bounded at a high level by static knowledge but molded by the dynamic knowledge found within the team and the environment.

In addition, there are specific aspects of the team sports setting that are dynamic and must be accounted for. First, sports teams must deal with the opposing team. The opposition's team directly affects how teams play on the field. New dynamic knowledge is created based on what the opposing team is doing. For example, if an opposing team's defensive strategy is overly aggressive throughout the game, the team then reacts to that to take advantage of the situation. When a basketball team switches their team defensive from man-to-man to zone, the realization of this switch from the other team is dependent on dynamic knowledge. Each of these examples demonstrates how dynamic sports are and how fast the environmental landscape can quickly change.

Another unique aspect of team sports is the influence of coaching. Coaching typically occurs in two different ways. First, coaching happens in practice and throughout this process a game plan is developed in response to an upcoming opponent. Second, coaching happens during a game in an ad hoc manner. Based on what the coach is observing in accordance with his or her own team and the opposing team, the coach makes on-the-fly adjustments in the overall strategy. This second type of coaching is mainly in response to the dynamic knowledge represented by the teams and their environment. Due to how the teams are playing and what they are doing on the field of play, the coach takes that dynamic knowledge and either continues with the same game plan or changes the game plan. The coach is a critical part of the team, and in many instances, the leader. The overall potential impact that a coach has on team cognition is understudied.

The opposing team and coaching are both dynamic aspects of team cognition and team sports that must be accounted for when studied. As these aspects are mainly dynamic, the theory of ITC is most appropriate for capturing the dynamic cognition associated with the team members and their environment. But as we can see, sports are not based on dynamic interactions alone. Static knowledge is engrained throughout many team sports aspects. This is another reason why an integrative approach considering both the shared knowledge perspective and the ecological perspective is needed. By using this approach, a researcher is able to account for both cognitive processing and shared knowledge. Both are paramount for sports and team cognition.

In conclusion, when comparing each team cognition perspective in the context of sports, it is apparent that both are useful and necessary. Each brings forth specific affordances that are necessary for the sports context. The shared knowledge perspective allows a better understanding of individual knowledge and how it is shared, which is critical to the performance of sports teams. Yet, the ecological perspective allows us to study sports teams at the level of the team. Knowing this, if a researcher seeks to completely understand how team cognition is developing and occurring, then they should account for the impact that both the individual and the team has on team cognition.

Also, sports are founded on the basis of both dynamic and static cognition. We know that the shared knowledge perspective is better at capturing static knowledge and the ecological perspective is better at capturing the dynamic cognitive processes. Once again, to best understand each type of cognition and its specific impact on team cognition, it is critical to apply both perspectives in concert. Although it might be easier to only use one perspective, in order to gather a holistic understanding of the activity of team cognition during sports from beginning to end, researchers need to integrate each perspective into their methodologies.

CONCLUSIONS

In conclusion, sports teams engage in both physical and cognitive activities. The two are intertwined and rely heavily on events in the environment and pushing and pulling from each teammate. Cognitive processing occurs at the team level and makes use of affordances in the environment. Individual and shared knowledge should not be discounted, as not all actions are directed by the environment. However, for very interdependent team sports (eg, football, basketball, hockey) the dynamic interplay among teammates is a very important source of information in the environment. ITC capitalizes on these interactions to monitor, assess, and improve teamwork through team communication and coordination.

A rich research agenda is suggested by ITC. Research is needed on how to best measure sports team interactions unobtrusively, including verbal and nonverbal communications. Then these patterns need to be statistically mapped on to effective teamwork in the various sport domains. Interventions need to be designed to improve team effectiveness through effects on team interactions.

Overall, the perspectives of shared mental models, ecological dynamics, and ITC need to be better integrated to capitalize on the strengths of each in the understanding and prediction of sports team effectiveness.

REFERENCES

Araujo, D., Silva, P., & Davids, K. (2015). Capturing group tactical behaviors in expert team players. In: J. Baker, D. Farrow (Eds.), *Routledge handbook of sport expertise* (pp. 209–220). Abingdon, Oxon: Routledge.

Austin, J. R. (2003). Transactive memory in organizational groups: the effects of content, consensus, specialization, and accuracy on group performance. *Journal of Applied Psychology, 88*(5), 866–878.

Blickensderfer, E., Cannon-Bowers, J. A., & Salas, E. (1999). The relationship between shared knowledge and team performance: a field study. In: K. A. Smith-Jenthsch, L. L. Levesque (C-chairs). Shared cognition in teams: predictors, processes, consequences. *Symposium conducted at the 14th annual meeting of the society industrial, organizational psychology.* Atlanta, GA.

Bourbousson, J., Poizat, G., Saury, J., & Sève, C. (2012). Temporal aspects of team cognition: a case study on concerns sharing within basketball. *Journal of Applied Sports Psychology, 24*(2), 224–241.

Cannon-Bowers, J. A., & Salas, E. (Eds.). (1998). *Making decisions under stress: implications for individual and team training* (pp. 447). Washington, DC: American Psychological Association.

Clemente, F., Couceiro, M., Martins, F., Mendes, R., & Figueiredo, A. (2013). Measuring collective behaviour in football teams: inspecting the impact of each half of the match on ball possession. *International Journal of Performance Analysis in Sport, 13*, 678–689.

Cooke, N. J., Gorman, J. C., Myers, C. W., & Duran, J. L. (2013). Interactive team cognition. *Cognitive Science, 37*(2), 255–285.

Cooke, N. J., Salas, E., Cannon-Bowers, J. A., & Stout, R. J. (2000). Measuring team knowledge. *Human Factors, 42*, 151–173.

Cooke, N. J., Salas, E., Kiekel, P. A., & Bell, B. (2004). Advances in measuring team cognition. In: E. Salas, & S. Fiore (Eds.), *Team cognition: Understanding the factors that drive process and performance* (pp. 83–106). Washington, DC: American Psychological Association.

Cooke, N. J., & Shope, S. M. (2004). Designing a synthetic task environment. In: S. J. Schiflett, L. R. Elliott, E. Salas, & M. D. Coovert (Eds.), *Scaled worlds: Development, validation, and application* (pp. 263–278). Aldershot: Ashgate.

Cooke, N. J., Stout, R., & Salas, E. (2001). A knowledge elicitation approach to the measurement of team situation awareness. In: E. McNeese, E. Salas, & M. R. Endsley (Eds.), *New trends in cooperative activities: Understanding system dynamics in complex environments* (pp. 114–139). Santa Monica: Human Factors and Ergonomics Society.

Correia, V., & Araujo, D. (2009). Tau influence on decision making in basketball. *Revista De Psicologia DePorte, 18*, 475–479.

Correia, V., Araujo, D., Cummins, A., & Craig, C. M. (2012). Perceiving and acting upon spaces in a VR rugby task: expertise effects in affordance detection and task achievement. *Journal of Sport & Exercise Psychology, 34*, 305–321.

Dyer, J. L. (1984). Team research and team training: a state-of-the-art review. *Human Factors Review, 26*, 285–323.

Endsley, M. R. (1995). Toward a theory of situation awareness in dynamic systems. *Human Factors, 37*, 32–64.

Fajen, B. R. (2007). Affordance-based control of visually guided action. *Ecological Psychology, 19*(4), 383–410.

Frencken, W., Lemmink, K., Delleman, N., & Visscher, C. (2011). Oscillations of centroid position and surface area of soccer teams in small-sided games. *European Journal of Sport Science, 11*(4), 215–223.

Giske, R., Rodahl, S. E., & Høigaard, R. (2015). Shared mental task models in elite ice hockey and handball teams: does it exist and how does the coach intervene to make an impact? *Journal of Applied Sport Psychology, 27*(1), 20–34.

Gorman, J. C., Cooke, N. J., & Amazeen, P. G. (2010). Training adaptive teams. *Human Factors, 52,* 295–307.

Gorman, J. C., Cooke, N. J., & Winner, J. L. (2006). Measuring team situation awareness in decentralized command and control environments. *Ergonomics, 49*(12–13), 1312–1325.

Hinsz, V. B., Tindale, R. S., & Vollrath, D. A. (1997). The emerging conceptualization of groups as information processors. *Psychological Bulletin, 121*(1), 43.

Ilgen, D. R., Hollenbeck, J. R., Johnson, M., & Jundt, D. (2005). Teams in organizations: from input-process-output models to IMOI models. *Annual Review of Psychology, 56,* 517–543.

Klimoski, R., & Mohammed, S. (1994). Team mental model: construct or metaphor? *Journal of Management, 20,* 403–437.

Kozlowski, S. W. J., Gully, S. M., Nason, E. R., & Smith, E. M. (1999). Developing adaptive teams: A theory of compilation and performance across levels and time. In: D. R. Ilgen, & E. D. Pulakos (Eds.), *The changing nature of performance: implications for staffing, motivation and development* (pp. 240–292). San Francisco: Jossey-Bass.

Marks, M. A., Mathieu, J. E., & Zaccaro, S. J. (2001). A temporally based framework and taxonomy of team processes. *Academy of Management Review, 26*(3), 356–376.

McPherson, S. L., & Kernodle, M. W. (2003). Tactics, the neglected attribute of expertise: problem representations and performance skills in tennis. In: J. L. Starkes, K. A. Ericsson (Eds.), *Expert performance in sports* (pp. 137–167). Champaign, IL: Human Kinetics.

Mohammed, S., Ferzandi, L., & Hamilton, K. (2010). Metaphor no more: a 15-year review of the team mental model construct. *Journal of Management, 36*(4), 876–910.

Mohammed, S., Hamilton, K., & Lim, A. (2009). The incorporation of time in team research: past, current, and future. In: E. Salas, G. G. Goodwin, & C. S. Burke (Eds.), *Team effectiveness in complex organizations: Cross-disciplinary perspectives and approaches* (pp. 321–348). New York: Routledge.

Moura, F., Martins, L., Anido, R., Barros, R., & Cunha, S. (2012). Quantitative analysis of Brazilian football players' organisation on the pitch. *Sport Biomechanics, 11*(1), 85–96.

Pedersen, H. K., & Cooke, N. J. (2006). From battle plans to football plays: extending military team cognition to football. *International Journal of Sport and Exercise Psychology, 4*(4), 422–446.

Reimer, T., Park, E. S., & Hinsz, V. B. (2006). Shared and coordinated cognition in competitive and dynamic task environments: an information-processing perspective for team sports. *International Journal of Sports and Exercise Psychology, 4,* 376–400.

Salas, E., & Cannon-Bowers, J. A. (2001). The science of training: a decade of progress. *Annual Review of Psychology, 52*(1), 471–499.

Salas, E., Cooke, N. J., & Rosen, M. A. (2008). On teams, teamwork, and team performance: discoveries and developments. *Human Factors, 50*(3), 540–547.

Salas, E. Dickinson, T. L., Converse, S. A., & Tannenbaum, S. I. (1992). Toward an understanding of team performance and training. In: R. W. Swezey, E. Salas (Eds.), *Teams: Their training and performance* (pp. 3–29). Westport, CT, US: Ablex Publishing Teams.

Silva, P., Garganta, J., Araujo, D., Davids, K., & Aguiar, P. (2013). Shared knowledge of shared affordances? Insights from an ecological dynamics approach to team cognition in sports. *Sports Medicine, 43,* 765–772.

Smith, M. R., Flach, J. M., Dittman, S. M., & Stanard, T. (2001). Monocular optical constraints on collision control. *Journal of Experimental Psychology, 27,* 395–410.

Tannenbaum, S. I., Salas, E., & Cannon-Bowers, J. A. (1996). Promoting team effectiveness. In: M. A. West (Ed.), *Handbook of work group psychology* (pp. 503–529). Chichester, UK: Wiley.

Section II

Individual Differences in Sport and Exercise Psychology

Chapter 7

Antecedents of Need Supportive and Controlling Interpersonal Styles From a Self-Determination Theory Perspective: A Review and Implications for Sport Psychology Research

Doris Matosic*, Nikos Ntoumanis**, Eleanor Quested**

*School of Sport, Exercise, and Rehabilitation Sciences, University of Birmingham, Birmingham, United Kingdom; **School of Psychology & Speech Pathology, Curtin University, Perth, Australia

Coaches play an important role in shaping athletes' sport experiences and use a range of strategies in an effort to motivate athletes. The coach's "typical" interpersonal style is reflective of the combination of strategies he/she usually adopts when communicating with athletes. The predominant interpersonal style adopted by the coach is a critical determinant of athletes' quality of sport experience and motivation, psychological need satisfaction, performance, and psychological well-being (see Duda and Appleton, Chapter 18; Mageau & Vallerand, 2003). Drawing from self-determination theory (SDT; Ryan & Deci, 2002), a considerable body of literature has substantiated the consequences of need supportive and controlling coaching (for a review in sport setting, see Ntoumanis, 2012). However, less attention has been paid to understanding the antecedents of these two interpersonal styles proposed by SDT. This chapter will serve to review the antecedents of need supportive and controlling motivational styles that have been identified in research undertaken in educational, parental, sport, workplace, and health contexts. Our overarching goal is to facilitate research and practice to foster adaptive coaching practices that will nurture more adaptive motivation and positive sport experiences for athletes.

Sport and Exercise Psychology Research. http://dx.doi.org/10.1016/B978-0-12-803634-1.00007-8

NEED SUPPORTIVE AND CONTROLLING INTERPERSONAL STYLES

SDT distinguishes between two broad interpersonal styles that hold relevance for the motivation and well-being of athletes. These styles are reflected in a set of distinct behaviors when adopted by individuals in a position of authority or leadership. The coaches' interpersonal style will facilitate motivation and well-being when it is supportive of athletes' psychological need to feel autonomy (ie, feeling a sense of free will, volition, and choice in relation to sport participation), competence (ie, feeling one is efficacious and can meet the challenges faced in sport), and a sense of relatedness (ie, feeling socially connected to the coaches and teammates). However, when coaches actively thwart these basic needs, coaching can be considered controlling (Bartholomew, Ntoumanis, Ryan, Bosch, & Thøgersen-Ntoumani, 2011). SDT proposes that coaches (or others in positions of authority/leadership) can support athletes' needs by creating a coaching environment that is high in autonomy support and interpersonal involvement, and has appropriate structure. A coaching style that is high in this trio of characteristics has been termed "need supportive" (Taylor & Ntoumanis, 2007). Autonomy support is evidenced when coaches provide opportunities for athletes to make meaningful choices, involve athletes in decision making, acknowledge athletes' perspective and feelings, and provide meaningful rationales for their requests (Ntoumanis, 2012). Interpersonal involvement is demonstrated when individuals in a position of authority or leadership show care and concern (Connell & Wellborn, 1991). A structured environment is evident when the coach provides guidance, direction, and organization that facilitate athletes' perceptions that they can meet the challenges of the activity and/or experience success. Thus, structure reflects coaches' provision of guidance and appropriate expectations in the learning process (Jang, Reeve, & Deci 2010; Skinner & Edge, 2002). In contrast, controlling coaching can be need thwarting and is evident when the coach intimidates athletes, exercises excessive personal control, uses rewards or praise in a controlling manner, and holds back on attention or support when athletes do not display required behaviors and when coaches actively undermine athletes' sense of self-worth (Bartholomew, Ntoumanis, & Thøgersen-Ntoumani, 2009).

Extensive research in sport (Bartholomew et al., 2011) and other life settings has examined the relations between need supportive (primarily the autonomy support component) and controlling styles with motivational processes as proposed by SDT. Need supportive coaching has been associated with the satisfaction of three basic needs, namely the need for athletes to feel autonomous in their actions, competent, and meaningfully related to others within the sport milieu (Adie, Duda, & Ntoumanis, 2012). A need supportive coaching style is also understood to be a critical determinant of behavior regulation that is autonomous (or self-determined), that is, motivation that reflects intrinsic interest, task enjoyment, or task utility (Amorose & Anderson-Butcher, 2007). In contrast, a controlling coaching style has been linked with psychological need thwarting (Balaguer et al., 2012). Controlling coaching is understood to be a key antecedent of controlled (or nonself-determined) type of athlete motivation, that is, motivation that reflects internal or external contingencies such as coercion, pressure, or guilt (Pelletier, Fortier, Vallerand, & Brière, 2001).

ANTECEDENTS OF NEED SUPPORTIVE AND CONTROLLING INTERPERSONAL STYLES

Despite repeated claims that SDT-based research in sport strives to foster more need supportive coaching and adaptive experiences for athletes, a paucity of attention has been paid to examining why coaches adopt need supportive and/or controlling styles. To date, only five studies have explored the antecedents of need supportive and controlling coaching in the sport domain (Iachini, 2013; Rocchi, Pelletier, & Couture, 2013; Stebbings, Taylor, & Spray, 2011; Stebbings, Taylor, Spray, & Ntoumanis, 2012; Stebbings, Taylor, & Spray, 2015). In the broader context of SDT, research on potential antecedent variables has been primarily undertaken in the educational and parental literatures (Deci, Spiegel, Ryan, Koestner, & Kaufmann, 1982; Grolnick, Price, Beiswenger, & Sauck, 2007; Reeve, 1998; Reeve et al., 2014). However, there has been no attempt to synthesize the evidence from these domains in an effort to further develop understanding of the primary determinants of coaches' interpersonal styles. Identifying the antecedents of motivationally adaptive versus maladaptive coaching styles could potentially explain why coaches adopt particular strategies to motivate their athletes (Occhino, Mallett, Rynne, & Carlisle, 2014). Importantly, such information could valuably contribute toward the design of interventions that aim to support coaches in fostering more motivationally adaptive styles of interaction.

The purpose of this chapter is to synthesize findings from the extant research concerning the antecedents of need supportive and controlling interpersonal styles proposed by SDT. We discuss specifically how these antecedents may impact upon the types of interpersonal style adopted. The implications for future research in the broader SDT literature, as well as applications in the coaching domain are also highlighted. As an outcome of this review, we identify additional potential antecedents of coaches' interpersonal style.

To initiate our review, a search was conducted using the computerized databases Medline, PsycINFO, Web of Science, and Scopus, encompassing articles published from 1969 to Apr. 2015. The terms used in the search strategy were: (antecedent* OR determinant* OR predictor* OR context* factor OR social* factor OR personal* factor OR belief* OR causality orientation OR pressure) AND (control* OR controlling OR autonomy support* OR autonomy support* behavior OR autonomy support* behavior OR control* behavior OR control* behavior OR teach* style OR motivating style OR parent* style OR coach* style OR teach* orientation OR parent* orientation OR coach* orientation OR interpersonal style* OR structure OR involvement OR need support) AND (self determination OR self-determination).

The first author received training on database searching and completed all of the searches independently. Inclusion criteria were determined a priori. An antecedent of controlling and need supportive styles was defined as any factor identified in the SDT literature as predicting one or both interpersonal styles. Participants in the included studies were individuals in a position of authority or leadership (ie, coaches, teachers, parents, supervisors, fitness instructors) of any age group, any experience, and either gender. Studies were excluded if one or more of the following criteria were not met: (1) SDT was not cited as a theoretical framework that underpinned the research presented in the manuscript; (2) if the study did not describe antecedents of need supportive (ie, autonomy support, and/or structure and/or interpersonal involvement) and/or controlling interpersonal styles, strategies, or behaviors; and (3) if the measures of need supportive and controlling interpersonal styles did not assess these variables as conceptualized by SDT (Fig. 7.1).

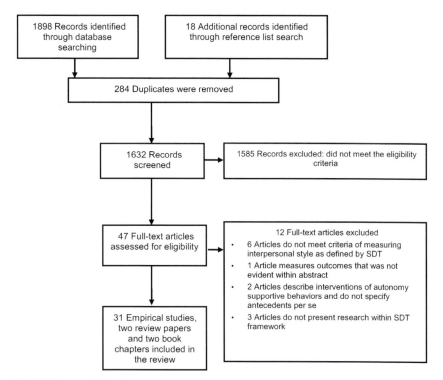

FIGURE 7.1   PRISMA flowchart describing the selection process in the systematic literature review (Moher, Liberati, Tetzlaff, & Altmann, 2009). The initial database search resulted in a total of 1898 articles. After duplicates were removed (n = 284), manuscript titles and abstracts were screened. Articles that did not meet inclusion criteria were removed (n = 1585). Postscreening, the full texts of the 29 remaining articles from the initial database search were assessed for eligibility using the same inclusion criteria. Seventeen articles were retained. A manual search from the reference lists of these full-text articles was subsequently conducted, adding 16 additional manuscripts and 2 book chapters. This selection process resulted in a total of 31 peer-reviewed articles with empirical data (25 cross-sectional, 1 longitudinal, and 5 experimental), 2 peer-reviewed review articles, and 2 book chapters that were included in this.

Coding of study characteristics was conducted by the first author and a sample of codings were checked by the second author. Studies were coded for type of publication (ie, published journal article, book chapter), design (eg, cross-sectional, longitudinal, experimental), role of participants (eg, coaches over athletes, parents over athletes, teachers over students, supervisors over employees, etc.), domain (ie, educational, home, sport, work, and health), antecedents tested (eg, perceived pressure from superiors, causality orientation), type of antecedent (ie, contextual or personal factors, perceptions of the others' motivation), measure of need supportive and/or controlling behaviors (eg, observation, self-report), and motivational style measured (ie, autonomy support, structure, involvement and/ or control; Table 7.1). Drawing from Mageau and Vallerand's (2003) motivational model of the coach–athlete relationship three broad categories of antecedents were also coded: contextual factors relevant to the coach, perceptions of others' behaviors and motivation, and personal factors (Fig. 7.2 for a summary).

With regard to domain, the majority of the included empirical articles (20 out of 31) explored antecedents within educational contexts. The sport literature represented 5 out of 31 of the reviewed studies, the home context represented 4 out of 31, work literature characterized 1 out of 31, and health context represented 1 out of 31 of the identified articles. Three antecedent variables were explored within more than one context. These were external pressure, perceptions of others' self-determined motivation, and self-determined motivation of the individual in a position of authority or leadership. For example, Rocchi et al. (2013) explored the external pressure antecedent in the sport literature, replicating the work of Pelletier, Seguin-Levesque, and Legault (2002) on external pressure in the education domain.

Studies adopted different methods to measure whether the leader's behavior was need supportive and/or controlling. Most ($n = 20$) of the studies reviewed utilized questionnaires completed by individuals in positions of authority or leadership (eg, teacher, parent, coach). In these studies those individuals' self-perceptions of the need supportive and controlling motivational styles that they adopted were measured using adaptations of established questionnaires, such as the Problems in School Questionnaire (Deci, Shwartz, Sheiman, & Ryan, 1981), the Interpersonal Behaviors Scale (Beaudry & Pelletier, 2008), the Health Care Climate Questionnaire (HCCQ; Williams, Grow, Freedman, Ryan, & Deci, 1996), or the Controlling Coach Behaviors Scale (CCBS; Bartholomew, Ntoumanis, & Thøgersen-Ntoumani, 2010). Three studies (Pelletier & Vallerand, 1996; Roth, Assor, Kanat-Maymon, & Kaplan, 2007; Roth & Weinstock, 2013) based measurement of autonomy supportive or controlling behaviors of the individual in a position of leadership upon perceptions of these styles by the individual with whom they were interacting. Those studies utilized a modified version of the teacher autonomy support scale developed by Assor, Kaplan, and Roth (2002). Three studies (Maulana, Opdenakker, Stroet, & Bosker, 2013; Sarrazin, Tessier, Pelletier, Trouilloud, & Chanal, 2006; Van den Berghe et al., 2013) utilized observation and included objective ratings of need supportive and controlling styl

TABLE 7.1 Description of Reviewed Studies

Study	Type of publication	Type of study (design)	Role of participants	Domain	Antecedents tested	Type of antecedent	Measure of the behavior/outcome predicted	Motivational style measured
Cai et al. (2002)	Journal article	Cross-sectional	Home educators, public school teachers, and university education students	Educational	Religious affiliation and frequency of church attendance	Personal factors	Self-report; Problems in School Questionnaire (PSQ; Deci et al., 1981)	Controlling and autonomy-supportive
Deci et al. (1982)	Journal article	Experimental	Undergraduate students that served as teachers	Educational	Pressure to maximize students' performance via control-inducing statements	Contextual	Experimental manipulation via informational (no-performance-standards) vs controlling (performance-standards) inductions measured by tape recorder analysis using objective ratings (eg, number of hints given), subjective rating (eg, extend of teacher interest in puzzle activity), and teacher's questionnaire (eg, how much do you enjoy being a teacher)	Controlling

Study								
Flink et al. (1990)	Journal article	Experimental	Fourth grade teachers	Educational	Pressure to maximize students' performance via control-inducing statements	Contextual	Mixed design: Self-report; PSQ (Deci et al., 1981) and experimental manipulation via pressure statement measured by videotape analysis using objective (eg, number of hints given) and subjective (eg, extend of teacher interest in the activity) rating	Controlling
Grolnick (2015)	Journal article	Cross-sectional	Parents (ie, mothers)	Home	Autonomous/controlled motivation	Personal factors	Self-report; Parent-School Interaction Questionnaire (PSIQ; Grolnick et al., 1997), frequencies of engagement in child's activity, Parenting Context Questionnaire (PCQ; Grolnick & Wellborn, 1988)	School, cognitive, and personal involvement
Grolnick and Apostoleris (2002)	Book chapter	Review	Parents (ie, mothers and fathers)	Home	Stress and social support, perceptions of the adolescents' "difficulty," internal pressures (eg, ego-involvement)	Contextual, perceptions of others' behaviors and motivation, and personal factors	Measured using variety of methods (eg, questionnaire, observation)	Controlling, autonomy-supportive

(Continued)

TABLE 7.1 Description of Reviewed Studies (cont.)

Study	Type of publication	Type of study (design)	Role of participants	Domain	Antecedents tested	Type of antecedent	Measure of the behavior/outcome predicted	Motivational style measured
Grolnick et al. (2002)	Journal article	Experimental	Parents (ie, mothers)	Home	Pressure to maximize children' performance via control-inducing statements; internal pressure (eg, ego-involvement)	Contextual, personal factors	Experimental manipulation via pressure statement measured by videotape analysis using verbal and nonverbal rating	Controlling
Grolnick et al. (1996)	Journal article	Cross-sectional	Parents (ie, mothers and fathers)	Home	Stress (eg, positive and negative life events), social support, and perceptions about adolescences' "difficulty"	Contextual, perceptions of others' behaviors and motivation	Interviews	Involvement, autonomy support, structure

				Home	Internal pressure (ie, high contingent self-worth, mind resistant to change) combined with external pressure (ie, evaluation)	Contextual, personal factors	Experimental manipulation via pressure statement measured by videotape analysis using verbal rating for controlling (eg, leading questions and giving answers) and autonomy supportive (eg, giving feedback and encouragement)	Controlling, autonomy-supportive
Grolnick et al. (2007)	Journal article	Experimental	Mothers and their fourth grade children					
Harackiewicz and Larson (1986)	Journal article	Experimental	Undergraduate students that served as supervisors	Workplace	Administration of rewards	Contextual	Experimental manipulation via controlling messages given by supervisor on what students should do	Controlling
Iachini (2013)	Journal article	Cross-sectional	Coaches	Coaching	Performance evaluations	Contextual	Self-report; Problems in Sports Questionnaire (PSQ; Amorose, 2008), modification of PCQ (Deci et al., 1981)	Autonomy-supportive

(Continued)

TABLE 7.1 Description of Reviewed Studies (cont.)

Study	Type of publication	Type of study (design)	Role of participants	Domain	Antecedents tested	Type of antecedent	Measure of the behavior/outcome predicted	Motivational style measured
Leroy et al. (2007)	Journal article	Cross-sectional	Fifth grade teachers	Educational	Obligations to comply with curriculum, colleagues' expectations and demands, administrative pressures, time constraints; entity vs incremental beliefs	Contextual and personal factors	Self-report; Learning Climate Questionnaire (Williams & Deci, 1996)	Autonomy-supportive
Maulana et al. (2013)	Journal article	Cross-sectional	Teachers	Educational	Cultural norms	Contextual	Observational study (videotape analyses) measured by observer ratings of several subdimensions of involvement in the classroom	Involvement

Ng et al. (2012)	Journal article	Cross-sectional	Exercise science students as fitness instructors	Health	Perceptions of exercisers' self-determined and nonself-determined motivation	Perceptions of others' behaviors and motivation	Self-report; Health Care Climate Questionnaire for autonomy-supportive (HCCQ; Williams et al., 1996); Controlling Coach Behaviors Scale for controlling (CCBS; Bartholomew et al., 2010)	Autonomy-supportive and controlling
Pelletier et al. (2002)	Journal article	Cross-sectional	Teachers (Grades 1–12)	Educational	Obligations to comply with curriculum, colleagues' expectations and demands, administrative pressures, time constraints; perceptions of students' self-determined and nonself-determined motivation	Contextual, perceptions of others' behaviors and motivation	Self-report; PSQ (Deci et al., 1981)	Autonomy-supportive

(Continued)

TABLE 7.1 Description of Reviewed Studies (cont.)

Study	Type of publication	Type of study (design)	Role of participants	Domain	Antecedents tested	Type of antecedent	Measure of the behavior/outcome predicted	Motivational style measured
Pelletier and Sharp (2009)	Journal article	Review	Teachers	Educational	Obligations to comply with curriculum, colleagues' expectations and demands, administrative pressures, time constraints; perceptions of students' self-determined and nonself-determined motivation	Contextual, perceptions of others' behaviors and motivation	Measured using variety of methods (eg, questionnaires, experimental manipulations)	Controlling, autonomy-supportive
Pelletier and Vallerand (1996)	Journal article	Experimental	Graduate students	Educational	Perceptions of students' self-determined and nonself-determined motivation	Perceptions of others' behaviors and motivation	Self-report and student perception; questionnaire included autonomy-supportive and controlling items developed from the SDT-based definition of those two behaviors	Autonomy-supportive and controlling

Pierro et al. (2009)	Journal article	Cross-sectional	Teachers (high school)	Educational	Self-regulatory orientation	Personal factors	Self-report; PSQ (Deci et al., 1981)	Controlling and autonomy-supportive
Reeve (1998)	Journal article	Cross-sectional	Students (future teachers)	Educational	Autonomous and controlled causality orientations	Personal factors	Self-report; PSQ (Deci et al., 1981)	Autonomy-supportive and controlling
Reeve (2002)	Book chapter	Review	Teachers	Educational	Obligations to comply with curriculum, colleagues' expectations and demands, administrative pressures, time constraints; perceptions of students' self-determined and nonself-determined motivation; controlled causality orientation	Contextual, perception of others' behaviors and motivation, and personal factors	Measured using variety of methods (eg, self-reports)	Autonomy-supportive, controlling

(Continued)

TABLE 7.1 Description of Reviewed Studies (*cont.*)

Study	Type of publication	Type of study (design)	Role of participants	Domain	Antecedents tested	Type of antecedent	Measure of the behavior/outcome predicted	Motivational style measured
Reeve (2009)	Journal article	Review	Teachers	Educational	Obligations to comply with curriculum, colleagues' expectations and demands, administrative pressures, time constraints; perceptions of students' self-determined and nonself-determined motivation; controlled causality orientation	Contextual, perception of others' behaviors and motivation, and personal factors	Measured using variety of methods (eg, questionnaires)	Autonomy-supportive, controlling
Reeve et al. (2014)	Journal article	Cross-sectional	Teachers	Educational	Cultural norms; normalcy, effectiveness, and implementation beliefs	Contextual, personal factors	Self-report; vignettes on autonomy-supportive and controlling style	Autonomy-supportive and controlling

Robertson and Jones (2013)	Journal article	Cross-sectional	Teachers	Educational	Autonomous motivation	Personal factors	Self-report: PSQ (Deci et al., 1981)	Autonomy-supportive
Rocchi et al. (2013)	Journal article	Cross-sectional	Coaches	Coaching	Obligations to comply with curriculum, colleagues' expectations and demands, administrative pressures; perceptions of athletes' self-determined and nonself-determined motivation	Contextual, perceptions of others' behaviors and motivation	Self-report; interpersonal behaviors scale (Beaudry & Pelletier, 2008)	Autonomy-supportive
Roth et al. (2007)	Journal article	Cross-sectional	Teachers, students (grades 3–6)	Educational	Autonomous motivation	Personal factors	Students' perceptions of autonomy-supportive behavior: scale developed by Assor et al. (2002) measuring autonomy-supportive teaching	Autonomy-supportive

(Continued)

TABLE 7.1 Description of Reviewed Studies (*cont.*)

Study	Type of publication	Type of study (design)	Role of participants	Domain	Antecedents tested	Type of antecedent	Measure of the behavior/outcome predicted	Motivational style measured
Roth and Weinstock (2013)	Journal article	Cross-sectional	High school students, teachers	Educational	Epistemological beliefs	Personal factors	Students' perceptions of autonomy-supportive behavior: scale developed by Roth et al. (2011) measuring teachers' perspective taking and teachers' provision of rationale	Autonomy-supportive
Sarrazin et al. (2006)	Journal article	Experimental	PE teachers, high school students	Educational	Perceptions of students' self-determined and nonself-determined motivation	Perceptions of others' behaviors and motivation	Observational study (videotape analyses) measured by observer ratings of verbal interactions of controlling and autonomy-supportive styles	Controlling, autonomy-supportive

Skinner and Belmont (1993)	Journal article	Cross-sectional	Teachers (grades 3–5)	Educational	Perceptions of students' behavioral engagement	Perceptions of others' behaviors and motivation	Self-report; involvement included items that tapped teachers' affection, attunement, dedication of resources, dependability; structure included items of clarity of expectations, contingency, instrumental help and support, and adjustment of teaching strategies; autonomy-supportive items tapped teacher's coercive behavior, respect, choice and relevance	Involvement, structure and autonomy support
Soenens et al. (2012)	Journal article	Cross-sectional	Teachers	Educational	Obligations to comply with curriculum, colleagues' expectations and demands, administrative pressures; time constraints; autonomous motivation	Contextual, personal factors	Self-report; psychological control scale-teacher self-report (Soenens et al., 2012)	Controlling

(Continued)

TABLE 7.1 Description of Reviewed Studies (*cont.*)

Study	Type of publication	Type of study (design)	Role of participants	Domain	Antecedents tested	Type of antecedent	Measure of the behavior/outcome predicted	Motivational style measured
Stebbings et al. (2011)	Journal article	Cross-sectional	Coaches	Coaching	Need satisfaction and well-being	Personal factors	Self-report; modified version of HCCQ for autonomy-supportive (Williams et al., 1996); CCBS for controlling (Bartholomew et al., 2010)	Autonomy-supportive and controlling
Stebbings et al. (2012)	Journal article	Cross-sectional	Coaches	Coaching	Opportunities for professional development, job security, work–life conflict	Contextual	Self-report; modified version of HCCQ for autonomy-supportive (Williams et al., 1996); CCBS for controlling (Bartholomew et al., 2010)	Autonomy-supportive and controlling
Stebbings et al. (2015)	Journal article	Longitudinal	Coaches	Coaching	Well-being (eg, positive affect, integration), ill-being (eg, negative affect, devaluation)	Personal factors	Self-report; modified version of HCCQ for autonomy-supportive (Williams et al., 1996); CCBS for controlling (Bartholomew et al., 2010)	Autonomy-supportive and controlling

Taylor and Ntoumanis (2007)	Journal article	Cross-sectional	PE teachers	Educational	Perceptions of students' self-determined and nonself-determined motivation	Perceptions of others' behaviors and motivation	Self-report; Teacher as Social Context Questionnaire (TASCQ; Wellborn et al., 1988)	Autonomy-supportive, structure, involvement
Taylor et al. (2008)	Journal article	Cross-sectional	PE teachers	Educational	Obligations to comply with curriculum, colleagues' expectations and demands, administrative pressures, time constraints; perceptions of students' self-determined and nonself-determined motivation; autonomous causality orientation	Contextual, perception of others' behaviors and motivation, and personal factors	Self-report; TASCQ (Wellborn et al., 1988)	Autonomy-supportive, structure, involvement

(Continued)

TABLE 7.1 Description of Reviewed Studies (*cont.*)

Study	Type of publication	Type of study (design)	Role of participants	Domain	Antecedents tested	Type of antecedent	Measure of the behavior/outcome predicted	Motivational style measured
Van den Berghe et al. (2013)	Journal article	Cross-sectional	PE teachers	Educational	Controlled causality orientation	Personal factors	Observational study (videotape analyses) measured by observer ratings of need-supportive teaching dimensions (autonomy support, structure, relatedness) and need-thwarting teaching dimensions (controlling, chaotic, cold)	Controlling, need supportive
Van den Berghe et al. (2014)	Journal article	Cross-sectional	PE teachers	Educational	Autonomous motivation	Personal factors	Self-report; TASCQ (Wellborn et al., 1988)	Autonomy support, structure, involvement

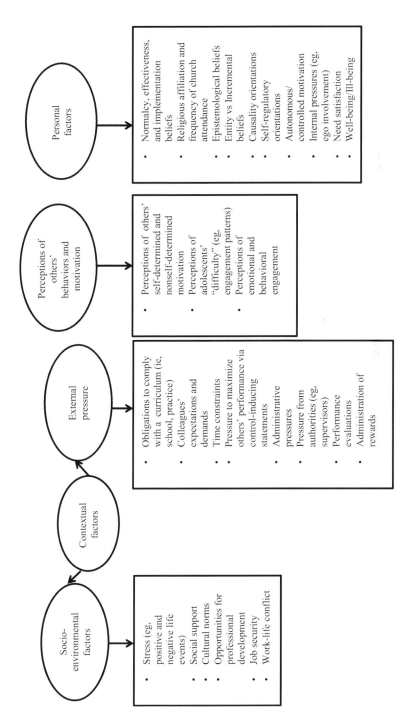

FIGURE 7.2   Summary of antecedents of controlling and need supportive behaviors identified within the SDT.

es via videotape coding. In the studies which employed an experimental design ($n = 4$), need supportive and controlling styles were manipulated via different tasks. For example, in one of the studies (Deci et al., 1982) undergraduate students were randomly assigned a role of an individual in a position of authority or leadership (eg, teacher) or a subordinate (eg, student). Teachers who were told they were responsible for their students performing up to the standard exhibited more controlling behaviors than teachers who were told there were no performance standards for their students' learning. One of the studies (Grolnick, Weiss, McKenzie, & Wrightman, 1996) used interview ratings with parents to measure autonomy support, involvement, and structure dimensions.

Drawing from the literature reviewed, we next present a detail report and explanation of the findings relevant for understanding of antecedents of coaches motivating styles. Additionally, we highlight the applications in the coaching domain and identify additional potential antecedents of coaches' interpersonal style. Specifically, the next sections are organized into three broad categories of antecedents, namely, contextual factors, perceptions of others' behaviors and motivation, and personal factors. We also present two subcategories (ie, social–environmental factors and external pressure) covered in the educational, parental, workplace, and sport domains of SDT.

CONTEXTUAL FACTORS

Contextual antecedents of need supportive and controlling motivational styles have received the most attention in the SDT literature (Deci et al., 1982; Flink, Boggiano, & Barrett, 1990; Pelletier et al., 2002; Pelletier & Sharp, 2009; Reeve, 2009; Taylor, Ntoumanis, & Standage, 2008). Our review suggested social–environmental factors and external pressures to be the predominant contextual factors in the literature.

Social–Environmental Factors

The themes within this category were identified in studies from the contexts of sport and parenthood and represent a variety of social–environmental factors that may have an influence on one's interpersonal style. For parents, stress (eg, negative and positive life events), and social support factors were identified as social–environmental contextual factors in the home context. Cultural norms were identified in the educational context; and job security, opportunities for professional development, and work–life conflict emerged from the sport context.

More specifically, in the parental literature, Grolnick et al. (1996) examined stress factors (eg, negative and positive life events), and social support as predictors of parenting style. Mothers who were exposed to more negative life events (eg, death in the family, illness, repossession of their home) were less likely to provide structure and autonomy support for their adolescents relative to those mothers experiencing positive events. Furthermore, Grolnick et al.

(1996) found no relation between stress factors and fathers' parenting style; however, fathers who reported higher social support were more involved (ie, participated in spontaneous and planned activities, spent time spent alone with their child, and others) with their adolescents.

In an observational study of an educational literature, teachers in individualistic (ie, Dutch classroom) and collectivistic cultures (ie, Indonesian classroom) by Maulana et al. (2013), teachers' involvement with students in lessons was found to differ across cultures in a manner that aligned with the typical findings from SDT-based crosscultural research. The findings suggest that teachers in individualistic societies see students as independent and autonomous and this was associated with the teachers allowing them to express their opinions, which is characteristic of an autonomy supportive teaching style. However, the findings suggest that teachers in collectivistic societies see students as class members rather than individuals resulting in less involvement (eg, closeness) with the students. This could be interpreted as suggesting teachers are less need supportive in collectivistic societies than in individualistic societies (Maulana et al., 2013). This notion is supported by Reeve et al. (2014) who found that teachers in collectivistic cultures are more controlling in their classroom because they believe controlling behavior is a cultural norm.

In the sport literature, Stebbings et al. (2012) examined coaches from various types and levels of sports and with job statuses ranging from full-time paid to part-time volunteer. Coaches in that study who experienced opportunities for professional development reported using autonomy supportive behaviors and also had high need satisfaction and psychological well-being. In contrast, coaches who experienced fewer opportunities for professional development were more likely to experience need thwarting and psychological ill-being, as well as the use of more controlling behaviors. This implies that opportunities to develop professionally may foster the coaches' sense of competence and autonomy, by increasing their knowledge and experience, and creating a sense that they are in control of their own development. Relatedness may also be fostered when engaging with their coaching peers during professional development activities. However, coaches who are not given these opportunities might feel isolated and prohibited from engaging with their coaching peers as well as from developing their coaching skills. This may ultimately be costly to the coaches' sense of relatedness and competence. Next, coaches who experienced greater job security reported higher need satisfaction and psychological well-being, as well as use of autonomy supportive behaviors when interacting with their athletes. Job security was not related to need thwarting and perceived controlling coach behaviors. Finally, coaches who experienced lower work–life conflict reported higher need satisfaction, psychological well-being, and the use of autonomy supportive strategies. Coaches who experienced higher work–life conflict reported higher need thwarting, psychological ill-being, and the use of controlling strategies. Experience of conflict between coaching and life demands may be related to coaches' experiencing an inability to function effectively in their coaching role, which may impact negatively upon the coaches' relationships with athletes, employers, and organizations as well as the coaches' use of more controlling strategies.

In summary, it is important to consider the nature of the social context and the cultural norms that coaches operate in when trying to understand the reason that they may engage in need supportive and controlling behaviors. Stressful and negative life events, poor opportunities for professional development, and job insecurity are likely to predict lower need satisfaction and less autonomous motivation among individuals in positions of authority or leadership. This review suggests these factors may be precursors to these individuals such as coaches utilizing less need supportive and more controlling strategies when interacting with their athletes. This is in contrast to individuals experiencing positive life experiences (eg, work–life balance), more opportunities for professional development and job security. In these circumstances, individuals in positions of authority or leadership are likely to be more need supportive and less controlling. Additionally, those individuals may be more controlling in collectivistic societies where they believe controlling behavior is a norm comparing to individuals in individualistic societies. Collectively, reviewed research suggests that organizations such as sport clubs should focus on creating a more positive environment for coaches, in part by providing them with job security, opportunities for professional development, and a healthy work–life balance.

External Pressures

Antecedents of interpersonal styles categorized as external pressures were obligations to comply with a curriculum (eg, school, practice), colleagues' expectations and demands, pressure from others to meet time constraints, pressure to maximize others' performance via control-inducing statements, administrative pressures, pressure from authorities (eg, supervisors), performance evaluations, and administration of rewards. This category was identified from the SDT literature in the areas of education (six empirical studies), parenthood (one empirical study), workplace (one empirical study), and more recently in the sport domain (two empirical studies). Illustrative examples are now provided in each case.

In the education literature (Pelletier & Sharp, 2009; Reeve, 2002, 2009), teachers were found to experience external pressure when feeling obligation to comply with the already established school curriculum, when experiencing expectations or demands from their colleagues and school administrators, as well as when operating under strict time constraints set by school authorities. Experiencing these pressures was directly associated with teachers' perceptions of themselves using more controlling strategies when interacting with their students (Soenens, Sierens, Vansteenkiste, Dochy, & Goossens, 2012).

In the early studies in the educational context, external pressure was manipulated via experimental study designs in which it was shown that teachers who were pressured by the experimenter to maximize their students' performance via control-inducing statements exhibited more controlling behaviors toward these students (eg, criticized; Deci et al., 1982; Flink et al., 1990). These findings were corroborated in more recent studies via teachers' self-reports of using less autonomy supportive and more controlling strategies in the classroom when experiencing external pressure, such as perceptions of pressure associated with colleagues, perceptions of pressure from the school administrators, and perceptions of pressure associated with the school curriculum (Leroy, Bressoux, Sarrazin, & Trouilloud, 2007; Pelletier et al., 2002; Soenens et al., 2012; Taylor et al., 2008). These studies showed that direct relations between external pressure and controlling behaviors were mediated by teachers' self-determined motivation. For example, external pressure such as time constraints, pressure from school authorities, or performance evaluations predicted lower autonomous motivation to teach (Leroy et al., 2007; Pelletier et al., 2002; Soenens et al., 2012; Taylor et al., 2008), which in turn predicted the teachers reporting using less autonomy supportive and more controlling behaviors toward their students (Deci et al., 1982; Taylor et al., 2008).

Similar findings have been reported in the parental literature (Grolnick, Gurland, DeCourcey, & Jacob, 2002). In this experimental study, external pressure toward mothers was created via control-inducing statements. Behaviors were observed (ie, videotaped) and analyzed using verbal rating for controlling (eg, mothers using leading questions and providing answers to their child) and autonomy supportive (eg, mothers providing feedback and support to their child) interactions. The results showed that mothers who were exposed to external pressure were more controlling and scored lower on using autonomy supportive strategies such as offering information and giving feedback, than mothers who experienced less external pressure.

Only one study with implications for the work place was relevant to the theme of external pressure. Harackiewicz and Larson (1986) revealed that experimental participants assigned as supervisors were more controlling in their supervision when their job included administering awards to maintain task enjoyment compared to supervisors whose job did not include rewarding others; the latter were less controlling (Harackiewicz & Larson, 1986). These findings suggest that in situations where supervisors administered rewards, they were less interested in the task enjoyment of those whom they supervised. However, in the events when their job did not include rewarding, supervisors might have felt more interested in their supervisees' task enjoyment, resulting in being less controlling.

In the sport literature, Rocchi et al. (2013) identified that basketball coaches were more likely to perceive themselves as low in autonomy support if they also had high perceptions of pressure from colleagues (ie, pressure from other coaches in terms of direct comparison), pressure associated with the practice curriculum (ie, perceived stress and impositions placed on them regarding how to run training sessions and what decisions to make about training) and administrative pressure (ie, pressure from club administration on how to run the team, select the team and fulfill requirements). Similarly, Iachini's (2013) study of high school coaches found that the more coaches perceived pressure from being evaluated for their athletes' performance, the less autonomy supportive they were toward their athletes. Collectively, the studies presented in this category imply that when experiencing external pressure, an individual in a position of authority or leadership (eg, coach) will tend to adopt more controlling and less autonomy supportive strategies to motivate others (Reeve, 2009).

In summary, evidence suggests that external pressure (eg, performance targets from club administrators) can undermine coaches' self-determined motivation and result in coaches' using more controlling behaviors (eg, using praise in a controlling way, punishment). Coaches will always have to deal with time constraints or performance evaluations (Pelletier & Sharp, 2009). However, this review highlights the importance of supporting coaches so that such circumstances do not internalize pressures and become controlling.

PERCEPTIONS OF OTHERS' BEHAVIORS AND MOTIVATION

Ten empirical studies found antecedents of leaders' interpersonal style to be their perception of other's behaviors (eg, engagement) and motivation. In the education literature, when perceiving students as highly self-determined to engage in classroom lessons, teachers reported that they tended to respond by using more structure, involvement, and autonomy supportive strategies (Pelletier et al., 2002; Pelletier & Vallerand, 1996; Reeve, 2002, 2009; Taylor & Ntoumanis, 2007; Taylor et al., 2008). Additionally, students who were perceived as showing higher emotional and behavioral engagement in the classroom received more autonomy support, structure, and involvement behaviors from their teachers (Skinner & Belmont, 1993). Two studies found that when perceiving students as not self-determined teachers tend to use controlling motivational strategies in their classrooms (Sarrazin et al., 2006; Soenens et al., 2012). For example, in an experimental study with graduate and undergraduate students being assigned as supervisors and supervisees, respectively, it was found that supervisors who believed that their supervisees were intrinsically motivated toward the experimental task were perceived as more autonomy supportive and less controlling than supervisors who considered their supervisees to be extrinsically motivated (Pelletier & Vallerand, 1996). Interestingly, Sarrazin et al. (2006) found similar results in a mixed method study that included self-reports from physical education teachers and high school students and objective coding of teacher behaviors from videotaped lessons. Teachers who had expectations of low self-determined motivation among their students were objectively rated as using more controlling strategies than teachers who had expectations of highly self-determined students.

In the parental literature, Grolnick et al. (1996) found that parents who perceived their adolescent as "difficult" (eg, tempered, moody, not engaged) reported providing less autonomy support and less involvement than parents who perceived their adolescents as less difficult (eg, more engaged, less moody).

Similarly, in the sport literature, high school coaches who perceived their athletes to be low in self-determined motivation, self-reported using less autonomy supportive behavior techniques toward these athletes than coaches who perceived their athletes to be more self-determined (Rocchi et al., 2013). In an experimental health context study of exercise science students being assigned the role of a fitness instructor, Ng, Thøgersen-Ntoumani, and Ntoumanis (2012) found that perceptions of exerciser self-determined motivation was associated with high instructor autonomy support, but only for male exercisers.

In sum, this review has revealed that coaches' perceptions of their athletes' self-determined motivation may be an important trigger of their adoption of a need supportive or controlling interpersonal style. The research suggests that coaches use more controlling strategies when perceiving that their athletes lack self-determined motivation. This may be because they feel pressure to "make" these athletes motivated because otherwise they may not meet the performance expectations of club administrators or others with expectations such as parents or sponsors. Hence, those coaches might use controlling strategies as means of ensuring that athletes reach the required standards (Pelletier & Sharp, 2009). On the other hand, the literature shows that perceiving athletes as self-determined may predict coaches' use of more need supportive strategies (Rocchi et al., 2013). When coaches can see that athletes are already self-determined, they may feel they have more freedom to be need supportive as the athletes' self-determined motivation is already in place. Ultimately, these findings highlight a common misunderstanding of the nature of self-determined motivation among the coaching community. It is important that coaches are educated to understand that need supportive coaching is in fact the more adaptive way to foster motivation, even among athletes low in self-determined motivation. When coaches are controlling they may witness an increase in athletes' levels of motivation, but this will not be self-determined motivation, it will most likely be introjected and/or external motivation. This is unlikely to sustain long term or be adaptive for the athletes' performance or well-being.

PERSONAL FACTORS

Seventeen empirical studies identified that personal factors (ie, beliefs or personal dispositions) played a role in determining interpersonal styles adopted by teachers, parents, or coaches. Personal factors identified in these studies were individuals' beliefs about effectiveness, implementation, and normalcy of implementation styles, religious affiliation and frequency of church attendance, individuals' epistemological and entity or incremental nature of the beliefs, causality orientations, self-regulation, and the individuals' self-determined motivation, internal pressures (eg, ego-involvement), psychological need satisfaction, and well-/ill-being.

Reeve et al. (2014) focused on three different beliefs teachers may have when orienting toward autonomy supportive and controlling interpersonal styles in relation to societal/cultural type. The study showed teachers will subscribe to a particular style depending on how effective, normative, and easy-to-implement they perceive this style to be. The effectiveness belief was higher among autonomy supportive teachers in individualistic societies. Teachers in collectivistic societies believed that a controlling style was more normative, and they reported that they used it more commonly in their classrooms. The ease of implementation belief predicted autonomy support in teachers in individualistic cultures, but not in collectivistic cultures.

Another type of belief, religious affiliation, was explored within the education literature as an antecedent of interpersonal styles (Cai, Reeve, & Robinson, 2002). This study of home educators and public school teachers found that religiously motivated and more frequent church attendees (ie, home educators) reported a preference toward motivating their children's learning in a more controlling manner than public school teachers. This suggests that religious beliefs may orient teachers toward a particular interpersonal style, although the evidence was correlational in nature.

One study has assessed personal epistemological beliefs (ie, beliefs about perception of knowledge characteristics and nature of knowing) as antecedents of interpersonal styles. In a study with high school teachers, it was found that students of teachers who were more absolute and objective (ie, the teachers believed knowledge is simple and allowed for single correct answers and self-evident truth) reported their teachers as less autonomy supportive. On the contrary, teachers who were more relativist and subjective (ie, believed knowledge is complex and changing and permit justifiable perspectives) were comparatively more autonomy supportive (Roth & Weinstock, 2013). This suggests that teachers with a relativist belief are more flexible in their approach and as such may be more willing and/or able to display other characteristics of autonomy support that also reflect flexibility. This could include demonstrating understanding of students' perspectives and providing students with opportunities for choice and decision making. In contrast, teachers with absolutist beliefs do not allow for flexibility in answers, and this is suggestive of more controlling behaviors.

Leroy et al. (2007) reported that the belief that academic abilities cannot change despite students' efforts (ie, entity belief) was negatively related to teachers' perception of autonomy supportive strategies. The belief that academic abilities can be improved through students' own efforts (ie, an incremental belief) did not have a direct relation with autonomy support.

This review identified three studies and two review chapters within educational context that had explored how causality orientations predict teacher's interpersonal style. SDT distinguishes between three types of causality orientations: autonomous, controlled, and impersonal (Deci & Ryan, 1985). Individuals with an autonomous causality orientation pursue volitional choices and experience higher self-determination and need satisfaction (Deci & Ryan, 1985; Taylor et al., 2008). Conversely, individuals with controlled causality orientation experience pressured behaviors, lower self-determination, and need thwarting (Deci & Ryan, 1985; Van den Berghe et al., 2013). Individuals with an impersonal causality orientation tend to experience inefficient behavior (Deci & Ryan, 1985). Overall, the reviewed studies found that causality orientations were significantly associated with interpersonal styles. Teachers with a controlled causality orientation embraced more controlling behaviors, whereas teachers with an autonomous causality orientation utilized more autonomy supportive behaviors (Reeve, 1998, 2002, 2009; Taylor et al., 2008; Van den Berghe et al., 2013). This may be because autonomous orientation allows teachers to function in self-determined ways. That is, autonomously orientated teachers feel more autonomous in their decisions, more competent when teaching and more related to their students, resulting in more autonomy supportive behaviors (Taylor et al., 2008). In contrast, control-oriented teachers may experience higher internal pressure to perform well and need thwarting; these experiences result in teachers displaying more controlling behaviors (Van den Berghe et al., 2013).

Other dispositional factors have recently been explored, beyond causality orientations. In a study by Pierro, Presaghi, Higgins, and Kruglanski (2009) in the educational literature, two self-regulatory orientations (ie, locomotion and assessment) were investigated as antecedents of the two interpersonal styles. Locomotion orientation refers to a trait of making something happen, whereas assessment orientation is a trait reflecting more critical evaluation. The results revealed that teachers who had more of an assessment orientation (such as comparing themselves with other people, thinking about their positive and negative characteristics, and critically evaluating their own and others' work), reported using less autonomy supportive behaviors and more controlling ones than teachers with a locomotion orientation (Pierro et al., 2009). High assessment teachers were found to be extrinsically motivated and used rewards and punishment to motivate their students, more than high locomotion teachers. The latter were more autonomously motivated and utilized more autonomy supportive strategies.

Furthermore, research studies identified in the review examined the degree of autonomous motivation of teachers as predictors of their autonomy supportive and controlling behaviors. The results indicated that autonomously motivated teachers reported the use of a more autonomy supportive teaching style (Robertson & Jones, 2013; Van den Berghe et al., 2014) and less use of a controlling style (Soenens et al., 2012). The results suggest that more autonomous motivation for teaching energizes and drives teachers to relate to students in a more autonomy supportive way. Moreover, Roth et al. (2007) revealed that teachers' self-reported autonomous motivation for teaching was positively related to students' perceptions of teacher's autonomy support. These findings highlight the importance of teachers feeling autonomously motivated. When this is the case, they are more likely to adopt an autonomy supportive style that is detectable by students.

In the parental literature, internal pressures such as high contingent self-esteem and ego-involvement have been identified as predictors of autonomy supportive and controlling behaviors. In two experimental studies by Grolnick and coworkers (2002, 2007), external pressure was manipulated via control-induced statements. Parents who were ego-involved in relation to their children's performance utilized more controlling than autonomy supportive strategies toward their children. Furthermore, parents with a mindset resistant to changes and those experiencing high contingent self-esteem also exhibited more controlling behaviors (Grolnick et al., 2007). The results suggest that parents who are ego-involved may utilize controlling behaviors in an effort to ensure their child's success, which they perhaps perceive will also reflect well on them. Hence, experiences of ego-involvement could be an antecedent of the creation of an ego-involving motivational climate, which is recognized in the SDT literature as a characteristic of controlling behaviors (Bartholomew et al., 2009). Furthermore, in a recent study, Grolnick (2015) found that autonomous motivation toward involvement in child's schooling (eg, knowing about school activities and events, going to school activities and events, and playing games that may help their children learn making the environment more positive) was positively related to the degree of involvement as well as experiences of positive affect during involvement.

In the sport literature, Stebbings et al. (2011) reported a positive relation between the coaches' need satisfaction and well-being and their use of autonomy supportive behaviors. These findings were extended in a longitudinal study by Stebbings et al. (2015) in which the coaches' psychological well-being (ie, positive affect and integration of coaching with one's sense of self) was positively associated with autonomy supportive coaching. This suggests that when coaches are excited and engaged in their coaching role and have internalized motives, they are more likely to provide their athletes with opportunities to make choices or feel volitional, compared to coaches who are less excited and engaged. Conversely, the study revealed that coaches who experienced psychological ill-being (ie, negative affect) reported being more controlling. Thus, when coaches are more distressed (eg, experiencing negative affect), they may be more likely to provide negative feedback and intimidate their athlete, compared to coaches who are not distressed.

In summary, although there is some evidence from other contexts, very few studies in the context of sport have researched personal factors as antecedents of controlling and need supportive behaviors. Personal factors have predominantly been examined in the parental and education literatures. Coaches' beliefs about need supportive and controlling behaviors (eg, in terms of how effective, normative and easy to implement they are) could predict the use of such behaviors (Reeve et al., 2014). As suggested by Reeve et al. (2014), these beliefs may be a potential mediator between external pressure and interpersonal style use. For example, pressures from club administration may shape the belief that a controlling style is the norm in the club, and this may encourage coaches to use controlling style strategies to motivate their athletes. In terms of beliefs about effectiveness and ease of implementation, providing training programs on effectiveness and implementation of need supportive behaviors may help coaches use need supportive strategies when interacting with their athletes.

Another type of belief that could be relevant to coach interpersonal styles identified in this review is the coaches' personal epistemological beliefs (Roth & Weinstock, 2013). Coaches who are more relativist about knowledge and believe that there are multiple perspectives on knowledge will more likely understand and enhance their athlete needs and self-determined motivation, ultimately adopting autonomy supportive strategies. On the contrary, coaches who are more absolutist believe knowledge is certain and objective, and will not allow flexibility for their athletes. These coaches may thwart their athlete needs and undermine their self-determined motivation, ultimately adopting controlling strategies.

Coaches who believe their athletes' abilities and skills cannot change regardless of their efforts (ie, entity belief) might focus on detecting athletes who are more "talented." In order to identify those athletes, they might conduct activities that focus more on athlete abilities, hence utilizing more ego-involving and controlling methods. However, coaches who believe athlete's abilities can be changed through their own effort (ie, incremental belief) may be less likely to utilize ego-involving methods. Exploring these beliefs among coaches may shed light on specific directions for designing coaching programs to facilitate need supportive behaviors.

Coaches may also experience ego-involvement, resistance to change, and contingent self-esteem (Grolnick & Apostoleris, 2002) as a result of feeling a threat to their sense of self when they want their athletes to perform to the standard at which they are being evaluated. In order to create a more adaptive environment that could serve to reduce the risks of coaches experiencing these internal and external pressures, sport administrators should regularly review their policies and practices to ensure that targets are agreed in a manner that is challenging to coaches rather than imposed in a way that is threatening. Moreover, it is clearly also important that sports administrators adopt a more need supportive and less controlling interpersonal style to ensure that the motivational climate surrounding coaches is adaptive. Furthermore, if clubs pressure coaches by placing emphasis on short-term outcomes, this is unlikely to be adaptive in the long term. Research suggests that this will have an undermining effect on the well-being of coaches and may create feelings of job insecurity (one of the predictors of controlling behaviors; Stebbings et al., 2012). According to SDT, if coaches also operate in a more need supportive environment, their well-being is likely to profit. Thus, when coaches experience high psychological well-being, they are more likely to use need supportive strategies and create more positive environment (Stebbings et al., 2011).

SUMMARY AND IMPLICATIONS FOR FUTURE RESEARCH

The factors that lead those in positions of power and/or influence to be need supportive and/or controlling when interacting with subordinates is a topic that has been explored in various life domains (parental, education), but less so in sport. This review has identified a number of potential areas for future research that may reveal additional potential antecedents of coaches' interpersonal style. To date, only one study grounded in SDT has explored personality traits (ie, narcissism) as predictors of autonomy supportive and controlling coach behaviors (Matosic et al., in press). The narcissistic leadership literature has focused mainly on the negative characteristics of narcissistic leaders, describing them as authoritarian, superior, not tolerating criticism, or reacting to perceived ego threat with aggression (Rosenthal & Pittinsky, 2006). In the context of sport, it has recently been found that coaches with narcissistic traits will embrace more a controlling than need supportive interpersonal style (Matosic et al., in press). Additional work on this topic is required by looking at other personality characteristics. For example, the same trend could follow in exploring the other two factors of the "dark triad" (ie, psychopathy, Machiavellianism), not just narcissism. The "dark triad" factors are found to share characteristics and all three entail characteristics such as self-promotion, lack of empathy, and aggressiveness. This suggests that such traits will potentially be positive predictors of controlling behaviors (Paulhus & Williams, 2002). Furthermore, it would be interesting to investigate the possibility of constructs from the Five-Factor model of personality (ie, extraversion, agreeableness, conscientiousness, neuroticism, openness to experience) as predictors of need supportive and controlling behaviors. For example, extraversion, agreeableness, and openness to experience are found to be positively related to supportive types of leadership, suggesting that they will also be associated with need supportive behaviors (Judge & Bono, 2000).

The literature reviewed in this chapter has also highlighted potential future directions on this topic from a methodological perspective. To date, no sport-specific studies have tested antecedents of coaching behaviors using an experimental design. Future studies could also replicate or expand upon experimental studies from other domains to determine whether similar antecedent variables are identified with regard to coaching. For example, replicating observational studies conducted in the educational literature could potentially determine the causes of need supportive and controlling interpersonal styles and answer why coaches engage in those specific behaviors (Sarrazin et al., 2006).

In summary, a number of antecedents of controlling and need supportive behaviors have been identified in the SDT literature across various life domains (eg, education, work, parenting, sport, health). This review has identified that these antecedents fall into three main categories, namely contextual factors, perceptions of subordinate's behaviors and motivation, and personal factors. The applicability of some of these antecedents to the coaches' interpersonal styles are discussed in this chapter, but such arguments need empirical testing to be better substantiated. Although there are still gaps in knowledge, the literature suggests that individuals in positions of authority or leadership, when feeling external and/or internal pressures will embrace a more controlling and less need supportive interpersonal style. Further exploration of antecedents of the two interpersonal styles is important to serve as a guideline in creating interventions for teachers, coaches, or parents to educate them in forming more positive environments. Ultimately, this will be more motivationally adaptive and will foster higher well-being and performance, both for their athletes and for the coaches themselves.

ACKNOWLEDGMENT

The research in this manuscript was supported by a PhD studentship awarded to the first author by the UK Economic and Social Research Council (Award No: ESJ50001X/1).

REFERENCES

Adie, J. W., Duda, J. L., & Ntoumanis, N. (2012). Perceived coach-autonomy support, basic need satisfaction and the well- and ill-being of elite youth soccer players: a longitudinal investigation. *Psychology of Sport and Exercise*, *13*(1), 51–59.

Amorose, A. J. (2008). *Development and validation of the problems in sport questionnaire*. Unpublished manuscript.

Amorose, A. J., & Anderson-Butcher, D. (2007). Autonomy-supportive coaching and self-determined motivation in high school and college athletes: a test of self-determination theory. *Psychology of Sport and Exercise*, *8*, 654–670.

Assor, A., Kaplan, H., & Roth, G. (2002). Choice is good, but relevance is excellent: autonomy-enhancing and suppressing teacher behaviours in predicting students' engagement in school work. *British Journal of Educational Psychology*, *72*, 261–278.

Balaguer, I., Gonzalez, L., Fabra, P., Castillo, I., Merce, J., & Duda, J. L. (2012). Coaches' interpersonal style, basic psychological needs and the well- and ill-being of young soccer players: a longitudinal analysis. *Journal of Sports Science*, *30*(15), 1619–1629.

Bartholomew, K. J., Ntoumanis, N., & Thøgersen-Ntoumani, C. (2009). A review of controlling motivational strategies from a self-determination theory perspective: implications for sports coaches. *International Review of Sport and Exercise Psychology*, *2*(2), 215–233.

Bartholomew, K. J., Ntoumanis, N., & Thøgersen-Ntoumani, C. (2010). The controlling interpersonal style in a coaching context: development and initial validation of a psychometric scale. *Journal of Sport & Exercise Psychology*, *32*, 193–216.

Bartholomew, K. J., Ntoumanis, N., Ryan, R. M., Bosch, J. A., & Thøgersen-Ntoumani, C. (2011). Self-determination theory and diminished functioning: the role of interpersonal control and psychological need thwarting. *Personality and Social Psychology Bulletin*, *37*(11), 1459–1473.

Beaudry, S., & Pelletier, L. (2008). Basic needs and psychological well-being: do all members of your social network contribute equally? *Poster session at the 9th annual convention of the Society for Personality and Social Psychology*. Albuquerque, NM.

Cai, Y., Reeve, J., & Robinson, D. T. (2002). Home schooling and teaching style: comparing the motivating styles of home school and public school teachers. *Journal of Educational Psychology*, *94*(2), 372–380.

Connell, J. P., & Wellborn, J. G. (1991). Competence, autonomy, and relatedness: a motivational analysis of self-system processes. *Minnesota Symposia on Child Psychology*, *23*, 43–77.

Deci, E. L., & Ryan, R. M. (1985). The general causality orientation scale: self-determination in personality. *Journal of Research in Personality*, *19*, 109–134.

Deci, E. L., Schwartz, A. J., Sheinman, L., & Ryan, R. M. (1981). An instrument to assess adults' orientations toward control versus autonomy with children: reflections on intrinsic motivation and perceived competence. *Journal of Educational Psychology*, *73*(5), 642–650.

Deci, E. L., Spiegel, N. H., Ryan, R. M., Koestner, R., & Kauffman, M. (1982). Effects of performance standards on teaching styles: behavior of controlling teachers. *Journal of Educational Psychology, 74*(6), 852–859.

Flink, C., Boggiano, A. K., & Barrett, M. (1990). Controlling teaching strategies: undermining children's self-determination and performance. *Journal of Personality and Social Psychology, 59*(5), 916–924.

Grolnick, W. S. (2015). Mothers' motivation for involvement in their children's schooling: mechanisms and outcomes. *Motivation and Emotion, 39*(1), 63–73.

Grolnick, W. S., & Apostoleris, N. H. (2002). What makes parents controlling? In: E. L. Deci, & R. M. Ryan (Eds.), *Handbook of self-determination research* (pp. 161–182). Rochester, NY: University of Rochester Press.

Grolnick, W. S., Benjet, C., Kurowski, C. O., & Apostoleris, N. (1997). Predictors of parent involvement in children's schooling. *Journal of Educational Psychology, 89*(3), 538–548.

Grolnick, W., Weiss, L., McKenzie, L., & Wrightman, J. (1996). Contextual, cognitive, and adolescent factors associated with parenting in adolescence. *Journal of Youth & Adolescence, 25*(1), 33–54.

Grolnick, W. S., Gurland, S., DeCourcey, W., & Jacob, K. (2002). Antecedents and consequences of mothers' autonomy support: an experimental investigation. *Developmental Psychology, 38*(1), 143–155.

Grolnick, W. S., Price, C. E., Beiswenger, K. L., & Sauck, C. C. (2007). Evaluative pressure in mothers: effects of situation, maternal, and child characteristics on autonomy supportive versus controlling behavior. *Developmental Psychology, 43*(4), 991–1002.

Grolnick, W., & Wellborn, J. (1988). *Parent influences on children's school-related self-system processes.* Paper presented at the annual meeting of the American Educational Research Association, New Orleans, LA.

Harackiewicz, J. M., & Larson, J. J. R. (1986). Managing motivation: the impact of supervisor feedback on subordinate task interest. *Journal of Personality & Social Psychology, 51*(3), 547–556.

Iachini, A. L. (2013). Development and empirical examination of a model of factors influencing coaches provision of autonomy-support. *International Journal of Sports Science & Coaching, 8*(4), 661–675.

Jang, H., Reeve, J., & Deci, E. L. (2010). Engaging students in learning activities: it is not autonomy support or structure but autonomy support and structure. *Journal of Educational Psychology, 102*, 588–600.

Judge, T. A., & Bono, J. E. (2000). Five-factor model of personality and transformational leadership. *Journal of Applied Psychology, 85*(5), 751–765.

Leroy, N., Bressoux, P., Sarrazin, P. G., & Trouilloud, D. (2007). Impact of teachers' implicit theories and perceived pressures on the establishment of an autonomy supportive climate. *European Journal of Psychology of Education, 22*(4), 529–545.

Mageau, G. A., & Vallerand, R. J. (2003). The coach-athlete relationship: a motivational model. *Journal of Sport Sciences, 21*, 883–904.

Matosic, D., Ntoumanis, N., Boardley, I. D., Sedikides, C., Stewart, B. D., & Chazisarantis, N. (in press). Narcissism and coach interpersonal style: a self-determination theory perspective. Scandinavian Journal of Medicine and Science in Sports. doi: 10.1111/sms.12635.

Maulana, R., Opdenakker, M. C., Stroet, K., & Bosker, R. (2013). Changes in teachers' involvement versus rejection and links with academic motivation during the first year of secondary education: a multilevel growth curve analysis. *Journal of Youth and Adolescence, 42*(9), 1348–1371.

Moher, D., Liberati, A., Tetzlaff, J., & Altman, D. G. (2009). Preferred reporting items for systematic reviews and meta-analyses: the PRISMA statement. *Annals of Internal Medicine, 151*(4), 264–269.

Ng, J. Y. Y., Thogersen-Ntoumani, C., & Ntoumanis, N. (2012). Motivation contagion when instructing obese individuals: a test in exercise settings. *Journal of Sport & Exercise Psychology*, *34*, 525–538.

Ntoumanis (2012). A self-determination theory perspective on motivation in sport and physical education: current trends and possible future research directions. In: G. C. Roberts, & S. C. Treasure (Eds.), *Motivation in sport and exercise* (pp. 91–128). (Vol. 3). Champaign, IL: Human Kinetics.

Occhino, J. L., Mallet, C. J., Rynne, S. B., & Carlisle, K. N. (2014). Autonomy-supportive pedagogical approach to sports coaching: research, challenges and opportunities. *International Journal of Sports Science & Coaching*, *9*(2), 401–415.

Paulhus, D. L., & Williams, K. M. (2002). The dark triad of personality: narcissism, Machiavellianism, and psychopathy. *Journal of Research in Personality*, *36*, 556–563.

Pelletier, L. G., & Sharp, E. C. (2009). Administrative pressures and teachers' interpersonal behaviour in the classroom. *Theory and Research in Education*, *7*(2), 174–183.

Pelletier, L. G., & Vallerand, R. J. (1996). Supervisors' beliefs and subordinates' intrinsic motivation: a behavioral confirmation analysis. *Journal of Personality & Social Psychology*, *71*(2), 331–340.

Pelletier, L. G., Fortier, M. S., Vallerand, R. J., & Brière, N. M. (2001). Associations among perceived autonomy support, forms of self-regulation, and persistence: a prospective study. *Motivation and Emotion*, *25*(4), 279–306.

Pelletier, L. G., Seguin-Levesque, C., & Legault, L. (2002). Pressure from above and pressure from below as determinants of teachers' motivation and teaching behaviors. *Journal of Educational Psychology*, *94*(1), 186–196.

Pierro, A., Presaghi, F., Higgins, T. E., & Kruglanski, A. W. (2009). Regulatory mode preferences for autonomy supporting versus controlling instructional styles. *British Journal of Educational Psychology*, *79*, 599–615.

Reeve, J. (1998). Autonomy support as an interpersonal motivating style: is it teachable? *Contemporary Educational Psychology*, *23*(3), 312–330.

Reeve, J. (2002). Self-determination theory applied to educational settings. In: E. L. Deci, & R. M. Ryan (Eds.), *Handbook of self-determination research* (pp. 183–204). Rochester NY: University of Rochester Press.

Reeve, J. (2009). Why teachers adopt a controlling motivating style toward students and how they can become more autonomy supportive. *Educational Psychologist*, *44*(3), 159–175.

Reeve, J., Vansteenkiste, M., Assor, A., Ahmad, I., Cheon, S. H., Jang, H., & Wang, C. K. J. (2014). The beliefs that underlie autonomy-supportive and controlling teaching: a multinational investigation. *Motivation and Emotion*, *38*(1), 93–110.

Robertson, L., & Jones, M. G. (2013). Chinese and US middle-school science teachers' autonomy, motivation, and instructional practices. *International Journal of Science Education*, *35*(9), 1454–1489.

Rocchi, M. A., Pelletier, L. G., & Couture, A. L. (2013). Determinants of coach motivation and autonomy supportive coaching behaviours. *Psychology of Sport and Exercise*, *14*(6), 852–859.

Rosenthal, S. A., & Pittinsky, T. L. (2006). Narcissistic leadership. *The Leadership Quarterly*, *17*(6), 617–633.

Roth, G., & Weinstock, M. (2013). Teachers' epistemological beliefs as an antecedent of autonomy-supportive teaching. *Motivation and Emotion*, *37*(3), 402–412.

Roth, G., Assor, A., Kanat-Maymon, Y., & Kaplan, H. (2007). Autonomous motivation for teaching: how self-determined teaching may lead to self-determined learning. *Journal of Educational Psychology*, *99*(4), 761–774.

Roth, G., Kanat-Maymon, Y., & Bibi, U. (2011). Prevention of school bullying: the important role of autonomy-supportive teaching and internalisation of prosocial values. *British Journal of Educational Psychology, 81*(4), 654–666.

Ryan, R. M., & Deci, E. L. (2002). An overview of self-determination theory. In: E. L. Deci, & R. M. Ryan (Eds.), *Handbook of self-determination research* (pp. 3–33). Rochester, NY: University of Rochester Press.

Sarrazin, P. G., Tessier, D. P., Pelletier, L. G., Trouilloud, D. O., & Chanal, J. P. (2006). The effects of teachers' expectations about students' motivation on teachers' autonomy-supportive and controlling behaviours. *International Journal of Sport and Exercise Psychology, 4*, 283–301.

Skinner, E. A., & Belmont, M. J. (1993). Motivation in the classroom: reciprocal effects of teacher behavior and student engagement across the school year. *Journal of Educational Psychology, 85*(4), 571–581.

Skinner, E. A., & Edge, K. (2002). Self-determination, coping, and development. In: E. L. Deci, & R. M. Ryan (Eds.), *Self-determination theory: extensions and applications* (pp. 297–337). Rochester NY: University of Rochester Press.

Soenens, B., Sierens, E., Vansteenkiste, M., Dochy, F., & Goossens, L. (2012). Psychologically controlling teaching: examining outcomes, antecedents, and mediators. *Journal of Educational Psychology, 104*(1), 108–120.

Stebbings, J., Taylor, I. M., & Spray, C. M. (2011). Antecedents of perceived coach autonomy supportive and controlling behaviors: coach psychological need satisfaction and well-being. *Journal of Sport & Exercise Psychology, 33*(2), 255–272.

Stebbings, J., Taylor, I. M., Spray, C. M., & Ntoumanis, N. (2012). Antecedents of perceived coach interpersonal behaviors: the coaching environment and coach psychological well- and ill-being. *Journal of Sport & Exercise Psychology, 34*(4), 481–502.

Stebbings, J., Taylor, I. M., & Spray, C. (2015). The relationship between psychological well- and ill-being, and perceived autonomy supportive and controlling interpersonal styles: a longitudinal study of sport coaches. *Psychology of Sport and Exercise, 19*, 42–19.

Taylor, I. M., & Ntoumanis, N. (2007). Teacher motivational strategies and student self-determination in physical education. *Journal of Educational Psychology, 99*(4), 747–760.

Taylor, I. M., Ntoumanis, N., & Standage, M. (2008). A self-determination theory approach to understanding the antecedents of teachers' motivational strategies in physical education. *Journal of Sport & Exercise Psychology, 30*(1), 75–94.

Van den Berghe, L., Soenens, B., Vansteenkiste, M., Aelterman, N., Cardon, G., Tallir, I. B., & Haerens, L. (2013). Observed need-supportive and need-thwarting teaching behavior in physical education: do teachers' motivational orientations matter? *Psychology of Sport and Exercise, 14*(5), 650–661.

Van den Berghe, L., Soenens, B., Aelterman, N., Cardon, G., Tallir, I. B., & Haerens, L. (2014). Within-in-person profiles of teachers' motivation to teach: associations with need satisfaction at work, need-supportive teaching, and burnout. *Psychology of Sport and Exercise, 15*(4), 407–417.

Wellborn, J., Connell, J., Skinner, E. A., & Pierson, L. H. (1988). *Teacher as social context: A measure of teacher provision of involvement, structure and autonomy support* (Tech. Rep. No. 102). Rochester, NY: University of Rochester.

Williams, G. C., & Deci, E. L. (1996). Internalization of biopsychosocial values by medical students: a test of self-determination theory. *Journal of Personality and Social Psychology, 70*(4), 767–779.

Williams, G. C., Grow, V. M., Freedman, Z. R., Ryan, R. M., & Deci, E. L. (1996). Motivational predictors of weight loss and weight-loss maintenance. *Journal of Personality & Social Psychology, 70*, 115–126.

Chapter 8

Why Self-Talk Is Effective? Perspectives on Self-Talk Mechanisms in Sport

Evangelos Galanis, Antonis Hatzigeorgiadis, Nikos Zourbanos, Yannis Theodorakis
Department of Physical Education and Sport Science, University of Thessaly, Trikala, Greece

The reciprocal relationships and the interactions between cognition, affect, and behavior lie in the core of the psychological inquiry. Despite the global acceptance of such a position, one aspect of human cognition and functioning that has been relatively neglected until recent years in the sport psychology literature is the role of what people say to themselves. Eventually, through the expansion of the field, the links between self-addressed statements and action captured researchers' attentions and nowadays the study of self-talk has been receiving increased research attention. In a simple way Hatzigeorgiadis, Zourbanos, Latinjak and Theodorakis (2014, p. 372) described self-talk as "what people say to themselves either silently or aloud, inherently or strategically, to stimulate, direct, react and evaluate events and actions." People talk to themselves a lot. What people say to themselves can refer to the past (evaluate and react to things that have happened) or the present/future (to stimulate and direct action). Most of the times this self-process happens inside their heads (silently), and this comes naturally (inherently/automatically); however, sometimes it occurs audibly (aloud) and many times, and particularly in achievement contexts such as sport, people talk to themselves for a purpose (strategically) and based on a plan to achieve certain outcomes.

The strategic use of self-talk in sport involves the use of cue words aiming at enhancing performance through the activation of appropriate responses. The principle underlying the use of self-talk strategies is that athletes provide to themselves appropriate instructions for action, and subsequently execute the appropriate action by simply following the self-instruction they have used, or reinforce

Sport and Exercise Psychology Research. http://dx.doi.org/10.1016/B978-0-12-803634-1.00008-X

themselves toward a desired outcome (Hatzigeorgiadis, Zourbanos, et al., 2014). There are robust findings supported through metaanalytic evidence that self-talk strategies in sport are effective in enhancing performance and facilitating learning (Hatzigeorgiadis, Zourbanos, Galanis, & Theodorakis, 2011); however, the variety of effects in different settings and populations has forwarded the need to understand how self-talk works, that is, the mechanisms underlying its effectiveness. Understanding the mechanisms of self-talk is significant because it will help improving interventions and, importantly, adapting interventions to match situational demands and individual needs.

At the apex level the social cognitive perspectives of human functioning provide the platform for the exploration of the links between thought and action. Bandura's (1986) social cognitive theory for the study of human behavior describes a model of reciprocal causation between behavior, personal, and environmental factors, reflecting the interaction between cognitive, affective, and physiological states. The reciprocal determinism approach has been very influential within the field of motivation postulating that the interaction of individuals' thought and affect energize, direct, and regulate behavior in achievement contexts.

More specific to the role of self-instruction is Zimmerman's (2000) approach to self-regulation. Zimmerman in the theory of self-regulation identified three cyclical phases, forethought, performance, and self-reflection. Within the performance phase, strategies such as self-instructional statements serve as discriminative stimuli to focus on key elements of the task (Schunk & Zimmerman, 2003), thus influencing performance and subsequently self-reaction including emotions in the self-reflection phase.

From an applied perspective, the development of self-instructional training that eventually led to the growth of self-talk strategies has been significantly influenced by psychotherapeutic approaches. Meichenbaum (1977) in his cognitive behavior modification model identified the important role of self-instructional training for treating cognitive and emotional disorders. Meichenbaum regarded self-statements as indices of individuals' beliefs and suggested that statements addressed to oneself can influence individuals' attentional and appraisal processes, thus regulating behavioral performance. Similarly, Ellis (1976), based on the assumption that intrusive thoughts lay at the core of anxiety and emotion, argued that thoughts are central to the formation and change of emotions. Restructuring the content or reducing the frequency of such thoughts during performance situations provided the foundation for cognitive and cognitive-behavioral approaches to reducing performance anxiety and subsequently improving performance. Overall, within a cognitive behavior therapy perspective, self-instructional training has been claimed to be useful in facilitating the learning of new skills and in enhancing the performance of adaptive responses (Rokke & Rehm, 2001). The theories already presented provide a foundation for the effectiveness of self-talk, but also for the potential mechanisms underlying the behavioral outcomes of self-talk, through the identification of attentional and motivational mechanisms, including cognitive and affective responses. Based on the aforementioned foundations and the effectiveness of self-talk strategies in educational and clinical psychology settings, the investigation of self-talk in sport eventually attracted significant research attention.

This chapter aims at providing an overview of the literature relevant to the identification of the self-talk mechanisms and offering a framework for the development of future research for the better understanding of the self-talk mechanisms. First, evidence supporting the effectiveness of self-talk in sport will be briefly presented to document the need for research on self-talk mechanisms. Subsequently, preliminary evidence regarding the potential factors explaining the effectiveness of self-talk strategies will be described and conceptual models that have been developed for the understanding of the mechanisms will be presented. Finally, theoretical perspectives that may accommodate research developments will be delineated and empirical evidence from the limited research on the self-talk mechanisms in sport will be reviewed, to support a proposed model mapping the constructs and the evidence surrounding the self-talk mechanisms research in sport.

EFFECTIVENESS OF SELF-TALK STRATEGIES

An overview of the self-talk literature in sport reveals that research has emphatically focused on the effectiveness of self-talk strategies for performance enhancement. This line of investigation involves conducting experiments and applying interventions using self-talk strategies and assessing the impact of using self-talk cues on performance. The reason for the popularity of this research is its direct applied value, as self-talk strategies appear to be effective in facilitating learning and enhancing performance, and such strategies can be immediately used in teaching, training, and competition settings.

In a review of the relevant literature, Theodorakis, Hatzigeorgiadis, and Zourbanos (2012) identified four levels at which the effectiveness of self-talk interventions have been investigated in sport: (1) effects on fundamental motor tasks (eg, vertical jump; Edwards, Tod, & McGuigan, 2008); (2) effects on components of performance in different sports (eg, basketball free-throw shooting; Perkos, Theodorakis, & Chroni, 2002); (3) effects on sport performance in noncompetitive settings (eg, running; Weinberg, Miller, & Horn, 2012); and (4) effects on sport performance in competitive settings (eg, swimming; Hatzigeorgiadis, Galanis, Zourbanos, & Theodorakis, 2014). The effectiveness of self-talk has been emphatically supported through a metaanalysis examining the effect of self-talk interventions on performance (Hatzigeorgiadis et al., 2011). The results revealed a moderate positive effect size ($d = 0.48$), thus providing robust evidences for the value of self-talk interventions. Examination of possible factors that may moderate the effectiveness of self-talk showed that self-talk was more effective in fine and novel tasks rather than gross and learned tasks, and in intervention, including some type of self-talk training rather than interventions where participants were asked to make use of self-talk cues without prior practice. Overall, there is now strong support for the benefits of using self-talk to facilitate learning and enhance performance in motor and sport settings.

A close look at the results from the different interventions suggests that different self-talk cues have different effects on task performance. Theodorakis, Weinberg, Natsis, Douma, and Kazakas (2000) proposed a self-talk type by task characteristics matching hypothesis. They speculated that instructional self-talk cues should be more suitable for fine tasks, whereas motivation self-talk cues should be more suitable for gross tasks. A series of experiments in task with different characteristics provided partial support for this matching hypothesis (Hatzigeorgiadis, Theodorakis & Zourbanos, 2004; Theodorakis et al., 2000). Importantly the matching hypothesis was partially supported through the results of the metaanalysis showing that instructional self-talk was more effective than motivational self-talk for fine tasks and that instructional self-talk was more effective for fine tasks rather than gross tasks (Hatzigeorgiadis et al., 2011).

Two more matching hypotheses have been proposed by Hatzigeorgiadis, Zourbanos, et al. (2014). The first suggests a self-talk type by learning stage matching, and the second, a self-talk type by performance setting matching. According to the former, it was claimed that for novel tasks, or for individuals in the early stages of learning, instructional self-talk will be more beneficial, whereas for well-learned tasks, or for individuals in the automated phase of performance, motivational self-talk will be more beneficial. A relevant study by Zourbanos, Hatzigeorgiadis, Bardas, and Theodorakis (2013) provided preliminary support for this hypothesis. In particular, it was found that in a handball-shooting task instructional self-talk had a larger effect than motivational self-talk when performing with the nondominant arm, whereas a marginal effect in favor of the motivational self-talk emerged for the dominant arm. According to the latter matching hypothesis, it was claimed that instructional self-talk should be beneficial in learning and training settings, whereas motivational self-talk will be more beneficial in performance and competition settings. Indirect evidence regarding this proposition have been provided by Hatzigeorgiadis, Galanis, et al. (2014) in an intervention aiming at testing the effectiveness of self-talk strategies in a competitive performance setting. Through an 8-week training program in the use of instructional and motivational self-talk, young swimmers developed their personal self-talk plans for the competition. Apart from the effectiveness of the intervention as this evidenced in the competition results, an examination of the content of the cues swimmers adopted revealed that the competition self-talk plans were, with minor exceptions, dominated by motivational self-talk cues.

Hatzigeorgiadis, Zourbanos, et al. (2014) argued that to develop effective interventions, researchers and practitioners should take into consideration the type of the task, the situational demands, and personal preferences. Taken together the findings previously reported suggest that different self-talk cues may be more or less effective in a given context, or that the same self-talk cues may be more or less effective in different contexts. This postulation suggests that self-talk may serve different purposes through the stimulation of different functions. As a result there is an increasing interest in exploring the mechanism that explain the facilitating effects of self-talk on task performance.

PRELIMINARY RESEARCH AND CONCEPTUAL MODELS

Preliminary evidence for the exploration of possible self-talk mechanisms has emerged through testimonials from athletes. In an early study with young tennis players, Van Raalte, Brewer, Rivera, and Petitpas (1994) explored the relationship between self-talk and performance based on observable self-talk and gestures. In follow-up discussions athletes reported that positive self-talk helped them to enhance their motivation and keep their calmness. In three studies using single-subject multiple-baseline design to test the effectiveness of self-talk in triathletes, tennis players, and football players, participants reported that self-talk helped them to feel more confident, improve their concentration, and direct their attention efficiently (Johnson, Hrycaiko, Johnson, & Halas, 2004; Landin & Hebert, 1999; Thelwell & Greenlees, 2003). Similar reports have been made by basketball players following a 12-week self-talk intervention (Perkos et al., 2002).

More systematic reports through interviews have been provided in three studies. Wayde and Hanton (2008) focused on the mechanisms through which self-talk operates. Athletes from a variety of sports stated that self-talk helped them to control their anxiety responses, increase their levels of effort and motivation, increase their concentration, and enhance their levels of self-confidence. Recently, Miles and Neil (2013) in an attempt to further elaborate on the mechanisms of self-talk interviewed elite cricket players based on video footage. The results showed that the use of instructional and motivational self-talk enhanced athletes' skill execution, self-efficacy, and focus of attention, and reduced performance anxiety. Finally, Cutton and Hearon (2014) in a case study mentioned that the self-talk of a world champion power lifter was associated with staying focused, regulating effort, maintaining motivation, and improving skills. Overall, these findings based on athletes' perceptions have offered initial viewpoints regarding the effects self-talk may have on several performance aspects, and have provided the basis for the further development of research onto the self-talk mechanisms.

Based on the previous prepositions, previous empirical evidence, and raw data collected from athletes' reports, Theodorakis, Hatzigeorgiadis, and Chroni (2008) forwarded a perceptual operationalization regarding the functions of self-talk. A series of qualitative and quantitative analyses led to the development of a multidimensional model and instrument depicting the self-talk functions (Function of Self-Talk Questionnaire; FSTQ). According to this model self-talk can serve to (1) improve attentional focus, (2) increase self-confidence, (3) regulate effort, (4) control cognitions and emotions, and (5) trigger automatic execution. Following the development of the FSTQ, studies explored differences in the functions of self-talk in relation to different self-talk cues' settings. In a study with physical education students, Hatzigeorgiadis (2006) compared the effects of instructional and motivational self-talk on a swimming task and the FSTQ dimensions. The results revealed that participants scored higher on the effort dimension of the FSTQ when using motivational self-talk, compared to when using instructional self-talk. In a similar investigation, Hatzigeorgiadis, Zourbanos, and Theodorakis (2007) examined the effects of a technical instruction and an anxiety regulation cue in a water polo precision task under evaluative conditions. The results revealed that participants scored higher on the cognitive and emotional control dimension of the FSTQ when using the anxiety regulation self-talk cue, than when using the technical instruction cue. These findings support the notion that in different situations self-talk may serve, at different intensity, different functions that may operate in tandem (Hardy, Oliver, & Tod, 2009).

For the better understanding of the possible mechanisms through which self-talk facilitates sport performance, Hardy et al. (2009) proposed a conceptual model with four dimensions of mechanisms that may explain the effects of self-talk on performance: first, a cognitive dimension of mechanisms referring to aspects such as information processing, concentration, attentional control, and attentional style; second, a motivational dimension of mechanisms, referring to self-efficacy and persistence; third, a behavioral dimension of mechanisms referring to technique improvement; and last, an affective dimension of mechanisms referring to regulation of affective states. This conceptualization shares certain characteristics with the mechanisms suggested through the functions of self-talk model presented earlier, but also introduces new elements and a more elaborate categorization of self-talk mechanisms. These models in combination with theoretical frameworks and perspectives underlying the potential impact of self-talk have been useful in fostering contemporary research for the study of self-talk mechanisms. The next sections review the up-to-date relevant research and provide a contemporary perspective toward the development of a comprehensive model of self-talk mechanisms.

A PROSPECTIVE MODEL OF SELF-TALK MECHANISMS

The scant research on the mechanisms underlying the effectiveness of self-talk so far has focused on two wider clusters of mechanisms: attentional and motivational. In this quest, several existing theoretical models have been used to develop research questions or interpret research findings. In addition, further theoretical frameworks can be adopted to accommodate findings pertaining to the self-talk mechanisms, but also provide the appropriate foundation for developing future research and inform applications. In the next section such frameworks will be presented with emphasis on those that can be linked to empirical evidence regarding the mechanisms explaining the self-talk performance relationship.

To facilitate the understanding of this section, a prospective model mapping the constructs and the theories that can be used to accommodate existing, but also future, research hypotheses and findings is presented in Fig. 8.1. Based on the premises of the theoretical foundations described at the beginning of this

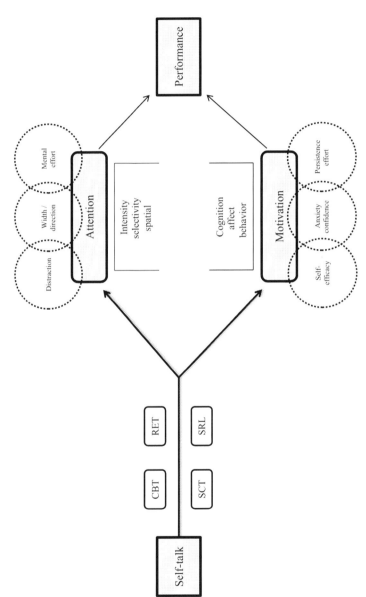

FIGURE 8.1 **A prospective model of self-talk mechanisms.** *CBT*, cognitive behavior therapy; *RET*, rational emotive therapy; *SCT*, social cognitive yheory; *SRL*, self-regulation learning.

chapter, and taking into consideration the model of Hardy et al. (2009), our current conceptualization includes two broad clusters of mechanisms mediating the effect of self-talk on performance, which reflect the relevant theories but mostly the existing self-talk literature in sport. The first cluster relates to an attentional interpretation of the facilitating effects of self-talk, comprising the different dimensions of attention (intensity-vigilance, selectivity-executive, and spatial-orienting), and including attentional constructs and theoretical perspectives that can be linked to the study of self-talk mechanisms: width and direction of attention, distractibility, and mental effort. The second cluster relates to a motivational interpretation of the facilitating effects of self-talk, comprising cognitive, affective, and behavioral aspects of motivation, and including constructs and theoretical perspectives that can be linked to the study of self-talk mechanisms: self-efficacy, self-confidence and anxiety, and effort and persistence.

Attentional Perspectives

Dimensions and Domains of Attention

Attention has been identified and widely acknowledged as a multidimensional cognitive ability. Posner and Petersen (1990) proposed a taxonomy of attention dimensions. They suggested that attention can be divided into three subsystems: orienting (orienting to sensory events), detecting (detecting signals for focal conscious processing), and alerting (maintaining an alert state). Based on Posner's model, Van Zomeren and Brouwer (1994) distinguished attention in two main domains: selectivity (attention can be directed to a certain location) and intensity (attention can be maintained to a certain location). In addition, the authors subdivided the selectivity aspect into focused and divided attention. Attempting a synthesis of Posner's and Van Zomeren and Brouwer's models, Sturm (2005) created a more inclusive framework for studying the dimensions of attention. The model describes three different dimensions of attention and their corresponding neuropsychological attention domains: (1) intensity, which includes alertness, sustained attention, and vigilance, (2) selectivity, which include selective, focused and divided attention, and (3) spatial attention.

Based on Sturm's taxonomy of the attentional dimensions, we have conducted a series of experiments to examine the effects of self-talk on attentional domains (Galanis, Hatzigeorgiadis, Zourbanos, Papaioannou, & Theodorakis, 2016), using the Test Battery for Perception and Attention Functions (WAF tests) of the Vienna Test System (VTS, Sturm, 2006). The WAF tests battery consist of six tests which reflect alertness and vigilance/sustained attention (intensity), selective, focused, and divided attention (selectivity), and finally spatial attention. A series of experiments were conducted to measure the six attentional domains involving in total 255 participants. A 5-days' experimental procedure was followed for each experiment, comprising three phases: baseline trial, attention training, and final assessment.

The first set of experiments examined the effects of self-talk strategy on attention intensity. In the first experiment, alertness, the ability of the individual to control arousal and response readiness (intrinsic and phasic), was tested in a combination of visual and audio tests. The results showed that the experimental group produced better reaction times compared to the control group in five out of the six tests. In the second experiment, vigilance, the ability of individuals to direct attention to one (or more) stimulus for a long time (with a low stimulus rate), was tested (visual test). In accordance to the first experiment, the results revealed that the experimental group had significantly faster reaction time than the control group.

The second set of experiments examined the effects of self-talk on attention selectivity. In the first experiment, selective attention, the ability of the individual to focus on a specific stimulus while irrelevant stimuli have to be ignored, was tested in two tests (visual and audio). In the second experiment, focused attention, the ability to focus on a specific stimulus, was tested in three tests (visual, audio, and crossaudiovisual). Finally, in the third experiment, divided attention, the ability of individuals to respond simultaneously to two (or more) different tasks, was tested in two tests (visual and crossaudiovisual tests). The results showed that for all seven tests of selective attention the experimental group performed better than the control group.

The third experiment examined the effects of self-talk on spatial attention, the ability of the individual to focus his/her attention on a location in the space in three tests (central cues, peripheral cues, and neglect). The results showed that in all three tests, participants of the experimental group displayed faster reaction times than participants of the control group. Overall, these findings involving direct tests of attentional performance provide strong evidence that the effects of self-talk on individuals' attentional functioning is a viable mechanism explaining the facilitating effects of self-talk strategies on task performance.

Width and Direction of Attention

Nideffer's (1976) theory of attentional style provides an interesting framework for the study of attention in sport in general and in relation to self-talk in particular. Nideffer identifies two dimensions of attention, direction and width. Direction denotes the target of the focus and may be internal or external. An internal focus involves directing attention inwards, for example, thoughts and feelings, whereas an external focus involves directing attention outwards, for example, the environment. Width denotes the range of attention and varies on a continuum from narrow (one or few sources of relevant stimuli) to broad (many sources of relevant stimuli). The two dimensions create a fourfold model of attentional focus: internal-narrow, internal-broad, external-narrow, and external-broad. In some sports, a particular type of attention is required to achieve quality performance, whereas in other sports, the focus of attention should shift from type to type to meet the demands of the situation/game progress. Even though the model has attracted relatively limited research attention, the shifting of attention aspect of the theory can be linked to the use of self-talk. In particular, self-talk strategies can be effective in facilitating athletes shifting the focus of attention to the attentional style appropriate to perform a skill, thus improving performance.

Indirect support for this hypothesis have been provided by Ziegler (1987) who examined the effects of a four-step verbal cueing program, each reflecting the attentional focus appropriate for different phases of a motion, on tennis forehand and backhand groundstrokes. The interventions aimed at shifting attention between narrow external and broad external. The results showed that the intervention was indeed effective in enhancing performance; however, no direct assessment of attentional focus was applied. Further indirect evidence regarding the effective directing of attention have been also reported from Landin and Hebert (1999) and Mallett and Hanrahan (1997) who developed interventions for tennis and sprinting, respectively. In these studies, however, the focus of attention did not shift in terms of width or direction, but in terms of target within a narrow internal focus. For example, Mallett and Hanrahan (1997) split a 100 m race into segments and developed a race plan using self-talk cues to direct attention to appropriate stimuli depending on the segment of the race. This evidence provides support to another potential attentional mechanism related to the regulation, directing and shifting, of attentional focus within sport. Similar indirect evidence from experiments using combination of self-talk cues to direct attention to different external targets has been reported by Hatzigeorgiadis et al. (2004), Theodorakis et al. (2000), and Zourbanos et al. (2013).

Internal and External Focus of Attention

A somewhat different conceptualization of the focus of attention direction that has attracted significant research attention in the motor learning domain is the internal–external focus of attention approach to learning and performance (Bernstein, 1996; Wulf & Prinz, 2001). Internal focus refers to focusing one's attention to the action itself, that is, the body and the movement of the limbs, whereas external focus refers to focusing one's attention to the effect of the action, that is, the outcome of the movement. The effectiveness of internal versus external focus has been central in this literature and an issue of great debate (Toner & Moran, 2015, 2016; Wulf, 2016). In favor of the external focus effectiveness, Wulf and Prinz (2001) have forwarded the constrained-action hypothesis, claiming that an internal focus of attention may restrict the automatic processes that would normally control a movement, whereas an external focus would promote an inherent self-organization process that will eventually facilitate learning and performance. In contrast, in favor of an interaction approach taking into consideration the skill level of athletes, Bernstein (1996) argued that, due to differences in automizations, an external focus will be more beneficial for skilled athletes. These propositions have received empirical support showing that different stages of skill acquisition require different cognitive processes, with a trend for increased proceduralization, linked to an external focus of attention, as expertise increases; whereas at earlier stages of learning, an internal focus may even help skill acquisition (Beilock & Carr, 2001; Beilock, Carr, MacMahon, & Starkes, 2002). In addition, Shusterman (2008) in his "somaesthetic awareness" approach argues that conscious processing strategies may be useful when adjusting or attempting to regain prior high levels of performance, as deliberate attention to aspects of movements may restore their efficiency.

Regardless of the focus of attention that is mostly relevant and effective for task performance, the use of self-talk strategies may strengthen the quality of the focus, either internal or external. In such a study, Bell and Hardy (2009) examined the effects of attentional focus on skilled performance in golf. They used three different attention foci reflecting on internal, proximal external, and distal external focus self-talk cues under two experimental conditions: neutral and anxiety condition. The results indicated a better performance in distal external focus self-talk rather that internal and proximal external focus self-talk in both neutral and anxiety conditions. In addition, proximal external focus compared to internal focus displayed better performance in both neutral and anxiety conditions. Importantly, a manipulation check revealed that participants in the three conditions reported greater focus on the respective type of attentional focus induced by the manipulation, thus supporting that self-talk influenced the strength of the focus.

To further explore the effectiveness of self-talk on improving internal and external focus of attention, two, still ongoing, experiments on an endurance cycling task are been conducted in our lab. Each experiment comprises three groups: (1) a group receiving no attention instruction, (2) a group receiving an internal/external attention instructions, and (3) a self-talk group receiving the same internal/external instruction and in addition are assigned an internal/external self-talk cue to further support the respective instruction. Preliminary analyses for the internal focus experiment that has been completed suggest that the internal focus self-talk group reported greater internal focus and performed better than the internal focus instruction only group, which reported greater internal focus and performed better than the control group (Charachousi, Christodoulou, Gourgoulias, Galanis, & Hatzigeorgiadis, 2015).

Internal and External Distraction

An important for the field of sport approach to the study of attention, which may be linked to the study of self-talk mechanisms, is the distraction approach (Moran, 1996). Nelson, Duncan, and Kiecker (1993) described a distraction as the occurrence of competing stimuli that may interfere with task-related stimuli and divert attention from its original focus. Moran (1996) argues that the study of distraction is not straightforward because it involves stimuli evolving from the environment and the self, but also their interaction. Moran subsequently referred to stimuli from the environment (such as noise, irrelevant visual stimuli, and environmental conditions) as external distractions, and to stimuli evolving from within (such as thoughts, mostly negative but also positive) as internal distractions. The study of external distractions has received more research attention, possibly due to methodological convenience of creating and manipulating such distractions (Eysenck & Keane, 1995). This research has adopted a cognitive psychology perspective through the examination of the impact of distractions to behavioral outcomes and performance. In contrast, the role of internal distractions, which encompass aspects of the self-talk phenomenon, has been less studied. Distractions have been linked with impaired performance and from information-processing perspective, this can be attributed to the detrimental effects of distraction to processing efficiency, as they occupy part of the working memory which could be used for task-processing purposes (Eysenck, 1992). A plausible hypothesis regarding the role of self-talk would be that self-talk strategies can help minimize the occurrence and the influence of distractions, both external and internal.

Regarding internal distractions, Hatzigeorgiadis et al. (2004) examined the effects of motivational and instructional self-talk on performance but also on the occurrence of interfering thoughts during task performance in two water-polo tasks (precision and power). The results showed that both self-talk types reduced the occurrence of interfering thoughts in both tasks. In addition, reductions in interfering thoughts were related to improvements in performance in one of the two tasks. This suggests that self-talk reduces internal distractions, however whether this relates to performance may depend on other factors such as the demands of the task. Similar findings were reported in another experiment involving a swimming task (Hatzigeorgiadis et al., 2007).

Regarding external distractions, recently completed research (Charachousi, Tsetsila, Tsimeas, Galanis, & Hatzigeorgiadis, 2014; Galanis, Hatzigeorgiadis, Sarampalis, & Sanchez, 2016) has provided useful preliminary data. In particular we have conducted two experiments, one in the lab and one in the field examining the effectiveness of self-talk on task performance under conditions of extreme, noncontinuous, sudden, high tone noise. In the lab experiment students were asked to complete a computer game, whereas in the field experiment female basketball players were tested on free-throw shooting. In both experiments participants of the experimental group, who received self-talk training, performed better than participants of the control group. The findings overall seem to support a protective effect of self-talk against distractions, both internal and external, thus suggesting that this is another viable attentional mechanisms of self-talk.

Mental Effort

An attentional approach that stems from the capacity models of attention is the mental effort approach (Kahneman, 1973). Kahneman described attention as a reservoir of mental energy from which resources are drawn to meet situational attentional demands for task processing. He then argued that mental effort reflects variations in processing demands. Among the assumptions underlying this approach of particular interest is that (1) mental effort increases with task difficulty/complexity, and (2) learning results in reduction of mental effort required performing a task and producing a certain outcome. Kahneman proposed that pupil dilation is the best physiological index to detect changes in mental effort, as it has proven effective in identifying between-tasks and within-tasks variation in pupil dilation reflecting the assumptions previously mentioned. Beatty and Lucero-Wagoner (2000) introduced the term "task-evoked pupillary responses" to describe dilations in the pupil due to cognitive processing of stimuli on a task, and stressed the importance of pupilometry as a measure reflecting brain activity and concomitant with cognitive processes.

In recently conducted experiments (Galanis, Hatzigeorgiadis, Sarampalis, & Sanchez, 2016), we have tried to explore the impact of self-talk on mental effort through pupilometry (eye tracker). We conducted two experiments involving a computerized fine motor task under conditions of different attentional demands manipulated through the generation of noise using a mixed, within and between, subject design. The analyses provided support for the integrity of our experiments. In accordance with the theory's assumptions, the pupil diameter decreased in the experimental trial compared to the baseline trial in both experiments (learning effect). In addition, the pupil size was greater in the second experiment when an audio distraction was introduced to increase the attentional demands. Moreover, it was revealed that the performance of the self-talk group was superior to that of the control group, whereas pupil dilation was smaller. These results seem to support an important performance effect through reduced mental effort that could be interpreted as a more *effortless attention effect* of self-talk. These findings albeit preliminary provide an exciting prospect and encourage further investigation of pupil dilation, as an index of mental effort, in relation to self-talk strategies and their underlying mechanisms.

Motivational Perspectives

Cognition: Self-Efficacy

Bandura's (1997) self-efficacy theory has been central in the field of human motivation and offers a sound framework that can partly accommodate the effects of self-talk on performance. Among the sources of self-efficacy, Bandura, in his original formulation of the theory, identified the small but potentially important role of verbal persuasion from others. Further considering the role of the verbal persuasion source, Hardy, Jones, and Gould (1996) argued for the importance of one's own self-persuasion through self-talk. Athletes can enhance their self-efficacy through statements addressed to themselves regarding their capabilities to attain certain outcomes. As self-talk has been linked to performance, self-efficacy may have an important mediating role in this relationship.

In a primary attempt to test this hypothesis, Hardy, Hall, Gibbs, and Greenslade (2005) examined the effects of instructional and motivational self-talk has on self-efficacy using a sit-up task. In general, the results revealed that both instructional and motivational self-talk were positively related to self-efficacy. Additionally, self-efficacy was positively related to sit-up performance, but neither self-talk dimension was related to performance. Hatzigeorgiadis, Zourbanos, Goltsios, and Theodorakis (2008) examined the effects of a self-talk intervention on self-efficacy and performance among young tennis players. The results revealed that the use of motivational self-talk significantly increased both self-efficacy and performance, compared to a control group. In addition, it was revealed that increases in self-efficacy were related to increases in performance, thus providing supporting evidence for the mediating role of self-efficacy. Similar findings have been reported by Zetou, Vernadakis, Bebetsos, and Makraki (2012) who examined the effects of instructional self-talk on the learning of a volley service skill and self-efficacy among young female volley players. The results indicated that the self-talk group displayed better performance and reported increased self-efficacy compared to a control group. Chang et al. (2014) examined the effects of self-talk on softball-throwing performance and self-efficacy. The results revealed that both instructional and motivational self-talk improved performance; in addition, they reported increases in self-efficacy for the motivational self-talk group. Overall, the self-efficacy hypothesis has received more research attention compared to other potential mechanisms, and considerable support as a plausible self-talk mechanism.

Affect: Anxiety and Self-Confidence

As identified in the previous section of the chapter, self-talk has been central to cognitive and cognitive-behavioral interventions for cognitive and emotional disorders, and behavior in general (Cognitive Behavior Therapy, Meichenbaum, 1977; Rational Emotive Behavior Therapy, Ellis, 1976). More emphatically Bernard, Ellis, and Terjensen (2006) identified the empowering aspect of self-talk on emotions in general and anxiety reduction in particular. Meichenbaum (1977) argued that self-statements will bring more adaptive thoughts and lead to more effective coping behavior under anxiety-inducing situations. In sport, performance anxiety and its treatment, through regulation of intensity or restructuring, is an issue of particular interest at both the applied and the research spectrums. Although self-talk has been identified as a potential strategy for reducing anxiety, research has been scarce.

In an intervention study with young tennis players, Hatzigeorgiadis, Zourbanos, Mpoumpaki, and Theodorakis (2009) found that the use of motivational self-talk following a 3-day self-talk training intervention resulted in improved performance and self-confidence, when performing under anxiety-inducing conditions. Importantly, a significant effect was identified for cognitive anxiety and a marginal effect for somatic anxiety, with participants of the interventions group reporting lower levels of anxiety than those of a control group. Further empirical evidence regarding effects of self-talk on anxiety, but also on emotion regulation in general, will strengthen our confidence for the popular, through anecdotal reports, belief regarding the role of self-talk for anxiety regulation, thus providing a basis for the mediating role of emotion regulation in the self-talk performance relationship.

Behavior: Effort and Persistence

Recent theorizing on perceptual interpretations of exertion and the regulation of effort, as these expressed through the psychobiological model of endurance performance (Marcora, Bosio, & Morree, 2008; Marcora, Staiano, & Manning, 2009), forwards another possible explanation for the facilitating effects of self-talk on performance, at least endurance performance, within a motivational perspective. According to the psychobiological model, exhaustion which limits the ability to sustain aerobic exercise is created by the conscious decision to terminate endurance task performance. The model suggests that perception of effort is a critical factor for endurance performance; hence, endurance performance might be affected by any physiological or psychological factor influencing perception of effort exhaustion (Marcora et al., 2008, 2009).

Blanchfield, Hardy, de Morree, Staiano, and Marcora (2014) examined the effect of a motivational self-talk intervention on cycling endurance performance, and ratings of perceived exertion. They found that the self-talk group had greater cycling time to exhaustion while reporting lower RPE during the task. In addition, no differences were recorded in facial EMG, which was assessed as a psychophysiological measure of perceived effort assessed during and near completion of the test, heart rate during and at completion of the test, and lactate concentration 3 min postcompletion. In a similar study, Barwood, Corbett, Wagstaff, McVeigh, and Thelwell (2015) reported that motivational self-talk during a 10 km cycling task resulted in increased power output, which were matched by increases in oxygen consumption, while no differences were observed in ratings of perceived exertion were stated.

Hatzigeorgiadis, Bartura, Argyropoulos, Zourbanos, and Flouris (2016) examined the effects of a motivational self-talk intervention self-talk on endurance cycling performance in extreme heat conditions. Participants were asked to cycle at a fixed perceived exertion rate (between 14 and 15 on the 6–20 Borg scale) for 30 min. The results revealed that self-talk group exhibited greater power output than the control group and the same pattern was revealed for oxygen consumption, while no differences were recorded for perceptual variables (perceived exertion, thermal comfort, and thermal sensation) and physiological variables (respiratory quotient, core, skin, and muscle temperature). In summary, the previous evidence provides support for a perceptual interpretation of the beneficial self-talk effects, as these recorded through enhanced input (effort, persistence) and subsequently output (covered distance, elapsed time), thus supporting the psychophysiological model of endurance performance and the fit of self-talk strategies within this model.

CONCLUSIONS AND DIRECTIONS FOR FUTURE RESEARCH

The study of self-talk mechanisms in sport is an emerging field of inquiry. The model described in this chapter is conceptually narrow because it was aimed at portraying the current literature; thus, we consider this as a provisional, but dynamic, model *under construction*. In comparison to the conceptual model proposed by Hardy et al. (2009), our model focuses on the sport literature that has directly examined potential mechanisms and this is why the clustering of some mechanisms appears different. The two models identify similar mechanisms; however, our model, based on the current state of research, in essence covers in a more thorough way, parts of the broader conceptual model introduced by Hardy et al. (2009). In particular, our model (1) focuses on the attentional aspect of cognitive mechanisms, and (2) examines cognitive, affective, and behavioral aspects of motivation. Hardy et al. (2009) identify the attentional processes as part of a wider cognitive mechanism, which however has attentional processes at its core. In addition, in Hardy et al.'s model affective aspects are identified as separate cluster of mechanisms. Research looking further into the emotion regulation aspect of self-talk will help to provide support for the integrity of the affective mechanisms underlying the effectiveness of self-talk. We believe that the relevant research is still in a premature stage to support with confidence a robust model of self-talk mechanisms. Thus, the model is subject to updates and modifications. Eventually, as research will grow, we expect that the two models will be integrated to accommodate the different perspectives and contribute to the development of a comprehensive model of self-talk mechanisms.

The approaches and the evidence reviewed in this chapter provide challenging research perspectives for the understanding of self-talk mechanisms and the self-talk phenomenon in total. Basic research seems to be a priority toward this direction. The advances in the self-talk literature can help designing and testing new hypotheses; basic research will help exploring these hypotheses and provide direction for field approaches. Within this frame, a multidisciplinary approach involving physiological and neurophysiological variables will greatly enhance our understanding and expand the field. Heart rate variability measures can help identifying self-talk related responses of the autonomic nervous system modulation, possibly linked to motivational and affective states. Investigation of gaze behavior and eye fixations through eye-tracker technology can help to explore hypotheses regarding the different dimensions and subdomains of attention, and the cognitive processes under different self-talk conditions, within the attentional theoretical frameworks linked to self-talk. Furthermore, portrayals of brain activity through electroencephalography (EEG) and functional magnetic resonance imaging (fMRI) can prove valuable tools for understanding how the brain regions activate when individuals talk to themselves, and whether different types of self-talk are related with different activation in the brain regions. Developments through basic research can then guide the applied field. Applied research has dominated the self-talk literature in sport and has provided useful directions for practice. However, it will be important to increase the focus on athletes and sport settings, through interventions testing hypotheses regarding the self-talk mechanisms and supporting the external validity of findings on the self-talk mechanisms. Finally, as research thus far has focused mostly on the examination of potential mechanisms as outcome measures, it will be important to eventually investigate full mediated relationships between self-talk, potential mechanisms, and performance.

The study of the mechanisms underlying the effectiveness of self-talk for enhancing sport performance is an exciting research endeavor. Understanding the mechanisms will help to develop effective interventions, considering personal, situational, and contextual factors. Most importantly, it is through the identification of mechanisms governing the effectiveness of self-talk that a comprehensive self-talk theory can be formed to guide research and inform practice. The model proposed in this chapter is intended as a dynamic platform for the development of systematic research on self-talk mechanisms. We expect that such research will inform further developments of this model, and facilitate the creation of a unified self-talk theory.

REFERENCES

Bandura, A. (1986). *Social foundation of thought and action: A social cognitive theory.* Englewood Cliffs, NJ: Prentice Hall.

Bandura, A. (1997). *Self-efficacy: The exercise of control.* New York: Freeman.

Barwood, M. J., Corbett, J., Wagstaff, C. R. D., McVeigh, D., & Thelwell, R. C. (2015). Improvement of 10-km time-trial cycling with motivational self-talk compared with neutral self-talk. *International Journal of Sports Physiology and Performance, 10,* 166–171.

Beatty, J., & Lucero-Wagoner, B. (2000). The pupillary system. In: J. T. Cacioppo, L. G. Tassinary, & G. G. Berntson (Eds.), *Handbook of psychophysiology* (pp. 14–162). Cambridge, UK: Cambridge University Press.

Beilock, S. L., & Carr, T. H. (2001). On the fragility of skilled performance: what governs choking under pressure? *Journal of Experimental Psychology, 140,* 701–725.

Beilock, S. L., Carr, T. H., MacMahon, C., & Starkes, J. L. (2002). When paying attention becomes counterproductive: impact of divided versus skill-focused attention on novice and experienced performance on sensorimotor skills. *Journal of Experimental Psychology, 8,* 6–16.

Bell, J. J., & Hardy, J. (2009). Effects of attentional focus on skilled performance in golf. *Journal of Applied Sport Psychology, 21,* 163–177.

Bernard, M. E., Ellis, A., & Terjesen, M. (2006). Rational-emotive behavioral approaches to childhood disorders: history, theory, practice and research. In: A. Ellis, & M. E. Bernard (Eds.), *Rational emotive behavioral approaches to childhood disorders* (pp. 3–84). New York: Springer.

Bernstein, N. A. (1996). Dexterity and its development. In: M. L. Latash, & M. T. Turvey (Eds., Transl.), *On Dexterity and its Development* (pp. 171–204). Mahwah, NJ: Lawrence Erlbaum.

Blanchfield, A., Hardy, J., de Morree, H. M., Staiano, W., & Marcora, S. M. (2014). Talking yourself out of exhaustion: effects of self-talk on perceived exertion and endurance performance. *Medicine and Science in Sport and Exercise, 46,* 998–1007.

Chang, Y. K., Ho, L. A., Lu, F. J. H., Ou, C. C., Song, T. F., & Gill, D. L. (2014). Self-talk and softball performance: the role of self-talk nature, motor task characteristics, and self-efficacy in novice softball players. *Psychology of Sport and Exercise, 15,* 139–145.

Charachousi, F., Tsetsila, P., Tsimeas, P., Galanis, E., & Hatzigeorgiadis, A. (2014). The effect of an intervention self-talk program on performance on free throws in distraction conditions. *Proceedings of the 13th National Congress of Sport Psychology* (p. 82). Trikala, Greece.

Charachousi, F., Christodoulou, E., Gourgoulias, K., Galanis, E., & Hatzigeorgiadis, A. (2015). Increases in internal focus of attention as a factor explaining the effectiveness of self-talk strategies. *Proceedings of the 23rd International Congress of Physical Education and Sport* (p. 89). Komotini, Greece.

Cutton, D. M., & Hearon, C. M. (2014). Self-talk functions: portrayal of an elite power lifter. *Perceptual and Motor Skills, 119*, 478–494.

Edwards, C., Tod, D., & McGuigan, M. (2008). Self-talk influences vertical jump performance and kinematics in male rugby union players. *Journal of Sports Sciences, 26*, 1459–1465.

Ellis, A. (1976). *Reason and emotion in psychotherapy*. New York: Lyle Stuart.

Eysenck, M. W. (1992). *Anxiety: The cognitive perspective*. Hove: Lawrence Erlbaum Associates Ltd.

Eysenck, M. W., & Keane, M. T. (1995). *Cognitive psychology: A student's handbook* (3rd ed.). Hove: Lawrence Erlbaum Associates Ltd.

Galanis, E., Hatzigeorgiadis, A., Sarampalis, A., & Sanchez, X. (2016). An effortless-attention interpretation of self-talk effectiveness: a look through the eye-tracker. Manuscript in preparation.

Galanis, E., Hatzigeorgiadis, A., Zourbanos, N., Papaioannou, A., & Theodorakis, Y. (2016). Self-talk and attention. Manuscript submitted for publication.

Hardy, L., Jones, G., & Gould, D. (1996). *Understanding psychological preparation for sport: Theory and practice of elite performers*. Chichester: Wiley.

Hardy, J., Hall, C. R., Gibbs, C., & Greenslade, C. (2005). Self-talk and gross motor skill performance: an experimental approach? *Athletic Insight, 7*(2). Available from www.athleticinsight. com/Vol7Iss2/SelfTalkPerformance.htm

Hardy, J., Oliver, E., & Tod, D. (2009). A framework for the study and application of self-talk in sport. In: S. D. Mellalieu, & S. Hanton (Eds.), *Advances in applied sport psychology: A review* (pp. 37–74). London: Routledge.

Hatzigeorgiadis, A. (2006). Instructional and motivational self-talk: an investigation on perceived self-talk functions [Special issue]. *Hellenic Journal of Psychology, 3*, 164–175.

Hatzigeorgiadis, A., Theodorakis, Y., & Zourbanos, N. (2004). Self-talk in the swimming pool: the effects of ST on thought content and performance on water-polo tasks. *Journal of Applied Sport Psychology, 16*, 138–150.

Hatzigeorgiadis, A., Zourbanos, N., & Theodorakis, Y. (2007). An examination on the moderating effects of self-talk content on self-talk functions. *Journal of Applied Sport Psychology, 19*, 240–251.

Hatzigeorgiadis, A., Zourbanos, N., Goltsios, C., & Theodorakis, Y. (2008). Exploring the functions of self-talk: the mediating role of self-efficacy on the self-talk—performance relationship in young tennis players. *The Sport Psychologist, 22*, 458–471.

Hatzigeorgiadis, A., Zourbanos, N., Mpoumpaki, S., & Theodorakis, Y. (2009). Mechanisms underlying the self-talk—performance relationship: the effects of self-talk on self-confidence and anxiety. *Psychology of Sport & Exercise, 10*, 186–192.

Hatzigeorgiadis, A., Zourbanos, N., Galanis, E., & Theodorakis, Y. (2011). Self-talk and sports performance: a meta-analysis. *Perspectives on Psychological Science, 6*, 348–356.

Hatzigeorgiadis, A., Galanis, E., Zourbanos, N., & Theodorakis, Y. (2014). Self-talk and competitive sport performance. *Journal of Applied Sport Psychology, 26*, 82–95.

Hatzigeorgiadis, A., Zourbanos, N., Latinjak, A., & Theodorakis, Y. (2014). Self-talk. In: A. Papaioannou, & D. Hackfort (Eds.), *Routledge companion to sport and exercise psychology: Global perspectives and fundamental concepts* (pp. 372–385). London: Taylor & Francis.

Hatzigeorgiadis, A., Bartura, K., Argyropoulos, C., Zourbanos, N., & Flouris, A. (2016). Performance in the heat: Effects of a self-talk intervention. Manuscript submitted for publication.

Johnson, J. M., Hrycaiko, D. W., Johnson, G. V., & Halas, J. M. (2004). Self-talk and female youth soccer performance. *The Sport Psychologist, 18*, 44–59.

Kahneman, D. (1973). *Attention and effort.* Engelwood Cliffs, NJ: Prentice Hall.

Landin, D. K., & Hebert, E. P. (1999). The influence of self-talk on the performance of skilled female tennis players. *Journal of Applied Sport Psychology, 11*, 263–282.

Mallett, C. J., & Hanrahan, S. J. (1997). Race modelling: an effective cognitive strategy for the 100 m sprinter? *The Sport Psychologist, 11*, 72–85.

Marcora, S. M., Bosio, A., & de Morree, H. M. (2008). Locomotor muscle fatigue increases cardio-respiratory responses and reduces performance during intense cycling exercise independently from metabolic stress. *American Journal of Physiology, 294*, 874–883.

Marcora, S. M., Staiano, W., & Manning, V. (2009). Mental fatigue impairs physical performance in humans. *Journal of Applied Physiology, 106*, 857–864.

Meichenbaum, D. H. (1977). *Cognitive behavior modification: An integrative approach.* New York: Plenum.

Miles, A., & Neil, R. (2013). The use of self-talk during elite cricket batting performance. *Psychology of Sport and Exercise, 14*, 874–881.

Moran, A. P. (1996). *The psychology of concentration in sport performance: A cognitive analysis.* New York: Freeman.

Nelson, J. E., Duncan, C. P., & Kiecker, P. L. (1993). Toward an understanding of the distraction construct in marketing. *Journal of Business Research, 26*, 201–221.

Nideffer, R. M. (1976). Test of attentional and interpersonal style. *Journal of Personality and Social Psychology, 34*, 394–404.

Perkos, S., Theodorakis, Y., & Chroni, S. (2002). Enhancing performance and skill acquisition in novice basketball players with instructional self-talk. *The Sport Psychologist, 16*, 368–383.

Posner, M. I., & Petersen, S. E. (1990). The attention system of the human brain. *Annual Review Neuroscience, 13*, 25–42.

Rokke, P. D., & Rehm, L. P. (2001). Self-management therapies. In: K. S. Donson (Ed.), *Handbook of cognitive-behavioral therapies* (pp. 173–210). New York, NY: Guilford Press.

Schunk, D. H., & Zimmerman, B. J. (2003). Self-regulation and learning. In: W. M. Reynolds, & G. E. Miller (Eds.), *Handbook of psychology: Educational psychology* (pp. 59–78). Hoboken, NJ: Wiley.

Shusterman, R. (2008). *Body consciousness: A philosophy of mindfulness and somaesthetics.* Cambridge: Cambridge University Press.

Sturm, W. (2005). *Aufmerkamkeitsstörungen [Attention deficit disorders].* Göttingen: Hogrefe.

Sturm, W. (2006). *Testmanual wahrnehmungs- und aufmerksamkeitsfunktionen [Test manual: Perception and attention functions].* Mödling: Schuhfried.

Thelwell, R. C., & Greenlees, I. A. (2003). Developing competitive endurance performance using mental skills training. *The Sport Psychologist, 17*, 318–337.

Theodorakis, Y., Weinberg, R., Natsis, P., Douma, I., & Kazakas, P. (2000). The effects of motivational versus instructional self-talk on improving motor performance. *The Sport Psychologist, 14*, 253–272.

Theodorakis, Y., Hatzigeorgiadis, A., & Chroni, S. (2008). Self-talk: it works, but how? Development and preliminary validation of the functions of self-talk questionnaire. *Measurement in Physical Education & Exercise Science, 12*, 10–30.

Theodorakis, Y., Hatzigeorgiadis, A., & Zourbanos, N. (2012). Cognitions: self-talk and performance. In: S. Murphy (Ed.), *Oxford handbook of sport and performance psychology* (pp. 191–212). New York: Oxford University Press.

Toner, J., & Moran, A. (2015). Enhancing performance proficiency at the expert level: considering the role of "somaesthetic awareness". *Psychology of Sport & Exercise, 16,* 110–117.

Toner, J., & Moran, A. (2016). On the importance of critical thinking: a response to Wulf's (2015) commentary. *Psychology of Sport & Exercise, 22,* 339–340.

Van Raalte, J. L., Brewer, B. W., Rivera, P. M., & Petitpas, A. J. (1994). The relationship between observable self-talk and competitive junior tennis players' match performances. *Journal of Sport and Exercise Psychology, 16,* 400–415.

Van Zomeren, A. H., & Brouwer, W. H. (1994). *Clinical neuropsychology of attention.* New York: Oxford University Press.

Wayde, R., & Hanton, S. (2008). Basic psychological skills usage and competitive anxiety responses: perceived underlying mechanisms. *Research Quarterly for Exercise and Sport, 79,* 363–373.

Weinberg, R., Miller, A., & Horn, T. (2012). The influence of a self-talk intervention on collegiate cross-country runners. *International Journal of Sport and Exercise Psychology, 10,* 123–134.

Wulf, G. (2016). Why did Tiger Woods shoot 28? A commentary on Toner and Moran (2015). *Psychology of Sport & Exercise, 22,* 337–338.

Wulf, G., & Prinz, W. (2001). Directing attention to movement effects enhances learning: a review. *Psychonomic Bulletin and Review, 8,* 648–660.

Zetou, E., Vernadakis, N., Bebetsos, E., & Makraki, E. (2012). The effects of self-talk in learning the volleyball service skill and self-efficacy improvement. *Journal of Human Sport & Exercise, 7,* 749–805.

Ziegler, S. G. (1987). Effects of stimulus cueing on the acquisition of groundstrokes by beginning tennis players. *Journal of Applied Behaviour Analysis, 20,* 405–411.

Zimmernam, B. J. (2000). Attaining self-regulation: a social cognitive perspective. In: M. Boekaerts, P. R. Pintrich, & M. Zeidner (Eds.), *Handbook of self-regulation* (pp. 451–502). San Diego, CA: Academic Press.

Zourbanos, N., Hatzigeorgiadis, A., Bardas, D., & Theodorakis, Y. (2013). The effects of self-talk on dominant and non-dominant arm performance on a handball task in primary physical education students. *The Sport Psychologist, 27,* 171–176.

Chapter 9

Personality-Trait-Like Individual Differences: Much More Than Noise in the Background for Sport and Exercise Psychology

Sylvain Laborde*, Mark S. Allen**

*Department of Performance Psychology, German Sport University Cologne, Cologne, Germany; University of Caen, France; **University of Wollongong, School of Psychology, Wollongong, Australia

INTRODUCTION

The notion of combining an individual differences approach to the standard experimental approach has been championed for a long time (Cronbach, 1957) and the argument is consistently renewed in psychological circles (Vogel & Awh, 2008). In this chapter we focus on interindividual variability in behavior, anchored in interindividual variability in perception, cognition, and neurophysiology. Sport and exercise psychology research often targets group-based differences (eg, experts vs novices, intervention vs control), and there is often a tendency to neglect the individual. For example, an experimental study might compare the average score of the pre–post difference of an experimental group to the average score of the pre–post difference of the control group. Using this approach, researchers are able to test hypotheses regarding how individuals function on average. This means that all people are considered on a level playing field and the differences between individuals (in the way they react to an intervention or control condition) are considered as error, noise, or a nuisance (Kanai & Rees, 2011; Vogel & Awh, 2008). Experimenters try to limit the role of individual differences by randomly allocating participants to different conditions—a procedure that became known as the randomized controlled trial. With a large enough sample, the likelihood that different experimental conditions will differ dramatically on individual differences (such as age or personality) decreases. However, that some individuals might respond better or worse to the treatment condition is lost using this approach.

Sport and Exercise Psychology Research. http://dx.doi.org/10.1016/B978-0-12-803634-1.00009-1

Psychological scientists are generally interested in the typical responses of the collective and not the particular responses of the individual. Our argument—that we wish to put forward in this chapter—is that the experimental approach to theory testing can be complemented by the individual differences approach (Vogel & Awh, 2008). Moreover, we propose that an understanding of personality-trait-like individual differences can be used to further advance theory, methods, and application. Indeed, intraindividual variability can be a particularly rich source of information that can, for example, explain why well-established interventions do not work for certain individuals—information that would be particularly valuable for practicing consultants sourcing treatments with the greatest potential to be effective for particular clients. The main goal of this chapter is to showcase the richness that can be obtained by taking into account such individual variability, and in particular, individual variability at the personality level.

Individual differences in personality might be used to explain, for example, why certain people react better to competitive pressure in sport, or why some people engage in and adhere to regular leisure-time physical activity. The Big Five (John, Naumann, & Soto, 2008) and by extension the Five-Factor theory of personality (McCrae & Costa, 2008) has been the dominant theoretical framework for personality trait research in psychology, and by extension sport and exercise psychology (Allen, Greenlees, & Jones, 2013; Allen & Laborde, 2014). Research has demonstrated, for example, that athletes with high levels of conscientiousness tend to be more successful (Piedmont, Hill, & Blanco, 1999) and that people with high levels of conscientiousness, extraversion and openness, and low levels of neuroticism are more likely to participate in regular physical activity (Rhodes & Smith, 2006; Wilson & Dishman, 2015). However, the Big Five model is just one of many approaches to the study of individual differences and sport and exercise psychology researchers have further explored how other characteristics of individuals such as perfectionism, optimism, mental toughness, trait anger, trait anxiety, emotional intelligence, hardiness, reinvestment, and narcissism relate to the way athletes and exercisers feel, think, and behave (for an overview, see Laborde, Breuer-Weissborn, & Dosseville, 2013; Mosley & Laborde, 2015a; Roberts & Woodman, 2015).

The psychological characteristics depicting typical responses of individuals have been grouped under the umbrella term "personality-trait-like individual differences" (PTLID; Laborde et al., 2013). This grouping is valuable because it provides researchers with a concept that acknowledges individual differences that do not belong to the Big Five conceptualization of personality, but that relate closely to personality trait theories—personality being defined as "psychological qualities that contribute to an individual's enduring and distinctive patterns of feeling, thinking and behaving" (Pervin & Cervone, 2010, p. 8). In addition, it allows researchers to clearly differentiate individual differences that are psychological in nature but do not reflect personality, like individual differences in working memory capacity (Wood, Vine, & Wilson, 2015), and exclude individual differences related to other personal characteristics (eg, age, sex, socioeconomic status). The PTLID concept was introduced to offer a practical framework for investigating unique patterns or combinations of individual differences (closely related to personality) and how they might relate to thought, affect, action, and motivation. PTLID are common to all athletes and exercisers, but all will differ (at least to some extent) in their particular pattern or magnitude of PTLID. Research has demonstrated that PTLID relate to athlete psychological functioning (see Mosley & Laborde, in press) and neurophysiological processes (Mosley & Laborde, 2015b) in pressure conditions. In addition, focusing on the global PTLID pattern instead of taking into account separate trait individual differences enables to get the "global picture" related to a phenomenon, as it as been shown with positive PTLID, chronotype, and sport participation through structural equation modeling (Laborde, Guillen, Dosseville, & Allen, 2015).

For the remainder of this chapter we will explore the potential benefits of PTLID for sport and exercise psychologists at three levels: theoretical, methodological, and applied. At the theoretical level, we explore the merits of incorporating PTLID components into existing theories to further develop and constrain theoretical predictions. At the methodological level, we discuss how variations from the group mean should be explored as more that simple measurement error and can help reduce the potential for a false positive or false negative finding in the testing of hypothetical predictions. At the applied level, we use examples to consider how an understanding of PTLID patterns and associated outcomes can enable practitioner psychologists to develop more targeted interventions that fit the needs of the particular athlete or exerciser.

THEORY DEVELOPMENT AND CONSTRAINT

The aim of scientific research—and by extension scientific theories—is to discover the laws that govern nature (Ashton, 2013). Psychologists typically focus on the universals governing human behavior. However, given the complexity of human behavior, psychologists (unlike physicists) are not ultimately targeting a "theory of everything" (Hawking, 2007) that will accurately predict behavior in all instances, but rather are seeking to uncover general laws that can offer insight into particular behaviors if and when they arise. Nevertheless, a good theoretical model (and even a psychological paradigm) lends itself to expansion and refinement, and those with good empirical support should be capable of integration into other conceptual models that also have good empirical support. Here, we argue that multiple theories (particularly from the domain of sport and exercise psychology) can be refined to offer more precise theoretical predictions through the integration of PTLID and PTLID models.

To illustrate how PTLID might benefit theoretical predictions, we offer the reader an example from human decision making—the Take-the-First heuristic. The Take-the-First heuristic (Johnson & Raab, 2003; Raab & Johnson, 2007)—based on the simple heuristics approach (Gigerenzer & Todd, 1999)—was developed in the context of tactical decisions in team handball and was later extended into other performance-related domains. The Take-the-First heuristic describes how options are searched for, how option generation is stopped, and how an option is chosen. It predicts that the first option people generate is generally the best when people have expertise in the activity (Johnson & Raab, 2003). Since the Take-the-First heuristic was initially developed, its main predictions have generally been supported through a number of independent research lines (Hepler & Feltz, 2012).

According to Take-the-First heuristic, options are generated sequentially based on experience, option similarity, and environmental factors. Later, the model was refined to include the PTLID of intuition and deliberation (Raab & Laborde, 2011). This experiment showed that more intuitive people made faster and better choices—relying more on the Take-the-First heuristic—than did more deliberative people. In short, the experiment demonstrated that combining a component of PTLID (intuition) to a model of option generation (Take-the-First) provided a more accurate prediction of decision making in a sport-based decision task. Later, the Take-the-First heuristic was further developed to incorporate a neurophysiological component—namely that described in the neurovisceral integration model (Thayer, Hansen, Saus-Rose, & Johnsen, 2009). In two studies, higher activity of the parasympathetic system was found to be associated with better decisions (Laborde & Raab, 2013). This development was then superseded through the addition of a PTLID, decision reinvestment (Laborde, Raab, & Kinrade, 2014). In this experiment, participants that had a tendency to consciously control and ruminate about poor decisions had greater parasympathetic activity and made slower decisions. Through these developments it was demonstrated that decision-making performance was best understood through combining an option generation model to a model of neurophysiological processes and PTLID.

This example illustrates the value of adding PTLID components to existing theoretical frameworks—offering more accurate predictions of human decision making—and similar findings have been reported in research on working memory (Laborde, Furley, & Schempp, 2015). To further expand on this, PTLID can predict not only individuals' current state (or their resting state) but also their reactivity to a given stimulus (magnitude or direction). This notion forms a central focus in the capability model of individual differences in EEG asymmetry (Coan, Allen, & McKnight, 2006). The authors found that PTLID were more resistant to measurement error during emotional challenges than during "resting" tasks. The capability model also provided a foundation for research into heart rate variability (Laborde, Lautenbach, & Allen, 2015). In this investigation, parasympathetic activity—calculated from the high-frequency analysis of heart rate variability (HF-HRV)—was found to act as a prerequisite for coping behavior (baseline HF-HRV), an outcome of coping behavior (task HF-HRV), and a process that accompanies coping behavior [reactivity (task–baseline) HF-HRV]. It was further observed that task and baseline levels of HF-HRV were connected to a PTLID (in this case, trait emotional intelligence).

That PTLID can predict biological reactivity to stressful conditions has been reported in a number of other research investigations. For example, people reporting high Type D personality characteristics (negative affectivity and social inhibition) show greater systolic blood pressure (Nyklicek, Vorselaars, & Denollet, 2011), greater cortisol reactivity to stress (Habra, Linden, Anderson, & Weinberg, 2003), and greater low frequency heart rate variability during stressful imagery experiences (Martin et al., 2010). Extraversion and neuroticism have also been found to relate to cardiac output reactivity, blood pressure reactivity, and heart rate reactivity during experimentally induced stress (Hughes, Howard, James, & Higgins, 2011; Jonassaint et al., 2009). Taken together, the studies demonstrate that psychophysiological responses are best understood by taking into account PTLID. The importance of PTLID is not limited to cognitive or neurophysiological theories but can also, for example, be extended to motor theories such as behavioral activation and motor control accuracy (Robinson & Bresin, 2015). Particular, Robinson and Bresin found that across a variety of affective priming conditions, people scoring high in the behavioral approach system had a better motor control (ie, smaller distances from targets) that people scoring low in the behavioral approach system. Essentially, the study demonstrated that PTLID (approach motivation) helps to better understand classical theories of action control (Miller, Galanter, & Pribram, 1960; van Galen & de Jong, 1995). In short, PTLID have an important role in theory development and we recommend current conceptual models (that are well supported in sport and exercise psychology) be developed to incorporate important PTLID components. Such developments are likely to provide a more rounded understanding of psychological phenomena in sport and physical activity.

METHODOLOGICAL ADVANCEMENT

Integrating PTLID into measurement can be useful because it allows researchers to control for potential confounding variables that might interact (in unknown ways) with the particular phenomena under study. Moreover, it can help researchers understand individual reactions to a treatment that would have otherwise been considered noise in the data. From the research exploring the Take-the-First heuristic (discussed in the previous section), it became clear that more accurate predictions on decision making could be made by controlling for individual differences in intuition and deliberation (Raab & Laborde, 2011). To explain, a small sample, randomized, controlled trial—that separates people into experimental and control groups—might (through chance) have a greater number of intuitive individuals in one condition, potentially contributing to a false acceptance or false rejection of the hypothesis under study. By including an assessment of intuition (at any point before or after the experiment), this potential confounding PTLID can be statistically controlled for (Cyders et al., 2014; Voracek, Reimer, & Dressler, 2010).

The benefit of PTLID is that they are relatively stable over time meaning that they can be measured with relative ease at any time before or after an experimental study. Indeed, research exploring PTLID such as reinvestment (Laborde et al., 2014c) and emotional intelligence (Laborde, Brüll, Weber, & Anders, 2011; Laborde et al., 2015b; Laborde, Lautenbach, Allen, Herbert, & Achtzehn, 2014) have been successful in connecting physiological reactions to stress (heart rate variability) to predicted outcomes after controlling for PTLID. The decision on the important PTLID to include in research designs should be determined by theory, and this further emphasizes the importance of theoretical models to incorporate PTLID. We now turn our attention to the importance of PTLID in applied practice.

APPLIED PRACTICE

At the beginning of this chapter we discussed how PTLID are often considered little more than simple noise in the data in experimental studies. To illustrate why this can be problematic for practicing consultants, we can use an example from sport-based personality research. In an investigation of dynamometer (physical strength) performance, it was found that emotions relate differently to performance, depending on the personality traits of the individual (Woodman et al., 2009). Moreover, the experiment demonstrated that anger had a greater positive effect on performance for participants with high levels of extraversion. It is easy to see how findings such as these can be of value to practicing psychologists—assuming these findings are independently and consistently replicated, a performance practitioner might consider targeting increases in anger as a means of facilitating performance, but would no doubt take into account the personality (extraversion) of the client before considering whether the intervention is likely to be successful.

An important finding from independent lines of PTLID inquiry is that although PTLID are relatively stable over time and across situations, they do appear open to modification either through life experiences or training. For example, participation in physical activity has been found to relate to more stable personality traits (Big Five) during adulthood and old age (Stephan, Sutin, & Terracciano, 2014), and emotional intelligence does appear open to modification through targeted emotional intelligence training (Barlow & Banks, 2014; Campo, Laborde, & Weckemann, 2015; Crombie, Lombard, & Noakes, 2011; Campo, Laborde & Mosley, in press). Since PTLID are associated with many positive health and performance outcomes (Roberts, Kuncel, Shiner, Caspi, & Goldberg, 2007), practitioners' understanding of the conditions under which PTLID can be developed or maintained is particularly important when targeting positive individual functioning in athletes and exercisers.

Lastly, an understanding of PTLID is important not only for the content of practitioner interventions but also for the manner in which those interventions are delivered (Allen et al., 2013). To explain, research has demonstrated that people with particular PTLID are better capable of interacting with others (Cuperman & Ickes, 2009) and this extends to the client–practitioner relationship. Clients with particular PTLID may be more or less responsive to intervention suggestions, or have an easier or more difficult time in developing a rapport with their consultant. An understanding of PTLID in client–consultant interactions can assist in maximizing the likelihood of intervention success. Further to this, as mentioned in previous work (Allen & Laborde, 2014; Laborde, Dosseville, Guillén, & Chávez, 2014), a consultant might consider administering a PTLID assessment measure (that offers numeric scores for PTLID components) when beginning work with a new client in order to deliberate on the best practices that fit the needs of the client (including their own mannerisms in engaging with that client) and also to consider the likelihood of success for particular interventions. Furthermore, applied research is needed to maximize the value of PTLID tests for consultation and intervention.

CONCLUSIONS

Sport and exercise psychology targets an understanding of the universals in human behavior that relate to sport and physical activity—for example, understanding the neurophysiological processes governing stress in competitive athletic situations, or understanding the environmental conditions that contribute to the development of obsessive and compulsive exercise behavior. However, we should not forget that every individual differs in PTLID patterns and magnitude. Consideration of this variability may be particularly beneficial for the development of the field not only at the theoretical level, but also at the methodological and applied levels. An understanding of PTLID can assist us in understanding what is hidden behind an average reaction—for example, why some people thrive and others nosedive in the presence of considerable competitive pressure. There are a number of steps that might be useful in developing this area of research inquiry: first, researchers might start to systematically explore what has been found in published research to date, and could use this information to start formulating potential conceptual frameworks. Then, they could start to identify the most important PTLID for particular contexts and populations. Finally, they could begin to reflect in more detail on the application of PTLID. To conclude, we can condense our main take-home message in the form of a metaphor—that bringing PTLID to the forefront of experimental research is a little like refining our ear to perceive the nice melody that appeared at first as being simple noise in the background.

REFERENCES

Allen, M. S., & Laborde, S. (2014). The role of personality in sport and physical activity. *Current Directions in Psychological Science, 23*, 460–465.

Allen, M. S., Greenlees, I., & Jones, M. V. (2013). Personality in sport: a comprehensive review. *International Review of Sport and Exercise Psychology, 6*, 184–208.

Ashton, M. (2013). Introduction. In M. Ashton (Ed.), *Individual differences and personality.* Amsterdam, The Netherlands: Elsevier, pp. xix–xxiv.

Barlow, A., & Banks, A. P. (2014). Using emotional intelligence in coaching high-performance athletes: a randomised controlled trial. *Coaching: An International Journal of Theory, Research and Practice, 7*, 132–139.

Campo, M., Laborde, S., & Weckemann, S. (2015). Emotional intelligence training: implications for performance and health. In A. M. Colombus (Ed.), *Advances in psychology research* (pp. 75–92). New York, NY: Nova Publishers.

Campo, M., Laborde, S., & Mosley, E. (in press). Emotional intelligence training in team sports: the influence of a season long intervention program on trait emotional intelligence. *Journal of Individual Differences*.

Coan, J. A., Allen, J. J., & McKnight, P. E. (2006). A capability model of individual differences in frontal EEG asymmetry. *Biological Psychology, 72*, 198–207.

Crombie, D., Lombard, C., & Noakes, T. D. (2011). Increasing emotional intelligence in cricketers: an intervention study. *International Journal of Sports Science & Coaching, 6*, 69–86, Available from <Go to ISI>://WOS:000288297400015.

Cronbach, L. J. (1957). The two disciplines of scientific psychology. *American Psychologist, 12*, 671–684.

Cuperman, R., & Ickes, W. (2009). Big Five predictors of behavior and perceptions in initial dyadic interactions: personality similarity helps extraverts and introverts, but hurts "disagreeables". *Journal of Personality and Social Psychology, 97*, 667–684.

Cyders, M. A., Dzemidzic, M., Eiler, W. J., Coskunpinar, A., Karyadi, K., & Kareken, D. A. (2014). Negative urgency and ventromedial prefrontal cortex responses to alcohol cues: fMRI evidence of emotion-based impulsivity. *Alcoholism, 38*, 409–417.

Gigerenzer, G., & Todd, P. M. (1999). *Simple heuristics that make us smart*. Oxford: Oxford University Press.

Habra, M. E., Linden, W., Anderson, J. C., & Weinberg, J. (2003). Type D personality is related to cardiovascular and neuroendocrine reactivity to acute stress. *Journal of Psychosomatic Research, 55*, 235–245, Available from http://www.ncbi.nlm.nih.gov/pubmed/12932797.

Hawking, S. (2007). *The theory of everything*. Mumbai, India: Jaico Publishing House.

Hepler, T. J., & Feltz, D. L. (2012). Take the first heuristic, self-efficacy, and decision-making in sport. *Journal of Experimental Psychology, 18*, 154–161.

Hughes, B. M., Howard, S., James, J. E., & Higgins, N. M. (2011). Individual differences in adaptation of cardiovascular responses to stress. *Biological Psychology, 86*, 129–136.

John, O. P., Naumann, L. P., & Soto, C. J. (2008). Paradigm shift to the integrative big five trait taxonomy: history, measurement, and conceptual issues. In O. P. John, R. W. Robins, & L. A. Pervin (Eds.), *Handbook of personality: Theory and research* (3rd ed., pp. 114–158). New York, NY: Guilford Press.

Johnson, J. G., & Raab, M. (2003). Take the First: option-generation and resulting choices. *Organizational Behavior and Human Decision Processes, 91*, 215–229.

Jonassaint, C. R., Why, Y. P., Bishop, G. D., Tong, E. M., Diong, S. M., Enkelmann, H. C., ... Ang, J. (2009). The effects of neuroticism and extraversion on cardiovascular reactivity during a mental and an emotional stress task. *International Journal of Psychophysiology, 74*, 274–279.

Kanai, R., & Rees, G. (2011). The structural basis of inter-individual differences in human behaviour and cognition. *Nature Reviews Neuroscience, 12*, 231–242.

Laborde, S., & Raab, M. (2013). The tale of hearts and reason: the influence of mood on decision making. *Journal of Sport & Exercise Psychology, 35*(4), 339–357, Available from http://www.ncbi.nlm.nih.gov/pubmed/23966445.

Laborde, S., Brüll, A., Weber, J., & Anders, L. S. (2011). Trait emotional intelligence in sports: a protective role against stress through heart rate variability? *Personality and Individual Differences, 51*, 23–27.

Laborde, S., Breuer-Weissborn, J., & Dosseville, F. (2013). Personality-trait-like individual differences in athletes. In C. Mohiyeddini (Ed.), *Advances in the psychology of sports and exercise* (pp. 25–60). New York, NY: Nova.

Laborde, S., Dosseville, F., Guillén, F., & Chávez, E. (2014a). Validity of the trait emotional intelligence questionnaire in sports and its links with performance satisfaction. *Psychology of Sport and Exercise, 15*, 481–490.

Laborde, S., Lautenbach, F., Allen, M. S., Herbert, C., & Achtzehn, S. (2014b). The role of trait emotional intelligence in emotion regulation and performance under pressure. *Personality and Individual Differences, 57*, 43–47.

Laborde, S., Raab, M., & Kinrade, N. P. (2014c). Is the ability to keep your mind sharp under pressure reflected in your heart? Evidence for the neurophysiological bases of decision reinvestment. *Biological Psychology, 100C*, 34–42.

Laborde, S., Furley, P., & Schempp, C. (2015a). The relationship between working memory, reinvestment, and heart rate variability. *Physiology & Behavior, 139*, 430–436.

Laborde, S., Lautenbach, F., & Allen, M. S. (2015b). The contribution of coping-related variables and heart rate variability to visual search performance under pressure. *Physiology & Behavior, 139*, 532–540.

Laborde, S., Guillen, F., Dosseville, F., & Allen, M. S. (2015). Chronotype, sport participation, and positive personality-trait-like individual differences. *Chronobiology International, 32*, 942–951.

Martin, L. A., Doster, J. A., Critelli, J. W., Lambert, P. L., Purdum, M., Powers, C., & Prazak, M. (2010). Ethnicity and Type D personality as predictors of heart rate variability. *International Journal of Psychophysiology, 76*, 118–121.

McCrae, R. R., & Costa, P. T. (2008). The Five-Factor theory of personality. In O. P. John, R. W. Robins, & L. A. Pervin (Eds.), *Handbook of personality: Theory and research* (3rd ed., pp. 159–181). New York, NY: Guilford Press.

Miller, G. A., Galanter, E., & Pribram, K. H. (1960). *Plans and the structure of behavior*. New York, NY: Henry Holt and Co.

Mosley, E., & Laborde, S. (2015a). Performing under pressure: influence of personality-trait-like individual differences. In M. Raab, B. Lobinger, S. Hoffmann, A. Pizzera, & S. Laborde (Eds.), *Performance psychology: Perception, action, cognition, and emotion*. Amsterdam, The Netherlands: Elsevier.

Mosley, E., & Laborde, S. (2015b). Performing with all my heart: heart rate variability and its relationship with personality-trait-like-individual-differences (PTLIDs) in pressurized performance situations. In S. Walters (Ed.), *Heart rate variability (HRV): Prognostic significance, risk factors and clinical applications* (pp. 45–60). New York: NY: Nova Publishers.

Mosley, E., & Laborde, S. (2015). Performing under pressure: influence of personality-trait-like individual differences. In M. Raab, B. Lobinger, S. Hoffmann, A. Pizzera & S. Laborde (Eds.), *Performance psychology: Perception, action, cognition, and emotion* (pp. 292–314). Amsterdam, the Netherlands: Elsevier.

Nyklicek, I., Vorselaars, A., & Denollet, J. (2011). Type D personality and cardiovascular function in daily life of people without documented cardiovascular disease. *International Journal of Psychophysiology, 80*, 139–142.

Pervin, L. A., & Cervone, D. (2010). *Personality: Theory and research* (11th ed.). New York, NY: Wiley.

Piedmont, R. L., Hill, D. C., & Blanco, S. (1999). Predicting athletic performance using the Five-Factor model of personality. *Personality and Individual Differences, 27*, 769–777.

Raab, M., & Johnson, J. G. (2007). Expertise-based differences in search and option-generation strategies. *Journal of Experimental Psychology, 13*, 158–170.

Raab, M., & Laborde, S. (2011). When to blink and when to think: preference for intuitive decisions results in faster and better tactical choices. *Research Quarterly for Exercise and Sport, 82*, 89–98.

Rhodes, R. E., & Smith, N. E. (2006). Personality correlates of physical activity: a review and meta-analysis. *British Journal of Sports Medicine, 40*, 958–965.

Roberts, R., & Woodman, T. (2015). Contemporary personality perspectives in sport psychology. In S. D. Mellalieu, & S. Hanton (Eds.), *Contemporary advances in sport psychology: A review* (pp. 1–27). New York, NY: Routledge.

Roberts, B. W., Kuncel, N. R., Shiner, R., Caspi, A., & Goldberg, L. R. (2007). The power of personality: the comparative validity of personality traits, socioeconomic status, and cognitive ability for predicting important life outcomes. *Perspectives on Psychological Science, 2*, 313–345.

Robinson, M. D., & Bresin, K. (2015). Personality and action control: BAS reward predicts motor control accuracy. *Personality and Individual Differences, 83*, 214–218.

Stephan, Y., Sutin, A. R., & Terracciano, A. (2014). Physical activity and personality development across adulthood and old age: evidence from two longitudinal studies. *Journal of Research in Personality, 49*, 1–7.

Thayer, J. F., Hansen, A. L., Saus-Rose, E., & Johnsen, B. H. (2009). Heart rate variability, prefrontal neural function, and cognitive performance: the neurovisceral integration perspective on self-regulation, adaptation, and health. *Annals of Behavioral Medicine, 37*, 141–153.

van Galen, G. P., & de Jong, W. P. (1995). Fitts' law as the outcome of a dynamic noise filtering model of motor control. *Human Movement Science, 14*, 539–571.

Vogel, E. K., & Awh, E. (2008). How to exploit diversity for scientific gain: using individual differences to constrain cognitive theory. *Current Directions in Psychological Science, 17*, 171–176.

Voracek, M., Reimer, B., & Dressler, S. G. (2010). Digit ratio (2D:4D) predicts sporting success among female fencers independent from physical, experience, and personality factors. *Scandinavian Journal of Medicine and Science in Sports, 20*, 853–860.

Wilson, K. E., & Dishman, R. K. (2015). Personality and physical activity: a systematic review and meta-analysis. *Personality and Individual Differences, 72*, 230–242.

Wood, G., Vine, S. J., & Wilson, M. R. (2015). Working memory capacity, controlled attention and aiming performance under pressure. *Psychological Research*, 1–8.

Woodman, T., Davis, P. A., Hardy, L., Callow, N., Glasscock, I., & Yuill-Proctor, J. (2009). Emotions and sport performance: an exploration of happiness, hope, and anger. *Journal of Sport & Exercise Psychology, 31*, 169–188.

Chapter 10

Promoting Acculturation Through Sport: An Ethnic-Cultural Identity Approach

Eleftheria Morela*,†, Antonis Hatzigeorgiadis*,
Xavier Sanchez**, Anne-Marie Elbe†

*Department of Physical Education and Sport Science, University of Thessaly, Trikala, Greece;
**Department of Medical and Sport Sciences, University of Cumbria, Lancaster, United Kingdom;
†Department of Nutrition, Exercise and Sports, University of Copenhagen, Copenhagen, Denmark

INTRODUCTION

Migration, a timeless phenomenon related to either seasonal or permanent movement of people, has been vital to human history, cultures, and civilizations. In 2013, the number of migrants worldwide was over 231 million—which accounts for 3% of the world population (United Nations, 2013). In light of constant economic, social, and political changes that occur globally, migration appears as a major challenge for many societies and thus has become a priority in the social–political agenda in most counties. The integration of migrants is of vital importance in order to maintain social cohesion—with emphasis on diversity management under conditions of equality and respect for human rights (Entzinger & Biezeveld, 2003).

The process of adjusting to a new culture and of eventually integrating migrants into their local communities and into the wider society in general has always been of fundamental importance. In recent years, the idea that sport participation can potentially be an effective socializing agent that facilitates the integration of migrants into the communities they live in has received political attention (Eitzen & Sage, 2003). For instance, 20 EU countries have lately been using sport as a way of increasing multicultural understanding (European Commission, 2004) and the EU White Paper on Sport demonstrates how sport can be used as an intervention strategy for the integration of migrants and minority groups (European Commission, 2007).

Sport and Exercise Psychology Research. http://dx.doi.org/10.1016/B978-0-12-803634-1.00010-8

Sport is discussed in connection with the migration phenomenon and with the process of adjusting to a new culture (Grove & Dodder, 1982). Eitzen and Sage (2003) stated that sport is among the few social activities that are globally recognized as a vehicle for bringing people together. Such claims can be attributed to certain characteristics of sport: (1) the large number of children and youth involved; (2) that sport participation is, at least for the vast majority of individuals, a volitional behavior; (3) the mixed demographic and socioeconomic backgrounds of those participating; and (4) its interactive and highly communicative nature. In addition, and in particular with regard to the integrative role of sport, it has been shown that contact and sharing across members of different groups may reduce negative intergroup attitudes (Allport, 1954) and enhance mutual acceptance (Amir, 1969); in particular, under conditions of both equality and the pursuit of shared goals among members (Brown, Vivian, & Hewstone, 1999). These conditions can be accommodated within the context of sport. Furthermore, according to the social identity theory (Tajfel, Billig, Bundy, & Flament, 1971), once people identify themselves as members of a group and find themselves within appropriate environments, they can develop a sense of collective identity, which subsequently influences their social behavior.

A growing body of research stresses that, in addition to improving physical health, sport plays a significant social and inclusive role in society (Seippel, 2002) as well as a positive role in personal and moral development (Bredemeir & Shields, 2006). More specifically, it has been argued that sport provides an arena for the development of social skills, such as cooperation and socialization (Wuest & Lombardo, 1994), intergroup relations (Wankel & Berger, 1990), and citizenship (Elley & Kirk, 2002). Especially team sports have been shown to promote the development of skills like trust (Priest, 1998), empathy (Moore, 2002), personal responsibility (Hellison, 2003), and cooperation (Miller, Bredemeier, & Shields, 1997). The need for individuals to work collaboratively in order to achieve the common team goal is believed to be the reason. Furthermore, team sports are believed to offer a strong feeling of belonging and identification. In addition to positive social effects, there is evidence that sport participation can lead to positive character building experiences (Bredemeir & Shields, 2006), and can be used as an effective tool for the enhancement of moral behaviors in athletes, as well as for the promotion of moral development in children (for a review, see Shields & Bredemeier, 2007).

Recently, there has been a growing policy interest in the use of sport as a potential method of developing social interaction and building citizenship in socially excluded individuals or groups, focusing mostly on disadvantaged and underrepresented young people (Kelly, 2011; Parnell, Pringle, Widdop, & Zwolimsky, 2015; Ryom & Stelter, 2015). Sport is promoted as a "positive activity" within mainstream policy for children and young people (HM Treasury, 2007). Indeed, engagement in sport activities is believed to facilitate social inclusion by both offering individuals a place to meet (Keller, Lamprocht, & Stamm, 1998) and giving them a sense of belonging, whether it is to a team, a club, or a wider community (Ennis, 1999).

The purpose of this chapter is to address the role of sport in the promotion of social integration among individuals and groups with different ethnic and cultural backgrounds in order to better understand the acculturation process and to identify factors that may facilitate the acculturation process through sport participation. Acculturation is defined as the process of cultural and psychological change that follows intercultural contact (Berry, 2003). To that end, the chapter will take an individual differences approach; that is, it will focus on specific identity factors (eg, ethnic and cultural identity) of both the dominant and nondominant sport participants. First, we will introduce relevant terminology, then describe Berry's integration framework. Subsequently, we will present empirical evidence based on the ethnic-cultural identity approach, and finally discuss directions for future research.

Social Inclusion and Exclusion

In ethnic and migration studies, social inclusion is often conceptualized in terms of social capital. The Organization for Economic Co-operation and Development (OECD, 2001) defined social capital as the "networks together with shared norms, values and understanding which facilitate cooperation within or among groups" (p. 41). In contrast, social exclusion is referred to as "the multiple and changing factors resulting in people being excluded from the normal exchanges, practices and rights of modern society" (Commission of the European Communities, 1993, p. 1). The long-standing belief in the potential of sport to promote tolerance and combat social exclusion (Committee for the Development of Sport, 1998) has led to the development of sport-based programs that might promote social inclusion in multicultural societies. However, social inclusion and social exclusion are challenged concepts (Levitas et al., 2007) and the processes through which the sports-based intervention programs might facilitate social inclusion require further investigation.

Acculturation

As mentioned earlier, acculturation is the process of cultural and psychological change that follows intercultural contact (Berry, 2003). Cultural changes refer to changes in a group's customs, and in their economic and political life, while psychological changes refer to changes in individuals' attitudes toward the acculturation process, their cultural identities, and their social behaviors in relation to the groups in contact (Phinney, 2003). These changes can take place in all groups and all individuals in contact. Berry (2006) argued that both migrants and host communities are influenced and transformed by their intercultural contact and that they have to find a way to adapt to cultural diversity. Therefore, intercultural relations are viewed as mutual and reciprocal, and all groups have to face two basic issues in the acculturation process based on the distinction between orientations toward one's own group, and those toward other groups (Berry, 1980). Accordingly, Berry (1997) proposed that there are two independent dimensions underlying the process of acculturation: *cultural maintenance* and *contact and participation*. *Cultural maintenance* refers to the degree to which people wish to maintain their heritage culture and identity. *Contact and participation* refers to the degree to which people seek involvement with the larger society. Findings from sport and migration studies support Berry's (1997) conceptual model for acculturation; migrants and minority groups use sport as a vehicle to either maintain their cultural identity or interact with the dominant culture (Hatzigeorgiadis, Morela, Elbe, & Sanchez, 2013). Subsequently, we briefly discuss findings within the sport literature that have either challenged or supported the dual cultural role of sport.

SPORT AND ACCULTURATION: CAN SPORT ENHANCE INTERCULTURAL RELATIONS?

The potential of sport to positively contribute to improving a range of social challenges is widely celebrated (Bloyce & Smith, 2010; Coalter, 2007): It is stated that sport participation can facilitate social inclusion (eg, reduce crime, develop communities, and improve health; Coalter, 2007). Sport has been described as, among others, an arena for equal opportunities and racial equality (Green & Hardman, 2000) and as a field wherein to reinforce understanding and respect of cultural diversity (Niessen, 2000). To date, research on the integrative role of sport in plural societies is limited, and findings seem ambiguous. A number of studies have supported the notion that sport can facilitate the relationships between groups (cultural interaction; eg, Rosenberg, Feijgin, & Talmor, 2003), while others indicate that sport is linked to both cultural interaction and cultural maintenance (Stodolska & Alexandris, 2004). Finally, some findings reveal that sport participation may lead to undesired outcomes and may even highlight ethnic and cultural differences and evoke tensions (Krouwel, Boostra, Duyvendak, & Veldboer, 2006). Therefore, we are going to present the most relevant findings with regards to the potential role of sport to either facilitate and/ or hinder the acculturation process.

A number of studies have supported the role of sport in facilitating and promoting cultural interaction across a diverse array of contexts, cultures, and participants. Among others, several studies have highlighted numerous benefits regarding sport participation in minority groups, such as overcoming social barriers and improving social networks with the majority group (Rosenberg et al., 2003; Guerin, Diiriye, Corrigan, & Guerin, 2003) as well as improving language skills (Ito, Nogawa, Kitamura, & Walker, 2011). Furthermore, it has been shown that sport participation can help individuals of minority groups adapt well to the stressful acculturation process, and feel included in the dominant society (Stack & Iwasaki, 2009). Sport can also, indirectly, increase structural integration, as individuals of minority groups are led to participate in other areas of society (Walseth & Fasting, 2004).

The previously mentioned studies have supported the role of sport in facilitating cultural interaction. However, according to Berry's (1980, 1997) framework, the goal of integration requires, in addition, the maintenance of cultural heritage. For individuals or groups who have preserved their cultural heritage, the cultural interaction provided through sport can facilitate integration. However, for individuals who have been absorbed by the dominant culture, integration involves seeking association with members of their own group to initiate or preserve links with their cultural traditions. In that context, a number of studies have supported the dual cultural role of sport. Their findings indicate that migrants can use sport activities to either interact with the dominant culture by taking part in activities with the mainstream population, or by socializing with their own community and preserving their ethnic values by participating in sports with individuals of the same ethnic background (Stodolska & Alexandris, 2004; Lee, 2005). It is not entirely clear whether the cultural maintenance and cultural interaction objectives can be accomplished in the same sport environment; this would mostly depend on the identity and the goals of the team members. However, research has identified both cultural functions (Allen, Drane, Byon & Mohn, 2010), and evidence suggests that, given the appropriate mixed composition of a team, the features of the sport environment can help promote integration through both cultural functions of sport.

However, there are findings that have challenged the role of sport as an inclusion agent; members of minority groups, occasionally, prefer to participate in sports with members of their own group, thus strengthening their sense of belonging and reinforcing their ethnic identity through homogeneous sport activities (Krouwel et al., 2006; Lee, Dunlap, & Scott, 2011). In addition, other researchers highlight that migrants, within the sport context, can feel marginalized and fail to develop friendships with their teammates (Walseth, 2008) because they experience social discrimination due to language barriers, unfamiliarity with the activities, and origin-related prejudice (Doherty & Taylor, 2007).

Furthermore, it is important to be aware that sport cannot automatically improve intercultural interaction and tolerance. Some findings even suggest that sport participation may lead to undesirable outcomes such as aggression, hostile attitudes, and polarity (Krouwel et al., 2006). Hatzigeorgiadis et al. (2013) listed a number of potential explanations for the inconsistent findings and address the limitations of these studies with regard to theoretical underpinning, study design, and sample size. Furthermore, Hatzigeorgiadis et al. (2013) discussed future research directions, which could enhance our understanding of the integrative role of sport.

Based on an extensive literature review, the previously mentioned researchers argued that a possible reason for the different findings with regard to the integrative role of sport can be the lack of and/or unclear use of a theoretical framework for investigating the phenomenon. Another important conclusion is that most of the studies were qualitative and hence aimed at generating rather than testing hypotheses. Furthermore, the number of participants in the qualitative studies was small, making inferences for a larger group impossible. In line with the lack of theoretical underpinning, the investigated factors were of an outcome nature (eg, did the participants improve their language skills, did more contact take place between groups, did sport participation increase?). These variables, however, do not assess the underlying variables responsible for successful acculturation, for example, in line with an individual differences approach. With regard to the small number of quantitative studies, it can be stated that they were basically descriptive, rather than hypothesis testing and provided limited information regarding the instruments and the measures developed to assess acculturation.

A further consequence evolving from the limited volume of research concerns the societal context within which acculturation occurs that might influence individuals' integration. Thus, the different (demographic) characteristics of the individuals participating in the acculturation process should be considered as well as the cultural environment of the host society and its background in receiving incoming individuals (eg, differences between or within continents, such as the United States, northern Europe, southern Europe) (Bourhis, Moise, Perreault, & Senecal, 1997). To date, these differences have not yet been addressed. As van Osch and Breugelmans (2012) recently suggested, perceived differences by the members of the involved groups may be a determinant of intergroup relations in culturally diverse societies. Accordingly, the role of sport may differ from group to group, given individual differences, and depending on the dominant cultural environment.

ETHNIC-CULTURAL IDENTITY FRAMEWORK: INDIVIDUAL DIFFERENCES APPROACH

Taking into consideration the shortcomings identified in the previous sections and trying to create a stable theoretical basis for developing improved and sound research on migrants' acculturation through sport, we propose the use of a framework that focuses on the underlying factors for acculturation in line with a focus on individual differences. This approach is based on Berry's (1980, 1997) seminal work, which proposes that migrants' integration involves the goal of interacting with the host society and adopting aspects of its culture (cultural interaction), while maintaining the links with the traditions and the heritage of the original culture (cultural maintenance). This two-dimensional model of acculturation for pluralistic societies is based on the principles of cultural maintenance and contact participation (Berry, 1980, 1997). This model describes different intercultural strategies based on the interaction of (1) individuals' wish to maintain their ethnic identity and (2) their desire to interact with the broader culture. When examined among the nondominant population, these are described and classified as *acculturation attitudes* and, when examined among the dominant population, as *acculturation expectations*.

With regard to *acculturation attitudes*, the impulse of nondominant groups to distance themselves from their original ethnic-cultural background and to seek absorption by the dominant culture is described as *assimilation*. In contrast, avoiding interaction with the host culture and remaining attached to the original ethnic identity is described as *separation*. Seeking to both maintain ethnic-cultural heritage and to interact with the dominant culture is described as *integration*, and is considered the most effective acculturation strategy. Finally, showing little interest in both interaction with the dominant culture and in maintaining one's original ethnic-cultural background is described as *marginalization*.

In addition, to the perspective of the incoming ethno-cultural group, this model identifies the importance of the host society's willingness to accept such populations, based on a similar two-dimensional model. Respectively, with regard to *acculturation expectations*, when the dominant group seeks the assimilation of migrants, this is described as *melting pot*; when separation is forced by the dominant group, this is described as *segregation*; when the dominant group seeks integration, this is described as *multiculturalism*; finally, when marginalization is imposed by the dominant group, this is described as *exclusion*. According to Berry (2011), this framework can be used to compare individuals and their ethno-cultural groups as well as the nondominant groups and the larger society, in order to enhance acculturation research.

In the acculturation literature, Berry's model, which has attracted the most interest, is considered the most effective in explaining, from a social–psychological perspective, the acculturation processes in multicultural societies (Bourhis et al., 1997). Ting-Toomey et al. (2000), taking into consideration Berry's framework about migrants' acculturation, presented an ethnic-cultural identity salience framework to facilitate understanding and provided a means for intercultural research. Within this conceptualization, ethnic identity is described as the importance attached to one's own ethnic background, its values and practices, and reflects the cultural maintenance dimension of Berry's model; whereas cultural identity is described as the importance attached to the broader cultural context and reflects the cultural interaction dimension of Berry's model. Both concepts address a specific aspect of individual differences, namely one's cultural/ethnic identity. Ting-Toomey et al.'s (2000) conceptual model comprises two dimensions of ethnic identity, which are a sense of *belonging* to a group and *feelings of fringe*, and two dimensions of cultural identity, which are *assimilation* and *lack of interaction*. Precisely, *belonging* is indicative of high ethnic identity. It refers to the sense of recognition and reveals the extent to which a person feels attached to his/her own ethnic group. The dimension *feelings of fringe* reflects low ethnic identity, and refers to the confusion a person feels concerning his/her ethnic identity. *Assimilation* reflects a high cultural identity and refers to the level of identification of individuals with the dominant culture they live in. Finally, *lack of interaction* reflects low cultural identity and refers to the absence of interaction among the members of different groups. Ting-Toomey et al. (2000) suggested that, depending on ethnic and cultural identity salience, individuals evaluate their group and the culture they live in, and may be more or less involved in ethnic or cultural practices.

Preliminary evidence for the use of the ethnic-cultural identity framework in sports literature was provided for the physical education context. Kouli and Papaioannou (2009) explored the relationship between motivational climate in physical education classes and ethnic-cultural identity among culturally diverse high school students in Greece. Findings revealed that task orientation and a mastery-oriented motivational climate, which places emphasis on learning and improving skills on the basis of self-referenced criteria, was related to cultural maintenance and to cultural interaction, which have been linked to integration. In contrast, ego orientation and a performance-oriented motivational climate, which place emphasis on outperforming others based on comparative criteria, were related to lack of interaction and feelings of fringe, which have been linked to marginalization and separation (Kouli & Papaioannou, 2009). These findings suggest that the environment in which the activity takes place, rather than the participation in the activity/sport per se, may well be the key to promoting integration through sport.

Based on an initiative by the European Federation of Sport Psychology (FEPSAC), a research program was developed to further explore the integrative role of sport, with particular interest in identifying the factors that may regulate the integrative power of sport for both host and migrant populations (Hatzigeorgiadis et al., 2013). This research program has, to date, involved five European countries (Denmark, Germany, Greece, Spain, and the United Kingdom), and progressed through a number of stages, from instrument development and exploratory descriptive data collection to the assessment of sport-related factors that may contribute to the promotion of sport as an integrative agent in multicultural and multiethnic societies. Currently, the research program is investigating if sport environment interventions can promote the integration of migrants. These studies have focused on individual differences of the participants and have investigated whether sport participation can affect the construction of ethnic-cultural identity and the acculturation process. The research was developed within the theoretical model provided by Berry (1980, 1997) and the conceptualization of the Ethnic-Cultural Identity Salience questionnaire developed by Ting-Toomey et al. (2000), as adapted for youth and used in the physical education context by Kouli and Papaioannou (2009).The key findings of this project are described and discussed next.

Elbe et al. (2012) examined sport factors related to the ethnic and cultural identity of young athletes with nondominant background in different European countries. The results showed differences among migrants in ethnic-cultural identity dimension as a function of sex and type of sport, with females and team sport athletes scoring higher on assimilation and lower on lack of interaction, thus showing a more integrative profile compared to male and individual sport athletes. The superiority of females over males on integrative patterns can be attributed to the greater importance female athletes place on the social aspects of sport participation (Flood & Hellstedt, 1991). In addition, team sport athletes experience greater interaction through their sport, due to the nature of the sport, and may have developed more socially adaptive attitudes. Lastly, a significant effect was identified for countries with several differences emerging across them on ethnic and cultural identity, suggesting that the structures of the different countries, and the tradition in receiving migrants should be considered for the interpretation of the findings.

Morela, Hatzigeorgiadis, Kouli, Elbe and Sanchez (2013) reported on the relationship between team cohesion and ethnic-cultural identity in young migrant athletes (aged 13–18) living, but not born, in Greece. Findings showed that cohesion negatively predicted feelings of fringe and lack of interaction, which suggests that sport participation, particularly in cohesive teams, can facilitate the development of an adaptive identity toward the goal of social integration in migrant adolescents, thus stressing the important role structures of the sport environment play in promoting participants' integration.

Elbe et al. (in press) examined the role of the team motivational environment in predicting ethnic and cultural identity in two heterogeneous samples: one from Spain, including young South American athletes playing on teams consisting of South Americans only, and one from Greece including migrants, mostly from Eastern Europe and the Balkans, participating in mixed teams. Considerable differences in the dimensions of ethnic and cultural identity were identified between the subsamples from the two countries. Examination of differences in ethnic and cultural identity between the two samples showed that migrants playing on mixed teams scored higher on feelings of fringe, but also on assimilation; but lower on lack of interaction, compared to migrants playing on pure migrant teams. These findings suggest that the athletes sampled in Greece were more confused about their ethnic identity and were seeking contact with the host culture, possibly through sport, whereas the participants in the sample in Spain had stronger ethnic identity and were interested in maintaining or strengthening this identity through sport participation. For migrants in mixed teams (Greece), a positive motivational environment (task motivational climate and autonomy support) was linked to an adaptive integrative profile, whereas no links emerged between motivational environment and ethnic-cultural identity for athletes playing on pure migrant teams (Spain). For the sample from Greece, findings supported that appropriate sport environments can promote integrative patterns of cultural identity. The lack of significant findings for the sample from Spain was attributed to the South American identity of the teams, which possibly strengthened ethnic belonging and weakened tendencies for interaction with the larger (Spanish) culture. These findings, once again, stress the need to consider the team composition (eg, how many dominants/nondominants) in addition to the environment that can be shaped from the coach in promoting the integrative role of sport.

As mentioned earlier in the chapter, research should also focus on the dominant culture and the attitudes of the receiving society toward acculturation. Morela, Hatzigeorgiadis, Elbe, Papaioannou, and Sanchez (2016) examined acculturation attitudes and perceptions of the host population as a function of sport participation and the role of motivational environment in the acculturation process of Greek adolescents. The findings showed that students who were participating in organized sport activities had more positive attitudes toward contact with individuals coming from different cultural backgrounds compared to their counterparts who did not engage in sports. In addition, the results revealed a significant effect for the city, with adolescents living in urban areas (Thessaloniki) appearing more receptive to migrant's interaction with the host culture than those who lived in the country (Trikala) where daily intercultural interactions are scarce. In addition, important findings emerged with regards to the structure of the sport environment, where mastery-oriented motivational climate and the satisfaction of the athlete's basic needs for autonomy, relatedness, and competence were positively related to the host community's attitudes toward migrants' acculturation. Overall, the findings of the present study suggest the participation in organized sport activities may contribute to shaping participants' attitudes toward acculturation but it seems to depend on the environment in which the activities take place. A sport environment manipulated in a way that encourages cooperation and socialization of all individuals and acknowledges athletes' feelings and attitudes can facilitate acculturation and promote multiculturalism in culturally diverse societies.

Research has identified team sport participation as a promising approach to socially integrating individuals from diverse cultural backgrounds (Hatzigeorgiadis et al., 2013). It has also been argued that sport participation may induce desired socio-moral outcomes, but that these outcomes depend on the environment within which sport takes place (Bredemeir & Shields, 2006). Adopting such a perspective, and based on the aforementioned findings, two interventions were recently developed and implemented. Ryom and Stelter (2015) investigated the participation of young migrants in football teams as a social tool to develop social capability, identity, and active citizenship in an area with major social challenges in Denmark. The study was conducted in Copenhagen's most diverse district Nørrebro, where approximately 24% of the population is of migrant background. A 2-year intervention study was conducted at a lower secondary school aiming to develop life skills and social resilience of young migrant boys by playing football and by being part of a sport team. The intervention included three weekly training sessions (1–1½ h), matches, and coach education in addition to a number of social activities outside of the football training. Qualitative interviews and observations showed that participants were able to develop their social capabilities in the school environment. By comparing the interviews before, during, and after the intervention, participants indicated a more profound understanding of the structure of the local society. Participants in the coach education stressed better self-confidence, commitment, and collaboration skills. The interviews also showed that social and cultural coherence was enhanced by the intervention. The results of this study indicated that football can be a tool to promote active citizenship and possibly also personal development in an area with major social challenges.

In the physical education context, Dankers and colleagues explored the extent to which team sport activities within multicultural PE classes in Denmark can facilitate the social inclusion of students with differing cultural backgrounds (Dankers, Elbe, Sanchez, Otten, & van Yperen, 2015). A 4-month physical education class intervention program targeting the class motivational climate was implemented. More specifically, by applying the TARGET framework (Ames, 1992), the physical education environment was manipulated in order to create a mastery motivational climate, characterized by cooperation, individual effort, and individual progress. During sport classes, pupils participated in a variety of new and cooperative team sport activities, engaged in individual decision-making processes, and performed exercises in small groups with sufficient time for task completion. To identify the impact of the intervention, pupils' perceptions of the motivational climate, perceived inclusion, and identification at the class level were assessed at pre- and postintervention. Results showed significant increases in perceptions of in-group identification and group inclusion in the intervention condition compared to the control condition. These findings suggest that mastery motivational climate perceptions may facilitate students' psychological integration in multicultural physical education settings.

The preliminary results of these two intervention studies shed light on the importance of manipulating the sport/physical activity environment in a specific way in order to promote integration goals and in line with participants' ethnic-cultural background. However, a more systematic investigation of sport environmental factors and participants' characteristics should be sought in order to fully understand and exploit the potential integrative role of sport in multicultural societies. Considering the lack of field work in the area and the identified limitations, some of the most basic future research directions are discussed in the next section.

FUTURE PERSPECTIVES

Sport seems an ideal setting for bridging the gap between people with different ethno-cultural backgrounds and for overcoming social and cultural barriers (Rosenberg et al., 2003). Despite the significance and intuitive appeal of such propositions, empirical evidence is still limited, especially in Europe, and the potential of sport as an integrative agent remains a scantly explored field.

The topic of this chapter addresses an issue of considerable importance for promoting intergroup relations in culturally diverse societies. The findings so far suggest that sport can play an important role in the acculturation process and can influence the ethnic-cultural identity construction, but that the outcome depends on the environment within which sport takes place. Recent studies conducted in European countries highlight the importance of using a solid theoretical framework based on individual differences when investigating the role of sport participation in the acculturation process of ethnically diverse individuals or groups. Through intercultural contact both minority groups and host communities can be influenced and transformed to adapt to a new multicultural reality (Berry, 2006). In Berry's bidimensional model, acculturation attitudes and perceptions are being examined from both the migrants' and dominant population's perspective, underlining that individual differences should be taken into consideration to better understand the complex process of acculturation.

The ambiguous research findings indicate that differences across various ethnic groups could be either accentuated or overcome in the sport arena; the effect of sport participation seems to depend on the dominant cultural environment and individual differences of the participants. Future research should consider individual differences (see Laborde and Allen, Chapter 9) such as ethnic-cultural identity, gender, nature and type of sport, and the fit between incoming and host populations when examining the integrative potential of sport. The role of sport may differ from group to group, and individuals with different characteristics probably face different challenges with regards to their sport participation. Therefore, intervention programs that address the different needs of individuals from different backgrounds should be developed to facilitate their participation in sport and to improve social integration and multiculturalism.

Successful acculturation should be among the priorities on the political agenda in contemporary multicultural societies. The potential of sport to promote intercultural interaction needs to be highlighted. Research in this field should be further developed and should be based on a solid theoretical background. It should take into consideration both the structures of sport teams (eg, team composition, team size, homogeneity and heterogeneity of members) and the attributes of the sport environment (eg, team dynamics, motivational orientations). Furthermore, it is essential to thoroughly consider individual differences and the characteristics of the dominant and nondominant populations involved. The examination of such factors will help in developing systematic research, as these factors may regulate the relationship between sport participation and acculturation, and will enhance our understanding of the potential role of sport in promoting integration and multiculturalism.

REFERENCES

Allen, J., Drane, D., Byon, K., & Mohn, R. (2010). Sport as a vehicle for socialization and maintenance of cultural identity: international students attending American universities. *Sport Management Review, 13*, 421–434.

Allport, G. W. (1954). *The nature of prejudice*. Cambridge, MA: Addison-Wesley.

Ames, C. (1992). Classrooms, goals, structures, and student motivation. *Journal of Educational Psychology, 84*, 261–327.

Amir, Y. (1969). Contact hypothesis in ethnic relations. *Psychological Bulletin, 71*, 319–342.

Berry, J. W. (1980). Acculturation as varieties of adaptation. In: A. Padilla (Ed.), *Acculturation: Theory, models and some new findings* (pp. 9–25). Boulder: Westview.

Berry, J. W. (1997). Immigration, acculturation, and adaptation. *Applied Psychology, 46*, 5–34.

Berry, J. W. (2003). Conceptual approaches to acculturation. In: K. Chun, P. Balls-Organista, & G. Marin (Eds.), *Acculturation: Advances in theory, measurement and applied research* (pp. 17–37). Washington, DC: APA Press.

Berry, J. W. (2006). Contexts of acculturation. In: D. L. Sam, & J. W. Berry (Eds.), *The Cambridge handbook of acculturation psychology* (pp. 27–42). New York, NY: Cambridge University Press.

Berry, J. W. (2011). Integration and multiculturalism: ways towards social solidarity. *Papers on Social Representations, 20*, 2.1–2.21.

Bloyce, D., & Smith, A. (2010). *Sport policy and development: An introduction.* London: Routledge.

Bourhis, R. Y., Moise, L. C., Perreault, S., & Senecal, S. (1997). Towards an interactive acculturation model: a social psychological approach. *International Journal of Psychology, 32*, 369–386.

Bredemeier, B. J., & Shields, D. L. (2006). Sports and character development. *President's Council on Physical Fitness and Sports, 7*, 1–8.

Brown, R., Vivian, J., & Hewstone, M. (1999). Changing attitudes through intergroup contact: the effects of group membership salience. *European Journal of Social Psychology, 29*, 741–764.

Coalter, F. (2007). *A wider social role of sport: Who's keeping the score?* New York: Routledge.

Commission of the European Communities. (1993). *Background report: Social exclusion-poverty and other social problems in the European community, ISEC/B11/93.* Luxembourg: Office for Official Publications of the European Communities.

Committee for the Development of Sport. (1998). *Social cohesion and sport.* Discussion paper by Ms Olivia Dorricott, CDDS, 14.

Dankers, S., Elbe, A.-M., Sanchez, X., Otten, S., & van Yperen, N. (2015). Promoting inclusion through team sport activities: a motivational climate intervention in multicultural physical education classes. In: O. Schmid, R. Seiler (Eds), *Sports psychology: Theories and applications for performance, health and humanity. Proceedings of the 14th FEPSAC Congress of Sport Psychology* (p. 48). Institute of Sport Science.

Doherty, A., & Taylor, T. (2007). Sport and physical recreation in the settlement of immigrant youth. *Leisure/Loisir, 31*, 27–55.

Eitzen, D. S., & Sage, G. H. (2003). *Sociology of North American sport* (7th ed.). New York: McGraw Hill.

Elbe, A.-M., Sanchez, X., Ries, F., Kouli, O., Pappous, A., & Hatzigeorgiadis, A. (2012). The integrative role of sport in multicultural groups: personal, motivational and team factors. In: R. Meeusen, J. Duchateau, B. Roelands, M. Klass, B. De Geus, S. Baudry, & E. Tsolakidis (Eds.), *17th annual Congress of the ECSS—Book of Abstracts* (p. 496). European College of Sport Science.

Elbe, A.-M., Hatzigeorgiadis, A., Morela, E., Ries, F., Kouli, O., & Sanchez, X. (in press). Acculturation through sport: different contexts different meanings. International Journal of Sport and Exercise Psychology.

Elley, D., & Kirk, D. (2002). Developing citizenship through sport: the impact of a sport-based volunteer programme on young sport leaders. *Sport Education & Society, 7*, 151–166.

Ennis, C. D. (1999). Creating a culturally relevant curriculum for disengaged girls. *Sport Education & Society, 4*, 31–49.

Entzinger, H., & Biezeveld, R. (2003). *Benchmarking in immigrant integration.* Rotterdam: Erasmus University.

European Commission. (2007). *White paper on sport.* Available from: http://ec.europa.eu/sport/white-paper/white-paper_en.htm

European Commission DG Education & Culture. (2004). *Sport and multiculturalism.* Available from http://www.iscaweb.org/files/Sport%20and%20Multiculturalism%20EU%202004.pdf

Flood, S. E., & Hellstedt, J. C. (1991). Gender differences in motivation for intercollegiate athletic participation. *Journal of Sport Behavior, 14*, 159–167.

Green, K., & Hardman, K. (Eds.). (2000). *Physical education: A reader.* Oxford: Meyer & Meyer sport (UK) Ltd.

Grove, S. J., & Dodder, R. A. (1982). Constructing measures to assess perceptions of sport functions: an exploratory investigation. *International Journal of Sport Psychology, 13*, 96–106.

Guerin, P. B., Diiriye, R. O., Corrigan, C., & Guerin, B. (2003). Physical activity programs for refugee Somali women: working out in a new country. *Women & Health, 38*, 83–99.

Hatzigeorgiadis, A., Morela, E., Elbe, A.-M., & Sanchez, X. (2013). The integrative role of sport in multicultural societies. *European Psychologist, 18*, 191–202.

Hellison, D. (2003). *Teaching responsibility through physical activity.* Champaign, IL: Human Kinetics.

HM Treasury. (2007). *Aiming high for young people: A ten year strategy for positive activities.* London: HM Treasury/Department for children, schools and families.

Ito, E., Nogawa, H., Kitamura, K., & Walker, G. J. (2011). The role of leisure in the assimilation of Brazilian immigrants into Japanese society: acculturation and structural assimilation. *International Journal of Sport & Health Science, 9*, 8–14.

Keller, H., Lamprocht, M., & Stamm, H. (1998). *Social cohesion through sport.* Strasbourg, France: Council of Europe.

Kelly, L. (2011). Social inclusion through sports-based interventions? *Critical Social Policy, 31*, 126–150.

Kouli, O., & Papaioannou, A. (2009). Ethnic/cultural identity salience, achievement goals and motivational climate in multicultural physical education classes. *Psychology of Sport & Exercise, 10*, 45–51.

Krouwel, A., Boostra, N., Duyvendak, J. W., & Veldboer, L. (2006). A good sport? Research into the capacity of recreational sport to integrate Dutch minorities. *International Review for the Sociology of Sport, 41*, 165–180.

Lee, Y. (2005). A new voice: Korean American women in sports. *International Review for the Sociology of Sport, 40*, 481–495.

Lee, K. J., Dunlap, R., & Scott, D. (2011). Korean American males' serious leisure experiences and their perceptions of different play styles. *Leisure Sciences, 33*, 290–308.

Levitas, R., Pantazis, C., Fahmy, E., Gordon, D., Lloyd, E., & Patsios, D. (2007). *The multidimensional analysis of social exclusion: Report prepared for the social exclusion unit.* Bristol: University of Bristol.

Miller, S. C., Bredemeier, B. J. L., & Shields, D. L. L. (1997). Sociomoral education through physical education with at-risk children. *Quest, 49*, 114–129.

Moore, G. (2002). In our hands: the future is in the hands of those who give our young people hope and reason to live. *British Journal of Teaching in Physical Education, 33*, 26–27.

Morela, E., Hatzigeorgiadis, A., Kouli, O., Elbe, A.-M., & Sanchez, X. (2013). Team cohesion and ethnic-cultural identity in adolescent migrant athletes. *International Journal of Intercultural Relations, 37*, 643–647.

Morela, E., Hatzigeorgiadis, A., Elbe, A.-M., Papaioannou, A., & Sanchez, X. (2016). *Acculturation through youth sport: the hosts' perspective.* Paper submitted for publication.

Niessen, J. (2000). *Diversity and cohesion: New challenges for the integration of immigrants and minorities.* Strasbourg, France: Council of Europe Publishing.

Organization for Economic Co-operation and Development. (2001). *The well-being of nations: The role of social and human capital.* Paris: OECD.

Parnell, D., Pringle, A., Widdop, P., & Zwolinsky, S. (2015). Understanding football as a vehicle for enhancing social inclusion: using an intervention mapping framework. *Social Inclusion, 3,* 1–9.

Phinney, J. (2003). Ethnic identity and acculturation. In: K. Chun, P. Organista, & G. Marin (Eds.), *Acculturation: Advances in theory, measurement, and applied research (63–81).* Washington, DC: American Psychological Association.

Priest, S. (1998). Physical challenge and the development of trust through corporate adventure training. *Journal of Experiential Learning, 21,* 31–34.

Rosenberg, D., Feijgin, N., & Talmor, R. (2003). Perceptions of immigrant students on the absorption process in an Israeli physical education and sport college. *European Journal of Physical Education, 8,* 52–77.

Ryom, K., & Stelter, R. (2015). The experience and effect of team sport in a migrant culture. In: O. Schmid, R. Seller, (Eds). *Sports psychology: Theories and applications for performance, health and humanity. Proceedings of the 14th FEPSAC Congress of Sport Psychology* (p. 49). Institute of Sport Science.

Seippel, O. (2002). Volunteers and professionals in Norwegian sport organizations: facts, visions and prospects. *Voluntas, 13,* 253–271.

Shields, D. L., & Bredemeier, B. L. (2007). Advances in sport mortality research. In: G. Tenenbaum, & R. C. Eklund (Eds.), *Handbook of sport psychology* (3rd ed., pp. 662–684). New York: John Wiley.

Stack, J. A. C., & Iwasaki, Y. (2009). The role of leisure pursuits in adaptation processes among Afghan refugees who have immigrated to Winnipeg, Canada. *Leisure Studies, 28,* 239–259.

Stodolska, M., & Alexandris, K. (2004). The role of recreational sport in the adaptation of first generation immigrants in the United States. *Journal of Leisure Research, 36,* 379–413.

Tajfel, H., Billig, M. G., Bundy, R. P., & Flament, C. (1971). Social categorization and intergroup behaviour. *European Journal of Social Psychology, 1,* 149–178.

Ting-Toomey, S., Yee-Jung, K., Shapiro, R., Garcia, W., Wright, T. J., & Oetzel, J. G. (2000). Ethnic/cultural identity salience and conflict styles in four US ethnic groups. *International Journal of Intercultural Relations, 24,* 47–81.

United Nations. (2013). International migration report 2013. Available from http://www.un.org/en/development/desa/population/migration/publications/wallchart/docs/wallchart2013.pdf

van Osch, Y., & Breugelmans, S. (2012). Perceived intergroup difference as an organizing principle of intercultural attitudes and acculturation attitudes. *Journal of Cross-Cultural Psychology, 43,* 801–821.

Walseth, K. (2008). Bridging and bonding social capital in sport-experiences of young women with an immigrant background. *Sport Education & Society, 13,* 1–17.

Walseth, K., & Fasting, K. (2004). Sport as a means of integrating minority women. *Sport & Society, 7,* 109–129.

Wankel, L. M., & Berger, B. G. (1990). The psychological and social benefits of sport and physical activity. *Journal of Leisure Research, 22,* 167–182.

Wuest, D., & Lombardo, B. (1994). *Curriculum and instruction: The secondary school physical education experience.* St. Louis, MI: Mosby Publishing.

Section III

Perspectives From Sport Psychology

Chapter 11

Doing Sport Psychology? Critical Reflections of a Scientist-Practitioner

Chris Harwood

School of Sport, Exercise and Health Sciences, Loughborough University, Loughborough, United Kingdom

INTRODUCTION

I've been privileged to have simultaneously experienced and served three key roles in sport psychology in my career so far; roles as an applied researcher, an educator/supervisor for students, and a practitioner that have become rather fused in my identity as a sport psychologist. During my PhD period (1993–97), I also made efforts to adhere to the scientist-practitioner model (see Frank, 1984; Lowman, 2012; Stoltenberg & Pace, 2007 for critical insights) and ensure that I was (1) a consumer of science with up-to-date knowledge of theories, methods, and techniques to inform interventions; (2) an evaluator of science who examined both the effects and the effectiveness of his interventions; and (3) a producer of science who disseminated ideas back to the profession and sought to advance pragmatic knowledge or theory refinement. Reflecting upon my attempts to achieve this cyclical "1, 2, and 3" process in my work, I would evaluate myself as being inconsistently successful. Indeed, I believe that the existence of pure scientist-practitioners is much less common nowadays. Having graduated from their PhDs or professional qualifications, sport psychologists find themselves doing either research or teaching, or engaged in consultancy work where there are many contextual, motivational, and resource constraints to living up to the prerequisites of being a scientist-practitioner. If we cannot achieve a growth in number of scientist-practitioners, then the next best thing is a greater proximity between applied research and practice, between scientists and practitioners. Improvements in science-to-practice work and the collaborative role of applied researchers and practitioners are exhorted by Lowman (2012) when making critical observations of the scientist-practitioner consulting psychologist:

Sport and Exercise Psychology Research. http://dx.doi.org/10.1016/B978-0-12-803634-1.00011-X

229

It [the article] asks what it means to be a scientist-practitioner in more than aspi-rational or superficial terms and notes the frequent gap between science and prac-tice and between practice and science. These gaps, it is argued, call for changed behavior on the part of both practitioners and of researchers. It is argued that the science-practitioner model can be differentiating in a highly competitive area of practice, that science can make its research more relevant to practice, and that practitioners have an important role to play in assuring the linkage of practice with research and theory. (Lowman, 2012, p. 151)

He goes on to note that "we need both good practice and good science to create a science-practitioner-driven discipline. We need both evidence-based practice and practice-based evidence to create and sustain that discipline" (Lowman, 2012, p. 155). This requires applied researchers to ask practitioners about those relevant "in the field" issues that they struggle with in terms of knowledge or skill; and it requires practitioners to consider working with ap-plied researchers on evaluating their interventions or gathering data on their own experiences as a practitioner such that pragmatic knowledge might be dis-seminated to the field in an improved and efficient manner.

In this chapter, I want to offer a series of constructive critical reflec-tions from my experiences doing sport psychology over the past 20 years and illustrate how I've attempted on more than a few occasions to create the bridge from science to practice and from practice to science. I will preface this by stating that as an applied sport psychologist I am a "developmental social psychologist" in terms of identity. Hence, my reflections to practi-tioners are based on the importance and value of social psychological in-terventions in sport. Likewise, I will also reflect on scientific knowledge gaps and opportunities that fall for social psychology researchers due to my background. Lastly, I also want to offer critical reflections from experi-ences of my third key role—that of educator and supervisor to students and practitioners—and what this means for the health of the profession. Permis-sion has been granted by the clubs and athlete–client to discuss examples of work for educational purposes.

REFLECTION NO. 1: TAKING CARE OF BUSINESS MEANS TAKING CARE OF TASK INVOLVEMENT

This first reflection extensively addresses my belief in the importance of in-tegrating achievement goal theory (Harwood & Hardy, 2001; Harwood & Swain, 2002; Harwood, Hardy, & Swain, 2000; Nicholls, 1989; Roberts & Treasure, 2012) into the business of research and everyday practice as a sport psychologist with clients. I believe that motivation is a psychological quality that is critical to take care of in much the same way as it is critical to take care of one's diet or fitness. Quality of motivation impacts health and where it is of poor quality, then it is a health risk in terms of sport experience, development, and performance. Indeed, as part of an interdisciplinary sport science team in a professional football academy, I have sat alongside nutritionists and physical trainers delivering diet and fitness education sessions to young parents. Each sport scientist passionately refers to the importance of portion sizes, vitamins, hydration, stretching, injury prevention, and subsequent parental roles to support the coach, child, and team. When it's my turn to talk about sport psychology, I practically acknowledge the high quantity of motivation and drive that they, as parents, and their children bring to the sport. However, it is the quality of their motivation—their personal beliefs about achievement and success, and that of their children, that will determine the quality of their experience and development through their journey at the club. We are talking about achievement goals here (Harwood, Spray, & Keegan, 2008), and practitioners will take better care of business in sport psychology with young athletes when they attend to this area. Likewise, applied researchers will support this business through the study of relevant questions that support and inform practitioner activity.

Achievement goal theory (Nicholls, 1984, 1989) focuses on the meaning of achievement to the achiever, and argues that we hold personal theories of achievement (or what constitutes success) about tasks in which we engage. We can view personal success and achievement in a task-involving or mastery-focused manner whereby self-improvement, learning, effortful engagement, curiosity, and increased understanding are self-referenced processes and outcomes that matter for occasioning a sense of personal competence (Duda, 1992; Roberts, 1992). Alternatively, we can view personal success in an ego involving or norm-referenced manner where superior (or less inferior) comparisons with others, demonstrations of higher ability relative to an external standard, or achieving a certain level with less normative effort expended are the criteria underpinning a sense of competence. These two contrasting definitions or conceptions of achievement, linked to the situation in which an athlete finds him/herself, are responsible for task or ego involvement—achievement goals that represent the meaning of achievement to the achiever on that task.

The starting gun for achievement goal research in sport was fired by Glyn Roberts and Joan Duda in the late 1980s and early 1990s, and *Motivation in Sport and Exercise* (Roberts, 1992) was a seminal text with contributions from Nicholls, Duda, Roberts, and Ames addressing the value, nature, consequences, and application of achievement goals in sport. The message was clear about the adaptive nature of task orientation and task involvement, and the more problematic and potentially maladaptive nature of ego orientation and ego involvement.

In my experience, when athletes discuss experiences of anxiety, anger/frustration, negative attention, low self-confidence, guilt/shame, and behavioral disengagement (eg, tanking; effort withdrawal), then it isn't too long until the consultation uncovers poor quality preexisting achievement goals or dominant personal theories of achievement. These are usually related to excessive ego involvement in a given situation or environment. Perhaps I am predisposed to thoroughly examining "achievement goals" in my athletes, but akin to the child in the film *The Sixth Sense*—"I see ego involvement ... everywhere!" During my PhD period, heavily influenced by Roberts (1992) and intensive research from a variety of scholars in the field, I focused on "achievement goal states" (Harwood & Swain, 1998, 2001; Swain & Harwood, 1996) and how we could apply field-based interventions to improve young athletes' quality of achievement goals in competitive situations (Harwood & Swain, 2002). In this latter single case design intervention, there was substantial practitioner work with athletes, coaches, and parents and a coordinated social approach toward helping athletes reform their conceptions of achievement in competition. Most notably, there were reported improvements in self-directed task involvement, reductions in social approval ego involvement, and enhancements in competitive cognitions around perceptions of challenge, threat, self-efficacy, and self-regulation.

What is noticeably disappointing about the intervening years since 2002 is the lack of field-relevant applied research in achievement goal theory, and particularly the lack of experimental or field-based achievement goal interventions. This statement is made in the context of a field that has become overly saturated with quantitative (largely cross-sectional) investigations that associate goals with antecedents or outcomes, without any focus on application or testing in the field (Harwood et al., 2008). It seems that researchers are more interested in seeing if their structural equation models statistically hold up, and then finding ways to tweak them, than "making the constructs sweat" in the real world of practice.

Perhaps I am partly responsible for this state of affairs due to turning points in my own career in 2002 and a sense that the field did not want to modernize by taking closer scrutiny of its constructs. I forwarded a critique of concepts and measurement issues in achievement goal theory that I saw as important for scholars to consider—and particularly with field application in mind (Harwood et al., 2000). This was rather comprehensively rebutted by respected motivation colleagues (Treasure et al., 2001), after which we reflected and revised terminology but persisted with our core messages in a final response (Harwood & Hardy, 2001). Soon after these publications, an opportunity arose to work as lead psychologist in a professional football club. As a result of this appointment, my academic commitments were reduced and I commenced a related line of research in team psychology and performance environments (Pain & Harwood, 2004, 2007, 2008, 2009). In the intervening years, the 2 × 2 achievement goal model from educational psychology (Elliot & McGregor, 2001) has overshadowed Nicholls's (1989) dichotomous model in terms of research interest in sport. However, I do not believe that this model has contributed extensively (or practically) to what we already knew about achievement goals in 1990s and early 2000s. For example, to an applied researcher working in the field, performance-avoidance goals are essentially reflective of individuals high in ego involvement who possess a low perception of their competence (at that moment; for that task) to favorably compare with others. This is not new, and we were already ascertaining that levels of perceived competence when ego involved (ie, the main differentiation between performance approach vs avoidance goals) was critical in judging the relative "healthiness" of ego involvement. Moreover, when striving to move achievement goal research forward in educational psychology, Vansteenkiste, Lens, Elliot, Soenens, & Mouratidis (2014) eruditely describe a $3 \times 2 \times 2$ model of goals where task-mastery, intrapersonal, and norm-referenced goals are considered not only in terms of valence but also motivational regulation. Specifically, the controlling versus autonomous regulatory reasons underpinning the adoption of the goal is considered (ie, the "why" behind the goal). These mastery, intrapersonal, and norm-referenced constructs bear a more than passing resemblance to the constructs of task-process, task-product, and ego involvement that were debated in 2000 and 2001 within sport psychology (Harwood & Hardy, 2001). Additionally, the notion of self-directed versus social approval goals (Harwood & Swain, 2002; Wilson, Hardy, & Harwood, 2006) concurs with the autonomous versus controlling nature of goal regulation posited by Vansteenkiste and coworkers. We were having the same debates and arguments in sport psychology 14 years earlier albeit without so rigorously integrating elements of self-determination theory (SDT; Deci & Ryan, 1985) into achievement goal theory. Perhaps I should have persisted more, or met with colleagues to determine a more palatable route for the future in achievement goals.

As it currently stands, my belief is that achievement goal research since the early 2000s has limped on slowly, meekly nudging forwards without attention to practical interventions or applied research questions that would make a practitioner want to sit up and read on. Applied implications sections in published achievement goal research have become rather "same" and repetitive. Importantly, there is no relevant published data on some of these newer constructs in sport settings, no matter how theoretically or pragmatically appealing these ideas appear to be. Nevertheless, there has been promising developments in applied research that have been assisted by achievement goal theory. The following sections serve to explain these in more critical detail.

Optimizing Motivational Climate and the 5Cs Approach

Where achievement goal theory has offered a great deal to the practice of coaching and parenting in sport lies in methods and strategies to optimize the motivational climate of an athlete (Ames, 1992). This relates to the perception of an athlete with respect to the situational goals (ie, criteria for achievement) that are emphasized by significant others (ie, coaches, parents, peers, officials, sport structure) in the immediate environment. In other words, those external parties or symbols that influence the athletes "personal theories of achievement" beyond the athlete's own achievement dispositions. Task-involving motivational climates consistently perform well in research compared to ego-involving climates on a variety of psychological indices (Harwood, Keegan, Smith, & Raine, 2015). The message from this research is the importance of getting the situational environment right for athletes. Attempts to apply the situational principles of achievement goal theory (with SDT) have been buoyant with applications of the Empowering Coaching program as part of the PAPA project (Duda, 2013; see Duda and Appleton, Chapter 18). This has involved a large-scale European-wide intervention focused on a 6-h workshop educating grass roots football coaches in the principles of AGT and SDT, including measures of self-reported and objective motivational climate to determine intervention effects on players (Tessier et al., 2013).

Beyond my PhD intervention, my focus on creating task-involving motivational climate in youth sport encompassed the development of a triangulated approach to psychosocial skills in youth football (Harwood, 2008a). After 2 years of working with the senior teams at the professional club in 2002, I initiated more work within the youth academy structure. I found the focus of the environment to be highly targeted toward technical, tactical, and physical skills. There was no mental skills identity, no dedicated room for the value of these in session plans, and clear strategy about the education, development, and monitoring of identified mental skills in the player pathway. I sought to develop a "community of practice" around mental skills whereby coaches, parents, and players could associate and identify with key psychosocial attributes that would help both football and personal development. I identified the 5Cs—commitment, communication, concentration, control, and confidence—as user-friendly terms, underpinned by theory, representing valued motivational, interpersonal, and self-regulatory qualities for young players. Importantly, work with coaches, players, and parents focused on discussing the behaviors that underpinned each C as experience taught me that psychology is easier to translate to these stakeholders when we consider specific behaviors for them to maintain or aspire toward. The resultant 5Cs program reported by Harwood (2008a) involved education across the academy age groups, but primarily targeted coaching efficacy—the confidence that coaches had in integrating strategies around the 5Cs in their natural coaching sessions. A key intervention strategy here was the development of a task-involving coaching climate for each of the 5Cs, and eight coaching directives were developed to facilitate the creation of such a climate. This is expanded upon in the next section.

In 1992, Carole Ames introduced the TARGET acronym (based on Epstein, 1989) as a mnemonic for optimizing the structure of teaching activities in the classroom. These have been transferred to sport as a means of helping coaches to structure a task-involving motivational climate:

Task—represents the design of tasks and activities that focus on learning and developing new skills, minimizing competition and social comparison.

Authority—incorporates athletes' participation in decision-making processes, with input on new drills, supporting their sense of participation and self-determination.

Reward—recognizes and acknowledges improvement, progress, and effort, individually and as a team.

Grouping—encourages heterogeneity and mixing of ability levels with co-operation of group members in trying to solve varying problems and challenges rather than competing with each other at any cost.

Evaluation—targets the provision of evaluative feedback around personal and team improvement, alongside quality of the work process, as opposed to who is superior at a given task.

Timing—challenges the coach to give sufficient time for athletes to master and develop without leaving tasks unfinished, as well as the timing of feedback (eg, immediately after seeing target behavior).

Working with the professional football coaches, I drew upon the principles offered by TARGET, but also considered the role of social learning theory (Bandura, 1977a) and the importance of supporting peers in the development of a task-involving climate (Ntoumanis & Vazou, 2005). I introduced eight directives or guidelines to coaches that could be used to a structure a coaching session that was task involving in nature while simultaneously focusing on the development of a specific C. These structural guidelines are housed within the acronym PROGRESS (Harwood & Anderson, 2015), which stands for:

Promote the C in the same way that coaches would introduce and value a technical or tactical skill. Provide the rationale for the C and how important it is to football.

Role-model the C through the appropriate model behavior as a coach. Bring the meaning of C to life by demonstrating or referring to excellent examples versus bad examples from football, or other sports.

Ownership of their learning. Involve players in decisions within the session about how they can demonstrate a C; allow them options to work at their own pace and to benefit from favorite drills and practices that showcase their strengths.

Grow the C by providing players with opportunities to practice the C, and then to train it in more open game situations when "pressure" can be added to test players.

Reinforce the C by praising those players who respond by demonstrating the chosen C skill or behavior, and by making courageous decisions.

Empower peer support by encouraging players to praise each other for positive efforts related to each C in order to build individual and collective confidence.

Support the supporter by acknowledging those players when praise a fellow peer, thereby closing the loop on a supportive peer climate around each of the Cs.

Self-review. Check-in with players on their levels of the C and empower them to keep working hard; use monitors to review collective efforts, and apply self-reflection and learning points at the end of the session.

The application of PROGRESS as part of 5Cs coach education has formed part of two well-received interventions (Harwood, 2008a; Harwood, Barker, & Anderson, 2015) with encouraging self-reported developments and positive coach, parent, and player feedback. Nevertheless, these mixed-method investigations were based entirely on subjective as opposed to objective data. Observational data is needed from the coach about how much they actually apply PROGRESS and the precise mechanisms by which they create a certain psychological climate in the coaching session (Tessier et al., 2013). Equally, more sophisticated measures of player psychosocial development with respect to the 5Cs should be considered in future.

This primary reflection has championed the importance of attending to the quality of motivation in young athletes, and improving the scientific body of knowledge to aid practitioners consistently in this area of work. There are several areas where I believe science and practice need to meet in the form of further applied research into achievement goals.

Future Science to Practice Research

One of the central areas of business with respect to achievement goals is the conduct of research that has clear practical, real-world value. For example, there is a premium on understanding the dynamics of personal theories of achievement during the childhood-to-adolescent transition (see Wylleman and Rosier, Chapter 14). As young athletes develop cognitively through childhood into puberty, they begin to fully differentiate the concepts of ability from effort, task difficulty, and luck and the role of these concepts in task achievement. They realize that ability is a capacity that sets the limit on what effort alone can accomplish, and they are more susceptible to wanting to prove their ability—where the meaning of achievement becomes about ego-involved peer comparison. Task involvement is therefore under threat and this may be a contributing factor to the attrition and drop-out rates of young people in sport around 11 years of age. However, importantly for sport psychologists, the mechanisms and processes that occur during this important transition toward adolescence have rarely been studied in youth sport. There are a number of questions for us to consider.

First, what are the implications for competitive sport contexts and achievement goals from developmental social neuroscience (Jetha & Segalowitz, 2012)? There is evidence that the emotional centers of the brain develop earlier during adolescence than the more rational, logical prefrontal areas. There is an emotional sensitivity to reward, a craving for the dopamine response, and an eagerness to "prove" and measure up to peers to gain peer acceptance during this period. Does the natural ego involving climate of sport interact with these developmental and neurological constraints to incite controlled forms of ego involvement in competition settings? It might follow that the young athlete sees the meaning of achievement only through the lens of demonstrating superior normative ability to peers, or at least minimizing lack of ability. Task involvement is heavily compromised or suppressed.

Second, what exactly are the necessary education and support mechanisms to stimulate the adolescent to consistently utilize mastery sources of competence information (eg, to draw success from losing; to draw learning from mistakes)? We require research that helps to inform practitioners in terms of putting a plan into place during this transition; a plan that counteracts the aforementioned developmental and neurological constraints. We need to understand exactly what needs to comprise a task-involving climate for such a climate to "stick" during this period. This is particularly important to those late maturing athletes who have seldom proved their ability levels to others, compared with early maturing athletes. How do we influence the personal theories of achievement for this group of success starved athletes? Conversely, how do practitioners help to prevent or manage a successful and "rewarded ego" *in the present* from becoming a "damaged ego" *in the future*? When young athletes win and are constantly rewarded for their normative success, they potentially become motivationally fragile when things go off plan. The early maturing "winner" seldom processes failure or makes the effort to learn about how and why they won, so when they start to fail, it is easy for them to be defined by their losses. They haven't learned how to cognitively process their achievements in a task-involved manner and "when the scaffolding of their wins gets removed, the matchstick house collapses." This is another period where once-talented adolescents seem to drop off the radar in sport and fail to transition to the potential that they may have had if they had better managed the quality of their motivation, attitude toward their success and achievement goals.

In sum, these are developmentally important questions for both achievement goal researchers and sport psychology practitioners in youth sport, yet few studies have explored these types of issue. What is clear is that task-involving climates are vital, and how they can be optimized in training, preperformance, during performance/time-outs, and postperformance in the context of healthy performance debriefing (Tannenbaum & Cerasoli, 2013) represent viable areas for further research.

REFLECTION NO. 2: WORKING ON SOCIAL-PERFORMANCE PROCESSES WITH ATHLETES AND TEAMS IS ENHANCED WHEN CONNECTED TO TANGIBLE SOCIAL PRODUCTS

This reflection represents an investigative proposition for applied researchers based on experiences of providing services in both team and individual sports. The origin of this reflection is grounded in social psychological theories of group productivity (Steiner, 1972) and stems from the value of helping athletes to understand the role of process losses in teams and how motivation, coordination, and performance improvements may stem from process gains (ie, proactive collaboration on behavioral processes to optimize team functioning). Driven by the principle of maximizing relevant resources and minimizing motivation and coordination losses in teams (Steiner), a great deal of applied work with teams nowadays targets the development of shared values, agreed behaviors, and codes of practice that enable the setting of efficient and functional individual and collective goals. A central point here is that values espoused by a team (Henriksen, Stambulova, & Roessler, 2010) are clearly enacted by agreed behaviors linked to the value. Words mean nothing; it is the actions behind those words that allow the performance of that value to be monitored and reviewed by a team. In my applied work in elite field hockey (Harwood, 2008b), youth football, and professional football (Harwood & Anderson, 2012), there have been specific behaviors related to team conduct, principles of play or mental performance identified and reviewed on an ongoing basis. Equally, work with individual athletes and their support team (eg, coach, trainer, and parent) has also included such attention to social-performance processes that enable optimal functioning (Harwood & Swain, 2002) and can be reviewed regularly.

A signature of my work with these teams and individuals has been the simultaneous work on tangible social products linked to the achievement of processes. Within elite field hockey and professional football, this took the form of weekly performance magazines that included team and individual appraisals of performance as well as other social components. In brief, these magazines tended to follow a formula of the following components (Harwood, 2008b).

1. Publication of team values, behavior codes, or principles of play
2. Player ratings of team performance in matches
3. Shared views of performance and special mentions to individual teammates
4. Humor (eg, through jokes, fun interview with a player, humorous stories about the match or training week)
5. Coach's corner (ie, report of the coach)
6. Sport psychologist reflection and priming (ie, report from the sport psychologist)

With the hockey team (Harwood, 2008b), all units of the team provided concise performance feedback to other units and individual players shared their own goals for the training week with team members based on their review of performance from the prior match.

Hockey's magazine was entitled *Hockey's the Winner*; in youth football, the magazine was entitled *Ahead of the Game*; whereas in professional football, our magazine was called *The Mental Toughness Review*. With respect to individual athletes and their support teams, I've created a quarterly team newsletter that allows the athlete and their team to contribute writing "columns" akin to a journalist in a newspaper. These columns reflected their recent work and experiences with the athlete, and served as a review process for the athlete and team. One such journalistic initiative with an elite tennis player was entitled *On the Rise* and was representative of his transitional process from junior to senior professional tennis. Indeed, this also served as a stimulus for him to write his own invited column in *The Times* newspaper about his exploits as a player on the circuit.

While these products have been met with reported client satisfaction following end-of-season consultancy evaluations and cooccurred with periods of objective performance improvements and positive team outcomes, there has been no scientific investigation of the process and product interaction on performance. I have an intuitive belief based on experience that these written products play a role in the cementing of processes within a consistent, adaptive psychological climate, and that this positively facilitates the effects of process-oriented work. However, I have no scientific data on the effects of the products per se, nor what particular subelements of the product (eg, performance ratings; shared views; humor; coach's corner) have the greatest impact or meaning for athletes.

A further reinforcement of my beliefs around the efficacy of these initiatives stemmed from recent work with a professional tennis player on a "return to play" plan following injury. As an example of the interdisciplinary sport science model of consulting (Poczwardowski, Sherman, & Ravizza, 2004), this involved a 6-week rehabilitation program in collaboration with the coach, physical trainer, physiotherapist, and governing body medical doctor. Work with the player was based on heightening perceptions of recovery efficacy and competition readiness in order to achieve a smooth transition back onto the professional tennis circuit. I proposed to the player the concept of a video diary and resilience documentary where he could plan, execute, and review his rehab sessions and on-court training days through visual methods. There were once again several processes at play here, driven conceptually by self-efficacy theory (Bandura, 1977b). First, he would engage in daily "set-up clips" where he would discuss his commitment goals for the day on camera; these would also tie in with his "strengths and accomplishments" reflections that he would record during (if appropriate) and at the end of day. His support team played both verbal persuasion and modeling roles by both encouragement and active participation in training sessions, as well as acting as "cameraperson" for the activities. While videotaping a selective range of sessions, there was special attention given to "Resilience TV viewing moments"—akin to moments on TV that are effortful and inspirational when watched. These were moments of adversity coping and demonstrations of toughness captured on camera that may have been spontaneous responses, or prospectively planned by the player in the knowledge that such a session was going to be a challenge. The player maintained an ongoing video archive of all his sessions and his self-reflections as the "return-to-play" process continued through the weeks. A final task offered to the player was to research a list of "mastery" or resilience-based quotes that resonated with him, and which served as additional motivational and attentional fuel for a given day. These could be from books, the Internet, or films. One such quote he cited from the movie *The Iron Lady* (Jones & Lloyd, 2011) that was delivered by Margaret Thatcher, the late British Prime Minister. It read:

> *Watch your thoughts, for they become words. Watch your words, for they become actions. Watch your actions, for they become habits. Watch your habits, for they become your character. And watch your character, for it becomes your destiny. What we think, we become. (Jones & Lloyd, 2011)*

As the interaction between these daily processes, interdisciplinary social support, and video products continued, I began to storyboard the resilience movie comprising of a highlights montage of his work ethic and accomplishments in the different "archived" activities—gym, pool, bike, physical simulation imagery on court, track work, on tennis court drills, and full court points. This visual script was then placed to music using Hans Zimmer's theme from the movie *Crimson Tide*. I had employed a similar approach to create a process-based movie product for the professional football team I had worked with in 2003. In that case I had employed visual segments and theme music from the movie *Gladiator* to create a 26-min product of the team's "season so far." In this individual tennis case, I constrained the movie to 4 min so that it could be viewed conveniently before training, practice, or matches as the player wished.

Throughout this entire process I met with the player weekly to review his progress acting as a supportive listener and sounding board, as well as establishing if there was any information for the support team with respect to facilitating the coming week's training. I also met with individual support team members to discuss the upcoming training week. In terms of intervention monitoring, twice weekly the player completed measures of positive and negative affect, recovery efficacy, competition readiness, and perceptions of social support. These measures showed sustained psychological well-being and positive progressions in all factors as the return to the circuit approached. The player had a successful return to competition and within 3 months had reached his highest international ranking. Nevertheless, despite the cooccurrence of objective competitive success and client satisfaction with the support, there remained no scientific consideration of which components may have contributed most to any of the positive psychological outcomes. Was it the social support and total team collaboration? The daily goal setting? The process of video-based self-reflection? The capturing of accomplishments on video? The effects of capturing more meaningful resilience episodes? The process plan itself from gym to court? Being autonomously part of a resilience movie that he is making of his rehabilitation? The movie itself and the music behind it? Was it all of these things in an integrated fashion? Scientifically, I don't know the answers to these questions. However, I do believe that the social-performance products in the form of the ongoing video, the video-based self-reflection archive, and the final movie enhanced the effects of the processes that served to generate such products. In turn, I would speculate that performance gains emerge more strongly as a function of the process and product interaction than processes alone.

Translations From Practice to Scientific Research

In terms of taking these practice-based insights into more scientific research, I drew upon my interest in team performance review processes to determine if open discussion of team functioning would enhance social and performance-related team factors. A series of studies in elite youth football were conducted on identifying and assessing components of optimal performance environments (Pain & Harwood, 2007, 2008). The Performance Environment Survey (PES) was developed as an empirically grounded assessment tool for players to rate various components of their environment (including physical, social, team, and psychological factors). The PES was applied by Pain and Harwood (2009) to collect week-by-week perceptions of the performance environment in an elite student–athlete football team. Following 6 weeks of data collection, the authors initiated a weekly open discussion/mutual sharing process about the performance environment using the collective mean scores of the PES from each of the prior match weeks. Using their collective ratings on the PES to different performance components as the product, players were facilitated to debrief openly and offer their reflections on the scores, in addition to discussing potential areas and strategies for improvement. Over the coming weeks, and during the postintervention retention phase, improvements in perceptions of trust and confidence in teammates, communication, and reported team performance emerged and were generally sustained. Qualitative social validation data also supported the value of the intervention in encouraging honesty and facilitating the confidence to make pertinent points with the facts laid down in front of the team that had been generated by the team (Pain & Harwood, 2009; Pain, Harwood, & Mullen, 2012).

In sum, this practice-to-science reflection encourages applied researchers and practitioners to consider interventions that employ processes and products, and to determine what are the most impactful and relevant components to intervention effectiveness.

REFLECTION NO. 3: UNIVERSITIES AND PROFESSIONAL ASSOCIATIONS NEED TO TAKE GREATER RESPONSIBILITY FOR THE APPROPRIATE TRAINING OF PRACTITIONERS

My final reflection is drawn from my interest and experience in education and supervision vis-a-vis the professional development of the neophyte sport psychology practitioner. It is the most subjective of my three reflections and therefore one with the greatest opportunity for more rigorous academic scrutiny. I want to locate the points I will make in due course by affirming how the breadth of competencies required of sport psychologists has evolved greatly in recent years. Knowledge, skills and experience are required in a range of competency fields (Fig. 11.1), with increasing demands in elite sport where organisational and political factors play more prominent roles. This professional evolution (eg, beyond the mere psychological skills training models of the 1980s and 1990s) subsequently shines the spotlight on professional development and training systems for quality assuring the service delivery of sport psychologists. Put simply, we are asked and challenged "to be more things to more people" and competent service delivery outcomes require a well-regulated professional system of training (BPS; British Psychological Society, 2011). This is what will ultimately differentiate sport psychologists from other less competent and unlicensed service providers.

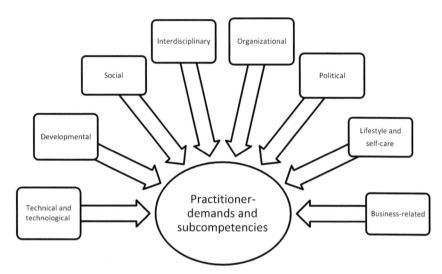

FIGURE 11.1   Fields of competency in sport psychology.

In my view, the education and professional development of sport psychology practitioners should mirror other healthcare professions when it comes to competency development and quality assurance of service. Miller (1990) proposes an assessment hierarchy of competence in clinical settings that has become known as Miller's Pyramid (Fig. 11.2). Taking this framework in mind, competency is progressed through several stages from: possessing factual knowledge of a relevant theory or issue (know); interpreting facts and knowing how to apply such knowledge to a given situation (know-how); demonstrating the application of knowledge and related technical skills in a simulation or practice setting (shows how); and applying knowledge, skills, and experience when performing in the real-world workplace of consulting (does). In the first

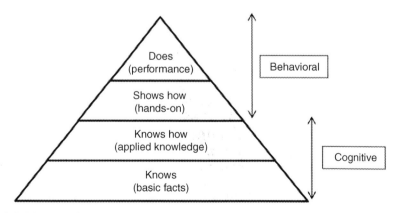

FIGURE 11.2   Miller's pyramid of clinical competence.

two stages, a student's cognitive skills are being assessed (typically in MCQs, essays, reports, presentations), whereas in the latter two stages behavioral observation and workplace assessment of skill applications are being employed. Through an accumulation of knowledge, skills, and experience of relevant theories, principles, and practices, the sport psychologist progresses from novice to expert in terms of professional authenticity (Rønnestad & Skovholt, 2003).

Miller's pyramid is valuable when being held up as a standard for evaluating the content and process of education and training programs for neophyte practitioners, and this is where issues of responsibility come into play. My reflection of being in the system of education and supervision of young sport psychology trainees in the United Kingdom is that education appears to be the responsibility of university institutions, whereas supervision is the responsibility of professional associations (eg, BPS; BASES—British Association of Sport and Exercise Sciences). University courses at BSc and MSc level should offer the "know," but how much they offer the "know how" depends greatly on the applied nature and assessment requirements of specific modules (and the specific skill sets of academic staff). For example, the principles of achievement goal theory may be taught and assessed (ie, know), but students may not be tasked with critically appraising how to develop a task-involving motivational climate in athletes from childhood-to-adolescence (ie, know how). In other words, opportunities to demonstrate relevant applied knowledge may be slim within university programs. Professional associations in the United Kingdom do not provide taught elements or mandate specific technical delivery skills training as part of their qualifications; the student is reliant on the supervisor relationship for essentially guidance, reflection, and mentoring. In effect, after completion of their MSc, student practitioners are "out on their own" doing the job and trying to make a living under the supervision of an individual they may meet only 6–12 times a year. You may have noticed what is missing here. Not only are there potential constraints and limitations in practically relevant "know how" education (that should be considered ethically before practicing), but there is potentially little or no "show how" in the training of student-practitioners. Indeed, my critical reflection is that there is a "practitioner skills gap" lying between education and supervision that exists because there is no training program for students. Students departing from their MSc degrees are consistently wanting more training (eg, practice intakes, observations) and "safe service delivery" experiences to build their confidence, yet with universities responsible for "know" and professional associations supervising what a practitioner "does," the canyon of untapped "know how" and "show how" looms large. This is the elephant in the room, and someone has to take responsibility for stating "there is massive elephant in this room … what are we going to do about it!?" One key research question that deserves attention is the degree to which neophyte practitioners feel that university undergraduate and postgraduate degrees adequately prepared them for supervised practice in the "real world"; and whether professional qualifications represented value for money in terms of content and process with respect to facilitating relevant, "real world" competency development following completion of postgraduate taught programs.

In the early 2000s, the teaching practice of applied sport psychology was enhanced by a number of universally helpful products for students and educators. Mark Andersen's *Doing Sport Psychology* (2000) and his follow-up text, *Sport Psychology in Practice* (2005) offered students insights into the person and process elements of sport psychology support in action. Practitioners were able to gain a greater feel for intake interviews, communication skills, application of philosophies, questioning skills, and simply conversational dialogue between client and sport psychologist within case work. These books also comprised chapters which targeted relevant themes (eg, career transitions; injury), populations, and contexts that practitioners would come across in the real, sometimes messy and complex, world of professional practice. Put simply, they were great for the practical "know" and "know how." In addition, in 2004, Judy Van Raalte, Al Petitpas, and the Springfield University staff produced *Three Approaches to Sport Psychology* (Virtual Brands, 2004), a video of three senior sport psychologists conducting a 25-min intake and consulting session with the same athlete. The beauty of this product lay not only in students being able to see a demonstration of a sport psychologist in practice (when this is not always easily accessible), but also the opportunity to debate the strengths and weaknesses/likes and dislikes of the stylistic approaches taken by the practitioners. Year after year the students on my course are split on the preferred style of how they would want to consult or be consulted (as a client) after watching this video. It represented an excellent starting point (and only a starting point) to get students thinking about their philosophy and model of practice with athlete-clients.

I believe the strengths of what these products offered to the teaching of students as part of their university education concurrently exposed the weaknesses and limitations of practitioner development in our system. In brief, they challenge academics to spend far more hours on practical training of students' communication skills, intake interviews, appraisal of cases and case formulations, as well as the practice of delivering techniques such as goal setting, imagery, cognitive restructuring, mindfulness, and other stress management strategies (to name but a few). When the students experience these videos, they are hungry for more practice. However, in my professional opinion and experience (and it is only my viewpoint), university courses and academics are seldom geared up to provide this "know how and show how"; many staff have not been practicing consultants and some are out of touch if ever they had been practitioners. Universities place other role-related demands on these staff (research; administration), and appropriately training the next generation of young practitioner psychologists is low on the list of university priorities in the United Kingdom. What this amounts to is a position where students enter the next stage of private supervision within a professional association qualification (ie, License; Registration) without a great deal of strategic confidence of delivery; yet the role of a supervisor in a professional association (eg, BPS; BASES) is not as a trainer whose responsibility it is for conducting multiple observations of practice and assessing via simulated case studies (known in the clinical world as Objective Structured Clinical Examinations; OSCEs, Harden & Gleeson, 1979). Hence, there emerges a practitioner skills/technical competencies gap and the unanswered question of "whose responsibility is it to train the practitioner."

This reflection is shared in order to encourage readers to hold the same mirror up to their own country's system of practitioner development, and ask if an appropriate job is being done by universities and professional associations together. In my view, we are in a tricky place at present with respect to the future health and well-being of applied sport psychology. Whoever provides the "knowledge, know how and show how," there is a need to ensure that:

1. The knowledge taught has relevance to the breadth of real-world practice competencies, and includes the cognate areas of sport science and sport medicine.
2. Counseling, interpersonal, and conflict management skills are well honed.
3. Students gain extensive practice in case formulations, OSCEs, and technical skill demonstrations.
4. Students receive formative feedback from staff vis-a-vis role plays and observations of practice that are set-up in safe learning environments.
5. Students experience working within an interdisciplinary sport science support team and appreciate their potential roles in a wider sport organization.

Few education and training systems in the world probably offer enough of this type of experience, although I believe Australia perhaps comes closest. I think I appreciate why this is the case, and why it may become more of the case in the future. Let me incisively expand on this point.

One of the major challenges to the profession of applied sport psychology currently is the effects of global pressure on academics in sport science to generate research income to justify their existence. Such research income generation is more readily available to "health-related" projects, many of which have little to do with sport, and even less to do with competitive sport. Yet, we see academics drift toward heath-based research as universities reward such work if it brings in money, no matter how much actual practical impact such research may exert. At the same time, institutions are in danger of forgetting their core business—the consumers in the form of students who come to study sports science, with sport psychology as one popular, core discipline at BSc and MSc level. In the majority of institutions in the United Kingdom, teaching income from student fees accounts for greater than 80% of the total income to a school or department; research income and rewards for research environment, impact and outputs are much "smaller players" in terms of the income side of the economics equation. Student satisfaction scores on university degrees represent important metrics to a university, and teaching content, quality, and processes should be taken seriously in terms of maintaining the health of student applications to degree programs. Students at 18 years of age who are interested in studying sport science and sport psychology (and their parents paying the fees) are more demanding of vocational and transferable skill development, and practical experiences on university programs. They want the knowledge, and they certainly want the "know how" if the degree is to be of intellectual and practical value in today's graduate marketplace. These students of sport science and sport psychology come to study sport and people who play sport with an interest in helping people in sport; they do not come to study the global health problem or the unhealthy, unmotivated individual who has no interest in seeing a tennis court or a swimming pool. Students signing up for sport science, kinesiology, or sport psychology generally want to be contributing to the development, performance, well-being, and science of athletes in sport—not the science of those populations who are not sport participants, nor have the drive to be. I do not make any apologies for being so frank here, given the resources available. With research and evidence-based teaching as a priority for degree courses, institutions need to be careful of keeping their teaching material and academic staff "up to date" and at the freshest forefront of applied research in sport. When staff migrate toward researching the physical health agenda, and when value to academics in applied research and practice in sport science is discounted, an institution risks deskilling and eroding its core business. Student and parent consumers will migrate to those programs that really do offer cutting-edge sport science, and which better prepare students as practitioners for the industry of sport.

At present, there is potential for a crisis of personnel to teach, prepare, and mentor the next generation of practitioner sport psychologists. Academic staff and educators at universities may not have the time, skill set, institutional mandate, or reward "incentives/criteria" to deliver cutting-edge "knowledge and know how" in applied sport psychology; equally, the current supervisors in professional associations are often academics (with practice as a hobby), and it is the full-time practitioner that is perhaps the most relevant individual to involve in the provision of supervision services to the neophyte consultant. This still leaves the matter of "training" and the hours devoted to "show how." Whose responsibility is this? I'll leave the reader to reflect on all of these points, to assimilate my subjective views, and to translate them into research questions that better examine the current state of affairs more objectively.

CONCLUSIONS

This chapter, based on the 2015 FEPSAC keynote, has offered three key reflections of my career so far as an inconsistent scientist-practitioner doing sport psychology. I hope that the reader sees the relevance of the scientist-practitioner model and its place in each of these three reflections. Importantly, I believe that the proximity of my roles as an applied researcher, educator/supervisor (not trainer!), and practitioner have enabled me to draw out these critical points, and I encourage those doing sport psychology to strive for greater impact in terms of research, practice, and teaching. We really do need applied researchers, educators, and practitioners to be a lot closer even if three different people are fulfilling these roles. One suggestion I offered at the end of this keynote was the potential for a special issue (in *Psychology of Sport and Exercise*, or another journal), which documented case studies of scientist-practitioner collaboration in applied sport psychology. In this way, applied researchers and practitioners may be challenged to work closely together on growing the evidence base of knowledge about real-world questions or issues. Indeed, this may also help institutions, professional associations, and national federations work more closely together on developing the profession of applied sport psychology in the long run.

REFERENCES

Ames, C. (1992). Achievement goals, motivational climate, and motivational processes. In: G. C. Roberts (Ed.), *Motivation in sport and exercise* (pp. 161–176). Champaign, IL: Human Kinetics.

Andersen, M. (2000). *Doing sport psychology*. Champaign, Illinois: Human Kinetics.

Andersen, M. (2005). *Sport psychology in practice*. Champaign, Illinois: Human Kinetics.

Bandura, A. (1977a). *Social learning theory*. Englewood Cliffs, NJ: Prentice Hall.

Bandura, A. (1977b). Self-efficacy: toward a unified theory of behavioral change. *Psychological Review, 84*, 191–215.

British Psychological Society (2011). *Qualification in sport and exercise psychology: Stage 2 candidate handbook*. Leicester: BPS.

Deci, E. L., & Ryan, R. M. (1985). *Intrinsic motivation and self-determination in human behavior*. New York: Plenum.

Duda, J. L. (1992). Motivation in sport settings: a goal perspective approach. In: G. C. Roberts (Ed.), *Motivation in sport and exercise* (pp. 57–91). Champaign, IL: Human Kinetics.

Duda, J. L. (2013). The conceptual and empirical foundations of Empowering Coaching™: setting the stage for the PAPA project. *International Journal of Sport and Exercise Psychology, 11*, 311–318.

Elliot, A. J., & McGregor, H. A. (2001). A 2 × 2 achievement goal framework. *Journal of Personality and Social Psychology, 80*, 501–519.

Epstein, J. (1989). Family structures and student motivation: a developmental 8 perspective. In: C. Ames, & R. Ames (Eds.), *Research on motivation in 9 education: Vol. 3. Goals and cognitions* (pp. 259–298). New York: Academic Press.

Frank, G. (1984). The Boulder Model: History, rationale, and critique. *Professional Psychology, 15*(3), 417–435.

Harden, R. M., & Gleeson, F. A. (1979). Assessment of clinical competence using an objective structured clinical examination (OSCE). *Medical Education, 13*, 41–54.

Harwood, C. G. (2008a). Developmental consulting in a professional soccer academy: the 5C's coaching efficacy program. *The Sport Psychologist, 22*, 109–133.

Harwood, C. G. (2008b). From researcher to water boy: reflections on in-depth consulting with an elite British student-athlete team. In: U. Johnson, & M. Lindwall (Eds.), *Svensk idrottspsykologisk förenings årsbok 2008 [Swedish yearbook of sport psychology, 2008]* (pp. 28–48). Sweden: Trydells Tryckeri AB.

Harwood, C. G., & Anderson, R. J. (2012). Professional practice issues when working with team sports. In: S. Hanton, & S. Mellalieu (Eds.), *Professional practice in sport psychology: A review* (pp. 79–106). London: Routledge.

Harwood, C. G., & Anderson, R. (2015). *Coaching psychological skills in youth football: Developing the 5Cs.* Stoke-on-Trent: Bennion-Kearny.

Harwood, C. G., & Hardy, L. (2001). Persistence and effort in moving achievement goal research forward: a response to Treasure and colleagues. *Journal of Sport and Exercise Psychology, 23,* 330–345.

Harwood, C. G., & Swain, A. B. (1998). Antecedents of pre-competition achievement goals in elite junior tennis players. *Journal of Sports Sciences, 16,* 357–371.

Harwood, C. G., & Swain, A. B. (2001). The development and activation of achievement goals in tennis I: understanding the underlying factors. *The Sport Psychologist, 15,* 319–341.

Harwood, C. G., & Swain, A. B. (2002). The development and activation of achievement goals within tennis II: a player, parent, and coach intervention. *The Sport Psychologist, 16,* 111–137.

Harwood, C. G., Hardy, L., & Swain, A. (2000). Achievement goals in competitive sport: a critique of conceptual and measurement issues. *Journal of Sport and Exercise Psychology, 22,* 235–255.

Harwood, C. G., Spray, C. M., & Keegan, R. (2008). Achievement goal theories in sport. In: T. S. Horn (Ed.), *Advances in sport psychology* (pp. 157–185). Champaign, IL: Human Kinetics.

Harwood, C. G., Barker, J. B., & Anderson, R. (2015a). Psychosocial development in youth soccer players: assessing the effectiveness of the 5C's intervention program. *The Sport Psychologist, 29,* 319–334.

Harwood, C. G., Keegan, R. J., Smith, J. M. J., & Raine, A. S. (2015b). A systematic review of the intrapersonal correlates of motivational climate perceptions in sport and physical activity. *Psychology of Sport and Exercise, 18,* 9–25.

Henriksen, K., Stambulova, N., & Roessler, K. K. (2010). Holistic approach to athletic talent development environments: a successful sailing milieu. *Psychology of Sport and Exercise, 11,* 212–222.

Jetha, M. K., & Segalowitz, S. J. (2012). *Adolescent brain development: Implications for behavior.* New York: Academic Press.

Jones, D. (Producer) & Lloyd, P. (Director) (2011). *The Iron Lady* [Motion picture]. United Kingdom: Pathe.

Lowman, R. L. (2012). The scientist-practitioner consulting psychologist. *Consulting Psychology Journal, 63*(4), 151–156.

Miller, G. E. (1990). The assessment of clinical skills/competence/performance. *Academic Medicine, 65,* S63–S67.

Nicholls, J. G. (1984). Achievement motivation: conceptions of ability, subjective experience, task choice, and performance. *Psychological Review, 91,* 328–346.

Nicholls, J. G. (1989). *The competitive ethos and democratic education.* Cambridge, MA: Harvard University Press.

Ntoumanis, N., & Vazou, S. (2005). Peer motivational climate in youth sport: measurement development and validation. *Journal of Sport & Exercise Psychology, 27,* 432–455.

Pain, M. A., & Harwood, C. G. (2004). Knowledge and perceptions of sport psychology within English soccer. *Journal of Sports Sciences, 22,* 813–826.

Pain, M. A., & Harwood, C. G. (2007). The performance environment in English youth soccer. *Journal of Sports Sciences, 25,* 1307–1324.

Pain, M. A., & Harwood, C. G. (2008). The performance environment in English youth soccer: a quantitative investigation. *Journal of Sports Sciences, 26,* 1157–1169.

Pain, M. A., & Harwood, C. G. (2009). Team building through mutual sharing and open discussion of team functioning. *The Sport Psychologist, 23,* 523–542.

Pain, M., Harwood, C. G., & Mullen, R. (2012). Improving the performance environment of a soccer team during a competitive season: an exploratory action research study. *The Sport Psychologist, 26,* 390–411.

Poczwardowski, A., Sherman, C. P., & Ravizza, K. (2004). Professional philosophy in the sport psychology service delivery: building on theory and practice. *The Sport Psychologist, 18*, 445–463.

Roberts, G. C. (1992). *Motivation in sport and exercise*. Champaign, IL: Human Kinetics.

Roberts, G. C., & Treasure, D. C. (2012). *Advances in motivation in sport and exercise* (3rd ed.). Champaign, IL: Human Kinetics.

Rønnestad, M. H., & Skovholt, T. M. (2003). The journey of the counselor and therapist: research findings and perspectives on professional development. *Journal of Career Development, 30*, 5–44.

Steiner, I. D. (1972). *Group processes and productivity*. New York: Academic Press.

Stoltenberg, C. D., & Pace, T. M. (2007). The scientist-practitioner model: now more than ever. *Journal of Contemporary Psychotherapy, 37*, 195–203.

Swain, A. B., & Harwood, C. G. (1996). Antecedents of state goals in age-group swimmers: an interactionist perspective. *Journal of Sports Sciences, 14*, 111–124.

Tannenbaum, S. I., & Cerasoli, C. P. (2013). Do team and individual debriefs enhance performance? A meta-analysis. *Human Factors, 55*, 231–245.

Tessier, D., Smith, N., Tzioumakis, Y., Quested, E., Sarrazin, P., Papaioannou, A., Digelidis, N., & Duda, J. L. (2013). Comparing the objective motivational climate created by grassroots soccer coaches in England, Greece and France. *International Journal of Sport and Exercise Psychology, 11*, 365–383.

Treasure, D. C., Duda, J. L., Hall, H. K., Roberts, G. C., Ames, C., & Maehr, M. L. (2001). Clarifying misconceptions and misrepresentations in achievement goal research in sport: a response to Harwood, Hardy and Swain. *Journal of Sport and Exercise Psychology, 23*, 317–329.

Vansteenkiste, M., Lens, W., Elliot, A. J., Soenens, B., & Mouratidis, A. (2014). Moving the achievement goal approach one step forward: toward a systematic examination of the autonomous and controlled reasons underlying achievement goals. *Educational Psychologist, 49*, 153–174.

Virtual Brands. (2004). Three approaches to sport psychology consulting [DVD], Wilbraham, MA.

Wilson, K., Hardy, L., & Harwood, C. G. (2006). Investigating the relationship between achievement goals and process goals in rugby union players. *Journal of Applied Sport Psychology, 18*, 297–311.

Chapter 12

Theoretical Developments in Career Transition Research: Contributions of European Sport Psychology

Natalia B. Stambulova

School of Health and Welfare, Halmstad University, Halmstad, Sweden

EVOLUTION OF THE EUROPEAN SPORT PSYCHOLOGY DISCOURSE ON CAREER TRANSITION

For the purpose of this chapter, I define the European sport psychology discourse on career transition (hereafter, the European discourse) as a historically constructed body of knowledge pertaining to athletes' careers and career transitions that European researchers and practitioners have been developing and sharing over time (Stambulova & Ryba, 2014). More specifically, the European discourse contains negotiated definitions of key concepts, identification of major career research foci internalized from sociocultural and sport contexts in European countries, and ways to theorize about and implement career transition knowledge—all supported by shared professional values and principles. Being involved in the development of this discourse for about 25 years allows me to trace its development through three major periods: (1) early research and theorizing (1960s to the mid-1990s), (2) establishment of major intellectual traditions and values (mid-1990s to the late 2000s), and (3) the structuring and contextualization of the knowledge (late 2000s to the present). Next I will briefly outline the historical context and content of each period, focusing on milestone events in cooperation of the European researchers that led to major theoretical developments within the European discourse.

Sport and Exercise Psychology Research. http://dx.doi.org/10.1016/B978-0-12-803634-1.00012-1

Early Research and Theorizing (1960s to the Mid-1990s)

European socio-political context during this period had evolved from the Cold War and political separation between the socialist block countries and the rest of Europe (1960–1980s) to major changes on the European map and socio-political context (eg, disintegration of the Soviet Union, Czechoslovakia, Yugoslavia and the socialist block as a whole, unification of Germany, formation of new independent countries) in the early 1990s. During the Cold War, political barriers limited information exchange and cooperation among researchers in Europe (Stambulova, 2009a). This might be the reason why two major lines in early career research in Europe were "unaware" of each other.

The first line (which is also the earlier one) represents athletic retirement research conducted in Sweden (Halldén, 1965), former Yugoslavia (Mihovilovic, 1968), former Czechoslovakia (Svoboda & Vanek, 1982), Greece (Koukouris, 1991), Hungary (Schaefer, 1992), Belgium (Wylleman, De Knop, Menkehorst, Theeboom, & Annerel, 1993), and Germany (Bussmann & Alfermann, 1994).[a] These studies were based mainly on frameworks and findings borrowed from North American transition research (Coakley, 1983; Schlossberg, 1981) and focused on reasons for retirement, coping or adaptation strategies, and athletes' integration in society. In contrast, the second line (initiated in the late 1980s) is represented by Russian research focused on the athletic career as a whole from its beginning to end. These studies were inspired by the Russian developmental psychology tradition (Vygotsky, 1896–1934) and resulted in two descriptive theoretical frameworks: the *synthetic athletic career model* and the *analytical athletic career model* (Stambulova, 1994). The synthetic model guided the description of an athletic career as a whole through a set of characteristics, such as duration of sport participation, sport event(s) in which the athlete had competed, achieved titles and results, perceived "benefits" and "costs" of sport involvement, career satisfaction, and perceived career success. In the analytical model, an athletic career was considered as a multiyear process with several stages and six normative transitions: (1) the beginning of sport specialization, (2) the transition to more intensive training in the chosen sport, (3) the junior-to-senior transition, (4) the amateur-to-professional transition, (5) the transition from peak to maintenance career stage, and (6) the transition to the postsport career. These two frameworks were seen as complementing ways to describe an athletic career, and both received solid empirical support in a series of Russian studies (Stambulova, 1993, 1994). However, these frameworks did not earn much popularity outside Russia, with the exception of the junior-to-senior transition identified in the analytical model. Pioneering Russian research on this transition (Stambulova, 1994; see also Stambulova, 2009a, 2009b) was followed by research in other European countries during the next developmental period of the European discourse.

---

[a] This is not an exhaustive list. I used mainly the bibliography of Lavallee, Wylleman, and Sinclair (2000).

Establishing Major Intellectual Traditions and Values (Mid-1990s to the Late 2000s)

A turning point in the development of career transition research in Europe and a consolidation of the researchers' efforts was the Ninth European Federation of Sport Psychology (FEPSAC) Congress, during which the Career Transition Special Interest Group (CT-SIG) was created. Paul Wylleman had initiated that meeting, and we were about 15 people interested in joining forces to advance our area of research and practice. The CT-SIG's activities were directed to the organization of career transition symposia at major international conferences, joint research projects, and publications. The CT-SIG cooperated with the FEPSAC Managing Council and prepared two FEPSAC Position Statements—"Career Transitions" (European Federation of Sport Psychology, 1995) and "Career Termination" (European Federation of Sport Psychology, 1997)—as well as a FEPSAC monograph, *Career Transitions in Competitive Sports* (Wylleman, Lavallee, & Alfermann, 1999). Dorothee Alfermann and I initiated the European Perspectives on Athletic Retirement Project, which involved researchers and samples from both West and East Europe and resulted in several joint publications (Alfermann, Stambulova, & Zemaityte, 2004; see also, Stambulova & Alfermann, 2009, for reflections on the project).

An important milestone of this period was the book *Career Transitions: International Perspectives*, edited by Lavallee and Wylleman (2000), in which European, North American, and Australian experts shared their research and applied experiences. The book covered theoretical considerations with an emphasis on the conceptual model of athletic career termination (Taylor & Ogilvie, 1994), research on athletic identity and other factors involved in athletes' adaptation during retirement, career assistance programs, and the theory-to-practice approach to transitions of special populations (eg, young athletes, disabled athletes). A solid contribution of this book was also a bibliography on career transition literature, with 270 annotated references. Taylor and Ogilvie's (1994) model, positioned in the book as the only sport-specific transition model, was soon after complemented by the athletic career transition model (Stambulova, 2003), which was based on research on various athletic transitions and recommended as a suitable framework to study a transition process and the factors involved.

The next two significant publications for the development of the European discourse came out in 2004, and both were involved in introducing a holistic lifespan perspective when considering athletes' career development. These were the *Psychology of Sport and Exercise* special issue "Career transitions" (Wylleman, Alfermann, & Lavallee, 2004a) and a book chapter that introduced the *developmental model of transitions faced by athletes* (Wylleman & Lavallee, 2004). The special issue contained one review article outlining the past, present, and future of career transition research, as well as five research articles devoted to various aspects of athletic retirement and careers in youth sport (all authored by European researchers). In the review article, "Career transitions in sport: European perspectives," Wylleman, Alfermann, and Lavallee (2004b) introduced the *developmental model of transitions faced by athletes* (Wylleman & Lavallee, 2004), as well as a conceptualization of the athlete as "a whole person." Although in 2004 the whole-person conceptualization and the holistic lifespan perspective were new trends, currently both are well established and widely used foundations for career transition research.

Structuring and Contextualization of the Knowledge (Late 2000s to the Present)

Two interrelated processes characterize the current period in the development of the European discourse: structuring the topic (ie, negotiating definitions, taxonomies, frameworks, principles of applied work) and contextualizing the athletic career knowledge (ie, considering athletes' careers as being constituted by the sociocultural contexts to which the athletes belong). A series of recent review papers published by European researchers (Alfermann & Stambulova, 2007; Park, Lavallee & Tod, 2013; Stambulova, 2010a) considered the topic from different perspectives and contributed with clarifications of the topic structure. Contextualization of career knowledge was stimulated by the cultural sport psychology literature (Ryba, Schinke, & Tenenbaum, 2010) and increased collaboration between career and cultural sport psychology researchers.

Major events and theoretical developments within the European discourse that mark the current period include (1) transformation of the developmental model of transitions faced by athletes into the *holistic athletic career model* (Reints, 2011; Wylleman, Reints, & De Knop, 2013), (2) introducing the *holistic ecological perspective* and relevant frameworks as a means to study the junior-to-senior transition (Henriksen, 2010), (3) a meta-review on the topic presenting major shifts in our understanding of athletes' career transitions and introducing the *assistance in career transition (ACT) model* (Stambulova, 2012), (4) the International Society of Sport Psychology (ISSP) position stand on athletes' career development and transitions with the first attempt to consider cultural traditions in athletic career research around the world (Stambulova, Alfermann, Statler, & Côté, 2009), (5) the book *Athletes' Career Across Cultures* (Stambulova & Ryba, 2013a) with further analysis of cultural discourses and an introduction of the *cultural praxis of athletes' careers* paradigm (Stambulova & Ryba, 2013b, 2014), and (6) involvement of career researchers in the development of the *EU Guidelines on Dual Careers of Athletes* (European Union, 2012), followed by the *Psychology of Sport and Exercise* special issue "Dual career development and transitions" (Stambulova & Wylleman, 2015a) and the EU funded (2015–16) project Gold in Education and Elite Sport (European Union, 2014; www.gees.eu; project leader: Paul Wylleman).

Prompted by the aforementioned review papers, key definitions (eg, athletic career, career transitions, career assistance) and a taxonomy of transitions (athletic and nonathletic, normative, nonnormative, and quasi-normative) were negotiated and established (Park & Lavallee, 2014; Stambulova, 2014, 2016; Stambulova & Wylleman, 2014). Alfermann and Stambulova (2007) also suggested a taxonomy of frameworks related to athlete careers consisting of *descriptive career-stage models, explanatory career transition models*, and *intervention models*. European researchers have contributed to all the model categories, and next I will discuss the major theoretical developments within the European discourse that guide career transition research and practice in Europe and beyond.

CURRENT THEORETICAL PILLARS IN EUROPEAN CAREER TRANSITION DISCOURSE

Conceptualizing an Athlete as a Whole Person

In the earlier decades of sport psychology, an athlete was conceptualized as an *athletic performer*, that is, a person who is involved in regular practice preparation for and practice and participation in sport competitions. Such conceptualization puts the major focus of sport psychology research and practice on performance enhancement, leaving other issues on the margins of the scholars' attention. However, the situation has changed since career researchers introduced the holistic lifespan perspective (Wylleman & Lavallee, 2004) and suggested conceptualization of an athlete as a *whole person*, that is, a person who practices sport within the scope of other life matters (eg, family, friends, studies, work; see also Chapter 14). This reconceptualization influenced applied work traditions, stimulating the development of *career assistance* as a professional discourse in applied sport psychology aimed at helping athletes with various sport and nonsport career issues (Stambulova & Wylleman, 2014; Wylleman & Reints, 2014).

Holistic Lifespan Perspective and Relevant Models

The holistic lifespan perspective was first articulated through the *developmental model of transitions faced by athletes* (Wylleman & Lavallee, 2004; Wylleman, Alfermann, & Lavallee, 2004b). In this model, stages and normative transitions in four layers of athletes' lifespan development—athletic, psychological, psychosocial, and academic-vocational—were defined and "roughly" aligned with chronological age markers. The layers were also shown to be "concurrent, interactive and reciprocal" (Wylleman, De Knop, & Reints, 2011, p. 66). *Athletic development* was described as having four stages—initiation, development, mastery, and discontinuation—with normative transitions between adjacent stages. Their timing depends on the athlete's type of sport, gender, and personal characteristics and circumstances. *Psychological development* was marked by stages of childhood (ages 12 and younger), adolescence (ages 13–18), and adulthood (ages 19 and older), with related transitions in the athletes' personal maturation. *Psychosocial development* was represented by the changes in the athletes' sport-related networks, including their parents, siblings, peers, coaches, and spouse/partner. *Academic-vocational development* was characterized by stages in the athlete's education (primary, secondary, higher education) and vocational career, with transitions defined by the relevant educational and vocational systems.

Recently, the four layers of athletes' development originally defined by the *developmental model of transitions faced by athletes* were complemented by the *financial level*, highlighting the roles of families, sport federations, national Olympic committees, sponsors, and employers as major financial supporters of athletes' careers. Some changes were also made in the *psychosocial* and *academic-vocational* layers. For example, support staff, teammates, and peer students were added to the athletes' network; and professional and semiprofessional statuses were added to the *academic-vocational* level—both corresponding to the mastery athletic stage. The model was also renamed the *holistic athletic career model* (Wylleman et al., 2013).

The earlier version of the model has been guiding a number of career studies in Europe and worldwide (Bruner, Munroe-Chandler, & Spink, 2008; Pummell, Harwood, & Lavallee, 2008; Wylleman, Reints, & Van Aken, 2012), facilitating a deeper analysis of an athlete's career and encouraging researchers and practitioners to establish links between the developmental layers and to strive for an optimal balance between an athletes' sport and nonsport life. It was also incorporated into the *EU Guidelines on Dual Careers of Athletes* (2012, p. 6) and contributed to the conceptualization of athletes' dual career development, transitions, and dual career support services. Since dual career transitions (ie, simultaneous transitions in sport and education or working life) are inevitably associated with challenges and changes in all other layers of an athlete's development (psychological, psychosocial, and financial), the use of the holistic lifespan perspective is a natural fit for research on dual career pathways and transitions (Stambulova & Wylleman, 2015b). For example, the overwhelming majority of articles included in the *Psychology of Sport and Exercise* special issue on dual career development and transitions (Stambulova & Wylleman, 2015a) shared the holistic lifespan perspective, with the authors using the holistic athletic career model as their framework (Debois, Ledon, & Wylleman, 2015; Ryba, Stambulova, Ronkainen, Bundgaard, & Selänne, 2015; Stambulova, Engström, Franck, Linnér, & Lindahl, 2015). This later version of the model is also currently employed as a theoretical framework in the European project Gold in Education and Elite Sport involving nine European countries and aiming at studying dual career competences (ie, relevant knowledge, skills, abilities, and attitudes) of 12- to 25-year-old athletes, as well as the competences of the dual career service providers who facilitate athletes' dual career development.

Athletic Career Transition Model

The athletic career transition model (Stambulova, 2003, 2009b) was designed to describe and explain a transition process through interactions of several transition components. In this model, the transition process is defined as *coping* with a set of *transition demands* or *challenges* using relevant *coping strategies* and taking into consideration internal (person-related) and external (environment-related) *resources* and *barriers*. The transition *outcomes* and relevant *pathways* are shown to be dependent on the effectiveness of coping. The model predicts two primary transition outcomes: a successful transition and a crisis-transition. A successful transition is the outcome of effective coping, with a good fit between transition demands on the one side and the athlete's coping resources and strategies on the other (the *most favorable transition pathway*). A crisis-transition is the outcome of ineffective coping, which can be caused by any of the following: lack of resources, excessive barriers, and ineffective coping strategies. According to the model, a crisis-transition might have two secondary outcomes: a "delayed" successful transition in the event of effective transition intervention (the *favorable transition pathway*), and an unsuccessful transition (the *unfavorable transition pathway*) associated with premature dropout, overtraining, substance abuse, or other negative consequences of not coping with the transition demands. Three types of career transition interventions related to *crisis prevention*, *crisis coping*, and *negative-consequences coping* are also outlined by the model. As the original author of this model, I can add that my thinking about the transition process changed over time from focusing mainly on the transition components and their interactions to emphasizing possible transition pathways and relevant intervention types.

Although the athletic career transition model was developed based on a series of Russian studies (Stambulova, 1994, 2000), later it was confirmed by research in other sociocultural contexts (Brown et al., 2015). Currently the model is used to study the junior-to-senior transition (Morris, Tod, & Oliver, 2015; Stambulova, Franck, & Weibull, 2012), dual career transitions (Brown et al., 2015; Stambulova et al., 2015), Olympic Games as a career transition (Schinke, Stambulova, Trepanier, & Oghene, 2015), and cultural transitions (Ryba, Stambulova, & Ronkainen, 2016).

Holistic Ecological Perspective and Relevant Models

The *holistic ecological perspective* in career transition research emphasizes "athletic career as a social affair" (Henriksen, Larsen, & Christensen, 2014) and shifts the researchers' focus from an individual athlete to the environment the athlete belongs to. It also encourages researchers to consider the talent/career development environment holistically, that is, as having micro and macro levels, athletic and nonathletic domains, and also a time dimension (ie, past, present, and future of the environment). This approach was developed and tested in the project called Successful Athletic Talent Development Environments in Scandinavia, in which three environments with a successful record of producing elite senior athletes from their respective junior pools—a Danish 49er sailing team, a Swedish track-and-field club in Växjö, and a kayak group from the Wang Elite Sport School in Norway—were studied (Henriksen, 2010; Henriksen, Stambulova, & Roessler, 2010a; 2010b; 2011). The theoretical contribution of this project consisted of two models (see the following paragraphs) aimed at describing an environment (eg, a club, team, or sport school) and explaining its success (or failure) in supporting young athletes in their junior-to-senior transition. Both frameworks were designed as working models to guide data collection (through analysis of documents, participant observation, and multiple interviews), with further transformation into empirical models reflecting unique features of each environment under study.

The first working model, the *athletic talent development environment (ATDE) model*, was designed as a descriptive framework. In this model the major components of the ATDE were structured as "nests" around young athletes (at the center of the model) into *micro* (eg, coaches, peers) and *macro* (eg, media) *levels*, and *athletic* and *nonathletic domains*; the model also guided researchers to explore how members of the ATDE perceived its past, present, and future. The model became a useful basis for investigating the various components of the ATDE and, more importantly, their relationships and functions in the talent development process. In the previously mentioned Scandinavian project, the empirical models (ie, created from the data) reflected unique combinations of their components, but also adhered to the basic tenets of the ATDE working model (Henriksen et al., 2010a, 2010b, 2011).

The second working model, the *environment success factors (EFS) model*, was designed as an explanatory framework, guiding researchers to consider *preconditions* (eg, financial and human resources of the ATDE), *processes* (ie, various activities the members of the ATDE are involved in, such as training camps, social events), and the ATDE's *organizational culture* (ie, artifacts, evident values, and basic assumptions) as major factors influencing the individuals' and teams' development, as well as the ATDE's success in facilitating athletes' junior-to-senior transition. In the aforementioned Scandinavian project, the EFS empirical models (ie, created from the data) helped uncover the "secrets" of each ATDE's success with some specific but also shared (eg, proximal role models, focus on long-term development; see more in Henriksen, 2010) features of the ATDEs involved.

In short, the theoretical contributions derived from the Scandinavian project helped complement the holistic lifespan thinking about an athlete's development with the holistic thinking about an athlete's environment. Currently, the holistic ecological perspective is used to study not only successful ATDEs (Pink, Saunders, & Stynes, 2015) but also less successful ATDEs (Henriksen et al., 2014). Therefore, this theoretical and research perspective opens up a new line in career assistance geared toward optimizing or "repairing" ATDEs to facilitate athletes' junior-to-senior transition.

Assistance in Career Transition (ACT) Model

Several review papers on career assistance and career assistance programs (Gordon, Lavallee, & Grove, 2005; Hackfort & Huang, 2005; Stambulova, 2010a;

Wylleman & Reints, 2014) and publications on applied strategies and tools (Lavallee, Nesti, Borkoles, Cockerill, & Edge, 2000; Stambulova, 2010b, 2011) called for structuring *career assistance* as a professional applied sport psychology discourse with defined goals and areas of expertise (eg, balancing lifestyle, educational, and vocational guidance, preparation for athletic retirement) and professional culture (ie, principles, values, frameworks, and strategies/tools shared by career practitioners). To integrate and structure the existing knowledge on applied work with athletes in career transitions, I proposed the assistance in career transitions (ACT) model as a set of guidelines on how to plan a career transition intervention (Stambulova, 2012) based on a meta-review of the career transition literature and my own expertise. The ACT model consists of eight interrelated components, set up as consecutive steps in a transition intervention planning: (1) foundations, (2) client's characteristics and cultural contexts, (3) goals, (4) life contexts to work in, (5) time frames, (6) basic methods, (7) perspectives and content, and (8) assessment.

Foundations in the ACT model refer to the basic competences for career assistance practitioners that enable them to help athletes in career transitions, such as familiarity with career development and transition models, access to a body of relevant research and applied principles, and command of necessary strategies and tools. Therefore, foundations can be seen as preconditions for a career transition intervention but they also contribute with theoretical and applied frameworks for the intervention (after the client data is collected and goals of the intervention are defined). To facilitate collecting information about the *client's characteristics and relevant contexts*, the ACT model recommends a structure, called the client's *form*. The client's form incorporates both the holistic lifespan and the holistic ecological perspective, while guiding the practitioner to explore (1) the client as a person (age, gender, psychological profile, etc.), (2) the client as an athlete (type of sport, level in sport, career stage, etc.), (3) the client's near social environment (eg, coach, teammates, parents, partner, peers, etc., and relationships with them) and non-athletic roles (eg, student, friend, worker, family member, etc.), and (4) client's near past (perception of preconditions for the present situation), present situation in sport and life, and perceived future. While processing this information, it is also recommended to consider wider sociocultural contexts (eg, national and sport cultures) that might contribute to the client's development. After such holistic information is collected and analyzed, *goals for the intervention* might be defined. In the ACT model the goals are formulated in a general manner (ie, helping athletes with preparation for and coping with athletic and non-athletic, normative and non-normative transitions), but should to be tailored to specific cases based on the analysis of the client's data.

After the goals are formulated and relevant theoretical frameworks and research are considered, the ACT model guides the practitioner in deciding about the *contexts to work in* (eg, sport and studies or sport and family life), the *time frame* for the intervention (eg, short term or long term), the *basic methods* to implement (ie, needs assessment, psychological education, psychological training, and counseling), and the *intervention perspectives and types* to be used. From the career assistance literature, two major perspectives (preventive/supportive and crisis/negative-consequences coping perspectives) and seven types of career transition interventions are identified in the ACT model. The *preventive/supportive perspective* covers interventions aimed at enhancing athletes' awareness of the forthcoming/current transition demands and aiding in timely development of all the necessary resources for effective coping. This perspective is represented by *career-planning interventions, lifestyle management interventions, life development interventions, identity development interventions*, and *cultural adaptation interventions*, with related professional strategies and tools. The *crisis/negative-consequences coping perspective* covers interventions that help athletes assess their crisis/traumatic situations and find the best available ways to cope and consists of *crisis-coping educational interventions* and *clinical interventions* (Lavallee, 2005; Stambulova, 2012, 2014; Stambulova & Wylleman, 2014). The final step in the ACT model encourages practitioners to plan *assessment of the intervention*, including measurements of the client's progress on intervention-related issues before, during, and after the intervention, as well as of any changes in the client's performance in sport and other activities, lifestyle, and well-being.

As seen from the previous description, the ACT model is a "general" or working model that is supposed to be transformed step-by-step into an *individualized* ACT model (or plan) based on the specific client's data. Metaphorically, the individualized ACT model can be seen as "a map" for the intervention, implying further concretization of each step during the actual work with the client that can be seen as "a territory" explored and managed by the practitioner. To my knowledge, during the last few years the model has been used mainly in applied sport psychology education to aid novice practitioners in planning their transitional work with athlete-clients (Stambulova, Johnson, & Linnér, 2014). The students reflected on the usefulness of the ACT model, but wider practical implementations of the model are needed to identify its advantages and limitations. It is also possible there will be further development of the ACT model, for example, when new theoretical and applied approaches in the career transition topic are in place.

Cultural Praxis of Athletes' Careers Paradigm

For a long time, career researchers were guided by thinking that the more their research findings and practical recommendations could be generalized, the better. Cultural praxis of athletes' careers encourages a new way of thinking: the more research findings and practical recommendations can be contextualized, the better. More broadly, the cultural praxis of athletes' careers is an emerging professional discourse outlining a set of challenges for career scholars to blend career theorizing, research, practice, and context to better match the diversity of athletes' careers across cultures. The development of this paradigm was heralded by several incremental steps in contextualizing the career topic, with European scholars leading the charge in this process. The discussion was initiated in the ISSP position stand on career development and transitions (Stambulova et al., 2009). The authors of the position stand analyzed similarities and differences in career research foci across cultures and articulated the idea that career researchers internalized their research topics from the sociocultural contexts to which they belonged. On the basis of this analysis, the authors identified four major cultural traditions in career research—North American, Australian, West European, and East European. The discussion on the role of context in career research was continued in a paper that introduced the idea of a "cultural mindset" in career research (Stambulova & Alfermann, 2009) published in the *International Journal of Sport and Exercise Psychology* special issue "Decolonizing methodologies: Approaches to sport and exercise psychology from the margins" (Ryba & Schinke, 2009). More specifically, the authors critically analyzed cross-cultural career research with its *etic* perspective on culture (ie, as an external entity) and articulated a need to consider cultural context as formative for an athlete's career development (ie, a shift to an *emic* perspective on culture). These two papers, together with publications in the rapidly developing field of cultural sport psychology (Ryba et al., 2010; Ryba & Wright, 2005; Schinke & Hanrahan, 2009), served as preconditions and inspiration for the book *Athletes' Careers Across Cultures* (Stambulova & Ryba, 2013a), where the cultural praxis of athletes' careers paradigm was first introduced.

This book contributed to the discourse with reviews of athletic career research and career assistance programs in sociocultural and sport system contexts in 19 countries, including 11 European countries (Belguim, Denmark, France, Germany, Greece, Ireland, Russia, Slovenia, Spain, Sweden, and the United Kingdom). The authors, who were leading career researchers and practitioners in their respective countries, were also cultural insiders representing emic perspectives on athletic careers. About 500 references were cited in the book, including 223 in national languages. The book's editors also identified three phases (metaphorically defined as "waves") in the process of incorporating culture in career research: cross-cultural, cultural mindset, and cultural praxis (Ryba & Stambulova, 2013). They also provided a comparative analysis of athletic careers across cultures, focusing on early careers/talent development, elite and dual careers, cultural transitions, and athletic retirement, and reached the following conclusion:

> *On the surface, the vast majority of athletes face rather similar challenges, but how these challenges are perceived and addressed heavily depends on the context in which the athlete is embedded. ... career stages established by career frameworks can be seen only as overarching categories having many variations behind and simplifying reality of athletes' career development. (Stambulova & Ryba, 2013b, p. 236)*

Further analysis in the book dealt with career research and careers assistance programs across cultures and resulted in identification of three dominant (North American, Australian, and European) and two emerging (Asian and South American) discourses in career research and practice worldwide (Stambulova & Ryba, 2014). The European discourse was shown to be "the most diverse in terms of research foci and theoretical frameworks, reflecting most probably the diversity of cultures behind it" (Stambulova & Ryba, 2014, p. 6). The cultural praxis of athletes' careers paradigm was the quintessence of *Athletes' Careers Across Cultures*. It was based on the authors' and editors' collective wisdom and emerged from the discussion of limitations in existing career research and practice in relation to the realities of modern sport (eg, increased globalization, professionalization, cultural diversity, and transnationalism).

More specifically, the cultural praxis of athletes' careers sets the following challenges: (1) to merge the holistic lifespan and holistic ecological perspectives in career projects to capture the whole spectrum of athletes' experiences in sport and beyond; (2) to contextualize all the steps in career projects, from providing culturally meaningful definitions of key concepts and using culturally adapted theoretical frameworks to contextualizing data interpretations and practical recommendations; (3) to strengthen the idiosyncratic approach in career research and assistance, with specific attention to diversity in career pathways, including marginalized athletic populations (eg, female or ethnic minority athletes); (4) to explore transnationalism in contemporary sporting culture and careers of transnational athletes; (5) to strengthen interdisciplinary career research reflecting the complexity of athletes' development in today's sports and world; (6) to promote participatory action research facilitating close collaboration between researchers, practitioners, and athlete-participants; and (7) to develop multicultural and transnational consulting, including international networks of existing career assistance programs. The cultural praxis of athletes' careers paradigm is still very new, and a good deal of time is needed to achieve the shift to cultural-praxis-type thinking in career researchers. Meanwhile, the impact of this paradigm is already visible in the dominance of the holistic perspective (see Chapter 14), implementation of participatory action research, and improved contextualization in the articles included in the *Psychology of Sport and Exercise* special issue on dual-career development and transitions (Blodgett & Schinke, 2015; Pink et al., 2015; Ryba et al., 2016).

Bridge to the Future

The overview of the European sport psychology discourse on career transition, with particular focus on its theoretical contributions, reveals its rich history and solid achievements. Conceptualization of an athlete as a whole person, the holistic athletic career model (Wylleman & Lavallee, 2004; Wylleman et al., 2013), the athletic career transition model (Stambulova, 2003, 2009b), the ATDE and ESF models (Henriksen, 2010), the ACT model (Stambulova, 2012), and the cultural praxis of athletes' careers paradigm (Stambulova & Ryba, 2013b, 2014) constitute the major theoretical contributions of European scholars that guide current career research and practice in Europe and continue to gain popularity worldwide. Meanwhile, there are still gaps to be addressed.

I see the first gap in the inconsistency between the "fixed" frameworks and the diversity and also fluidity of cultural contexts of which the athletes are a part. Research findings on athletes' careers across cultures have revealed that "real careers are much more diverse and richer than any theoretical framework can show us" (Stambulova & Ryba, 2013b, p. 242). Therefore, the "general" models should be culturally adapted (to national and/or specific sport contexts) or used as working models to guide the data collection, followed by their transformation into empirical models that grasp the nuances of career development or the transition process in a specific athletic population and context. This approach has already been found to be useful within the holistic ecological research, and it might also be applied in the holistic lifespan research, for example, through adaptations of the holistic athletic career model (ie, specifying stages and relevant age markers) and the athletic career transition model (ie, specifying demands, resources, barriers, coping strategies, etc.) in relation to a particular career pathway or transition and sociocultural and sport contexts (Brown et al., 2015; Debois et al., 2015). Culturally adapted (empirically based) frameworks might facilitate development of contextualized career assistance services.

The second gap is relevant to career scholars' cultural competences (ie, cultural awareness and reflexivity, knowledge and skills; see more in Ryba, Stambulova, Si, & Schinke, 2013), given that "many sport and exercise psychology professionals are intuitive or naive cultural or crosscultural researchers lacking awareness of how all aspects of their projects are culturally infused" (p. 137). To consider athletes' careers in various contexts and from different perspectives, development and use of diverse research methodologies and designs are highly desirable. However, the researchers need to be able to properly position their projects methodologically and also within *cross-cultural psychology* (ie, with an etic perspective on culture), *cultural psychology* (ie, with an emic perspective on culture), or *cultural praxis* (ie, theorizing, research, and practice constituted by cultural contexts relevant to the project participants). Further, the researchers should be encouraged to position themselves within the projects, reflecting on how their background and experiences contributed to their project planning, data collection, and interpretations.

The third gap is visible in the disproportion between the large body of empirical findings on athletic retirement and the availability of data on other athletes' transitions. Therefore, new research trends are needed, for example, studies on quasi-normative transitions that are predictable only for select categories of athletes, such as elite, professional, or transnational (Schinke et al., 2015). Examples of quasi-normative transitions include the transition to the residential high performance center (Verkooijen, Van Hove, & Dik, 2012), cultural transitions

(Blodgett & Schinke, 2015; Ryba et al., 2016), Olympic Games as a career transition (Wylleman et al., 2012), injury as a career transition (Ivarsson, Stambulova, & Johnson, 2015), and others. These and other new trends (eg, dual-career transitions) should be developed further and appropriately positioned within the existing system of athletic career knowledge (Stambulova, 2016) to facilitate further structuring of the career topic.

Last but not least, there is still a gap between career research and assistance. The *career assistance applied sport psychology discourse* should be further developed through publications introducing existing and newly developed tools and strategies with case examples demonstrating their implementation. For example, within the Gold in Education and Elite Sport project there are plans to identify the required competences of dual career service providers and create a repository of relevant applied frameworks, strategies, and tools. As an educator, I would also love to see a textbook on career assistance that can be used in applied sport psychology education that promotes career assistance among new generations of sport psychology practitioners.

REFERENCES

Alfermann, D., & Stambulova, N. (2007). Career transitions and career termination. In G. Tenenbaum, & R. C. Eklund (Eds.), *Handbook of sport psychology* (3rd ed., pp. 712–733). New York: Wiley.

Alfermann, D., Stambulova, N., & Zemaityte, A. (2004). Reactions to sports career termination: a cross-national comparison of German, Lithuanian, and Russian athletes. *Psychology of Sport and Exercise, 5*, 61–75.

Blodgett, A. T., & Schinke, R. J. (2015). "When you're coming from the reserve you're not supposed to make it": stories of aboriginal athletes pursuing sport and academic careers in "mainstream" cultural contexts. *Psychology of Sport and Exercise, 21*, 115–124.

Brown, D. J., Fletcher, D., Henry, I., Borrie, A., Emmett, J., Buzza, A., & Wombwell, S. (2015). A British university case study of the transitional experiences of student-athletes. *Psychology of Sport and Exercise, 21*, 78–90.

Bruner, M. W., Munroe-Chandler, K. J., & Spink, K. S. (2008). Entry to elite sport: a preliminary investigation into the transition experiences of rookie athletes. *Journal of Applied Sport Psychology, 20*, 236–252.

Bussmann, G., & Alfermann, D. (1994). Drop-out and the female athlete. In D. Hackfort (Ed.), *Psycho-social issues and interventions in elite sport* (pp. 90–128). Frankfurt, Germany: Lang.

Coakley, J. J. (1983). Leaving competitive sport: retirement or rebirth? *Quest, 35*, 1–11.

Debois, N., Ledon, A., & Wylleman, P. (2015). A lifespan perspective on the dual career of elite male athletes. *Psychology of Sport and Exercise, 21*, 15–26.

European Union. (2012). EU guidelines on dual careers of athletes: Recommended policy actions in support of dual careers in high-performance sport. Available from http://ec.europa.eu/sport/news/20130123-eu-guidelines-dualcareers_en.htm

European Federation of Sport Psychology. (1995). Position statement "Career transitions". *FEPSAC Bulletin, 2*, 9–10.

European Federation of Sport Psychology. (1997). Position statement "Career termination". *FEPSAC Bulletin, 1*, 5–6.

European Union. (2014). *Gold in Education and Elite Sport*. European Union's Erasmus + Sport Project. Available from www.gees.eu

Gordon, S., Lavallee, D., & Grove, J. R. (2005). Career assistance program interventions in sport. In D. Hackfort, J. Duda, & R. Lidor (Eds.), *Handbook of research in applied sport and exercise psychology: International perspectives* (pp. 233–244). Morgantown, WV: Fitness Information Technology.

Hackfort, D., & Huang, Z. (2005). Considerations for research on career counseling and career transition. In D. Hackfort, J. Duda, & R. Lidor (Eds.), *Handbook of research in applied sport and exercise psychology: International perspectives* (pp. 245–255). Morgantown, WV: Fitness Information Technology.

Halldén, O. (1965). The adjustment of athletes after retiring from sport. In F. Antonelli (Ed.), *Proceedings of the first international congress of sport psychology* (pp. 730–733). Rome, Italy: Pozzi.

Henriksen, K. (2010). *The ecology of talent development in sport*. Doctoral dissertation, University of Southern Denmark, Odense, Denmark.

Henriksen, K., Larsen, C. H., & Christensen, M. K. (2014). Looking at success from its opposite pole: the case of a talent development golf environment. *International Journal of Sport and Exercise Psychology, 12*, 134–149.

Henriksen, K., Stambulova, N., & Roessler, K. K. (2010a). Holistic approach to athletic talent development environment: a successful sailing milieu. *Psychology of Sport and Exercise, 11*, 212–222.

Henriksen, K., Stambulova, N., & Roessler, K. K. (2010b). Successful talent development in athletics: considering the role of environment. *Scandinavian Journal of Medicine and Science in Sports, 20*, 122–132.

Henriksen, K., Stambulova, N., & Roessler, K. (2011). Riding the wave of an expert: a successful talent development environment in kayaking. *The Sport Psychologist, 25*, 341–362.

Ivarsson, A., Stambulova, N., & Johnson, U. (2015). Injury as a career transition: experiences of a Swedish elite handball player. In O. Schmid, R. Seiler (Eds.), *Proceedings of the 14th European congress of sport psychology* (pp. 241–242). Bern, Switzerland: University of Bern, Institute of Sport Science.

Koukouris, K. (1991). Disengagement of advanced and elite Greek male athletes from organized competitive sport. *International Review for the Sociology of Sport, 26*, 289–306.

Lavallee, D. (2005). The effect of a life development intervention on sports career transition adjustment. *The Sport Psychologist, 19*, 193–202.

Lavallee, D., Nesti, M., Borkoles, E., Cockerill, I., & Edge, A. (2000a). Intervention strategies for athletes in transition. In D. Lavallee, & P. Wylleman (Eds.), *Career transitions in sport: International perspectives* (pp. 111–130). Morgantown, WV: Fitness Information Technology.

Lavallee, D., & Wylleman, P. (Eds.). (2000). *Career transitions in sport: International perspectives*. Morgantown, WV: Fitness Information Technology.

Lavallee, D., Wylleman, P., & Sinclair, D. (2000b). Career transitions in sport: an annotated bibliography. In D. Lavallee, & P. Wylleman (Eds.), *Career transitions in sport: International perspectives* (pp. 207–258). Morgantown, WV: Fitness Information Technology.

Mihovilovic, M. (1968). The status of former sportsmen. *International Review of Sport Sociology, 3*, 73–93.

Morris, R., Tod, D., & Oliver, E. (2015). An analysis of organizational structure and transition outcomes in the youth-to-senior professional soccer transition. *Journal of Applied Sport Psychology, 27*, 216–234.

Park, S., & Lavallee, D. (2014). Transition. In R. C. Eklund, & G. Tenenbaum (Eds.), *Encyclopedia of sport and exercise psychology* (pp. 763–767). Thousand Oaks, CA: Sage.

Park, S., Lavallee, D., & Tod, D. (2013). Athletes' career transition out of sport: a systematic review. *International Review of Sport and Exercise Psychology, 6*, 22–53.

Pink, M. A., Saunders, J., & Stynes, J. (2015). Reconciling the maintenance of on-field success with off-field player development: a case study of a club within the Australian Football League. *Psychology of Sport and Exercise, 21*, 98–108.

Pummell, B., Harwood, C., & Lavallee, D. (2008). Jumping to the next level: a qualitative examination of within-career transition in adolescent event riders. *Psychology of Sport and Exercise, 9*, 427–447.

Reints, A. (2011). *Validation of the holistic athletic career model and the identification of variables related to athletic retirement*. Doctoral dissertation, Vrije Universiteit Brussel, Belgium.

Ryba, T.V., & Schinke, R.J. (Eds.). (2009). Decolonizing methodologies: approaches to sport and exercise psychology from the margins [Special issue]. *International Journal of Sport and Exercise Psychology, 7* (3), 359–379.

Ryba, T. V., Schinke, R. J., & Tenenbaum, G. (Eds.). (2010). *The cultural turn in sport psychology*. Morgantown, WV: Fitness Information Technology.

Ryba, T. V., & Stambulova, N. (2013). The turn to a culturally informed career research and assistance in sport psychology. In N. B. Stambulova, & T. V. Ryba (Eds.), *Athletes' careers across cultures* (pp. 1–16). New York, NY: Routledge.

Ryba, T. V., Stambulova, N., & Ronkainen, N. (2016). *The work of cultural transition: An emerging model. Frontiers in Psychology, 7*, doi: 10.3389/fpsyg. 2016.00427

Ryba, T. V., Stambulova, N., Ronkainen, N., Bundgaard, J., & Selänne, H. (2015). Dual career pathways of transnational athletes. *Psychology of Sport and Exercise, 21*, 125–134.

Ryba, T. V., Stambulova, N., Si, G., & Schinke, R. J. (2013). The ISSP position stand: culturally competent research and practice in sport and exercise psychology. *International Journal of Sport and Exercise Psychology, 11*, 123–142.

Ryba, T. V., & Wright, H. K. (2005). From mental game to cultural praxis: a cultural studies model's implications for the future of sport psychology. *Quest, 57*, 192–212.

Schaefer, U. (1992). *Retirement and adjustment process of top level athletes*. Doctoral dissertation, Hungarian University of Physical Education and Sport, Budapest, Hungary.

Schinke, R. J., & Hanrahan, S. (Eds.). (2009). *Cultural sport psychology*. Champaign, IL: Human Kinetics.

Schinke, R. J., Stambulova, N., Trepanier, D., & Oghene, O. (2015). Psychological support for the Canadian Olympic boxing team in meta-transitions through the national team program. *International Journal of Sport and Exercise Psychology, 13*, 74–89.

Schlossberg, N. K. (1981). A model for analyzing human adaptation to transition. *The Counseling Psychologist, 9*(2), 2–18.

Stambulova, N. (1993). Two ways of psychological description of sports career. In S. Serpa, J. Alves, V. Ferreira, V. Pataco (Eds.), *Proceedings of the eigth ISSP world congress of sport psychology* (pp. 762–764). Lisbon, Portugal: ISSP.

Stambulova, N. (1994). Developmental sports career investigations in Russia: a post-Perestroika analysis. *The Sport Psychologist, 8*, 221–237.

Stambulova, N. (2000). Athlete's crises: a developmental perspective. *International Journal of Sport Psychology, 31*, 584–601.

Stambulova, N. (2003). Symptoms of a crisis-transition: a grounded theory study. In N. Hassmén (Ed.), *SIPF yearbook 2003* (pp. 97–109). Örebro, Sweden: Örebro University Press.

Stambulova, N. (2009a). European perspectives on career development and transition research and practice. *Japanese Journal of Sport Psychology, 36*, 57–60.

Stambulova, N. (2009b). Talent development in sport: a career transition perspective. In E. Tsung-Min Hung, R. Lidor, & D. Hackfort (Eds.), *Psychology of sport excellence* (pp. 63–74). Morgantown, WV: Fitness Information Technology.

Stambulova, N. (2010a). Professional culture of career assistance to athletes: a look through contrasting lenses of career metaphors. In T. V. Ryba, R. J. Schinke, & G. Tenenbaum (Eds.), *The cultural turn in sport psychology* (pp. 285–314). Morgantown, WV: Fitness Information Technology.

Stambulova, N. (2010b). Counseling athletes in career transitions: the five-step career planning strategy. *Journal of Sport Psychology in Action, 1,* 95–105.

Stambulova, N. (2011). The mobilization model of counseling athletes in crisis-transitions: an educational intervention tool. *Journal of Sport Psychology in Action, 2,* 156–170.

Stambulova, N. (2012). Working with athletes in career transitions. In S. Hanton, & S. Mellalieu (Eds.), *Professional practice in sport psychology: A review* (pp. 165–194). London, England: Routledge.

Stambulova, N. (2014). Career transitions. In R. C. Eklund, & G. Tenenbaum (Eds.), *Encyclopedia of sport and exercise psychology* (pp. 110–115). Thousand Oaks, CA: Sage.

Stambulova, N. (2016). Athletes' transitions in sport and life: positioning new research trends within existing system of athlete career knowledge. In R. Schinke, K. McGannon, & B. Smith (Eds.), *The Routledge international handbook of sport psychology* (pp. 519–535). New York, NY: Routledge.

Stambulova, N., & Alfermann, D. (2009). Putting culture into context: cultural and cross-cultural perspectives in career development and transition research and practice. *International Journal of Sport and Exercise Psychology, 7,* 292–308.

Stambulova, N., Alfermann, D., Statler, T., & Côté, J. (2009). ISSP position stand: career development and transitions of athletes. *International Journal of Sport & Exercise Psychology, 7,* 395–412.

Stambulova, N., Engström, C., Franck, A., Linnér, L., & Lindahl, K. (2015). Searching for an optimal balance: dual career experiences of Swedish adolescent athletes. *Psychology of Sport and Exercise, 21,* 4–14.

Stambulova, N., Franck, A., & Weibull, F. (2012). Assessment of the transition from junior to senior sports in Swedish athletes. *International Journal of Sport & Exercise Psychology, 10,* 1–17.

Stambulova, N., Johnson, U., & Linnér, L. (2014). Insights from Sweden: Halmstad applied sport psychology supervision model. In L. Tashman, & G. Cremades (Eds.), *Becoming a sport, exercise and performance psychology professional: International perspectives* (pp. 276–284). New York, NY: Routledge.

Stambulova, N., & Ryba, T. V. (Eds.). (2013a). *Athletes' careers across cultures.* New York, NY: Routledge.

Stambulova, N., & Ryba, T. V. (2013b). Setting the bar: towards cultural praxis of athletes' careers. In N. Stambulova, & T. V. Ryba (Eds.), *Athletes' careers across cultures* (pp. 235–254). New York, NY: Routledge.

Stambulova, N., & Ryba, T. (2014). A critical review of career research and assistance through the cultural lens: towards cultural praxis of athletes' careers. *International Review of Sport and Exercise Psychology, 7,* 1–17.

Stambulova, N., & Wylleman, P. (2014). Athletes' career development and transitions. In A. Papaioannou, & D. Hackfort (Eds.), *Routledge companion to sport and exercise psychology* (pp. 605–621). London, England: Routledge.

Stambulova, N., & Wylleman, P. (Eds.). (2015a). Dual career development and transitions [Special issue]. *Psychology of Sport and Exercise, 21,* 1–134.

Stambulova, N., & Wylleman, P. (2015b). Editorial. *Psychology of Sport and Exercise, 21,* 1–3.

Svoboda, B., & Vanek, M. (1982). Retirement from high level competition. In: *Proceedings of the fifth world congress of sport psychology* (pp. 166–175). Ottawa, Canada: Coaching Association of Canada.

Taylor, J., & Ogilvie, B. C. (1994). A conceptual model of adaptation to retirement among athletes. *Journal of Applied Sport Psychology, 6,* 1–20.

Verkooijen, K. T., Van Hove, P., & Dik, G. (2012). Athletic identity and well-being among youth talent athletes who live at a Dutch elite sport center. *Journal of Applied Sport Psychology, 24,* 106–113.

Wylleman, P., Alfermann, D., & Lavallee, D. (Eds.), (2004a). Career transitions in sport [Special issue]. *Psychology of Sport and Exercise, 5*(1), 1–88.

Wylleman, P., Alfermann, D., & Lavallee, D. (2004b). Career transitions in sport: European perspectives. *Psychology of Sport and Exercise, 5,* 7–20.

Wylleman, P., De Knop, P., Menkehorst, H., Theeboom, M., & Annerel, J. (1993). Career termination and social integration among elite athletes. In S. Serpa, J. Alves, V. Ferreira, V. Pataco (Eds.), *Proceedings of the eigth world congress of sport psychology* (pp. 902–906). Lisbon, Portugal: ISSP.

Wylleman, P., De Knop, P., & Reints, A. (2011). Transitions in competitive sports. In N. L. Holt, & M. Talbot (Eds.), *Lifelong engagement in sport and physical activity* (pp. 63–76). New York, NY: Routledge.

Wylleman, P., & Lavallee, D. (2004). A developmental perspective on transitions faced by athletes. In M. Weiss (Ed.), *Developmental sport and exercise psychology: A lifespan perspective* (pp. 507–527). Morgantown, WV: Fitness Information Technology.

Wylleman, P., Lavallee, D., & Alfermann, D. (Eds.). (1999). *Career transitions in competitive sports.* Biel, Switzerland: FEPSAC.

Wylleman, P., & Reints, A. (2014). Career assistance programs. In R. C. Eklund, & G. Tenenbaum (Eds.), *Encyclopedia of sport and exercise psychology* (pp. 105–108). Thousand Oaks, CA: Sage.

Wylleman, P., Reints, A., & De Knop, P. (2013). A developmental and holistic perspective on athletic career development. In P. Sotiaradou, & V. De Bosscher (Eds.), *Managing high performance sport* (pp. 159–182). New York, NY: Routledge.

Wylleman, P., Reints, A., & Van Aken, S. (2012). Athletes' perceptions of multilevel changes related to competing at the 2008 Beijing Olympic Games. *Psychology of Sport and Exercise, 13,* 687–692.

Chapter 13

Holistic Perspective on the Development of Elite Athletes

Paul Wylleman*, Nathalie Rosier**

*Research Group Sport Psychology and Mental Support (SPMB),Department of Movement and Sport Sciences, Faculty of Physical Education and Physiotherapy and Faculty of Psychology and Educational Sciences, Vrije Universiteit Brussel, Brussels, Belgium; **Faculty of Physical Education and Physiotherapy, Vrije Universiteit Brussel, Brussels, Belgium

During the past decades, the topic of career transitions developed into a well-researched and well-established domain of sport psychology. While sport psychologists' interest was initially geared toward the individual (psychological) factors influencing athletic retirement—or the "end-of-career" transition—the focus of researchers steadily broadened leading up to the current developmental and holistic perspective taken on a spectrum of transitions faced by talented and elite athletes (Stambulova & Wylleman, 2015). Witnesses to this development include not only the increasing number of research-driven articles (Bruner, Munroe-Chandler, & Spink, 2008; Debois, Ledon, Argiolas, & Rosnet, 2012; Pummell, Harwood, & Lavallee, 2008; Tekavc, Wylleman, & Cecić Erpič, 2015), but also the many thematic symposia and presentations at international congresses (continuously since the 1995 FEPSAC Congress), special journal issues (Wylleman, Alfermann, & Lavallee, 2004; Stambulova & Wylleman, 2015), thematic chapters and books (Alfermann & Stambulova, 2007; Lavallee & Wylleman, 2000; Ryba & Stambulova, 2013; Wylleman, Lavallee, & Theeboom, 2004), (organizational) guidelines (FEPSAC, 2003a,b; European Union, 2012) as well (applied) recommendations aimed at assisting (former) athletes to cope with career transitions (Murphy, 1995; Stambulova, 2010; Wylleman, Rosier, & De Knop, 2015).

In light of this broad interest, the purpose of this chapter is to provide in first instance a brief overview of sport psychology research into the concept of career transitions, followed by the description of a conceptual model providing a developmental and holistic perspective on the occurrence of multilevel transitions as faced by talented and elite athletes. In second instance, this conceptual model will be used to illustrate the influence of three transitional challenges athletes may face at different points in their career, namely the junior-to-senior transition, participation in the Olympic Games, and the end of the athletic

Sport and Exercise Psychology Research. http://dx.doi.org/10.1016/B978-0-12-803634-1.00013-3

career. Finally, the chapter will conclude with perspectives for future research on career transitions faced by talented, elite, and retiring athletes.

Taking into account the different foci on career transitions used by researchers and applied sport psychologists, both this chapter and Chapter 12 are very complementary. More specifically, in her chapter Stambulova not only builds upon this chapter by elaborating on recently developed frameworks such as the holistic ecological perspective and the cultural praxis of athletes' careers paradigm, but also provides an insight into the assistance in career transitions (ACT) model, which provides a hands-on approach to some of the transitional challenges as described in this chapter.

A DEVELOPMENTAL AND HOLISTIC PERSPECTIVE ON CAREER TRANSITIONS

Athletic retirement is not only inevitable to all elite athletes but may also be accompanied by a period of emotional, cognitive, and social turmoil (Wippert & Wippert, 2008; Wylleman, De Knop, Menkehorst, Theeboom, & Annerel, 1993). It should therefore not be surprising that this "end-of-career" transition already attracted sport psychologists' interest four decades ago (Haerle, 1975; Hallden, 1965; Mihovilovic, 1968), revealing that former (professional) athletes experienced a range of negative or traumatic experiences (eg, alcohol and substance abuse, acute depression, eating disorders, identity confusion, decreased self-confidence, attempted suicide) during, as well as after, athletic retirement (Blinde & Stratta, 1992; Sinclair & Orlick, 1993). It is interesting to note that later research relativized the traumatic character of elite athletes' career termination (Alfermann, 2000; Wylleman et al., 1993).

Research on the causes for retirement and on the factors mediating the adjustment process to postathletic life (Alfermann & Gross, 1997; Webb, Nasco, Riley, & Headrick, 1998) made it clear that this "end-of-career" transition was actually a transitional process consisting of different stages (ie, phase of preretirement, phase of retirement, and phase of postretirement) rather than a singular event (Lavallee, 2000). By using Sussman's (1972) Analytical model, and especially Schlossberg and coworkers' model of Human Adaptation to Transition (Charner & Schlossberg, 1986; Schlossberg, 1981, 1984), sport psychologists had to link up with conceptual frameworks from outside of sport in order to study this transitional process (Baillie & Danish, 1992; Coakley, 1983; McPherson, 1980; Parker, 1994; Sinclair & Orlick, 1994; Swain, 1991). Schlossberg's model enabled not only to define a career transition as "an event or nonevent which results in a change in assumptions about oneself and the world and thus requires a corresponding change in one's behavior and relationships" (Schlossberg, 1981, p. 5), but also described three interacting sets of factors (ie, the athlete's characteristics, the athlete's perception of the particular transition, and the characteristics of the pre- and posttransition environments) influencing the transitional process of retirement.

As more empirical data on (elite) athletes became available, researchers were able to develop sport-specific career transition models. For example, Taylor and Ogilvie's (1998) model conceptualized the career transition process in terms of causal factors initiating the transitional process, developmental factors related to transition adaptation, coping resources affecting the responses to career transitions, the quality of adjustment to career transition, and the possible treatment issues for distressful reactions to career transition. With her Athletic Career Transition model, Stambulova (2003) stipulated further that a career transition actually challenged athletes to find an effective fit between the demands of the transition and their coping resources and strategies: the closer the fit, the higher the probability for athletes to experience a successful transition. If, however, athletes are ineffective in coping, have a lack of resources, or are unable to analyze the transitional situation, then athletes await a possible crisis transition (Stambulova, 2000). It is important to note that these models were not only important to research, but also initiated the development of sport-specific interventions amongst applied sport psychologists.

As continued research broadened the knowledge base on the transitional process faced by athletes, so did sport psychologists' insight in, and understanding of the types and occurrence of transitions. In function of their degree of predictability, a distinction was now being made between normative transitions that are generally predictable and anticipated (eg, athletic retirement) and nonnormative transitions that are generally unpredicted, unanticipated, and involuntary in nature (eg, an injury). By taking into account the predictability of transitions, sport psychologists started to identify transitions occurring during the athletic career. As (especially) normative "within-career" transitions (eg, the junior to senior transition, initiating a dual "study and elite sport" career, a first-time Olympic participation) were being considered (Wylleman et al., 2004a; Wylleman, Verdet, Lévêque, De Knop, & Huts, 2004), sport-specific career transition models developed into a representation of a succession of normative transitions (and stages). For example, Stambulova's (1994) analytical athletic career model identified five normative stages (ie, preparatory stage, stage of the start into specialization, stage of intensive training in the chosen sport, culmination stage, the final stage and career end). Interesting to note is that in this way, the conceptualization of career transitions started to converge toward that of talent development, where, for example, Salmela (1994) considered three normative career stages—initiation, development, and perfection.

Building upon research on the development of athletes' interpersonal relationships (Wylleman, 2000; Wylleman, De Knop, Verdet, & Cecić Erpič, 2007), elite student-athletes' dual career (Wylleman et al., 2004c), and former elite athletes (Wylleman et al., 1993), Wylleman introduced the developmental model of transitions faced by athletes (Wylleman & Lavallee, 2004). This "lifespan" model combined a developmental (ie, initiation into postathletic career) with a holistic perspective (ie, athlete's multilevel development) reflecting domain-specific normative transitions in athletes' psychological, psychosocial,

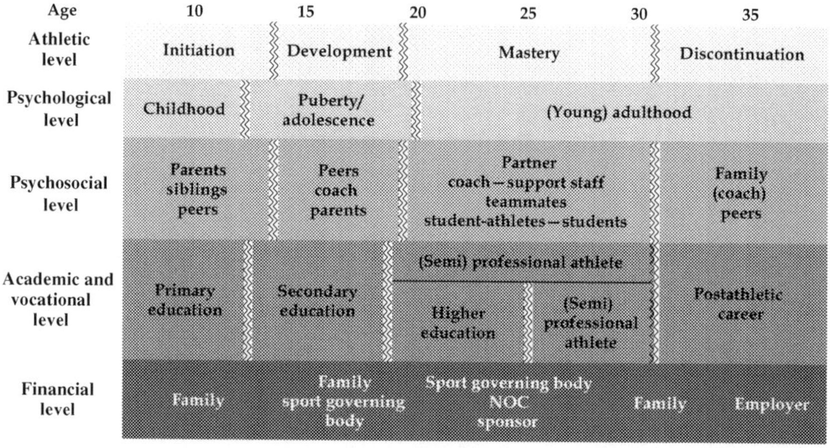

Age	10	15	20	25	30	35
Athletic level	Initiation	Development	Mastery		Discontinuation	
Psychological level	Childhood	Puberty/adolescence	(Young) adulthood			
Psychosocial level	Parents siblings peers	Peers coach parents	Partner coach–support staff teammates student-athletes–students		Family (coach) peers	
Academic and vocational level	Primary education	Secondary education	(Semi) professional athlete		Postathletic career	
			Higher education	(Semi) professional athlete		
Financial level	Family	Family sport governing body	Sport governing body NOC sponsor		Family	Employer

FIGURE 13.1 The Holistic Athlete Career model representing transitions and stages faced by athletes at athletic, psychological, psychosocial, academic/vocational, and financial levels. Note. A *dotted line* indicates that the age at which the transition occurs is an approximation.

and academic and vocational development. During the past years, the model was further developed leading up to the current Holistic Athletic Career (HAC) model outlining stages and normative transitions in athletes' developments in athletic and nonathletic domains (Wylleman, Reints, & De Knop, 2013a) (Fig. 13.1).

This HAC model represents the concurrent, interactive, and reciprocal nature of the development of athletes in five domains (ie, athletic, psychological, psychosocial, academic/vocational, and financial). The top layer represents transitions and stages athletes face in their athletic development, namely (1) the initiation stage during which young athletes are introduced to organized competitive sports (from about 6 to 7 years of age); (2) the development stage during which young athletes are recognized as being talented bringing with it an intensive level of training and competitions (from about 12 to 13 years of age); (3) the mastery stage reflecting athletes' participation at the highest competitive level (from about 18 to 19 years of age); and (4) the discontinuation stage entailing elite athletes' transition out of competitive sports (from 28 to 30 years of age). The second layer reflects the major transitions and stages in athletes' psychological development, including childhood, adolescence, and (young) adulthood. The third layer is indicative of transitions and stages occurring in athletes' psychosocial development and denotes those individuals who are perceived by athletes as being (most) significant during that particular transition or stage (eg, parents, coach, peers, lifetime partner). The fourth layer represents stages and transitions at academic (primary education/elementary school, secondary education/high school, higher education) and vocational level. For elite athletes, vocational development may also start after secondary education, and may involve a full-/part-time occupation in the field of professional sports.

The final layer illustrates the way in which the involvement of athletes may be financially supported throughout, as well as after, their athletic career. With family support being significant in the beginning, and for some elite athletes also again before and during retirement, the supportive role of sport-governing bodies, national Olympic Committees, and/or (private) sponsors is clearly present from the end of the development into the mastery stage. By presenting the concurrent, interactive, and reciprocal nature of these normative transitions, the Holistic Athletic Career model shows that normative transitions do not only coincide, but also influence athletes' development and success at every level. It should be noted that, while normative in nature, the specific ages at which these transitions occur can vary.

This model added to the conceptualization of career transitions because it shows that athletes will not only face within-career transitions at athletic level, but actually at different levels of development. Furthermore, as it provides sport psychologists with a conceptual framework of multilevel transitional demands (and possible resources) athletes may face (Alfermann & Stambulova, 2007; Stambulova, 2000), the HAC model was used not only in research (Bruner et al., 2008; Debois, Ledon, & Wylleman, 2014; Pummell et al., 2008; Reints, 2011; Tekavc et al., 2015; Wylleman, Reints, & Van Aken, 2012), but also in the (continued) development of athlete career support provision (eg, Scotland, France, the Netherlands, Belgium) (Bouchetal Pellegri, Leseur, & Debois, 2006; Wylleman, Reints, & De Knop, 2013a), and the development of guidelines on dual careers in Europe (European Union, 2012).

Taking into account that the athletic career can possibly span 15–25 years (Sosniak, 2006; Wylleman et al., 1993), a strong need exists for sport psychologists to increase and deepen their knowledge on the transitional challenges faced by talented, elite, and former elite athletes. In order to illustrate the relevance of specific career transitions, and more particularly of the reciprocal nature of concurrent multilevel transitions, the next section will describe three examples of transitional challenges.

EXAMPLES OF CAREER TRANSITIONS FACED BY OLYMPIC ATHLETES

While Olympic athletes will face different normative and nonnormative transitions, the following three major normative transitions were chosen as representative for a developmental perspective to an Olympic athlete's career. These transitions are an institutionalized part of the fabric of competitive sports and are thus seen by former Olympians as having had a significant influence on their (post) athletic career (Redgrave & Townsend, 2001). It should be noted of course that while all three transitions apply directly to Olympic athletes, the junior–senior transition and athletic retirement are also relevant to non-Olympians. We refer to the HAC model (Fig. 13.1) as a visual aid to the description of the transitions and the challenges faced by athletes.

"Junior-to-Senior" Transition

When making the transition to senior level, athletes face concurrently transitions at the athletic level, the psychological level (from adolescence to young adulthood), and the academic level (from secondary to higher education). As this requires them to cope with an accumulation of transitional challenges, it should not be surprising that, on average, only one junior elite athlete in three actually makes a successful transition into the senior elite ranks (Australian Sports Commission, 2003; Bussmann & Alfermann, 1994; Vanden Auweele, De Martelaer, Rzewnicki, De Knop, & Wylleman, 2004) and that successfully completing the junior–senior transition takes novice senior athletes on average 2.1 years (Australian Sports Commission, 2003).

As final year juniors, athletes have a final opportunity to perform to their best level within their own age-category at, for example, Youth Olympic Games or World Junior Championships, and in this way also gain a better starting position to obtain a (semi) professional contract, or be selected for the senior team the following season. This period of increased—and perhaps self-imposed—performance expectations may lead final-year juniors not only to experience (increased) frustration, anxiety, stress (and even burnout) (Bruner et al., 2008; Pummell et al., 2008; Rosier, Wylleman, De Bosscher, & Van Hoecke, in review; Schinke, 2014), but also into physical overload, overtraining, or athletic injury (Australian Sports Commission, 2003; Lorenzo, Borrás, Sánchez, Jiménez, & Sampedro, 2009; MacNamara & Collins, 2010; Orchard & Seward, 2002).

In comparison to the junior category, first-year senior athletes are faced with more mature and experienced senior athletes (as teammates and as rivals) and higher frequencies and standards of training and competition (Bruner et al., 2008; Lorenzo et al., 2009; Pummell et al., 2008). Going from being (one of) the best as junior to achieving lower levels of achievement as first-year senior athletes (Bussmann & Alfermann, 1994) may have a strong impact on athletes' self-image and athletic identity (Brewer, Van Raalte, & Petitpas, 2000). The need for novice senior athletes to invest more time in their athletic involvement at the senior level will also impact their development at other levels (eg, social relationships, academic endeavors), possibly reducing athletes' feelings of enjoyment and motivation (Pummell et al., 2008; Stambulova, Franck, & Weibull, 2012). This may make them feel "entrapped in" rather than "attracted to" senior elite level (Cresswell & Eklund, 2007; Raedeke & Smith, 2001).

As athletes make the concurrent transition from adolescence into young adulthood, they face the challenge to develop their identity. This requires from them greater independency, responsibility, and discipline (Rosier et al., 2015), as well as stronger self-regulatory and coping skills to cope with (unexpected) situations, higher expectations, and pressures (Wylleman et al., 2013a) and adopt the everyday lifestyle of an elite athlete (eg, healthy food intake, recuperation, good sleeping habits, time management) (Stambulova, Alfermann, Statler, & Côté, 2009).

At the psychosocial level, athletes' relations with significant others also develop or change: the involvement and expectations of coaches (eg, for more self-discipline) and training partners or teammates (eg, for high-quality training) may increase (Lorenzo et al., 2009). Because athletes may move into a professional (sport) academy, private accommodation, or student housing, they will face the challenge of leaving family, friends, and club and of having to adapt to a new psychosocial environment (eg, new coach, new teammates). While parental roles and involvement may thus change (Wylleman et al., 2007), the reduction in daily parents–child interactions in combination with the maturation into (young) adulthood may actually improve parent–child relationships (Lefkowitz, 2005). Athletes' strong focus on and involvement in their elite sport career may impact (negatively) their friendships and lead to possible feelings of isolation (Pummell et al., 2008; Rosier et al., 2015). For these (young) adults, romantic relationships may become an important part of their lives (Wylleman & Lavallee, 2004), leading to an increase of support from a significant other, while at the same time possibly requiring athletes to cope with extra expectations and pressure (Stambulova et al., 2012).

Athletes will not only transit out of secondary education, but many continue their dual career by combining an academic career in higher education with an elite athletic career (Wylleman, Reints, & De Knop, 2013b). The challenges at academic level will be different from those in secondary education and could include, among others, taking more charge of their own academic career, being more self-regulated (eg, attending classes, rescheduling exams, investing time in studying), or coping with changing social environments (eg, student life) (De Knop, Wylleman, Van Hoecke, & Bollaert, 1999). The value attributed to an academic education in view of the risks and disadvantages of elite sport (eg, a career-ending injury, lack of financial stability) has led to an increased importance awarded to support systems providing elite athletes with a maximum of possibilities to develop the required competences in order to successfully start and complete a dual career (De Brandt, Wylleman, & Van Rossem, 2015; European Union, 2012; Stambulova & Wylleman, 2015).

Other athletes may, however, also discontinue their academic career and choose for a vocational career as (professional, full-time) athlete, or for a dual career involving elite sport and another (part-time) occupation. In the first case, athletes will be faced with the transitional challenges of more, and of an increased focus on, training sessions and competitions, which requires not only more time to recuperate, but leads—perhaps unexpectedly—also to being more available for social activities (eg, with family, friends) (Rosier et al., 2015). In the latter case, athletes will need to be able to prioritize and plan within a working context, ensuring them with flexibilities (eg, time off from work for competitions, training camps abroad).

Finally, athletes will also face a transition at financial level. More particularly, as not all first-year senior athletes will have a financial security via a contract as (semi) professional athlete, most will not be in the position to be self-sufficient. In fact, many novice senior athletes will require continued financial support from significant others (eg, parents, partner) (Reints, 2011), thus having a possible debilitating influence on elite athletes' perception and development into independence and self-control.

Olympic Games as Transition

As successfully competing (and possibly excelling) at the Olympic Games is seen by many elite athletes as the pinnacle of their athletic career (Redgrave & Townsend, 2001), researchers have focused on the significance of psychological preparation and support for Olympic excellence (Greenleaf, Gould, & Dieffenbach, 2001; Gould, Greenleaf, Guinan, & Chung, 2002; Pensgaard & Duda, 2002; Wylleman, Harwood, Elbe, Reints, & de Caluwé, 2009). While strongly aspiring to it, competing at the Olympic Games presents first-time Olympians, with specific transitional challenges (Wylleman et al., 2012). In fact, viewed from a developmental as well as a holistic perspective, novice Olympians are confronted with a diversity of (sometimes new) demands.

These may include transitional challenges at the athletic level such as (late) changes in physical and technical preparation and in training routines (frequency and load), as well as coping with jet lag and climate change (Wylleman et al., 2012). Because these issues are perceived to affect athletes' mental functioning (eg, tiredness), support will generally be provided to specifically prepare athletes physically and mentally for the effects of jet lag (Waterhouse, Reilly, & Atkinson, 1997) and fatigue (Hung, Lin, Lee, & Chen, 2008). Post-Olympic Games, athletes can find themselves, in comparison to other major competitions, taking a longer break away from their sport in view of the need to reestablish a more balanced mental functioning (eg, returning to their daily routines, focus on goals in other domains of interest or studies).

Athletes perceive also challenges at the psychological level. As first-time Olympians, they can experience a stronger self-confidence as they identified greatly with the role of Olympian before, during, as well as post-Olympic Games (eg, being part of the Olympic family). Other challenges may include changes in athletic identity and self-awareness, both of which can influence athletes' personal lives.

At psychosocial level, athletes can experience a clear decrease in their interactions with their parents, family, partner, and/or peers, and this before as well as during the Olympic Games. They need to be able to adapt to an exciting, yet restricted psychosocial (ie, residing at the holding camp before the Olympic Games, their own Olympic team house in the Olympic village) and social environment (ie, living in the Olympic village) (Gould et al., 2002; Jowett & Cramer, 2009). In fact, research revealed that performance success was influenced, among others, by a positive social environment (eg, more support from family and friends), including satisfaction with housing in the Olympic village (Gould, Guinan, Greenleaf, Medbery, & Peterson, 1999; Greenleaf et al., 2001). This secluded environment also affects athletes at psychological level: The continuous buildup (and sometimes long wait) before being able to start competing requires athletes not only to cope with precompetition pressure and tension, but will also make them face the major challenge of boredom (eg, "sleep-eat-train-recuperate" routine, avoiding any energy-draining activities in the Olympic village). This feeling is strengthened by the imposed rules to avoid, among others, disruptions to their own routines or those of Olympic teammates, lack of focus for the upcoming competition, or physical and/or mental overload due to the many distractions at hand in the Olympic village (Blumenstein & Lidor, 2007; Greenleaf et al., 2001; Hodge & Hermansson, 2007). This may lead novice Olympians to actively look for more and more intense interactions within their own Olympic team, or on the other hand, to actively withdraw from general social interactions, thus creating for themselves a "safe haven."

Due to its highly mediatized character, novice Olympians may receive greater than usual postcompetition attention from their psychosocial environment on their return from the Olympic Games. Coming from a more secluded environment, the increased contact with parents, family, partner, and/or peers after returning home can lead to an "inundation" of social requirements (eg, parties, press meetings, sponsorship activities) (Kristiansen, Hanstad, & Roberts, 2011). For some, this may be a challenge as they were actually looking to settle back down in to their own, pre-Games' daily routines. This (perceived) lack of being able to control their own personal time and space may be overwhelming, resulting in feelings of isolation and loneliness, possibly leading to social seclusion or psychological maladjustment (Tracey & Corlett, 1995; Storch, Storch, Killiany, & Roberti, 2005). In consequence, first-time Olympians may find themselves in having a strongly reduced contact with their (Olympic) coach and thus be confronted with the need to reestablish their working relationship or communication process with their coach (Antonini Philippe & Seiler, 2006).

First-time Olympians will also be confronted with challenges at the academic, vocational, and financial levels. More specifically, as elite student-athletes, they may choose to decrease their academic efforts in the period prior to, and increase them when returning from the Olympic Games. This requires athletes to plan ahead—generally 2 academic years before the Olympic Games—as they will need to plan how many study credits to take and whether or not to participate in exams (or other academic activities which require their presence at the university). Interesting to note is that, due to the need to get selected for the Olympic Games and the national Olympic team, the pre-Olympic year, rather than the actual Olympic year, may be more difficult to combine with academic activities. For those athletes in a dual career "elite sport and vocational profession," a similar need for reduction in load may require novice Olympians to engage in discussions with their employer. This need should be absent for those with a professional full-time contract as elite athlete. Finally, for some elite athletes, successful participation at Olympic level may also lead to financial revenue (eg, sponsorship, remuneration for starting in a competition or for a public appearance), thus increasing their financial self-support after the Olympic Games (eg, by moving away from the parental home into their own apartment).

Athletic Retirement

On average, 5–7% of elite athletes may annually retire from elite sport at an age that varies depending upon the sport (North & Lavallee, 2004; Wylleman et al., 1993). For example, North and Lavallee (2004) found that elite athletes from gymnastics, diving, swimming, ice skating, and judo planned to retire in the 24–30 year age category, while those from sailing, golf, equestrian, and shooting saw this transition well after age 40.

Discontinuation from elite sports confronts retiring elite athletes possibly with a diversity of challenges (Alfermann & Stambulova, 2007; Cecić Erpič, Wylleman, & Zupančič, 2004; Lavallee, Sugnhee, & Tod, 2010; Lavallee & Wylleman, 2000; Murphy, 1995; Scanlan, Ravizza, & Stein, 1989; Stephan, Torregrosa, & Sanchez, 2007; Taylor & Ogilvie, 2001). These may include, for example, experiencing a sense of loss of personal competence and mastery, of social recognition, and of enjoyment. Dealing with changes also includes coping with changes at physical level and in subjective well-being. These challenges could be aggravated as athletes have to develop their identity to a new life(style) as the "not-elite athlete" and thus being "like everyone else" trying to cope with a future that requires new skills and competences. As they had to withdraw from the sport atmosphere, they may also have to cope with missing numerous satisfying social relationships resulting from competing in international elite sport, and thus be confronted with the need to renew their social network (ie, relationships with peers). In this way, retiring elite athletes will have (to learn) to adapt to a new social status, possibly having to deal with family issues (eg, parenthood), as well as to have to take on other vocational responsibilities in order to start a new professional career (in or outside sports).

Different factors may play a role in the decision-making process of retiring from elite and Olympic level sport: Some are related to sport (eg, stagnation, nonselection, injuries, lack of financial support), others are clearly linked to the athlete's (current or future) development (eg, need for financial security, other vocational development, starting a family). This entails that the way in which athletes need to cope with athletic retirement may differ. In fact, about 80% of athletes are reported to experience a successful transition, whereas about 20% perceive it as a crisis (Stambulova & Wylleman, 2014). The way in which this transitional challenge is experienced is greatly influenced by the way in which retiring athletes perceive to be in control over (eg, are able to cope with) the process of retirement as well as by athletes' (perceptions of their) resources at hand to cope with these challenges (Alfermann & Stambulova, 2007). These resources could include a proactive retirement planning (eg, before the start of the last season, during the pre-Olympic year), a voluntary discontinuation of the athletic career (eg, after the Olympic Games, when ending a contract as professional athlete), having different personal roles (eg, as partner, as retiring athlete, as employee, as novice coach), and enjoying support from their psychosocial network (eg, family, coach, peers) and sport organizations.

For some, this "end-of-career" transition may include a clear-cut change in how they engage in life. Athletes retiring with an especially high athletic identity are thus more likely to adapt poorly to career termination, especially if there is a clear lack of support (eg, career support) (Gardner & Moore, 2006). This identity crisis may lead to a lack of optimal psychological well-being and behavioral deactivation, resulting in dysphoric mood and a heightened sense of hopelessness, potentially falling prey to major depression or even suicidal behavior (Baum, 2006; Chartrand & Lent, 1987; Gardner & Moore, 2006). Although the rate of retirees experiencing depressive symptoms is found to be fairly similar to that of the general population, the impact of these symptoms may become compounded by high levels of physical pain (eg, due to long-term sport-related physical strain and injuries). This may put retired athletes at a higher risk of significant difficulties with sleep, social relationships, finances, and exercise and fitness, or even at an increased risk for suicide (Schwenk, Gorenflo, Dopp, & Hipple, 2007). It should be noted that the macrosocial context (eg, culture, sport system) can also impact the retirement process (Alfermann, Stambulova, & Zemaityte, 2004; Stambulova, Stephan, & Jäphag, 2007).

Challenges facing retirees when building up a new professional career are not always straightforward (eg, increase in responsibilities, changing financial situation, working within fixed hours) and can also be related to the phenomenon of "occupational delay" (Naul, 1994). Few retired athletes may have had the opportunity to actively employ their knowledge and skills gained in higher education (eg, via summer jobs, vocational or in-service training, part-time employment) during their (professional full-time) sport career. The "delay" between acquiring this knowledge and these skills, and the duration of the period after retirement during which they could put them to use, may be so long that these competences are not strong enough anymore for retired athletes to successfully start a vocational career, or to attain vocational success. Retirees may have to return to higher (postgraduate) education, or to basic vocational training in order to gain (up-to-date or new) professional knowledge and skills.

Once entering the job market, retired athletes may also find themselves "at the bottom of the ladder." In comparison to their nonathletic peers they may not only be paid lower wages than could be expected on the basis of their age (and athletic achievements), but also be confronted with younger aged coworkers or colleagues who have seniority over them. Former elite athletes may thus not only need motivational readiness, but also interpersonal skills in order to integrate in such a new professional setting.

These challenges may lead some retirees to actually turn to their parents and/or family-of-origin for (financial) support, or even to return to their parental home possibly leading up to interpersonal (or intergenerational) problems. Taking into account these challenges, it should not be surprising that not only vocational training and finding a job are among the top reasons for athletes to terminate their sport career (Bussmann & Alfermann, 1994), but also that vocational training is an important part of career support services enhancing the quality of the postathletic career (Reints & Wylleman, 2009).

CONCLUSIONS

Career transitions research has undeniably known a strong development during the past decades. Researchers have been able to formulate and empirically test sport-specific models that allow for a more detailed understanding and analysis of transitional challenges athletes may face (eg, the Holistic Athletic Career model, the Athletic Career Transition model). Specifically, as the (normative) "whole person/whole career" conceptualization has created a greater awareness for the different concurrent, interactive, and reciprocal transitions, elite athletes face in different domains of life during as well as after their athletic career, more insight has also be gained into the process of transitions.

When considering future avenues of research, it should be noted that research into career transitions has in itself reached a point of transition. In analogy to an hourglass, most empirical data has up until now largely been funneled toward model development and thus reached the most narrow point of the hourglass. And as with an hourglass, these models will now have to face the challenge of funneling out and opening new lines of research.

A first avenue open to researchers relates to the type and process of transitions. While an understanding of the occurrence of multilevel normative transitions has been gained, a need exists to study in more detail the occurrence of nonnormative transitions, that is, idiosyncratic transitions that are generally unpredicted, unanticipated, and involuntary in nature and that do not occur in a set plan or schedule (Schlossberg, 1981). Based on current knowledge, researchers should not only focus on athletic nonnormative transitions (eg, injury, unexpected deselection) but also on nonnormative transitions occurring at other levels of development (eg, sudden loss of a significant other, failing exams at university).

More research is also required on the transitional challenges former elite athletes face when starting out into the postathletic retirement stage. Since successful adaptation to the postsport career was found to generally last between 8 and 18 months (Stambulova & Wylleman, 2014; Stephan et al., 2007), there is a concrete need to gain an overview of, and insight into the multilevel (non) normative transitions retirees face during (as well as after) this period. This focus of research should also allow to investigate whether deliberate, voluntary, proactive planned decisions related to their own future plans, lead retired elite athletes to continue to perceive their retirement as positive, and to convert into another vocational career.

A need also exists to take a more "micro" perspective at the actual process of transitions in order to identify possible "within-transition" stages or transitions. For example, the transitional challenge of elite student-athletes from secondary to higher education has been shown to consist of three different within-transition stages: namely, finalizing the last year of secondary education, the stage between leaving secondary and accessing higher education, and the first year in higher education (De Brandt et al., 2015). In a similar vein, athletic retirement has been shown to be perceived by former elite athletes as consisting of the stages of planning the career end, the actual retirement, the start of the postathletic career, and the reintegration into society (Wylleman, De Knop, & Reints, 2011). Researchers are therefore encouraged to deconstruct transitions in order to identify their constituent parts.

A second avenue of research relates to the individuals facing transitional challenges and the context in which these transitions occur. Specifically, it is worthwhile to consider athletes' age, gender, and competences (De Brandt et al., 2015; Tekavc et al., 2015). Researchers could focus, for example, on the age-related effect of the transition into international-level competition (eg, female gymnastics vs male volleyball players), the role of gender in the occurrence and perception of transitional challenge of parenthood by elite athletes, or the impact of the (un)availability of dual-career support services on elite student-athletes' athletic achievements.

With regard to the contextual characteristics, researchers could focus on the type and organization of sport, as well as on the significance of culture (Chapter 12). With regard to the latter, a clear step has already been taken as the holistic perspective is being amalgamated with approaches developed in cultural sport psychology into a new paradigm coined the cultural praxis of athletes' careers (Stambulova & Ryba, 2014). This development should certainly enable researchers to focus more on conducting multicultural research and to include more culture-relevant variables in their studies on career transitions. The current career transitions models should be studied in light of the specific characteristics of the type (eg, early vs late specialization) and organization (eg, level of financial support awarded to elite athletes) of sport.

A third avenue of future research is explicitly linked to the provision of applied sport psychology services. More particularly, this could include the use of, for example, the HAC model in order to investigate the competences (ie, knowledge, skills, attitude, experience) required by talented and elite athletes in order to prepare for, and cope with, the different multilevel transitional challenges they could encounter. These findings could lead to the development of a support program, for example, for talented athletes who are educated about (future) transitions and proactively learn to cope with transitional challenges (eg, entering senior level, starting in higher education, becoming a parent) (De Brandt et al., 2015; Wylleman, 1999).

A final avenue for future research relates to the fact that not only athletes are confronted with transitional challenges. In fact, there is a clear need to gain an understanding of the transitions faced by other elite sport populations. First, researchers should focus on (elite) coaches and gather empirical data on, for example, the multilevel challenges faced by young adult coaches developing toward the mastery coach level, or of the adult former elite athlete starting out in the coaching profession as part of her postathletic career. The "whole person/whole career" approach, as provided by the HAC model, could assist researchers in ensuring a developmental and holistic perspective on the transitional challenges faced by (developing and elite) coaches. This conceptual approach, which has already been used with another elite sport population, namely applied sport psychologists working with elite and Olympic athletes (De Caluwé, Wylleman, & Borgoo, 2009), could also be employed with, for example, athletes' parents (Lally & Kerr, 2008).

As they are not only "signposts along a long and continuous learning process" (Bloom, 1985, p. 537) but can become turning points "at which talent may be derailed or may flourish" (Dweck, 2009, p. xii), research into career transitions has become a vital part of the field of sport psychology: not only does it provide insight into the career development of (retired) athletes, but it adds also a new conceptual (ie, developmental, holistic) perspective on psychological (eg, self-regulation), psychosocial (eg, parental behaviors), and social processes (eg, dual careers, vocational development, financial management) with which athletes and others (eg, coaches, support staff, parents) in (competitive) sport are confronted.

In conclusion it can be said that, during the past decades, the domain of career transitions not only successfully outgrew the "initiation" stage, characterized by a descriptive approach, but developed, via specific lines of research, conceptualizations and career transition models, strongly into and throughout the "development" stage. It is hoped that this chapter, and the suggested avenues of research, will enable researchers and applied sport psychologists to bring it fully into the "mastery" stage.

ACKNOWLEDGMENT

In memory of Anke Reints who passed away unexpectedly and untimely during the writing of this chapter.

REFERENCES

Alfermann, D. (2000). Causes and consequences of sport career termination. In D. Lavallee, & P. Wylleman (Eds.), *Career transitions in sport: International perspectives* (pp. 45–58). Morgantown, WV: Fitness International Technology.

Alfermann, D., & Gross, A. (1997). Coping with career termination: It all depends on freedom of choice. In R., Lidor, M., Bar-Eli, (Eds.), *Proceedings of the ninth world congress on sport psychology* (pp. 65–67). Netanya: Wingate Institute for Physical Education and Sport.

Alfermann, D., & Stambulova, N. (2007). Career transitions and career termination. In G. Tenenbaum, & R. C. Eklund (Eds.), *Handbook of sport psychology* (3rd ed., pp. 712–733). New York: Wiley.

Alfermann, D., Stambulova, N., & Zemaityte, A. (2004). Reactions to sport career termination: a cross-national comparison of German, Lithuanian, and Russian athletes. *Psychology of Sport and Exercise*, 5(1), 61–75.

Antonini Philippe, R., & Seiler, R. (2006). Closeness, co-orientation and complementarity in coach-athlete relationships: what male swimmers say about their male coaches. *Psychology of Sport and Exercise, 7*(2), 159–171.

Australian Sports Commission. (2003). *How do elite athletes develop? A look through the "rear-view mirror." A preliminary report from the National Athlete Development Survey (NADS).* Canberra, Australia: Australian Sports Commission.

Baillie, P. H. F., & Danish, S. J. (1992). Understanding the career transition of athletes. *The Sport Psychologist, 6*, 77–98.

Baum, A. (2006). Eating disorders in the male athlete. *Sports Medicine, 36*(1), 1–6.

Blinde, E. M., & Stratta, T. (1992). The "sport career death" of college athletes: involuntary and unanticipated sports exit. *Journal of Sport Behavior, 15*, 3–20.

Bloom, B. S. (1985). Generalizations about talent development. In B. S. Bloom (Ed.), *Developing talent in young people* (pp. 507–549). New York: Ballantine.

Blumenstein, B., & Lidor, R. (2007). The road to the Olympic Games: a four-year psychological preparation program. *Athletic Insight, 9*(4), 15–28.

Bouchetal Pellegri, F., Leseur, V., & Debois, N. (2006). *Carrière sportive. Projet de vie [Athletic career. Life project]*. Paris: INSEP-Publications.

Brewer, B. W., Van Raalte, J. L., & Petitpas, A. J. (2000). Self-identity issues in sport career transitions. In D. Lavallee, & P. Wylleman (Eds.), *Career transitions in sport: International perspectives* (pp. 29–43). Morgontown, WV: Fitness International Technology.

Bruner, M. W., Munroe-Chandler, K. J., & Spink, K. S. (2008). Entry into elite sport: a preliminary investigation into the transition experiences of rookie athletes. *Journal of Applied Sport Psychology, 20*(2), 236–252.

Bussmann, G., & Alfermann, D. (1994). Drop-out and the female athlete: a study with track-and-field athletes. In D. Hackfort (Ed.), *Psycho-social issues and interventions in elite sport* (pp. 89–128). Frankfurt: Lang.

Cecić Erpič, S., Wylleman, P., & Zupančič, M. (2004). The effect of athletic and non-athletic factors on the sports career termination process. *Psychology of Sport and Exercise, 5*(1), 45–59.

Charner, I., & Schlossberg, N. K. (1986). Variations by theme: the life transitions of clerical workers. *The Vocational Guidance Quarterly, 34*, 212–224.

Chartrand, J. M., & Lent, R. W. (1987). Sport counseling: enhancing the development of the student-athlete. *Journal of Counseling, 66*, 164–167.

Coakley, J. J. (1983). Leaving competitive sport: retirement or rebirth? *Quest, 35*, 1–11.

Cresswell, S. L., & Eklund, R. C. (2007). Athlete burnout: a longitudinal qualitative study. *The Sport Psychologist, 21*(1), 1–20.

De Brandt, K., Wylleman, P., & Van Rossem, N. (2015). The dual career of elite student-athletes: a competency profile. In: *During the 14th FEPSAC European congress of sport psychology.* Bern, Switzerland: FEPSAC—University of Bern, July 16–19.

De Caluwé, D., Wylleman, P., & Borgoo, P. (2009). Career development and competence profile of European sport psychologists. In: *Proceedings of the 12th world congress of sport psychology* (p. 62). Marrakesh, Morocco: ISSP, June 17-21.

De Knop, P., Wylleman, P., Van Hoecke, J., & Bollaert, L. (1999). Sports management—a European approach to the management of the combination of academics and elite-level sport. In: S. Bailey (Ed.), *Perspectives—The interdisciplinary series of Physical Education and Sport Science: Vol. 1. School sport and competition* (pp. 49–62). Oxford: Meyer & Meyer Sport.

Debois, N., Ledon, A., Argiolas, C., & Rosnet, E. (2012). A lifespan perspective on transitions during a top sports career: a case of an elite female fencer. *Psychology of Sport and Exercise, 13*(5), 660–668.

Debois, N., Ledon, A., & Wylleman, P. (2014). A lifespan perspective on the dual career of elite male athletes. *Psychology of Sport and Exercise*, *21*, 1–12.

Dweck, C. S. (2009). Foreword. In F. D. Horowitz, R. F. Subotnik, & D. J. Matthews (Eds.), *The development of giftedness and talent across the life span* (pp. xi–xi10). Washington DC: American Psychological Association.

European Union. (2012). EU guidelines on dual careers of athletes: Recommended policy actions in support of dual careers in high-performance sport. Available from http://ec.europa.eu/sport/news/20130123-eu-guidelines-dualcareers_en.htm

FEPSAC. (2003a). FEPSAC Position Statement #3 "Sports Career Transitions. In E. Apitzsch, & G. Schilling (Eds.), *Sport psychology in Europe. FEPSAC—An organisational platform and a scientific meeting point* (pp. 101–102). Biel: European Federation of Sport Psychology.

FEPSAC. (2003b). FEPSAC Position Statement #5 "Sports Career Termination. In E. Apitzsch, & G. Schilling (Eds.), *Sport psychology in Europe. FEPSAC—An organisational platform and a scientific meeting point* (pp. 96–97). Biel: European Federation of Sport Psychology.

Gardner, F., & Moore, Z. (2006). *Clinical sport psychology*. Champaign, IL: Human Kinetics.

Gould, D., Guinan, D., Greenleaf, C., Medbery, R., & Peterson, K. (1999). Factors affecting Olympic performance: perceptions of athletes and coaches from more and less successful teams. *The Sport Psychologist*, *13*, 371–395.

Gould, D., Greenleaf, C., Guinan, D., & Chung, Y. (2002). A survey of U.S. Olympic coaches: factors influencing athlete performances and coach effectiveness. *The Sport Psychologist*, *16*, 229–250.

Greenleaf, C., Gould, D., & Dieffenbach, K. (2001). Factors Influencing Olympic Performance: interviews with Atlanta and Negano US Olympians. *Journal of Applied Sport Psychology*, *13*(2), 154–184.

Haerle, R. K. (1975). Career patterns and career contingencies of professional baseball players: an occupational analysis. In D. W. Ball, & J. W. Loy (Eds.), *Sport and social order* (pp. 461–519). Reading, MA: Addison-Wesley.

Hallden, O. (1965). The adjustment of athletes after retiring from sport. In: F. Antonelli (Ed.), *Proceedings of the first international congress of sport psychology* (pp. 730–733). Rome: International Society of Sport Psychology.

Hodge, K., & Hermansson, G. (2007). Psychological preparation of athletes for the Olympic context: the New Zealand Summer and Winter Olympic Teams. *Athletic Insight*, *9*(4), 1–19.

Hung, T., Lin, T., Lee, C., & Chen, L. (2008). Provision of sport psychology services to Taiwan archery team for the 2004 Athens Olympic Games. *International Journal of Sport and Exercise Psychology*, *6*(3), 308–318.

Jowett, S., & Cramer, D. (2009). The role of romantic relationships on athletes' performance and well-being. *Journal of Clinical Sport Psychology*, *3*(1), 58–72.

Kristiansen, E., Hanstad, D. V., & Roberts, G. C. (2011). Coping with the media at the Vancouver Winter Olympics: "We all make a living out of this.". *Journal of Applied Sport Psychology*, *23*(4), 443–458.

Lally, P., & Kerr, G. (2008). The effects of athlete retirement on parents. *Journal of Applied Sport Psychology*, *20*(1), 42–56.

Lavallee, D. (2000). Theoretical perspectives on career transitions in sport. In D. Lavallee, & P. Wylleman (Eds.), *Career transitions in sport: International perspectives* (pp. 1–27). Morgantown, WV: Fitness International Technology.

Lavallee, D., & Wylleman, P. (2000). In D. Lavallee, & P. Wylleman (Eds.), *Career transitions in sport: International perspectives*. Morgantown, WV: Fitness International Technology.

Lavallee, D., Sugnhee, P., & Tod, D. (2010). Career termination. In S. J. Hanrahan, & M. B. Andersen (Eds.), *Routledge handbook of applied sport psychology. A comprehensive guide for students and practitioners* (pp. 242–249). New York, NY: Routledge.

Lefkowitz, E. S. (2005). Things have gotten better: developmental changes among emerging adults after the transition to university. *Journal of Adolescent Research, 20*(1), 40–63.

Lorenzo, A., Borrás, P. J., Sánchez, J. M., Jiménez, S., & Sampedro, J. (2009). Career transition from junior to senior in basketball players. *Revista de Psicologia Del Deporte, 18*(Suppl.), 309–312.

MacNamara, Á., & Collins, D. (2010). The role of psychological characteristics in managing the transition to university. *Psychology of Sport & Exercise, 11*(5), 353–362.

McPherson, B. D. (1980). Retirement from professional sport: the process and problems of occupational and psychological adjustment. *Sociological Symposium, 30*, 126–143.

Mihovilovic, M. (1968). The status of former sportsmen. *International Review of Sport Sociology, 3*, 73–93.

Murphy, S. M. (1995). Transitions in competitive sport: maximizing individual potential. In S. M. Murphy (Ed.), *Sport psychology interventions* (pp. 331–346). Champaign, IL: Human Kinetics.

Naul, R. (1994). The elite athlete career: sport pedagogy must counsel social and professional problems in life development. In D. Hackfort (Ed.), *Psycho-social issues and interventions in elite sport* (pp. 237–258). Frankfurt: Lang.

North, J., & Lavallee, D. (2004). An investigation of potential users of career transition services in the United Kingdom. *Psychology of Sport and Exercise, 5*(1), 77–84.

Orchard, J., & Seward, H. (2002). Epidemiology of injuries in the Australian Football League, seasons 1997–2000. *British Journal of Sports Medicine, 36*, 39–44.

Parker, K. B. (1994). Has-beens" and "wanna-bes": transition experiences of former major college football players. *The Sport Psychologist, 8*, 287–304.

Pensgaard, A. M., & Duda, J. L. (2002). If we work hard, we can do it: a tale from an Olympic (gold) medallist. *Journal of Applied Sport Psychology, 14*(3), 219–236.

Pummell, B., Harwood, C., & Lavallee, D. (2008). Jumping to the next level: a qualitative examination of within-career transition in adolescent event riders. *Psychology of Sport and Exercise, 9*(4), 427–447.

Raedeke, T. D., & Smith, A. L. (2001). Development and preliminary validation of an athlete burnout measure. *Journal of Sport & Exercise Psychology, 23*, 281–306.

Redgrave, S., & Townsend, N. (2001). *A golden age*. London, UK: BBC Worldwide Ltd.

Reints, A. (2011). *Validation of the holistic athletic career model and the identification of variables related to athletic retirement*. Doctoral dissertation, Brussel, Belgium: Vrije Universiteit Brussel.

Reints, A., & Wylleman, P. (2009). Career development and transitions of elite athletes. Paper presented at the *Symposium Managing elite sports: a multidisciplinary perspective on the management of elite sports in Flanders*. Barcelona, Spain: Centre d'Alt Rendiment (C.A.R.) Sant Cugat, November 16.

Rosier, N., Wylleman, P., De Bosscher, V., & Van Hoecke, J. (in review). Four perceptions on the changes elite athletes experience during the junior-senior transition. *International Journal of Sport and Exercise Psychology*.

Ryba, T. V., & Stambulova, N. B. (2013). The turn towards a culturally informed approach to career research and assistance in sport psychology. In N. B. Stambulova, & T. V. Ryba (Eds.), *Athletes' careers across cultures* (pp. 1–16). London: Routledge.

Salmela, J. H. (1994). Phases and transitions across sports career. In D. Hackfort (Ed.), *Psychosocial issues and interventions in elite sport* (pp. 11–28). Frankfurt: Lang.

Scanlan, T. K., Ravizza, K., & Stein, G. L. (1989). An in depth study of former elite figure skaters: 1. Introduction to the project. *Journal of Sport & Exercise Psychology, 11*, 54–64.

Schinke, R. (2014). Adaptation. In R. C. Eklund, & G. Tenenbaum (Eds.), *Encyclopedia of sport and exercise psychology* (pp. 10–11). Thousand Oaks, CA: SAGE Publications.

Schlossberg, N. (1981). A model for analyzing human adaptation to transition. *The Counseling Psychologist, 9*, 2–18.

Schlossberg, N. (1984). *Counseling adults in transition: Linking practice with theory*. New York: Springer.

Schwenk, T. L., Gorenflo, D. W., Dopp, R. R., & Hipple, E. (2007). Depression and pain in retired professional football players. *Medicine and Science in Sports and Exercise, 39*(4), 599–605.

Sinclair, D. A., & Orlick, T. (1993). Positive transitions from high-performance sport. *The Sport Psychologist, 7*(2), 138–150.

Sinclair, D. A., & Orlick, T. (1994). The effects of transition on high performance sport. In D. Hackfort (Ed.), *Psycho-social issues and interventions in elite sports* (pp. 29–55). Frankfurt: Lang.

Sosniak, A. (2006). Retrospective interviews in the study of expertise and expert performance. In K. A. Ericsson, N. Charness, P. J. Feltovich, & R. R. Hoffman (Eds.), *The Cambridge handbook of expertise and expert performance* (pp. 287–302). New York: Cambridge University Press.

Stambulova, N. (1994). Developmental sport career investigations in Russia: a post- perestroika analysis. *The Sport Psychologist, 8*, 221–237.

Stambulova, N. (2000). Athletes' crises: a developmental perspective. *International Journal of Sport Psychology, 31*, 582–601.

Stambulova, N. (2003). Symptoms of a crisis-transition: a grounded theory study. In N. Hassemen (Ed.), *SIPF Yearbook 2003* (pp. 97–109). Örebro, Sweden: Örebro University Press.

Stambulova, N. (2010). Professional culture of career assistance to athletes: a look through contrasting lenses of career metaphors. In T. V. Ryba, R. J. Schinke, & G. Tenenbaum (Eds.), *Cultural turn in sport psychology* (pp. 285–314). Morgantown, WV: Fitness International Technology.

Stambulova, N., & Ryba, T. (2014). A critical review of career research and assistance through the cultural lens: towards cultural praxis of athletes' careers. *International Review of Sport and Exercise Psychology, 7*, 1–17.

Stambulova, N., & Wylleman, P. (2014). Athletes' career development and transitions. In A. Papaioannou, & D. Hackfort (Eds.), *Routledge companion to sport and exercise psychology: Global perspectives and fundamental concepts* (1st ed., pp. 605–620). London: Routledge.

Stambulova, N., & Wylleman, P. (2015). Dual career development and transitions. *Psychology of Sport and Exercise, 21*, 1–3.

Stambulova, N., Stephan, Y., & Jäphag, U. (2007). Athletic retirement: a cross-national comparison of elite French and Swedish athletes. *Psychology of Sport and Exercise, 8*(1), 101–118.

Stambulova, N., Alfermann, D., Statler, T., & Côté, J. (2009). ISSP position stand: career development and transitions of athletes. *International Journal of Sport and Exercise Psychology, 7*, 395–412.

Stambulova, N., Franck, A., & Weibull, F. (2012). Assessment of the transition from junior-to-senior sports in Swedish athletes. *International Journal of Sport and Exercise Psychology, 10*(2), 79–95.

Stephan, Y., Torregrosa, M., & Sanchez, X. (2007). The body matters: psychophysical impact of retiring from elite sport. *Psychology of Sport and Exercise, 8*(1), 73–83.

Storch, E. A., Storch, J. B., Killiany, E. M., & Roberti, J. W. (2005). Self-reported psychopathology in athletes: a comparison of intercollegiate student-athletes and non-athletes. *Journal of Sport Behavior, 28*, 86–98.

Sussman, M. B. (1972). An analytical model for the sociological study of retirement. In F. M. Carp (Ed.), *Retirement* (pp. 29–74). New York: Human Sciences.

Swain, D. A. (1991). Withdrawal from sport and Schlossberg's model of transitions. *Sociology of Sport Journal, 8*, 152–160.

Taylor, J., & Ogilvie, B. C. (1998). Career transition among elite athletes: is there life after sports? In J. M. Williams (Ed.), *Applied sport psychology: Personal growth to peak performance* (pp. 429–444). Mountain View, CA: Mayfield.

Taylor, J., & Ogilvie, B. C. (2001). Career termination among athletes. In R. N. Singer, H. A. Hausenblas, & C. M. Janelle (Eds.), *Handbook of sport psychology* (2nd ed., pp. 672–691). New York, NY: Wiley & Sons.

Tekavc, J., Wylleman, P., & Cecić Erpič, S. (2015). Perceptions of dual career development among elite level swimmers and basketball players. *Psychology of Sport and Exercise*, 1–15.

Tracey, J., & Corlett, J. (1995). The transition experience of first-year university track and field student athletes. *Journal of the Freshman Year Experience*, 7(2), 81–102.

Vanden Auweele, Y., De Martelaer, K., Rzewnicki, R., De Knop, P., & Wylleman, P. (2004). Parents and coaches: a help or harm? Affective outcomes for children in sport. In Y. Vanden Auweele (Ed.), *Ethics in youth sport*. Leuven: Leuven, Belgium: Lannoocampus.

Waterhouse, J., Reilly, T., & Atkinson, G. (1997). Jet-lag. *Lancet*, 350, 1609–1614.

Webb, W. M., Nasco, S. A., Riley, S., & Headrick, B. (1998). Athlete identity and reactions to retirement from sports. *Journal of Sport Behavior*, 21, 338–362.

Wippert, P. -M., & Wippert, J. (2008). Perceived stress and prevalence of traumatic stress symptoms following athletic career termination. *Journal of Clinical Sport Psychology*, 2(1), 1–16.

Wylleman, P. (1999). A career assistance program for elite and student-athletes. In: *During the workshop career transitions*. Copenhagen, Denmark: Olympic Team Denmark, December 8.

Wylleman, P. (2000). Interpersonal relationships in sport: uncharted territory in sport psychology research. *International Journal of Sport Psychology*, 31, 1–18.

Wylleman, P., & Lavallee, D. (2004). A developmental perspective on transitions faced by athletes. In M. Weis (Ed.), *Developmental sport and exercise psychology: A lifespan perspective* (pp. 507–527). Morgantown, WV: Fitness International Technology.

Wylleman, P., De Knop, P., Menkehorst, H., Theeboom, M., & Annerel, J. (1993). Van topsporter naar ex-topsporter. De noodzaak tot het optimaliseren van het beëindigen van de topsport-carrière [From elite athlete to former elite athlete. The need to optimize the discontinuation of the elite sport career]. In: K. Rijsdorp et al. (Ed.), *Handboek voor lichamelijke opvoeding en sportbegeleiding* [*Handbook for physical education and sport support*] (p. IV.3.Wyll.1–IV.3.Wyll.24). Deventer: Van Loghum Slaterus.

Wylleman, P., Alfermann, D., & Lavallee, D. (2004a). Career transitions in sport: European perspectives. *Psychology of Sport and Exercise*, 5(1), 7–20.

Wylleman, P., Lavallee, D., & Theeboom, M. (2004b). Successful athletic careers. In C. Spielberger (Ed.), *Encyclopedia of applied psychology* (pp. 511–517). (Vol. 3). New York: San Diego, CA: Elsevier Ltd.

Wylleman, P., Verdet, M. -C., Lévêque, M., De Knop, P., & Huts, K. (2004c). Athlètes de haut niveau, transitions scolaires et rôle des parents [Elite athletes, academic transitions and parental roles]. *STAPS*, 64, 71–87.

Wylleman, P., De Knop, P., Verdet, M. -C., & Cecić Erpič, S. (2007). Parenting and career transitions of elite athletes. In S. Jowett, & D. E. Lavallee (Eds.), *Social psychology of sport* (pp. 233–248). Champaign, IL: Human Kinetics.

Wylleman, P., Harwood, C. G., Elbe, A. M., Reints, A., & de Caluwé, D. (2009). A perspective on education and professional development in applied sport psychology. *Psychology of Sport and Exercise*, 10(4), 435–446.

Wylleman, P., De Knop, P., & Reints, A. (2011). Transitions in competitive sports. In N. L. Holt, & M. Talbot (Eds.), *Lifelong engagement in sport and physical activity* (pp. 63–76). New York, NY: Routledge.

Wylleman, P., Reints, A., & Van Aken, S. (2012). Athletes' perceptions of multilevel changes related to competing at the 2008 Beijing Olympic Games. *Psychology of Sport and Exercise*, 13(5), 687–692.

Wylleman, P., Reints, A., & De Knop, P. (2013a). Athletes' careers in Belgium. A holistic perspective to understand and alleviate challenges occurring throughout the athletic and post- athletic career. In N. Stambulova, & T. Ryba (Eds.), *Athletes' careers across cultures* (pp. 31–42). New York NY: Routledge—ISSP.

Wylleman, P., Reints, A., & De Knop, P. (2013b). A developmental and holistic perspective on athletic career development. In P. Sotiriadou, & V. De Bosscher (Eds.), *Managing high performance sport* (pp. 159–182). New York: NY: Routledge.

Wylleman, P., Rosier, N., & De Knop, P. (2015). Transitional challenges and elite athletes' mental health. In J. Baker, P. Safai, & J. Fraser-Thomas (Eds.), *Health and elite sport: Is high performance sport a healthy pursuit?* (pp. 99–116). London and New York: Routledge.

Chapter 14

Serial Winning Coaches: People, Vision, and Environment

Clifford J. Mallett*, Sergio Lara-Bercial**

*School of Human Movement and Nutrition Sciences, The University of Queensland, Brisbane, Australia; **School of Sport, Carnegie Faculty & International Council for Coaching Excellence, Leeds Beckett University, Leeds, United Kingdom

INTRODUCTION

The vocation of sports coaching is a relatively new in comparison to, say, the professions of medicine, law, and teaching. In the past few decades, the vocation of sports coaching has continued to develop toward professionalization across the world. Indeed, this progression toward professionalization is more advanced in some countries compared to others. However, as an emerging profession, the field of sports coaching has a limited empirical base to inform this process of professionalization. This limited empirical base is understandable in light of its recent emergence as an established vocation. Nevertheless, a key criterion for becoming a profession is an adequate research base (Duffy et al., 2011). Hence, a key intention of this study was to contribute in meaningful ways to the empirical base about the development of successful high-performance coaches.

Within the context of high-performance sports, coaches are central actors in the coach–athlete–performance relationship (Cushion, 2010; Lyle, 2002; Mallett, 2010). It is their responsibility to guide athletes' performances in the international sporting arena and they are held accountable to produce winning outcomes (Kristiansen & Roberts, 2010; Mallett & Côté, 2006). Therefore, they are performers in their own right (Gould, Guinan, Greenleaf, & Chung, 2002). However, high-performance sport coaching (Olympic and professional sports) is dynamic, complex, and at times characterized by chaos (Purdy & Jones, 2011). Adding to this complexity, the work of coaches in elite sport has become increasingly more demanding and complex, reflecting transformations in society and sport itself (Kristiansen & Roberts, 2010; Mallett, 2010). High-performance coaches face ever-growing challenges to succeed in their daily practice due to a number of factors; for example, increased international competition, the importance of the stakes relative to the country's investment in elite

Sport and Exercise Psychology Research. http://dx.doi.org/10.1016/B978-0-12-803634-1.00014-5

sport, the lack of adequate resources or the opposite—the appropriate coordination and maximization of the abundance of resources available.

The recruitment and development of these coaches of elite athletes and teams is challenging and typically serendipitous, especially in light of the changing nature of high-performance coaches' work and the increasing demands placed on them to produce winning performances in this turbulent and uncertain environment (Mallett, 2010). Typically, coaches are employed because of their playing success (Gilbert, Côté, & Mallett, 2006; Trudel & Gilbert, 2006) and appointed without adequate training (Mallett, Rossi, Rynne, & Tinning, 2016). It is noteworthy that the recruitment of executives across professions has also been reported as random and unsystematic (Fernández-Aráoz, Groysberg, & Nohria, 2009), and at best, relies on subjective preference and trait-based personality tests (Fernández-Aráoz, Groysberg, & Nohria, 2009; Singer, 2005). This ad hoc approach to recruitment and appointment is most likely the case with high-performance coaches in many countries.

High-performance coaches who do not produce winning results are often sacked during or at the end of the competitive season. The sacking of professional coaches is commonplace and costs sporting organizations significant money [eg, $n = 31$ sacked Australian football coaches (=25%) have cost clubs almost $11 million AUD in payouts over the last 5 years; personal communication David Parkin, Australian Football League]. This example of coach sackings is not confined to Australia but occurs also in other parts of the world; for example, in England where football coaches have been sacked before the season has commenced and often after only a few weeks into the competitive season. This high turnover of high-performance coaches has significant implications for player and team development, organizational growth, and the financial security of sporting clubs. This volatility in coach employment is a major issue for the professionalization of sports coaching. We argue that there is a lack of a significant quantum of research to inform how organizations might make better decisions in the identification, recruitment, and development of high-performance coaches. Furthermore, much of the research that has been conducted does not provide much insight into knowing the coach in any depth; therefore, this superficial understanding of the coach is limited in making appropriate decisions to produce successful coach–athlete–performance outcomes.

Currently, the identification, recruitment, and development of the next generation of high-performance coaches in many countries are sketchy at best. In the appointment of executive leaders, personality assessment is often a core feature of the process using popular tools (eg, "Big Five" model) that target the broad and decontextualized qualities of people. However, this broad understanding of people is limited. Contemporary views of personality suggest that person-based psychology and its assessment should consider a more comprehensive and integrated portrait. Understanding coaches, as people, requires a deeper understanding of the person that also includes why they do what they do and how they make sense of their lived experiences (past, present, and future) in terms of time and place (McAdams & Pals, 2006). To enhance our understanding of the practices of highly successful people across various contexts, a more comprehensive and nuanced examination of what underpins their successes is imperative; that is, why they behave the way they do. In this chapter, some significant research findings will be revealed and discussed to provide an insight into what we have learned from these highly successful sport coaches and how this understanding might inform coach identification, recruitment, and development.

So, what we do know already about successful coaches? Several research studies have yielded interesting insights into the developmental experiences of successful coaches (Gilbert et al., 2006; Erickson, Côté, & Fraser-Thomas, 2007; Jiménez-Sáiz, Lorenzo-Calvo, & Ibañez-Godoy, 2008; Nash & Sproule, 2009; Rynne & Mallett, 2012; Werthner & Trudel, 2006); their most valued characteristics (Ruiz-Tendero, & Salinero-Martín, 2011); their motivations (McLean & Mallett, 2012) and perceived needs (Allen & Shaw, 2009); how they draw from the knowledge and experience provided by sport scientists (Reade, Rodgers, & Spriggs, 2008); and their psychological makeup, skills, and coping strategies (Olusoga, Maynard, Hays, & Butt, 2012; Thelwell, Weston, Greenlees, & Hutchings, 2008). Studies gathering athletes' interpretations of their coaches' practices have also been conducted (Purdy & Jones, 2011). Specifically, empirical accounts of coaches' personalities have typically referred to broad traits or similar constructs (Becker, 2009; Lee, Kim, & Kang, 2013; Nash & Sproule, 2009; Norman & French, 2013; Olusoga et al., 2012). This research has highlighted some consistent findings (eg, diligent; typically played the sport they coached; learn mostly through experience and influenced by more knowledgeable others; relevance of life histories to how they coach). However, from a whole person perspective, this focus on broad traits provides an incomplete psychological portrait of coaches. Methodologically, these studies have typically focused on either the coach or athlete perspectives and conducted mostly with samples from the United States, Canada, the United Kingdom, and Australia. Furthermore, much of this research has been focused on the "what" of coaching practice (eg, behaviors, traits) and provides limited understanding of the person-in-context. There is a paucity of research that has examined: (1) consistently successful international coaches from around the world, (2) coach–athlete dyad perspectives, and (3) an examination of who they are (eg, meaning making) beyond what they do (attributes, behaviors).

The notion of a more comprehensive understanding of a person dates back to Allport (1937) and his view that in knowing someone we should explore the socially constructed meanings that people attach to one's lived experiences and the settings in which they take place; that is, to know someone beyond traits is to understand their subjective identities and how they tell their story that, in turn, provides a more holistic portrait.

There have been recent shifts toward frameworks for person-based psychology that considers the interplay between the individual and the social (McAdams & Pals, 2006; Mischel & Shoda, 2008). These frameworks for developing a coherent understanding of the person synthesize the dynamic interplay between biological contributions, traits, motives, and personal stories, within a broader sociocultural context (McAdams, 1995). This return to a holistic understanding of a person offers an opportunity for a deeper understanding of personality development that could be generative for future research in coach identification, recruitment, and development. Embracing an integrative perspective of coaches' multilayered personality is logically aligned with the area of sport leadership and more broadly within sport and exercise psychology (Coulter, Mallett, Singer, & Gucciardi, 2016).

McADAMS'S INTEGRATED FRAMEWORK OF PERSONALITY

Personality is a person's "unique variation of the general evolutionary design for human nature, expressed as a developing pattern of dispositional traits, characteristic adaptations, and integrative life stories complexly and differentially situated in culture" (McAdams & Pals, 2006, p. 212). In recent times, there has been a return by researchers to appreciating an understanding of the whole person including contextual, biological, and experiential factors that were originally foregrounded by Allport (1937) and his contemporaries. The complementarity of phenomenological experience and normative assessments is consistent with Allport's well-known ideographic and nomothetic distinctions in studying the person. In the past two decades, several theorists (Mayer, 2005; McAdams & Pals, 2006; McCrae & Costa, 1997; Mischel & Shoda, 2008) have developed integrative models that capture the complexities of personality. For example, McAdams (1995, 2013, 2015) developed a metatheory of personality development that drew upon both the research fields of developmental and personality psychology, two fields in which people typically operate in "discursive silos" with limited dialogue between them (McAdams, 2015). This integrated framework for understanding the whole person (psychological self) was expressed in terms of three broad metaphors: the self as social actor, motivated agent, and autobiographical author. These three interrelated and increasingly more complex layers of a person permit a deeper understanding of why we do what we do (McAdams & Cox, 2010). Moreover, these three layers draw upon three epistemological frames (positivist, critical realist, and phenomenological paradigms) that represent conceptually different layers of personality (McAdams & Pals, 2006) that enable an examination of the person-in-context. Typically, these "discursive tribes" (eg, developmental psychology and personality psychology; positivist and constructivist) do not "talk" with each other and subsequently limit the potential of a comprehensive understanding of people.

Social Actor

From birth we play the role of *social actors*. Initially, genetics lay the foundation for people as social actors, whose actions are constantly evaluated by self and others. Indeed, people are performative in the social interactions of daily life (McAdams, 2013) and these judgments of social performance are framed relative to others (eg, self-regulation, societal norms). Over time, people's behavioral signature (McAdams, 2013) is characterized by these broad and partly inherited dispositional traits (McAdams & Olsen, 2010). These behavioral signatures reflect peoples' social reputation in specific roles such as coaching and across contexts. Traits provide a broad and generally stable "skeleton" or outline for understanding people's personalities. However, traits are broad and decontextualized, which limits a deep understanding of people in specific roles such as coaching (McAdams, 2013). So, when we say we know someone, relying on traits is insufficient in knowing their deeply held goals and values and how they make sense of the lived experiences in telling their story about who they are and who they are becoming.

Motivated Agent

White (1965) refers to the *age 5–7 shift* that highlights a psychosocial transition from early- to mid-childhood, which has significant implications for personality development (McAdams, 2015). From this transition, children's personalities from about 7–9 years undergo further transformation toward that of a *motivated agent* (Bandura, 1989; Erikson, 1963; Harter, 2006; Piaget, 1970; Sameroff & Haith, 1996). Children's psychosocial development during this transformation enables them to choose where and how to invest their time and effort (McAdams, 2013). Social forces are more influential at this layer of personality than the social actor's traits and are expressed in terms of personal goals, values, ideologies, and cognitive style (McAdams, 2015; Singer, 2005). McAdams (1995) also refers to this layer of personality as characteristic adaptations, reflecting the influences of social forces on personality development. Peoples' motivational and intentional lives, and how they differ in relation to a wide range of social-cognitive, and developmental adaptations embedded in time, place, and social role characterize this aspect of personality; children begin to express what they want to achieve, what they want to avoid, and what they value in their lives.

Narrative Identity

Around late adolescence and early adulthood, people become an *autobiographical author* (McAdams & Olsen, 2010). In McAdams's (1995) integrated personality framework, this third and final layer is concerned with how people make sense of their past life experiences and their imagined future in creating a coherent story about themselves. It is noteworthy that not all stories are coherent within and across all three layers (McAdams, 2015). Nevertheless, this often cohesive, purposeful life narrative and identity builds upon the foundation of the two previous layers (social actor and motivated agent). In telling their story, people reflect upon "why the actor does what it does, why the agent wants what it wants, and who the self was, is, and will be as a developing person in time" (McAdams, 2013, p. 273). Comparatively, social and cultural forces shape the autobiographical author's unique story more than the first two layers (McAdams, 2013). "The internalized and evolving stories reconstruct the past and imagine the future in order to describe how we have become the people that we are becoming" (McAdams, 2015, p. 270); that is, a person's narrative identity is a first-person account of the author's subjective understanding of how he came to be and who he is becoming (McAdams & Pals, 2006).

PURPOSE OF STUDY

The International Council for Coaching Excellence (www.icce.ws) established the Innovation Group of Lead Agencies in 2011. This group brings together a number of leading coaching organizations from all over the world with the purpose of advancing coach education and development in a number of key priority areas. High-performance (HP) coaching is one of those areas. The HP Sub-Committee, led by ICCE President Mr John Bales (Canada), recognized these challenges and agreed to initiate a research project entitled "Serial Winning Coaches" (SWC). The SWC project aimed to study those coaches who have, repeatedly and over a sustained period of time, coached teams and athletes to gold medals at the highest level of competition such as the Olympic Games, the World Championships, or major professional leagues. Therefore, the purpose of the research study was to profile SWC in order to facilitate the identification, recruitment, and development of high-potential HP coaches in the future, as well as better support the further development of HP coaches already working in elite sport. Essentially, they were interested in what can we learn from consistently successful high-performance sport coaches? Therefore, the primary aim of this study was to examine some of the world's most successful international coaches using McAdams's integrated personality framework. Specifically, we sought to investigate the personality of these serial winning coaches from a whole person perspective using different ways of knowing that reflect each of McAdams's three personality layers. This unique way of investigating these coaches will enable us to learn more about how these serial winning coaches typically behave, why they behave the way they do, and how they make sense of their life experiences that informs their unique identities. In reviewing all data sets, we seek to identify a metastory that captures the essence of who these coaches are, their goals, values, and how these understandings shape their narrative identities.

METHOD

A key aim of this research is to identify some common qualities and understandings of their personality but also to identify some unique stories about these highly successful high-performance coaches that will be informative to coach developers. Hence, the search is not for a "magic recipe" or "ideal profile" but to contribute in meaningful ways to an empirical base to inform policy and practice in coach identification, recruitment, and development.

Methodology

Idiographic and nomothetic research approaches can provide complementary information about understanding both the uniqueness of these individual coaches and then collectively as a unique cohort. However, the discussion of each of these coaches as unique people is beyond the scope of this chapter; therefore, the focus of this chapter is to use a nomothetic approach to search for some common elements. Nevertheless, we are mindful of some potential variation within this group; indeed, there is most likely "outliers" among the group of "outliers." From these various case studies of SWC, we collected multiple data sets to enhance understanding of a highly successful coaches (intrinsic) and to also facilitate understanding of people who are consistently successful in the international arena (instrumental) (Stake, 1994). This study was designed and conducted across several research paradigms. The use of questionnaires (traits and strivings) and a semistructured interview embraced an eclectic mix of positivist, critical realist, and phenomenological paradigms that matched the conceptually distinctive layers of personality (McAdams & Pals, 2006). The integration of data from these multiple case studies enabled the identification of common traits and strivings but also the creation of a metastory that captured the core themes from the semistructured interviews.

Participants

A purposive sample of several of the world's most successful coaches was recruited for this project. These coaches were recruited through the Innovation Group of Leading Agencies (IGLA) of the International Council for Coaching Excellence (ICCE). Fourteen SWC, who among them had won 128 gold medals and major trophies, participated in this study. These "outliers among outliers" had won major international championships with many athletes/teams and in multiple contexts. In this research, 14 serial winning coaches (SWC) from 11 countries (10 sports, including 5 team sports and 1 combat sport) contributed to multiple data sets that were complemented with data from some of their successful athletes. The criteria for athletes ($n = 17$; 12 male and 5 female) were that she/he won a gold medal or title with coach and worked with that coach in last 5 years and for a minimum of 2 years. At least one athlete for 10 of the 14 coaches participated in the study. The coaches did not know which athlete participated in the study. The 14 SWC were all male, and had been successful in different contexts (eg, coached men and women; different leagues/countries), with an average age of 55 years (range = 44–67) and had coached for an average of 25 years (range = 7–43). All coaches were married (one remarried) and had children. All but one coach was university-educated. Eight SWC were ex-internationals and 5 competed at the national level. All experienced short apprenticeships into high-performance sport after playing their sport.

Procedure

Institutional ethics was obtained for this study prior to data collection. The participant coaches voluntarily agreed to participate in this study. They were purposively selected (Patton, 2002) because they fulfilled the criteria of repeatedly and over a sustained period of time, and in different settings, coached teams and athletes to gold medals at the highest level of competition such as the Olympic Games or the World Championships. The coach participants completed both measures and were interviewed (range = 60–180 min). The athlete participants completed the observer rater NEO-FFI-3 and participated in an interview about the coach. Data were transcribed verbatim, producing 650 pages of text (double-spacing). Through the extensive network of contacts available via the participating organizations, the researchers were able to access a unique sample of SWC based on the previous criteria. Likewise, a total of 20 gold medal or major trophy winners coached by the SWC were recruited for the study. This was an exclusive and select sample of consistently successful coaches and their athletes in a study of high-performance sport coaching.

Measures

The primary aim of this study was to elicit information about the SWC personality across a number of layers as well as their daily practices, the education and development routes they took in their journey to success, and the key challenges facing HP coaches in the future. For this purpose, the following methods were employed.

NEO-FFI-3. The NEO Five-Factor inventories (self and observer reports) are commonly used trait measures within contemporary psychology research (McAdams & Pals, 2006). Specifically, the NEO-FFI-3 (Costa & McCrae, 2010) is a self-report measure that collects data specific to the first layer of personality—self as social actor (McAdams & Pals). The 60-item NEO-FFI-3 (self and observer reports) assesses the established Five-Factor model of personality—openness, conscientiousness, extraversion, agreeableness, and neuroticism (McCrae & Costa, 1997; McAdams & Pals, 2006). For each item, respondents are asked to rate the degree to which they agree that the description is true of the coach (self and observers reports) (1 = strongly disagree to 5 = strongly agree). The NEO-FFI-3 has high internal consistency ($\alpha = 0.78$–0.86), sound factor structure, and convergent validity with the longer 240-item NEO-Personality inventory (NEO-PI-3; McCrae & Costa, 2007). Earlier versions of the NEO-FFI have received satisfactory support for its validity, including convergence with other measures of personality (McCrae & Costa, 1997). The NEO-PI-3, which is the longer version of the NEO-FFI-3, has been used in sport contexts (Allen, Greenlees, & Jones, 2011; Hughes, Case, Stuempfle, & Evans, 2003).

Personal strivings. This strivings measure (Emmons, 1989) captures information related to the second layer of McAdams and Pals (2006) integrated framework of personality—motivated agent. Respondents are asked to consider what they typically are trying to do in everyday behavior. Participants respond to the stem: "On a daily basis I typically try to …"; for example, "appear knowledgeable," "avoid appearing indecisive." These strivings represent an underlying organization of how individuals think about their goals. A *striving assessment* matrix is created on the basis of respondents considering each striving and rating them along a continuum from 1 (not very) to 5 (very) on the following: how committed are you this behavior? How important is this striving to you? How likely is it that you will be successful in doing it? How challenging is this striving be for you? How much satisfaction does it bring to you when you achieve it? Motivational themes can be abstracted from this matrix striving content.

Semistructured interview. SWC and the athletes they coach participated in semistructured interviews. The semistructured interview was an attempt to examine the third layer of McAdams integrated model of personality—autobiographical author. Indeed, the interviews attempted to explore the personal narratives of these coaches that underpinned their traits and motives. Through the interviews, we sought to confirm, refute, and enhance the information provided by the psychometric questionnaires as well as elicit new information regarding practical examples of their daily behaviors and the strategies they use to successfully navigate the HP environment. The aim of the interview is to understand the different ways in which coaches have experienced their lives in and out of sport and how it might contribute to who they are and how and why they coach. The interviews also contained specific questions in a number of areas such as the learning and development opportunities accessed by SWC, the vital steps in their journey to coaching glory and the key challenges facing HP coaches in the future. In addition, athletes were also asked to identify the main differences, positive and negative, they saw between the SWC and other coaches they had worked with in the past or what they understood had been the main changes they had noticed in the SWC over the years.

Data Analysis

The data analysis was based on McAdams and Manczak's (2011) three-phase sequence termed "logic of person perception" (p. 41). This data analytical approach integrated findings across the three "levels" of understanding the participants—from macro (broad and decontextualized traits) to micro (personalized life story). Importantly, the data analysis was concerned with describing and understanding psychological individuality rather than searching for potential (mal)adaptive functioning. Initially, analysis was performed on data for the first layer (personality traits), which was followed by analysis of the motives (second layer). Then an analysis that integrated the findings for the first two layers was conducted. The next phase of data analysis included an analysis of the third layer (life narrative), which was subsequently integrated with the first two layers to produce an assimilated and comprehensive story about the coach (Singer, 2005). Self and observer scores for personality traits were interpreted for each trait domain and personality style graphs were plotted following established scoring procedures (Costa & McCrae, 2010). The authors abstracted key motivational themes (eg, avoidance/achievement goals) based on participants' strivings based on Emmons's (1989, 2003) analytical procedure. The two authors repeatedly discussed the codes and themes until they reached at least 85% consensus (Smith, 2000). The authors analyzed the data following the principles of thematic analysis described by Braun and Clarke (2006) to reveal patterns within the data. Owning to its theoretical freedom, thematic analysis provides a flexible and useful research tool, which can support researchers in yielding a rich and complex account of data. The authors followed the six-step approach proposed by Braun and Clarke, which included a period of familiarization with the data through repeated readings of the data sets; a phase of initial generation of codes; categorizing the general codes into themes; reviewing the themes; defining and refining the themes; and the final production of the full report from which this section of the chapter has been developed (Mallett & Lara-Bercial, 2016). The coaches' and athletes' interview data were coded separately after which key themes from both data sets were compared. The broad themes that emerged were similar, yet there were noteworthy nuances within the themes, which we draw attention in the results and discussion sections. Nevertheless, it is acknowledged that there is always potential for some confirmatory bias in the analytical process, which the authors were cognizant of and attempted to minimize (Patton, 2002). Strategies to minimize researcher bias included multiple readings of the text by both authors, and then the extraction of major themes that were discussed until consensus was reached.

RESULTS AND DISCUSSION

Social Actor—Personality Traits

Coach self-reports. When compared to other adult men, the SWC self-reports offer the following information. The most distinctive features of this serial winning coaching cohort are this group's standings on the factors of conscientiousness (C), neuroticism (N), and extraversion (E) (Table 14.1).

Observer—reports of coaches (athletes). Ten of the 14 participant coaches received observer reports from athletes with whom they were recently successful over the last 5 years prior to data collection. Of these 10 coaches, 4 received 2 athletes' observer reports; hence, there were 14 athlete observer reports in total.

TABLE 14.1 NEO-FFI-3 Serial Winners' Scores

Scale	Raw score	T score	Range
(N) Neuroticism	12	40	Low
(E) Extraversion	32	58	High
(O) Openness	28	51	Average
(A) Agreeableness	28	46	Average
(C) Conscientiousness	40	63	High

There were consistencies between the scores and the overall range for the self-reports and observer reports. This consistency provided some validity to the self-reported scores of the coaches. Nonetheless, an examination of the scores for N factor showed that the eight athletes' averaged scores (four received two athlete reports) reported that the coaches were less emotionally stable than self-reported. The athletes overall reported the coaches as average N. In terms of E scores there some variability with five athletes' scores reporting their coaches as High. Similarly, five of the 10 athletes' differentially rated their coaches on Openness—some higher and others lower but overall average. Four of the 10 athletes' scores were inconsistent with the coaches' scores for A. All four rated their coaches less agreeable, which meant they were comparatively Low. The most consistent coach–athlete scores were reported for the Conscientiousness factor. Seven of the 10 athletes' scores were consistent but the other three athletes' scores rated their coaches as more conscientious than coach-reported.

Overall, it is suggested that the coaches' self-reported scores were consistent with their athletes. Nevertheless, the participant athletes perceived their coaches as less emotionally stable and less agreeable, which warrants some consideration in making sense of the results of the coaches' self-reports.

Distinctive trends in personality style. Coach scores for Conscientiousness, Neuroticism, and Extraversion—and their interaction—produce a noticeable profile that places this cohort as clear optimists (well-being), directed individuals (impulse control), and go-getters (activity). This combination of personality styles (for well-being, impulse control, and activity) builds a picture of most coaches within this SWC group that (1) takes life in its stride, with a positive orientation focused on the future; and (2) has a clear vision of what each wants and needs to be done in this regard—accompanied by a will and zeal to work and focus hard to reach set targets.

More generally, this cohort is able to deal with stress in an adaptive manner, and focus on problem-solving solutions and actions instead of dwelling on life's challenges. They generally control their anger and frustration—if anything, showing an ability to suppress negative emotions and harness these for their own benefit and pursuits. They display a mix of creative instincts, enjoy topical discussion with others, and are attracted to educating and working alongside colleagues. In this socially desirable context, they are confident decision makers and often see themselves as leaders who can mobilize people. These coaches are aspiring learners with an ongoing thirst for knowledge. Their approach to learning advocates a collection of individuals who either enjoy the creative nature of problem solving, or instead, stick to more traditional rules of engagement. Lastly, these coaches are clear achievement strivers, who channel tiresome efforts into others for (1) the selfless development, growth, and achievements of the athlete, and/or (2) the promotion of their own personal needs and recognition as a coach.

In providing a foundational structure to these SWC, the broad, comparative, and decontextualized traits (McAdams, 1995) portray an understanding of how they typically present themselves in the public domain. As a group, these coaches present themselves as conscientious, extraverted, and emotionally stable, which is consistent with some of the literature (Olusoga et al., 2012; Thelwell et al., 2008). Nonetheless, traits are limited in what they tell us about people. Specifically, we are unclear about people's motives, goals, and values that drive their actions. What do they want to achieve and why? To answer these and related questions requires a shift to another epistemological lens to examine the second and third layers of their personality.

Motivated Agent—Strivings

In assessing the SWC personal strivings, the focus was on understanding these coaches as motivated agents, specifically, what they want in their life and how that is expressed in their coaching practice. These strivings provide some understanding of their motivational agendas that underpin their coaching behaviors and coaching priorities. A thematic content analysis (Patton, 2002) revealed several key motivational themes from the strivings, guided by Emmons's (1989) structure (Singer, 2005). In assessing personal strivings, the emphasis is on what the coaches are trying to do rather than what are they like (Traits). McAdams (2015) suggests that the influence of traits on goals is modest, partly because they represent different layers of personality development. The influence of social and cultural forces on the motivated agent is much stronger compared to dispositional traits (McAdams, 2015).

Content of Strivings

Approach versus avoidance. Overall, the SWC were very much approach oriented. Their daily strivings included, "be enthusiastic toward my job," "be energized," "have fun," "complete tasks and meet deadlines," "control training intensity," and to "help athletes with skills." These coaches are positive in their outlook and possessed a strong sense of purpose and overall striving for achievement. Their strivings suggested they were optimistic, sought opportunities, and were solution and future focused. This strong approach theme correlates with trait profiles associated with upbeat optimists (low N, high E) and go-getters (high E, high C). Bleidorn et al. (2010) suggested that people high in conscientiousness tend to be associated with strivings focused on achievement and power. Comparatively, there were very few avoidance strivings (eg, "to not lose control," "not be withdrawn").

Agency versus communion. From the trait profiles (average A, high C), we did not know whether the SWC were more driven in helping others (ie, getting along; McAdams, 2015) or for own needs or self-promotion (ie, getting ahead; McAdams, 2015). The content of these strivings provided some insight into the motives and goals of these SWC in terms of what was the source of their conscientiousness. Overall, the two-thirds of the strivings of these SWC reflected strong agency (eg, for self-improvement, learning; "to learn something new about my job everyday," "challenge my thinking every day"); however, there was a commitment to the service of others for a clear purpose (eg, "be fair," "do something good for someone I know and someone I don't know") albeit less strong than agentic strivings. This strong theme of agency correlates with trait profiles associated people who have clear direction (low N, high C). Perhaps the SWC seek to be the best performers they can be to enhance athlete/ team performance outcomes.

Motivational Themes

Learning and personal growth. A central motivational theme centered on learning and personal growth (eg, "engage, support and learn from support staff"). This personal growth was considered important for both coach and athlete (eg, "permanent ongoing education"). Many strivings were focused on self-improvement, which demonstrates the high degree of agency in becoming the best they could be (eg, "learn something new about my job every day"; "discover something new"). This strong sense of purpose (eg, "to achieve my objectives") also reflected in their commitment to the service of others (ie, athletes and support staff; eg, "promote teamwork"; "support my kids and athletes"); that is, they were also athlete-centered and realistic (demand but be supportive).

Achievement. Another key motivational theme was associated with achievement (eg, "perform my potential"; "be successful"). They valued their work as highly important and challenging and the sense of accomplishment was a driving force (ie, high levels of internal motivation). This strong task focus with clarity of purpose (eg, "clear daily goals") is associated with the drive to be successful. Moreover, this drive for success was driven by an approach for success rather than avoidance strivings (eg, "try not to be negative," "build confidence daily"). These strivings, which suggest a high degree of confidence in their method, were consistent with the low-average N and high C.

Power. The third motivational theme that emerged was power, the ability to positively influence others (eg, "teach something to my children every day"), also emerged as a strong motivational theme and consistent with the high E, and average A (Leader Style of Interactions). Central to this motive for power was the holistic development of athletes (average A, high C). For example, "have the athletes move one step closer to their performance" and "build athletes' confidence daily." Furthermore, the strivings reflected the need for personal development (eg, "balance work and family," "look after own health") to create the best environment for the athletes to thrive (eg, "be positive within positive surroundings").

In summary, these strivings reveal that these coaches are driven by (1) personal growth and development for self and others; that is, *getting along* (McAdams, 2015); (2) to be highly successful and achieve through thorough planning and contingency plans that internally fueled their desire to challenge themselves; and (3) lead through the positive influence over others (ie, power); that is, *getting ahead* (McAdams, 2015).

Commitment-investment. These coaches reported a strong commitment to most of their strivings, which they also considered important. Unsurprisingly, there was a high degree of personal investment in sport and specifically the development of athletes. These strivings are consistent with the high scores for conscientiousness and, for example, Style of Learning (high C, low to high O; good students, by-the-bookers) and the need for achievement.

Ease-effort. Ratings from the perceived challenge and likelihood of success related to the stated strivings are related to the theme of ease-effort. The scores for these aspects of the strivings are consistent with the style of Well-Being (up-beat optimist) and a directed Style of Impulse Control (low N, high C).

Desirability reward. The coaches' scores for how satisfied they feel when their strivings are achieved related to the desirability-reward theme. The high scores for satisfaction and the many strivings related to enhancing performance reflected the strong drive for success. From the trait profile (high E, average A), they enjoy the company of others and the ability to lead others to successful outcomes (Style of Interactions).

These SWC are highly motivated for success. Nevertheless, little is known about why they are driven to improve themselves. Why is it so important for them to be successful? What does it mean for them to be coaches within the context of their own lives? How do they make sense of their lived experiences and the person they seek to become; in other words, what are their narrative identities?

Coach (and Athlete) Narratives

Fourteen serial winning coaches and 17 of their athletes (coached by 10 of the coaches) participated in semistructured interviews. The authors and in some cases author-led trained researchers conducted the interviews in the various countries. Interviews were audio recorded, transcribed verbatim, and where necessary, translated into English. These were returned to participant coaches for review and editing but they did not request any changes.

In this section, we provide an overview of the key findings. However, presenting a thorough and detailed account of each of the themes and subthemes elicited by the interviews is beyond the scope of this chapter. After summarizing the key themes that emerged, the authors highlight and discuss, in some depth, a few themes deemed to be of special significance either because of their novelty; or because they affirm and/or challenge previous research findings or public opinion of what serial winning coaches are like and do; or because of the potential impact of these findings in the thinking and practice in how high-performance coaches are recruited, developed, and managed in the future. We use coach and athlete data to illustrate these key themes.

As previously stated, although the emergent themes and narratives might suggest a simplistic overview of the coach–athlete–performance relationship, we underscore both the complexity and diversity of elite coaching experiences and how coaches and athletes made sense of these events. Identifying a stereotypical serial winning coach is likely impossible; however, the research has identified some common and also several unique qualities and practices and the underlying forces that contributed to making these coaches highly successful. At the request of the IGLA group, the researchers focused on the following broad questions in the interviews:

1. What are serial winning coaches like (personality traits, values, and beliefs)?
2. What do serial winning coaches do (practices and behaviors)?
3. How did serial winning coaches develop into the coaches they are today?

What are serial winning coaches like? There were consistencies between data collected from all three layers of a person: NEO-FFI-3 (Costa & McRae, 2010), the strivings matrix (Emmons, 1989), and coaches' and athletes' interviews. These emergent themes are presented in Table 14.2.

What do serial winning coaches do? The data revealed three key themes about what serial winning coaches do: vision, people, and environment. First, a clearly articulated vision of what is necessary to win was perceived as central to success. Seeing the "big picture," understanding its complexity while being able to simplify it into manageable components and developing and implementing pertinent strategies to make this vision a reality was underscored. Monitoring and regulating action plans was pivotal to achieve that end. Second, the importance of selecting and developing a high-performing and cohesive group of people who exude confidence (including the athletes and the support team) was reported. This confidence or belief in all actors was framed as the ability of the coach to instill belief in: *me* (get all in the program to believe in the coach); *you* (develop higher levels of confidence in athletes and the support team that they could succeed); and *us* (the realization in all involved of the power of the group to achieve more by working together). Third, SWC created a functional work environment, which facilitated the achievement of actors' goals (coach, athlete, and organization). These SWC developed a high-performing culture, in which everyone understood and bought into the communicated vision and

TABLE 14.2 Comparative Analysis (Coach vs Athlete) of SWC Personality Traits, Values and Beliefs, and Key Skills

Coach data themes	Athlete data themes
Personality traits	
SWC described themselves as:	Athletes described their coaches as:
• having a very strong work ethic	• having a very strong work ethic
• confident	• confident
• being thirsty for knowledge	• knowledgeable
• socially competent	• socially competent
• endorsing a positive approach to problem solving	• endorsing a positive approach to problem solving
Values and beliefs (the way the world should be)	
SWC believed that:	Athletes thought that their coaches:
• coaching should be athlete-centered and holistic	• were athlete- and team-centered
• coaches must uphold high moral standards	• upheld very high moral standards
• sustained success requires an adequate work-life balance	• valued all involved
	• had an appropriate work-life balance
Key skills required to succeed	
• Effective communication	• Effective communication
• Teaching	• Managing
• Planning	• Motivating
• Managing	• Planning
• Decision making	• Relationship building
• Relationship building	

invested necessary (human and material) resources, to maximize the chances of success. The congruent data and emergent themes from both coaches and athletes are combined and presented in Table 14.3.

A detailed discussion of what SWC are like and do is not possible in this chapter. Nonetheless, in the following section we attempt to consider the findings previously described to offer a tentative explanation of what we believed to be central to success in a high-performance environment as described by these SWC and their athletes. When considered as a whole, coach and athlete data were consistently pointing in the direction of the relational nature of high-performance coaching as a fundamental factor to success. We will thus shift the focus to this point and the impact of the nature of the coach–athlete–performance relationship on performance outcomes.

High-performance coaching is highly relational. A large part of the role of the high-performance coach revolves around the management of the performance team, including but not limited to athletes, other coaches, and support staff (Lyle, 2002; Mallett, 2010). We concluded that it is the ability of the SWC

TABLE 14.3 What Serial Winning Coaches Do: Main Themes and Subthemes Emerging from Coach and Athlete Interviews

Vision	• Developing and enacting a clear philosophy • Ability to see into the future • Capacity to simplify complexity • Thorough action planning • Constant reviewing and adjusting
People	• People selection (athletes and staff) • Believe in *me* (the coach) • Believe in *you* (the athlete) • Believe in *us* (the team and organization) • Managing the high-performance entourage
Environment	• Building the organization (influencing upwards) • Creating the culture (norms and ways of working) • Providing stability and dependability

to build and manage a "high-performing" coalition of people that facilitated success. The members of this coalition must have the required skills to fulfill their roles, the motivation to succeed, and the desire to compromise personal pride or gain for the benefit of medium- to long-term success (ie, selflessness). From this perspective, high-performance coaching is clearly relational. It is about people supporting other people to achieve exceptional outcomes. Two main themes emerge from this parallel analysis of the data: the role of emotional intelligence as a springboard to a plethora of positive outcomes; and the evolving shift in the nature of the coach–athlete–performance team relationship toward a "benevolent dictatorship."

Emotional intelligence as a springboard to management, learning, and coping. Chan and Mallett (2011) underscored the importance of emotional intelligence in successfully dealing with interpersonal challenges in highly contested sporting environments. The International Sport Coaching Framework (ICCE, ASOIF, & LBU, 2013), based on the work of Côté and Gilbert (2009) and Gilbert and Côté (2013), proposed that as well as having appropriate professional knowledge (ie, of the sciences and the sport), coaches must also possess interpersonal (ie, how to connect with people) and intrapersonal (ie, self-awareness) knowledge and skills. Moreover, Côté and Gilbert posited that effective coaching is the consistent and integrated application of these three types of knowledge to facilitate athletes' developmental outcomes, including performance. Both coaches and athletes corroborated these assumptions.

From the high degree of congruence between coach and athlete NEO-FFI data, it was established that SWC have an enhanced level of self-awareness, a key component and mediator of emotional intelligence (Chan & Mallett, 2011; Gilbert & Côté, 2013). Interviewed athletes also reported their coach as having an enhanced level of self-awareness and emotional intelligence. For instance, an athlete talked about how his coach "wasn't always nice, but knew exactly when he was and when he wasn't and plays whatever role he thinks is going to get the job done on that day" (Athlete 11). Another female athlete (Coach 10) openly said that her relationship with her coach and her performance was hindered:

> *until the coach became more self-aware of some of his behaviours and how they affected us. We were constantly in fear of him and it took us two years to gather the courage to talk to him about it. He has done a lot of self-reflection since and we went on to win gold (Athlete 12).*

Coaches reported that high levels of emotional intelligence were necessary to adapt their behavior to each individual rather than using a one-size-fits-all to relationship building and/or conflict management. They also reported that emotional intelligence played a role in anticipating problems and putting the steps in place to avoid them before they occur (Olusoga et al., 2012).

Within this context, and as expressed in Athlete 12's previous quote, optimal levels of self-awareness seem to protect coaches against their own behavior that unwittingly can have potentially detrimental effects on athletes' performance. It is also plausible that enhanced levels of self-awareness are linked to the ability of this group of coaches to be effective and efficient learners. Having a clear idea, through introspection and self-reflection, of one's own strengths and areas for improvement could provide the impetus needed to seek ways to fill a gap in knowledge or skill.

As aforementioned, high-performance coaching is a social activity in a highly pressurized context. Long and irregular hours, prolonged international commitments, close yet hierarchical relationships with athletes and staff, within a highly contested and at times unpredictable setting, among other factors were identified by SWC as a potential "recipe for disaster" (Coach 10). The majority of SWC expressed a view that high-performance coaching is not a profession for the faint hearted and that steps need to be taken to ensure that the coach remains healthy and fit to lead and manage the group. Coach 7 put it this way "I learnt the hard way. I became very ill and had to drastically change my approach to things, find ways to switch off and manage pressure better. I am never going there again." While high-performance coaching can obviously lead to proud and memorable moments in a coach's career, it is clear that the mental and physical well-being of the high-performance coaches can be compromised by the very nature of the job. Aspiring high-performance coaches should be made aware of these risks and the antecedents. Increased self-awareness, as suggested by Longshore (2015), may have potential therapeutic and protective properties to buffer against the inevitable stresses of high-performance sport and help coaches cope (Olusoga et al., 2012).

The coach as a benevolent dictator. Although coaches and their athletes generally agreed with the nature of the coach–athlete–performance relationship, they emphasized different elements of the coach–athlete dyad. Coaches viewed their coaching style as collaborative and facilitative, whereas the athletes generally viewed the coaches as a "benevolent dictator."

I think the consequences [of tough decisions] are, he feels massive pressure to get it right and it's people's lives. People are there, [athletes] are there giving up their all of their twenties and some of their thirties because they love [sport], but when you have to make selection decisions it's people's lives. And that's tough especially for the Olympics. He's not a robot with no emotion. He understands that that affects people, but they're decisions that have to be made and he makes them in the best interest of [national sport] and he justifies that, but it's still tough for him. (Athlete 11)

The athletes acknowledged that while coaches were keen to demonstrate some eagerness to listen and take athletes' opinions on board to build a partnership between athlete and coach, athletes recognized that the final decision was the coach's and that that was his role. The term "benevolent" however, indicated that athletes felt the coach had their best interest at heart the majority of the time (Jowett & Clark-Carter, 2006). Coaches repeatedly stated that they always tried to put themselves in the shoes of the athlete. This need to show empathy was something these coaches learned as athletes. Through the interviews, coaches were mindful that the daily decisions they make affect people. However, coaches stressed that, while being considerate to athletes and others in the way decisions were made and communicated, they were paid to make those decisions and live with the consequences. These SWC were described as ruthless, yet not heartless decision makers because they cared about others.

Consequently, SWC are not just transactional leaders, but transformational in how they conducted their business. This is consistent with previous literature (Chan & Mallett, 2011; Din & Paskevich, 2013; Hodge, Henry & Smith, 2014; Kellet, 2009). Indeed, sustained success at the highest level of competition depended on the ability of the coach to transform athletes and teams into self-driven, self-regulated, and self-reliant actors—this agency was identified in the strivings data. Coaching at this level (it could be argued at any level) is interpreted much more as a partnership between coach and athlete rather than a dominant hierarchical power relationship. This paradigm shift in the way high-performance coach–athlete relationships are construed and function has been reported in the literature (Davis & Jowett, 2014; Hodge et al., 2014; Mallett, 2005). Nonetheless, this (when appropriate) collaborative approach to leadership between coach and athlete at the elite level has not been commonly reported and especially in terms of contributing to successful performance outcomes. These collective studies provide increasing support for this paradigm shift in fostering successful coach–athlete–performance relationships. A fundamental part of this partnership building relies on coaches' respect for athletes as people:

Yes, and coaching, but not only as a person, but also as a human being. And also some sort of a manager, because he wants … at some point my management quit, for example, and he searched for a new management for me, so he wants the best for me and then ... of course it is not part of his job, but he wants ... he just does that. I think that is the bond you have or something, but he is very ... yes, how should I say this... he is very involved with you. And sometimes more than you know. And he treats everybody of our team like that, so to speak. (Athlete 7)

Within this context, several athletes identified the persuasive skills of their coaches to build a collaborative environment, which was characterized by open and transparent communication, consensus decision making, and support for athlete initiative in problem solving. A number of athletes expressed how they had struggled with this idea of collaboration as they had always worked under more controlling and directive coaches who told them what to do and when to do it, which problematizes the notion of collaboration or autonomy-support in decision making (Mallett, Rabjohns, & Occhino, 2015; Occhino, Mallett, Rynne, & Carlisle, 2014). Essentially, athletes referred to their coach as someone who had their best interest at heart, sought consensus, but in the end made decisions, some of which may have been unpopular. Furthermore, athletes accepted that the final decision rested with their coach but endorsed the shift away from coaches whose practice was "my way or the highway."

Look, from my own experience, if I was a coach this is what I would do. The more dictator-like coaches, the reputation of the guys from the Balkans, that kind of coach doesn't work at all, they are going to become extinct because sportsmen need to be happy too and enjoy what we do and what we like doing. When we stop enjoying ourselves, we cannot perform at our best and you can tell very easily when you go to a session happy because you know you are going to have a great time, that you are going to have a dynamic session, that you are not going to have a coach making you run or punishing for just about any silly thing for small stuff ... when you are happy is when you are going to perform better and also improve more. (Athlete 3)

Another key element of the effective coach–athlete collaborative approach was the ability of the coach to find the appropriate balance between challenge and support to facilitate growth and development. These data associated with collaboration are related to key themes from the strivings data around personal growth and learning as well as power to influence others. The importance of creating simulated pressure was emphasized; however, supporting athletes through that process was deemed vital to success. Likewise, eliminating athletes' sense of entitlement (eg, taking staff and fellow athletes, resources, and status for granted), especially in an era where financial support for some athletes is vast and some of them enjoy celebrity-like status, are daily problems faced by SWC. Coaches also felt that the current trend in which athletes' every want is catered for by the coaches, support staff, and the organization had the potential to undermine athletes' agency, independence, and initiative (Mallett, 2005) and to likely produce docile athletes (Denison, 2007). Coaches felt this docility potentially mitigated against the development of self-reliance, which they viewed as fundamental to success; we termed this notion *athlete grounding*.

Furthermore, the belief that athletes should be solely focused on training and performance and not be "bothered" with potential distractions (eg, family, friends, study) was not supported. Coaches stressed the need to understand that athletes "have other things going on in their lives" (Coach 6) and that providing the time to deal with them can actually enhance performance rather than take away from it. Athletes generally supported this view.

How did serial winning coaches develop their craft? The final element of the study related to the developmental pathway of the coaches. Two main lines of enquiry were pursued in this respect. The first revolved around the educational pathways of the coaches and the second delved into the most significant events and milestones in their career.

Coach education pathways and opportunities. Contrary to some previous accounts (Trudel, Gilbert, & Werthner, 2010), SWC strongly valued formal education, be it academic or sport-specific, as a platform or foundational stage of learning from where to grow (Araya, Bennie, & O'Connor, 2015; Demers, Woodburn, & Savard, 2006; Mallett & Dickens, 2009). All but one of the SWC were university-educated. Regardless of the discipline studied (eg, sport science), they all reported the significant contribution of their formal education to provide foundational skills to succeed in professional coaching (Allen & Shaw, 2009). Formal education, especially early on in their careers, provided SWC with mental models and reference points they could use to attempt to define what their objectives were and how they would go about achieving them. It also provided "thinking tools" they could use to interpret events unfolding in front of their eyes. In addition, SWC emphasized the power of nonformal (eg, clinics, seminars) and informal learning opportunities (eg, dialogue with others or self-reflection). Collectively, these formal, nonformal, and informal learning opportunities were valued by the SWC, yet their relative contribution seemed to vary over time and at different stages of their coaching career as previous research has shown (Côté, 2006; Mallett, Trudel, Lyle, & Rynne, 2009; Mallett, Rynne, & Billett, 2016).

SWC viewed themselves as curious and having an insatiable thirst for knowledge (Valée & Bloom, 2005), which is generally consistent with their trait profile (conscientious and most with a high degree of openness) and strivings (eg, agentic, personal growth, and centrality of learning). What underpinned these themes of conscientiousness, personal growth, and learning was the desire to be better and know more (*to get ahead*). This led them to seek additional learning opportunities in the guise of coaching clinics and study visits and were avid readers of electronic and hard-copy material, especially early in their careers (Mallett et al., 2014). They also confessed to being avid consumers of their own sport, watching it as much as they could afford. This ongoing obsession to learn as much as they could was underpinned by their need to prove themselves competent (Deci & Ryan, 1985; McLean & Mallett, 2012).

Various forms of informal learning were reported. All coaches identified that direct engagement in coaching practice was the most influential on their coach development (Jiménez-Sáiz, Lorenzo-Calvo, & Ibañez-Godoy, 2008). Catalysts for learning were the athletes and other coaches. In particular, the importance of athletes for stimulating learning is a novel finding. Although this finding makes intuitive sense, the role of athletes in high-performance coach learning has received little attention in the literature (Rynne & Mallett, 2016). Gilbert and Trudel (2001) reported the significance of issue setting (how issues were identified and framed) to stimulate reflective practice, albeit with youth coaches. Nevertheless, the notion that athletes stimulate coach learning is implicit in Gilbert and Trudel's notion of issue setting. SWC viewed athletes as invaluable sources of information. Observing athletes in training and competition striving to find solutions to problems allowed coaches to think through the same issues and find novel solutions (if not outright copy those found by the athletes themselves). Engaging athletes in a regular process of consultation was also viewed as capital to obtaining "insider information" that otherwise would remain hidden. Coaches and athletes stressed that this was not an easy process as there was a fine line between athletes liking being consulted and them thinking the coach had run out of ideas or was directionless. This consultative process was especially so, particularly for athletes more used to didactic and controlling approaches with previous coaches.

Nevertheless, for any learning to take place, a deep level of self-reflection and self-awareness was deemed necessary (Werthner & Trudel, 2006). Structured self-reflection was not considered essential, although necessary, when dealing with technical and tactical debriefs (ie, formal meetings with staff and players). As an example of unstructured regular self-reflection, Coach 3 said "you never stop thinking about it when you go home; about the things you could have done better to impact the outcome." SWC reported that solitary introspection contributed to regulating coaching practice. This is in keeping with the earlier theme of self-awareness as a springboard to other positive outcomes and the striving to influence others in this process.

All SWC stressed how a number of significant others (eg, mentors, family) had been very influential in their learning. Mentors were highlighted as one of the greatest influences on SWC development and importantly they identified the capacity of the "developing coach" to retain decision-making power, even if wrong, was necessary for enhanced growth and learning (Bloom, Crumpton, & Anderson, 1999). Sometimes, this mentor was just someone they admired and tried to emulate, but no direct contact was necessary other than observation and writings of these "mentor" coaches.

In addition, most coaches were former elite athletes themselves (Côté, Erickson & Duffy, 2013; Gilbert et al., 2006). Eight of the 14 had been international athletes, five had been national level athletes, and only one had not played his sport at a high level. An elite playing background was not considered the main reason for elite coaching success, but coaches stressed it had afforded them a frame of reference as both a player as well as a coach (Rynne, Mallett, & Tinning, 2010). It also provided an expedited transition into high-performance coaching (Rynne, 2014). Specifically, this previous elite athlete experience provided not only credibility with the players and a very practical knowledge of their sport, but a way to better relate to what their athletes were going through (Côté & Gilbert, 2009; Erickson et al., 2007; Occhino, Mallett, & Rynne, 2013; Rynne et al., 2010).

In sum, the obsessive pursuit of knowledge was central to these coaches' ongoing success. Their personal agency and meaningful engagement in learning situations guided learning and growth. This obsessive pursuit of knowing more is consistent with the trait profiles and striving themes of these coaches. Among other things, the next section will propose an explanation for the SWC's quest for knowledge and the constant need to demonstrate competence.

Coach critical life events and milestones. Becoming a high-performance coach and specifically a serial winning high-performance coach was characterized by a combination of four underpinning factors that are worthy of discussion. These included: (1) parental influences—work ethic, lifelong learning, and altruism; (2) early desire to coach; (3) "serial insecurity"; and (4) serendipity and risk taking.

First, SWC attributed their strong work ethic, engagement in lifelong learning, as well as their passion for coaching, to parental influences. In other words, having been brought up in an environment that valued these qualities had impacted their approach to work. Nine coaches reported how the work ethic exhibited by their parents had had a significant impact in the way they approached their sport and the subsequent obsessive engagement in lifelong learning, initiated by a valued university education that was considered essential to success. In addition, half the SWC attributed their altruistic nature, their desire to help others, to their parents who worked in the "helping professions" (eg, teaching, nursing). For instance, Coach 3 stated that, "he had the teaching gene in him" because his mother was a teacher.

Second, SWC identified both an early desire to coach (from a very early age) and the recognition by a significant other (a teacher or one of their coaches) that (1) they wanted to coach, and (2) that there was a "special talent" or disposition for coaching. Coach 4 recalled how older coaches used to mock him because he was attending coaching clinics while still playing the sport or how his teammates would come to him for advice instead of going to the coach. He also spoke about how his coach would sit down with him and run things past him. Coach 7 retold the story of how he always felt he was the teacher or coach in the field and that he brought it upon himself to coach his teammates during games and practices and that it just felt natural. For the majority of the coaches, their previous elite athlete experience provided a "foot in the door" to elite coaching opportunities (Erickson et al., 2007; Rynne, 2014), which they embraced.

Third, many of the SWC identified their need to constantly prove themselves as a key driver for their progression and consistent success. Consistent with the high scores for the conscientiousness trait in the NEO-FFI and the very strong achievement striving, coaches and their athletes reported the extremely high work capacity of the serial winners and their very strong drive to win. Two main factors were identified as underpinning their significant drive for success: *grounded self-belief* (coaches' self-belief based on previous successes and on how much work has gone into preparing for a specific competition); and *reasonable self-doubt* (a nagging feeling at the back of the coaches' mind that they either were not good enough to win again or that they still had something to prove). These interrelated factors seemed to spur the coaches onto continued effort and buffered against potential complacency. Remarkably, for such an accomplished group of people, and in line with Carter and Bloom (2009) and Mallett and Coulter (2016), a high number of the SWC recounted experiences of "unfinished business" as athletes that somehow they had managed to "put right," or were trying to, as coaches. Painful losses or an overall sense of not having fulfilled their potential as athletes seemed to have driven the careers of some of these coaches. These statements point toward a underlying drive for these coaches to consistently need to prove themselves, a certain level of what we have called "serial insecurity," which were significant forces in driving their motivating them to continue to strive and thrive in the high-performance environment.

> *I'd say is I've been on a journey that in some ways has been driven a little bit by fear of not being good enough—I want to be great, I don't know why but I do. I don't want to be great last year; I want to be great this year. I was voted "coach of the decade" by [sports magazine] and that summer I was sitting with my Dad, before I went to the Olympics, and he said "what decade was that again?" I said "it was last decade" and he said "that's what I'm saying." (Coach 2)*

The SWC's "serial insecurity" also reflects the very nature of high-performance sport in which coaches' and athletes' self-efficacy and perceived competence are put to the test on a daily basis. SWC expressed that to be able to cope with this constant pressure, developing "a thick skin" and learning to embrace the "insecurity" and allowing it to drive you forward was vital (Coach 2).

Finally, although most SWC were doing rudimentary "coaching work" prior to commencing their coaching careers, their foray into formal coaching was typically serendipitous and opportunistic. For example, Coach 4 spoke of how he received a phone call while he was about to jump on the team bus as the captain of the national team to go to the European Championships when he was asked if he wanted to coach a specific senior team. Put on the spot, the SWC decided to "hang up his boots" there and then and to start his coaching career as of that moment. For others, their athletic careers were cut short due to critical life incidents. For instance, Coaches 10 and 13 spoke about road accidents, which finished their playing career or sidelined them for a substantial period of time. It was during these critical periods that they either started considering a career as a coach or actually started coaching. Associated with this notion of serendipity was the opportunistic risk-taking, considered necessary for coaching development and success. This risk-taking element was present in most SCW career pathways. These risks included leaving stable employment, dropping pay or status to become a head coach in a different setting, retiring early from playing to coach as the opportunity arose, taking a coaching job in a faraway country just to get started. Some were calculated risks, some were perceived as outright "leaps of faith," but it was apparent that a certain element of serendipity and potential risk, in addition to their strong work ethic and passion, was a feature of these consistently successful career coaches. Incidentally, Coach 4 went on to win a national and European title in his first season as a coach. This is not to say that the coaches had got lucky or had not worked hard. These coaches were ready, willing, and able to take their chance when it came along: A winning coach is a "predator of opportunity" (Coach 13).

Author—Coaches' Personal Narratives

In general terms, SWC told underlying plots in their stories. For ease of understanding, we provide a generic "title" for two major characterizations and then go on to offer a rationale and description for both. Every coach is different and they differentially share aspects of both primary narratives. We are solely attempting to generate a coherent story that best represents this group of coaches.

The righteous avenger. There is a strong sense that many of these coaches are on a personal crusade of atonement fueled by perceived past failings that are omnipresent. They are trying to put "right" the perceived "wrongs" of the past. For example, unfulfilled ambitions as an athlete due to personal shortcomings or critical life-events and a near-pathological "serial insecurity" drives them to work relentlessly hard to achieve their goals. However, single Olympic or championship success does little to feel atonement for past failings. Even repeated success (winning) does little to stifle their quest for some redemption. They always need a new adventure to aim for and see themselves as the heroes who will save the day. This obsession with their past inadequacies might manifest in potentially blinding egos, which they need to keep under control to ensure it does thwart succeeding in their quest. This is a precarious balance, which can only be sustained through high levels of emotional intelligence, self-awareness, and persuasive power (at times manipulation) to bring the performance team (athletes, coaches, and support staff) along with them on this quest. Nevertheless, these adventurers operate from a moral high ground and strive to do the right thing for themselves and others. Finally, these coaches understand that no adventure worth a big reward is risk-free and demonstrate a tendency to take risks when the opportunity arises in order to achieve their goals. As we have seen, some of these risks can be fairly calculated, while others are outright leaps of faith.

The higher-purpose altruist. Coaches fitting this description tended to believe that their actions where driven by a higher purpose, such as the nation's pride or fulfilling the dreams of the athletes and their families. They carry out their work with a sense of duty and responsibility and understand the inevitability of the personal suffering attached to the job (eg, lack of family time; stress and pressure; public scrutiny) as part of the package and something to be proud of. While guided by a strong sense of right and wrong, in pursuing this higher purpose, these coaches exhibit a certain ruthlessness and steely determination to achieve their goals that may appear as detached or impersonal, particularly when it is necessary to make a difficult decision. A higher proportion of coaches in our sample would fit within the adventurer profile than the altruist, and yet the two plots can coexist within the same coach.

In addition, the researchers found that the two types of SWC shared a common narrative that we termed the *grounded realist*. The grounded realist is the part of these coaches' persona that allows them to normalize the exceptional set of circumstances surrounding the life and work of a high-performance coach: a highly pressurized job, public scrutiny, long hours, time spent away from home, the immediacy and potency of results, managing a large group under pressure, etc. The grounded realist is able to keep these factors in perspective and rather than fight them, embrace them, and use them to his advantage. This coach is also able to find ways to keep doing the normal things and preserve their life outside the sport (stay in touch with family and friends, hobbies, etc.), as well as staying in good physical and mental shape in order to be able to do the job to the best of their ability. All in all, the grounded realist provides the conditions that allow the coach to continue to perform; in other words, it underpins the longevity of the coach, which is requisite to become a SWC.

IMPLICATIONS AND CONCLUSIONS

Recommendations for Coach Recruitment

The premium placed on the identification, recruitment, and development of elite athletes should be afforded to those charged with the responsibility for delivering athlete success—the high-performance coaches. These coaches should be identified, recruited, and developed appropriately. For some sports, this essential component of sustained high performance takes the shape of carefully designed succession plans. In most sports, however, it seems the appointment of high-performance coaches remains ad hoc, unplanned and haphazard. Organizations seeking to develop high-performance coaches are encouraged to design talent identification and development programs akin to those of athletes and informed by empirical evidence.

From the perspective of the key stakeholders, an important outcome of this research was to learn more about what makes these coaches so successful to inform both policy and practice in the identification, recruitment, and development of the next generation of high-performance coaches. Indeed, these coach developers sought a comprehensive and flexible profiling system for high-performance coaches. The significance of a deeper understanding of the person behind the coach was a key finding in this research. To assist coach developers in introducing and implementing such a comprehensive profiling system might require the support of specially trained psychologists, but could lead to the identification of potential coaches who have an insatiable drive and who are: athlete-centered; able to create a vision and communicate that vision; capable of leading and managing large groups of people; lifelong learners; highly resilient and prepared to take risks.

A point of special interest identified by this study is the long-term potential of the coaches and their prospect of longevity in the job. One area of interest is assessing prospective coaches' resilience (eg, "thick skin"). In addition, those looking to recruit high-performance coaches would be advised to evaluate the coaches' ability to maintain an appropriate work–life balance for self and others in the program. Being able to do so allowed SWC to remain fresh and energetic, and to cultivate better relationships with their families and the athletes themselves. Of course, as Coach 7 indicated when he said that "on average I spend 200 days away from home with my athletes, but I still think I have a pretty good work–life balance," that balance is relative and each individual has to find what works for them. SWC stressed the value of quality time with friends and family, time for self around some kind of hobby, and the importance of remaining in good physical shape. In profiling prospective coaches, gaining an insight into how they manage this could prove very useful. It may not be the make-or-break of hiring a coach, but it may be something that the employing organization can support the coach with over time for the benefit of the athletes, the coach, and the organization itself.

Recommendations for Coach Education and Development

From the analysis of the SWC data, the authors would like to put forth the following recommendations to coach developers:

- At the highest level of coaching, a solid educational grounding seemed to matter for SWC. This is supported by other studies of high-performance coaches (Araya et al., 2015; Mallett et al., 2014; Mallett & Dickens, 2009; Olusoga et al., 2012). SWC felt that their formal training accelerated the amount of on-the-job learning they could do. So, although interpreted mostly as a starting point and foundation for the journey, organizations supporting young high-performance coaches should encourage, facilitate, and support engagement in this process of formal education. In saying that, SWC stated clearly that they were not supportive of "token coach education" and that formal and nonformal development opportunities should be carefully thought out and be pitched at the right level for the coach.
- Coaching courses should support the acquisition of new knowledge, yet for coach education to fulfill its role, coaches must be provided with time, opportunities, and support during or in between courses to take stock of current

knowledge, digest new knowledge, and look for ways to translate it into practical applications. Individual and guided self-reflection appears critical for this to happen. By the admission of the SWC, high-performance coaches are never the finished article. In a way, those developing high-performance coaches should make explicit attempts to connect formal and informal learning in seamless ways, for instance, through the careful design of learning tasks that require the application of a recently acquired knowledge base to a specific and real situation the coach is trying to resolve (ie, issue setting; Gilbert & Trudel, 2001).

- In connection with the previous items, coach development should be embedded in the reality of the job and appropriately supported via a mentor, a "more capable" assistant, peer groups, social networks, and vast amounts of guided and nonguided self-reflection. SWC strongly supports the value of the mentoring process, yet stresses that throughout this process, the developing coach should retain decision-making capability and power in order to develop accountability and accelerate learning.

- In appropriate countries, sports, and specific settings, a "coach loan" system similar to that of professional team sport players might be generative in coach development. Emerging high-performance coaches would thus be loaned out to other organizations where the coach could "cut his/her teeth" and learn safely on the job until they are ready to come back to the institution of origin.

- The development of the program management capabilities of the coach should be enhanced at every opportunity. SWC invariably reported that the management of large operations and groups was a key feature of "modern" coaching and that it would become even more important in the future.

- SWC corroborated the suggestion that high levels of emotional intelligence were pivotal to successful management of elite athletes and programs (Chan & Mallett, 2011; Côté & Gilbert, 2009). A first step would be to support coaches in developing heightened levels of self-awareness. Recently, Longshore (2015) has demonstrated how mindfulness training, a technique that revolves around the development of moment-awareness, can improve emotional control, reduce stress, and help build better coach–athlete relationships in high-performance coaches. Supporting coaches in understanding what makes them who they are and how they behave via exercises similar to the strivings questionnaire (Emmons, 1989, 2003) or the life story interview may be generative in fostering self-awareness. Likewise, consistent amounts of guided and nonguided self-reflection will enhance the coaches' self-awareness and their critical thinking ability (always questioning what you and others do and looking for a better way), which SWC remarked as key to sustained success.

- Finally, as already mentioned, SWC place great emphasis in achieving a relative work–life balance. Coach education and development for high-performance coaches should devote time and resources to support that current and prospective coaches understand the value of this proposition and develop strategies to fulfill it.

Role of the Sport Psychologist

Sport psychologists can play a leading role in supporting high-performance coaches and those recruiting and developing them. With regards to recruitment, sport psychologists are well placed to support a more comprehensive profiling process, recommended earlier, to promote an effective coach–organizational fit. Along these lines, sport psychologists can play a significant part in supporting sporting organizations define more clearly who they are, their philosophy and vision, and the kind of people they need to maximize adaptive outcomes for all actors within the sporting context.

When high-performance coaches are considered (and consider themselves) as performers in their own right (Gould et al., 2002), it is easy to see the potential role of sport psychologist in supporting the development of coaches. However, an agentic coach should drive this coach–sport psychologist partnership. Based on the results of this study, we see two major areas where sport psychologists can make a contribution. First, sport psychologists can support coaches to achieve deeper levels of self-awareness. This process of self-awareness augmentation can lead to coaches gaining a deeper understanding of who they are, what drives them, and what triggers certain feelings, emotions, reactions, and behaviors. It can also help coaches recognize possible issues earlier and the potential consequence of different ways of dealing with them before they happen. It may also improve the ability of the coach to understand athletes better and be able to empathize with their needs and wants. Positioning coaches as performers is central to coaches understanding themselves and reflecting upon how they act and subsequently impact on athletes. An antecedent of leading others is first, knowing thyself. Enhanced self-awareness has the potential to mediate many positive or adaptive coach and athlete outcomes: for example, stress reduction and coping; emotional regulation; higher levels of emotional intelligence; and increased management capacity.

Second, we have shown how throughout the data collection process, SWC emphasized the need to achieve an adequate, yet relative, work–life balance. Sport psychologists can help coaches recognize the need for this balance and then work with them to support them to find this balance. Given that the SWC tended to believe this is something they had learned over the years and, in some cases, the hard way, this may be especially helpful for young aspiring coaches who may be more inclined to spouse an "all-out" or "win or bust" theory of success.

Guided self-reflection, personal counseling/coaching, rest and regeneration diaries, and mindfulness training might be just a few of the ways in which sport psychologists can support the development of high-performance coaches. Perhaps working with coaches, in preference to athletes, might be more beneficial to the coach–athlete–performance relationship.

Recommendations for Future Research

On the basis of the findings from this research study, we propose some ideas for future research. First, more research is required to continue to build an empirical base in knowing coaches better. This research is important to assist coach developers and sports psychologists in supporting the learning and development of high-performance coaches. Indeed, improving the quality of coaches will importantly contribute to more than successful performance outcomes—it will contribute to the holistic development of young people, which is a key purpose of sport (Côté & Gilbert, 2009). Second, we support the complementarity of ideographic and nomothetic approaches to knowing a person in sport settings (Coulter et al., 2016). McAdams's (1995) three-layered approach to knowing a person integrates multiple data sets from different epistemological frames that provide a more comprehensive portrait of people that gives a deeper understanding of people and their behaviors. These integrated accounts of coaches might be extended to include data from additional and relevant layers that also shape personality development. For example, examine the relational dynamics between key actors in the sport setting as well as the sociocultural context in which they operate (eg, ethnographic accounts) to gain a deeper understanding of the whole person in context (Sheldon, Cheng, & Hilpert, 2011).

ACKNOWLEDGMENTS

First, we acknowledge Mr John Bales, President of the ICCE, who initiated the idea of the SWC project. Second, we recognize the support of The Innovation Group of Leading Agencies of the International Council for Coaching Excellence (ICCE) that commissioned this study. This group brings together select national coaching agencies from all over the world to advance coaching in key priority areas. In a few instances, these national leaders conducted the interviews in their respective countries. We acknowledge the IGLA members for their contribution: Mr Christoph Dolch (Trainerakademie Köln, Germany); Mr Adrian Bürgi and Mr Mark Wolff (BASPO Switzerland); Ms Lorraine Lafreniere (Coaches Association of Canada); Mr Frederic Sadys (INSEP France); Mr Graham Taylor (UK Sport); Mr Ian Smyth (Leeds Beckett University); Mr Arjen Von Stoppel (NOC*NSF Netherlands); Mr Erling Rimeslatten (Olympiatoppen Norway); Ms Darlene Harrison (Australian Sport Commission); Mr Chris Bullen (High Performance Sport New Zealand); and Ms Desiree Vardhan (SASCOC, South Africa). Third, we acknowledge the contributions of doctoral student Tristan Coulter (The University of Queensland & Queensland University of Technology, Australia) and Professor Jefferson Singer (Connecticut College, USA) for their introduction to McAdams's work and advice on integrating multiple data sets from different epistemological frames in knowing a person.

REFERENCES

Allen, J. B., & Shaw, S. (2009). Women coaches' perceptions of their sport organizations' social environment: supporting coaches' psychological needs? *The Sport Psychologist, 23*, 346–366.

Allen, M. S., Greenlees, I., & Jones, M. V. (2011). An investigation of the five-factor model of personality and coping behaviour in sport. *Journal of Sports Sciences, 29*, 841–850.

Allport, G. W. (1937). *Personality: A psychological interpretation.* New York: Holt, Rinehart, & Winston.

Araya, J., Bennie, A., & O'Connor, D. (2015). Understanding performance coach development: perceptions about a postgraduate coach education program. *International Sport Coaching Journal, 2*(1), 3–14.

Bandura, A. (1989). Human agency in social-cognitive theory. American Psychologist 44, 1175–1184.

Becker, A. (2009). It's not what they do, it's how they do it: athlete experiences of great coaching. *International Journal of Sports Science and Coaching, 4*(1), 93–119.

Bleidorn, W., Kandler, C., Hulsheger, U. R., Riemann, R., Angleitner, A., & Spinath, F. M. (2010). Nature and nurture of the interplay between personality traits and major life goals. *Journal of Personality and Social Psychology, 99*, 366–379.

Bloom, G. A., Crumpton, R., & Anderson, J. E. (1999). A systematic observation study of the teaching behaviours of expert basketball coach. *The Sport Psychologist, 13*, 157–170.

Braun, V., & Clarke, V. (2006). Using thematic analysis in psychology. *Qualitative Research in Psychology, 3*(2), 77–101.

Carter, D. A., & Bloom, G. A. (2009). Coaching knowledge and success: going beyond athletic experiences. *Journal of Sport Behavior, 32*, 419–437.

Chan, J. T., & Mallett, C. J. (2011). The value of emotional intelligence for high performance coaching. *International Journal for Sport Science and Coaching, 6*, 315–328.

Costa, P. T., & McCrae, R. R. (2010). *NEO inventories: Professional manual.* Odessa, FL: Psychological Assessment Resources.

Côté, J. (2006). The development of coaching knowledge. *International Journal of Sports Science and Coaching, 1*, 217–222.

Côté, J., & Gilbert, W. (2009). An integrative definition of coaching effectiveness and expertise. *International Journal of Sport Science and Coaching, 4*, 307–323.

Côté, J., Erickson, K., & Duffy, P. (2013). Developing the expert performance coach. In D. Farrow, J. Baker, & C. MacMahon (Eds.), *Developing elite sport performance: Lessons from theory and practice* (2nd ed., pp. 17–28). New York: Routledge.

Coulter, T., Mallett, C. J., Singer, J., & Gucciardi, D. F. (2016). Personality in sport and exercise psychology: integrating a whole person perspective. *International Journal of Sport and Exercise Psychology, 14*(1), 23–41.

Cushion, C. (2010). Coach behaviour. In J. Lyle, & C. Cushion (Eds.), *Sports coaching: Professionalism and practice* (pp. 44–61). London: Elsevier.

Davis, L., & Jowett, S. (2014). Coach-athlete attachment and the quality of the coach-athlete relationship: implications for athlete's well-being. *Journal of Sports Sciences, 32*, 1454–1464.

Deci, E. L., & Ryan, R. M. (1985). *Intrinsic motivation and self-determination in human behavior.* New York: Plenum.

Demers, G., Woodburn, A. J., & Savard, C. (2006). The development of an undergraduate competency-based coach education program. *The Sport Psychologist, 20*, 162–173.

Denison, J. (2007). Social theory for coaches: a Foucauldian reading of one athlete's poor performance. *International Journal of Sports Science & Coaching, 2*, 369–383.

Din, C., & Paskevich, D. (2013). An integrated research model of Olympic podium performance. *International Journal of Sport Science and Coaching, 8*, 431–444.

Duffy, P., Hartley, H., Bales, J., Crespo, M., Dick, F., Vardhan, D., & Curado, J. (2011). Sport coaching as a "profession": challenges and future directions. *International Journal for Coaching Science, 5*(2), 93–123.

Emmons, R. A. (1989). The personal striving approach to personality. In L. A. Pervin (Ed.), *Goal concepts in personality and social psychology* (pp. 87–126). Hillsdale, NJ: Erlbaum.

Emmons, R.A. (2003). The psychology of ultimate concerns: Motivation and spirituality in personality. The Guildford Press, New York, NY.

Erickson, K., Côté, J., & Fraser-Thomas, J. (2007). Sport experiences, milestones, and educational activities associated with high-performance coaches' development. *The Sport Psychologist, 21,* 302–316.

Erikson, E. (1963). Childhood and society. W. W. Norton, New York.

Fernández-Aráoz, C., Groysberg, B., & Nohria, N. (2009). The definitive guide to recruiting in good times and bad. *Harvard Business Review, 87*(5), 74–84.

Gilbert, W., & Côté, J. (2013). Defining coaching effectiveness: a focus on coaches' knowledge. In W. Gilbert (Ed.), *Handbook of sports coaching.* London: Routledge.

Gilbert, W., & Trudel, P. (2001). Learning to coach through experience: reflection in model youth sport coaches. *Journal of Teaching in Physical Education, 21,* 16–34.

Gilbert, W., Côté, J., & Mallett, C. (2006). Developmental paths and activities of successful sport coaches. *International Journal of Sports Science and Coaching, 1,* 69–76.

Gould, D., Guinan, D., Greenleaf, C., & Chung, Y. (2002). A survey of U.S. Olympic coaches: variables perceived to have influenced athlete performances and coach effectiveness. *The Sport Psychologist, 16,* 229–250.

Harter, S. (2006). The self. In N. Eisenberg (Ed.), W. Damon & R. M. Lerner (Series Eds.), *Handbook of child psychology* (Vol. 3). *Social, emotional and personality development* (pp. 505–570). New York: Wiley.

Hodge, K., Henry, G., & Smith, W. (2014). A case study of excellence in elite sport: motivational climate in a world champion team. *The Sports Psychologist, 28,* 60–74.

Hughes, S. L., Case, H. S., Stumemple, K. J., & Evans, D. S. (2003). Personality profiles of Iditasport ultra-marathon participants. *Journal of Applied Sport Psychology, 15,* 256–261.

ICCE, ASOIF, & LBU. (2013). International sport coaching framework: version 1.2. Champaign, IL: Human Kinetics.

Jiménez-Sáiz, S. L., Lorenzo-Calvo, A., & Ibañez-Godoy (2008). Development of expertise in Spanish elite basketball coaches. *International Journal of Sport Science, 5*(17), 19–32.

Jowett, S., & Clark-Carter, D. (2006). Perceptions of empathic accuracy and assumed similarity in the coach-athlete relationship. *British Journal of Social Psychology, 45,* 617–637.

Kellet, P. (2009). Organisational leadership: lessons from professional coaches. *Sport Management Review, 2,* 150–171.

Kristiansen, E., & Roberts, G. C. (2010). Young elite athletes and social support: coping with competitive and organizational stress in "Olympic" competition. *Scandinavian Journal of Medicine & Science in Sports, 20,* 686–695.

Lee, Y., Kim, S., & Kang, J. (2013). Coach leadership effect on elite handball players' psychological empowerment and organizational citizenship behavior. *International Journal of Sport Science and Coaching, 8,* 327–342.

Longshore, K. (2015). Mindfulness training for coaches: a mixed methods exploratory study. *Journal of Clinical Sport Psychology, 9,* 116–137.

Lyle, J. (2002). *Sports coaching concepts: a framework for coaches.* London: Routledge.

Mallett, C. (2005). Self-determination theory: a case study of evidence-based coaching. *The Sport Psychologist, 19,* 417–429.

Mallett, C. J. (2010). High performance coaches' careers and communities. In J. Lyle, & C. Cushion (Eds.), *Sports coaching: Professionalism and practice* (pp. 119–133). London: Elsevier.

Mallett, C. J., & Côté, J. (2006). Beyond winning and losing: guidelines for evaluating high performance coaches. *The Sport Psychologist, 20*, 213–221.

Mallett, C. J., & Coulter, T. J. (2016). The anatomy of a successful Olympic coach: actor, agent, and author. *International Sports Coaching Journal.*

Mallett, C. J., & Dickens, S. (2009). Authenticity in formal coach education: online postgraduate studies in sports coaching at The University of Queensland. *International Journal of Coaching Science, 3*(2), 79–90.

Mallett, C. J., & Lara-Bercial, S. (2016). Serial winning coaches' project report—innovation group of leading agencies of the International Council for Coaching Excellence. Leeds Beckett: UK.

Mallett, C. J., Trudel, P., Lyle, J., & Rynne, S. (2009). Formal versus informal coach education. *International Journal of Sport Science & Coaching, 4*, 325–334.

Mallett, C. J., Rynne, S. B., & Billett, S. (2016). Valued learning experiences of early career and experienced high-performance coaches. *Physical Education and Sport Pedagogy, 21*(1), 89–104.

Mallett, C. J., Rabjohns, M., & Occhino, J. L. (2016). Challenging coaching orthodoxy: a self-determination theory perspective. In P. Davis (Ed.), *The psychology of effective coaching and management* (pp. 167–182). London: Nova Publishers.

Mallett, C.J., Rossi, T., Rynne, S., Tinning, R. (2016). In pursuit of becoming a senior coach: the learning culture for Australian Football League coaches. Physical Education and Sport Pedagogy 21, 24–39.

Mayer, J. D. (2005). A tale of two visions: can a new view of personality help integrate psychology? *American Psychologist, 60*, 294–307.

McAdams, D. P. (1995). What do we know when we know a person? *Journal of Personality, 63*, 365–396.

McAdams, D. P. (2013). The psychological self as actor, agent, and author. *Perspectives on Psychological Science, 8*, 272–295.

McAdams, D. P. (2015). *The art and science of personality development.* New York: Guilford.

McAdams, D.P., Olson, B.D. (2010). Personality development: continuity and change over the life course. Annual Review of Psychology 61, 517–542.

McAdams, D. P., & Cox, K. (2010). Self and identity across the life span. In R. Lerner, A. Freund, & M. Lamb (Eds.), *Handbook of life span development.* New York: Wiley.

McAdams, D. P., & Manczak, E. (2011). What is a "level" of personality? *Psychological Inquiry, 22*, 40–44.

McAdams, D. P., & Pals, J. L. (2006). A new Big Five: fundamental principles for an integrative science of personality. *American Psychologist, 61*, 204–217.

McCrae, R. R., & Costa, P. T. (1997). Personality trait structure as a human universal. *American Psychologist, 52*, 509–516.

McCrae, R. R., & Costa, P. T. (2007). *NEO inventories: Professional manual.* Odessa, FL: Psychological Assessment Resources.

McLean, K., & Mallett, C. J. (2012). What motivates the motivators? *Physical Education and Sport Pedagogy, 17*(1), 21–35.

Mischel, W., & Shoda, Y. (2008). Toward a unified theory of personality: integrating dispositions and processing dynamics within the Cognitive-Affective Processing System (CAPS). In O. P. John, R. W. Robins, & L. A. Pervin (Eds.), *Handbook of personality* (3rd ed., pp. 208–241). New York: Guilford.

Nash, C. S., & Sproule, J. (2009). Career development of expert coaches. *International Journal of Sports Science & Coaching, 4*(1), 121–138.

Norman, L., & French, J. (2013). Understanding how high performance women athletes experience the coach-athlete relationship. *International Journal of Coaching Science, 7*(1), 3–24.

Occhino, J., Mallett, C. J., & Rynne, S. B. (2013). Dynamic social networks in high performance football coaching. *Physical Education and Sport Pedagogy, 18*(1), 90–102.

Occhino, J. L., Mallett, C. J., Rynne, S. B., & Carlisle, K. N. (2014). Autonomy-supportive pedagogical approach to sports coaching: research, challenges and opportunities. *International Journal of Sport Science and Coaching, 9*, 401–416.

Olusoga, P., Maynard, I., Hays, K., & Butt, J. (2012). Coaching under pressure: a study of Olympic coaches. *Journal of Sports Sciences, 30*, 229–239.

Patton, M. Q. (2002). *Qualitative research and evaluation methods.* Thousand Oaks, CA: Sage.

Piaget, J. (1970). Piaget's theory. In: Mussen, P. (Ed.), Carmichael's manual of child psychology. John Wiley, New York.

Purdy, L., & Jones, R. (2011). Choppy waters: elite rowers' perceptions of coaching. *Sociology of Sport Journal, 28*, 329–346.

Reade, I., Rodgers, W., & Spriggs, K. (2008). New ideas for high performance coaches: a case study of knowledge transfer in sport science. *International Journal of Sports Science and Coaching, 3*, 335–354.

Ruiz-Tendero, G., & Salinero-Martín, J. J. (2011). *International Journal of Sport Science, 7*(23), 113–125.

Rynne, S. B. (2014). "Fast track" and "traditional path" coaches: affordances, agency and social capital. *Sport Education and Society, 19*(3), 299–313.

Rynne, S. B., & Mallett, C. J. (2012). Understanding the work and learning of high performance coaches. *Physical Education and Sport Pedagogy, 17*, 507–523.

Rynne, S. B., & Mallett, C. J. (2016). High performance coaching: demands and development. In R. Thelwell, C. Harwood, I. Greenlees (Eds.), *The psychology of coaching: A contemporary review.* London: Routledge.

Rynne, S., Mallett, C. J., & Tinning, R. (2010). The learning of sport coaches in high performance workplaces. *Sport Education and Society, 15*, 331–346.

Sameroff, A.J., Haith, M.M. (Eds.) (1996). The five to seven year shift: The age of reason and responsibility. University of Chicago Press, Chicago, IL.

Sheldon, K. M., Cheng, C., & Hilpert, J. (2011). Understanding well-being and optimal functioning: applying the Multilevel Personality in Context (MPIC) model. *Psychological Inquiry, 22*, 1–16.

Singer, J. (2005). *Personality and psychotherapy: Treating the whole person.* New York: Guilford.

Smith, C. P. (2000). Content analysis and narrative analysis. In H. T. Reis, & C. M. Judd (Eds.), *Handbook of research methods in social and personality psychology* (pp. 313–335). New York, NY: Cambridge University Press.

Stake, R. E. (1994). Case studies. In N. K. Denzin, & Y. S. Lincoln (Eds.), *Handbook of qualitative research* (pp. 236–247). Thousand Oaks, CA: Sage.

Thelwell, R. C., Weston, N. J. V., Greenlees, I. A., & Hutchings, N. (2008). Stressors in elite sport: a coach perspective. *Journal of Sports Sciences, 26*, 905–918.

Trudel, P., & Gilbert, W. (2006). Coaching and coach education. In D. Kirk, D. Macdonald, & M. O'Sullivan (Eds.), *The handbook of physical education* (pp. 516–539). London: Sage.

Trudel, P., Gilbert, W., & Werthner, P. (2010). Coach education effectiveness. In J. Lyle, & C. Cushion (Eds.), *Sport coaching: Professionalisation and practice* (pp. 135–152). London: Elsevier.

Vallée, C. N., & Bloom, G. A. (2005). Building a successful program: perspectives of expert Canadian female coaches of team sports. *Journal of Applied Sport Psychology, 17*, 179–196.

Werthner, P., & Trudel, P. (2006). A new theoretical perspective for understanding how coaches learn to coach. *The Sport Psychologist, 20*, 198–212.

White, S.H. (1965). Evidence for a hierarchical arrangement of learning processes. Advances in Child Behaviour 2, 187–220.

Chapter 15

Sexual Harassment and Abuse in Sport: Implications for Sport Psychologists

Kari Fasting

Department of Cultural and Social Studies, Norwegian School of Sport Science, Oslo, Norway

INTRODUCTION

Most people will agree that participation in sport is a very positive activity and that the sporting field is a safe arena. Accordingly, it is difficult for people to believe that there are individuals in the sporting environment who harass and abuse athletes. But research over the past 20 years has shown that sexual harassment and abuse (SHA) do occur in sport, which also has led to a more critical analysis of the quality of sporting environments, and their impact on young people (Fasting, Brackenridge, & Sundgot-Borgen, 2003, 2004; Fasting, Chroni, & Knorre, 2014; Kirby, Greaves, & Hankivsky, 2000; Leahy, Pretty, & Tenenbaum, 2002; Stirling & Kerr, 2009; Volkwein, Schnell, Sherwood, & Livezey, 1997). According to the World Health Organization (WHO), both sexual harassment and sexual abuse are examples of violence (Krug, Dahlberg, Mercy, Zwi, & Lozano, 2002). Violence particular against girls and women is a worldwide problem. It occurs in all regions, countries, societies, and cultures. It affects women and men irrespective of income, class, race, or ethnicity. Because sport in many ways is a mirror of society, we should therefore not be surprised that SHA also occurs in sport.

There are many different concepts used in this area such as sexual assault, sexual violence, gender-based violence, sexual intimidation, sexual exploitation, sexual harm, and maltreatment. Violence in sport also takes many different forms. Sometimes the same behaviors have different names, depending on the language and the culture of a country: gender and sexual harassment; sexual abuse; physical abuse; bullying; emotional and psychological abuse; neglect; child labor and trafficking; by-standing; and homophobia, to mention some of the names. The literature also is "blurred," because sometimes these concepts are used interchangeably. This chapter, therefore, starts with an explanation of

Sport and Exercise Psychology Research. http://dx.doi.org/10.1016/B978-0-12-803634-1.00015-7

some of the concepts and how they are used in connection with sport. Thereafter, a short overview of what we know about the prevalence, the forms, the impact, the risk factors, and the perpetrators of gender-sexual harassment and abuse (GSHA) in sport is presented. The last part of the chapter focuses on prevention and protection initiatives, before it closes with the implications of this knowledge for sport psychologists.

DEFINITIONS

Historically, empirical definitions of sexual harassment have been derived from students' and employee's descriptions of their experiences of harassment. According to Gruber and Fineran (2008), sexual harassment was originally formulated as behavior by males who used organizational power or cultural privilege to coerce sexual favors from women. This initial formulation has expanded both theoretically and legally over the decades to include gender- or sexually focused behaviors, and more recently, same-sex harassment involving the use of sexual threats, taunts, or attacks. Hunt, Davidson, Fielden, and Hoel (2010, p. 657) write that "there is no one definition of sexual harassment, either in terms of behavior or the circumstances in which it occurs." Common for most definitions is that they refer to that the experienced behavior is unwanted or threatening, troublesome, insulting or offensive. A frequently used model was published 20 years ago by Gelfand, Fitzgerald, and Drasgow (1995). They classified sexually harassing behaviors into three related, yet conceptually distinct, dimensions: *gender harassment, unwanted sexual attention,* and *sexual coercion.* Gender harassment refers to a broad range of verbal and nonverbal behaviors not aiming at sexual cooperation but conveying insulting, hostile, and degrading attitudes about women or men. Ridiculing is often a form of gender harassment, like telling a boy "you throw like a girl." Environments that allow insulting and degrading behaviors or remarks about one's gender contribute to a culture that can have a very negative effect on the people in that particular sport, whether they are athletes, coaches, or sport psychologists.

Unwanted sexual attention, which is the core in the definitions of sexual harassment, refers to a wide range of verbal and nonverbal behaviors that are offensive and unwanted, and that are not reciprocated. In the position statement to the International Olympic Committee (IOC) sexual harassment is defined as follows:

> *Sexual harassment refers to behaviour towards an individual or group that involves sexualised verbal, non-verbal or physical behaviour, whether intended or unintended, legal or illegal, that is based upon an abuse of power and trust and that is considered by the victim or a bystander to be unwanted or coerced.* (International Olympic Committee, 2007)

It is common to distinguish between verbal, nonverbal, and physical sexual harassment. Verbal sexual harassment may include unwanted intimate questions relating to one's body, clothes, or private life, including "jokes" with a sexual innuendo, and proposals for sexual services or sexual relationships. Nonverbal sexual harassment might take the form of staring at people, or showing pictures of objects with sexual allusions. Physical sexual harassment is unwanted or unnecessary physical contact of a sexual nature, such as "pinching," pressing oneself onto the body of others, or attempting to kiss or caress another person.

Sexual coercion refers to the extortion of sexual cooperation in return for job-related considerations (or in relation to sport in return for sport-related consideration, such as, for example, to be a member of a national team). An important difference between definitions of sexual harassment and sexual abuse is that abuse is characterized by nonconsensual sexual contact or acts. Further, abuse can involve a person being tricked, forced, or coerced into a sexual act that they do not want, or to which they are not mature enough to consent. Attempted rape and rape are examples of sexual abuse. Depending on the age of the victim, the definition may change. A behavior that might be labeled as harassment toward an adult might be abuse if experienced by a child. And legally, childhood may include those athletes up to age 18. Thus, a gray zone exists in defining harassment and abuse in terms of age. It is also true in viewing the continuum of negative actions from sex discrimination through sexual harassment to sexual abuse (Brackenridge, 1997). However, making a distinction between harassment and abuse can be useful in trying to understand what sometimes happens between coaches and young athletes.

"Grooming" is a tool that potential abusers may use to gain a position of trust (usually with a minor) from which to carry out the abuse. Grooming someone for sexual abuse involves slowly gaining the trust of the person before breaking down barriers against sexual involvement. Young athletes being groomed in this way can feel trapped into obedience: Their compliance is assured or compelled by threats of being dropped from the team, or by being given or by withholding of privileges (Bringer, Brackenridge, & Johnston, 2001).

The United Nations (UN) and the European Union (EU) often use the term "gender-based violence" as an umbrella term. In the European Commission's report on gender equality in sport from 2014 (European Commission, 2014) gender-based violence is defined as "violence directed against a person because of that person's gender (including gender identity/expression) or as violence that affects persons of a particular gender disproportionately" (p. 47). Another umbrella concept that is used in relation to children and youth is "maltreatment." With reference to Crooks and Wolfe (2007), Stirling and Kerr (2010) write that:

> *Relational maltreatment occurs when there is a pattern of abusive or neglectful*
> *behaviors within a critical relationship—a relationship in which one individual*
> *is dependent, fully or in part, on another individual for her or his sense of safety,*
> *trust and fulfillment of needs. (p. 305)*

The authors mention coach–athlete relationships as an example; they recognize physical abuse, sexual abuse, emotional abuse, and neglect as the four forms of relational maltreatment.

Viewed from an international perspective, the legislative protection given to athletes and members of the support personnel varies greatly. According to the United Nations (2006), 90 nation states have some form of legislation prohibiting sexual harassment; however, depending on the country in question, sports organizations may or may not be covered by these various laws. In most countries, the penal code applies to sexual abuse, though the age of consent varies internationally. Sport organizations may also have their own rules and laws, but a general rule is that the police should handle violations of the penal code.

In legal terms, the penal code in the United States of America recognizes two kinds of sexual harassment: quid pro quo and hostile environment (Holland & Cortina, 2015). Applied to sexual harassment in sport, a quid pro quo relationship exists when benefits are granted or withheld depending on an athlete's willingness or refusal to submit to the sexual demands from a person in authority. A coach, for example, might drop an athlete from the team because the coach's sexual advances are refused. A hostile environment exists when a person's conduct is severe enough to disturb an athlete and interfere with the athlete's ability to perform. A hostile environment can affect more than the targeted person—for example, a team member who witnesses repeated incidents, even if not directed at that person, might also be considered a victim of sexual harassment.

WHAT DO WE KNOW FROM RESEARCH ON SHA?

The first studies on SHA in sport were published about 25 years ago, and most of the studies have been prevalence studies, but there is a marked variety of approaches to the subject, both theoretical and methodological. In addition to prevalence, quantitative studies have focused on the athletes' perceptions of sexual harassment (Auweele et al., 2008), prevalence in relation to sport types (Fasting et al., 2004), prevalence in relation to sport performance level (Fasting, Brackenridge, & Knorre, 2010), prevalence in relation to coaching behavior (Sand, Fasting, Chroni, & Knorre, 2011), and female athletes' experiences of sexual harassment in sport compared to women outside sport (Fasting et al., 2003). In another recent quantitative study, Parent, Lavoie, Thibodeau, Hebert, and Blais (2015) in Quebec have surveyed consensual sexual contact between coaches and young athletes 14–17 years of age, a context of authority that constitutes sexual abuse under the Canadian law. In addition, qualitative studies have been used to gather descriptions of harassment experiences, athletes' responses to sexual harassment, and the impact that these experiences have had for them (eg, Fasting, Brackenridge, & Walseth, 2002, 2007; Krauchek & Ranson, 1999). From these studies, the risk factors described later in this chapter have been developed (Brackenridge, 2001; Cense & Brackenridge, 2001). Though we have much more knowledge now compared to 15 years ago, we still do not know very much, and more empirical research is needed. There are many reasons for this; for example, the area is politically sensitive, and it is often difficult to gain access to the athletes, in addition to methodological and ethical issues.

One of the major problems with some of the first quantitative prevalence studies was the low response rates. This is often common for surveys in general, but more so with sensitive themes. Another question is the validity of the results because athletes often are asked about situations that happened to them many years ago. This is also true for qualitative interviews. There is a general problem with retrospective studies, but in this field, there can be more traumatic reasons for underreporting. It has been indicated that unwanted sexual behaviors are underreported because many repress the events, are ashamed or embarrassed, or want to avoid incrimination of people they know (Koss, 1992, 1993). It is also often impossible to compare the different studies, due to the difference in sampling procedures, the methodological approaches, the vocabulary and connotative meanings of questionnaire items, the anonymity and confidentiality of disclosures, the statistical analyses employed, and so forth (Timmermann, 2003).

Another problem often discussed in sexual harassment research is that women will report experiencing unwanted sexually harassing behaviors, but not label those experiences as sexual harassment (Welsh, 2009). For example, in a comparative study among American, Brazilian, Canadian, and Israeli female students, there was a huge discrepancy between the prevalence of sexual harassment objectively (also often referred to as legally) and subjectively defined and measured (Barak, 1997). Overall, 89.3% of Brazilians experienced sexual harassment in comparison to 72.8% of the Americans. When the same students reported their experiences subjectively by answering the question: "Have you been sexually harassed?" the percentages dropped to 6.1% among the Brazilians and to 4.4% among the Americans. Stirling and Kerr (2009) also found in an interview study that some athletes who had experienced sexual abuse seem not to look upon themselves as victims, because they thought the sexually abusive behavior experienced to be normal in sport, and according to Parent et al. (2015) therefore probably would not self-report them in a questionnaire.

With all this taken into account, it is not surprising that the studies on prevalence of sexual harassment in sport varies between 0.4% and 92%. The first number refers to the study from Quebec mentioned earlier, a representative study among 6450 boys and girls 14–17 years of age that were asked about sexual harassment from a coach the last 12 months (Parent et al., 2015). The last number refers to a study among 213 female athletes in Zimbabwe with a mean age of 26 years (Madzivivre, Mkumbuzi, Nyaundi, Benza, & Mupaso, 2006). They included also vandalism, stalking, and bullying in the concept of sexual harassment and referred to a sport setting in general. The prevalence of sexual abuse also varies, but here the numbers are lower. It varies from 2% to 49%. The first number refers to a large study in the United Kingdom covering 6000 students 18–22 years old asking questions about their experiences before they were 16 years of age, whereas the second number (49%) refers to the study just mentioned from Zimbabwe.

In the first and so far last prevalent study in Norway, even though it was conducted 15 years ago, the sample consisted of 660 elite female athletes, defined as athletes who were members of a junior, development, or senior national team, 15–39 years of age, representing 58 sport disciplines. The Norwegian Olympic, Paralympic and Confederation of Sport (NIF) financed this study, and a representative sample of the Norwegian female population of the same ages as the athlete group, a total of 785 females who were not elite athletes, received the same questionnaire, and both samples had a very high answering percentage (87% respective 73%). Sexual harassing behaviors were measured through 11 questions from lighter to more serious forms of sexually harassing behaviors such as attempted rape and rape. The percentage of female athletes who had experienced one or more of these kinds of behaviors was 28. The survey found no difference between the prevalence of sexual harassment experienced by athletes in a sports context and that experienced by the control group of women in an educational or workplace setting. Most of the participants had been harassed by men, but some had also been harassed by women. This study further revealed that sexual harassment seemed to occur in all sports (Fasting et al., 2004). The authors concluded that "sexual harassment is a societal problem and therefore also, as a consequence, a problem for Norwegian sport ... There is however, no reason to conclude that sport in general is worse than in other arenas" (Fasting, Brackenridge, & Sundgot-Borgen, 2000, p. 30). The Canadian study mentioned earlier among those 14–17 years old confirms this result because the authors concluded that athletes at the time of the study were not at greater risk of experiencing sexual abuse by a coach than nonathletes (Parent et al., 2015). The Norwegian questionnaire was followed up with 25 qualitative interviews with female elite-level athletes who had been harassed or abused. In all, 15 of these athletes had participated in the Olympic Games, world championships, or world cup competitions. These interviews revealed that most of the female athletes' sexual harassing experiences were from male coaches.

Some years later, I did a study for the Czech Olympic Committee. Here sexual harassment was measured with those three items that were most frequently answered in the Norwegian study. Altogether 45% of the Czech athletes had experienced sexual harassment. This study found that the probability of being harassed by someone inside a sport setting increased from 33% for those playing the sport purely for the exercise to 55% for athletes at the elite level (Fasting et al., 2010). As mentioned before, it is very problematic to compare different studies, but one study of incidents of sexual harassment among sports students in three European countries—the Czech Republic, Greece, and Norway—measured sexual harassing behavior in exactly the same way. This study found that sexual harassing behaviors experienced in sport were reported far more often in the Czech Republic (42%) and Greece (44%) than in Norway (24%). Therefore, the marked differences in the prevalence were attributed to the differences in social structures between the three countries; that is, differences in gender hierarchy in society, in gender equality laws, and in the severity and rigor of enforcing laws prohibiting sexual harassment within and outside sports (Fasting, Chroni, Hervik, & Knorre, 2011).

Most of the studies have taken place in Western countries (Chroni & Fasting, 2009; Fasting et al., 2011; Fejgin & Hanegby, 2001; Jolly & Decamps, 2006; Nielsen, 2001; Tomlinson & Yorganci, 1997). Until a few years ago there was only anecdotal information about the prevalence and experience of GSHA in Africa, but in addition to the study mentioned previously from Zimbabwe, at least four projects from respectively South Africa (van Niekerk & Rzygula, 2010), Zimbabwe (Muchena & Mapfuno, 2010), Nigeria (Elendu & Umeakuka, 2011), and Kenya have been published. The latest from 2014 was a study among 339 university female athletes in Kenya, which found that 64% had experienced sexual harassment incidences (Rintaugu, Kamau, Amusa, & Toriola, 2014).

Gender

Most of the published work on SHA in sport has focused on male harassment of females, particularly male coach–female athlete, but some research has shown female–female and male–male harassment (Fasting et al., 2000; Fasting & Knorre, 2005; Hartill, 2009; Shire, Brackenridge, & Fuller, 2000). Hartill (2005) focuses on this when he wrote already 10 years ago that "sport researchers, to date, have been driven by the male perpetrator–female victim paradigm," and that "this focus has influenced the type of research that has been conducted and has inadvertently contributed to the further silencing of the sexually abused male" (p. 287). This has been true until recently and was confirmed in a review article from 2012 titled "Sexual abuse in sport: What about boys?" by Parent and Bannon (2012). Hartill (2005) has also stressed that victimization and the way it is experienced in sport are different for boys than for girls. However, in 2004 Toftegaard Nielsen analyzed 160 criminal court cases concerning sexual abuse in sport in Denmark. A surprising result was that 65% of the victims were boys in these cases. The study from the United Kingdom mentioned earlier found that more young women than young men reported sexual harassment (34% and 17%), but more boys than girls reported sexual abuse (5% and 2%). In the study of youth in Canada previously mentioned, there were the expected gender differences with respect to experiences of sexual abuse from a coach—more female than male victims—but with respect to sexual harassment female and male athletes had experienced similar rates of sexual harassment by a coach within the last 12 months (Parent et al., 2015, p. 17).

Forms

We have relatively little detailed knowledge about what types of SHA athletes have experienced. This is because sexual harassment behaviors both in quantitative and qualitative studies often are grouped into categories such as verbal, nonverbal, and physical harassment. Based on these studies, it seems that verbal harassment in the form of ridiculing (gender harassment), sexual hints, and jokes are most common, but many female athletes also experience physically sexual harassing behavior. However, there is relatively little detailed knowledge about how these experiences are articulated or performed. The stories and processes behind unwanted experiences are of particular interest given that the context and individual interpretation are crucial aspects of sexual harassment (Volkwein et al., 1997). In other words, the same behavior could be welcomed among some athletes but could be uncomfortable for others. Equally, the same behavior could lead to different reactions from the same athletes depending on the differences in the sporting or social context.

The survey of Norwegian female elite-level athletes revealed that the three most commonly reported experiences in sport were: "ridiculing of your sport performance and of you as an athlete because of your gender or your sexuality" (22%); "unwanted physical contact, body contact" (21%); and "repeated unwanted sexually suggestive glances, comments, teasing and jokes, about your body, your clothes, your private life, etc." (16%) (Fasting et al., 2000). A study from Belgium among Flemish female student-athletes found that more than one in five had experienced the following from their coach: "flirting with you or others in your team," "making a sexual remark about you," and "staring at your breasts/ your buttocks/your pubic area" (Auweele et al., 2008). Nina experienced the following example of verbal sexual harassment from a Norwegian male coach:

> *He says things in a way that maybe is meant as a joke, but sometimes I get very hurt by it. He can for example say something about that I have too small 'boobs' or comments on other parts of my body ... and it doesn't at all have anything to do with the sport I am competing in. (Fasting et al., 2002, p. 42)*

The following are two examples of unwanted physical contact from a Norwegian respective a Czech male coach told by Mari and Simona:

> *... when we didn't perform well, then the punishment was that we should sit on his lap. I remember I thought it was disgusting. He touched us and was really very disgusting. I don't understand today that we accepted it at all. We had a drill where we had to sprint, and the one who came last had to sit on his lap, so everyone were running like hell... (Fasting et al., 2002, p. 42)*

> *It happens quite often that people try to hug people, but with this particular coach it is very clear that it was in a sexual context, so you have to be really insistent to keep him away from yourself. I experienced it as unpleasant ... It mainly happens during the training where he uses opportunities like when someone is coming to practice*

and he comes to hug and says I'm really glad to see you. But during the hug he can move his hands on the body, which is unpleasant. (Fasting & Knorre, 2005, p. 44)

Impacts and Risks

The impact of SHA can be serious for the athlete, but also for the sport itself, because clubs and sports associations may lose both members and sponsors. For athletes and nonathletes, studies have shown many individual consequences of exposure to gender, sexual harassment and abuse (GSHA): anxiety, fear, a sense of vulnerability and helplessness, fear of rape, decreased ability to concentrate, poor sports performance, depression, lower self-esteem, negative effects on family life, absence from work or studies, feelings of guilt and shame, negative effects on social activities, and the premature end of their sporting career (Fasting et al., 2002).

Some abused athletes have developed posttraumatic stress disorders. Relational difficulties with trust and intimacy are also commonly observed as reported by an athlete who was sexually abused by her coach:

It's been years where I haven't been able to be close to a boy. I just don't trust them. So, for someone that I cared about, you know, I'd throw it away, because, you know, I just don't trust them. (Leahy & Fasting, 2014, p. 8)

Other reported health consequences are physical complaints such as fatigue, headaches, sleep disturbance, weight loss or gain, gastrointestinal disturbances and nausea, fatigue, and neck and back pain (Dansky & Kilpatrick, 1997; Duffy, Wareham, & Walsh, 2004; Rintaugu et al., 2014).

Unfortunately, athletes often do not report incidents of SHA. In one of the first studies in the area by Kirby et al. (2000) in Canada, some of the reasons given for a reluctance to report harassment were fear of being dropped from the team, fear of not being believed, feeling ashamed or embarrassed, loyalty to the coach or team, and not knowing to whom to talk.

The importance of education, ethical guidelines, and a reporting system is important if the athletes will dare to report harassment and abuse, and the role of the sport psychologist may be important here, which I will come back to at the end of the chapter.

Risk factors can be related not only to the coach and athlete, but also to the sport itself—in relation to both the culture and structure of the sport organization. Examples of risk factors for the athletes are poor relationships with their parents, so the perpetrator has a chance to get close to the victims, during trips, during massage, at the coach's home, and during drives to and from practice. This can afford the coach complete control of her/his life, and she/he may be totally dedicated to the coach or authority figure who assumes the status of a father figure (Brackenridge, 2001; Cense & Brackenridge, 2001). Concerning the sport culture, the following risk factors have been identified: has an autocratic authority system, involves close personal contact with athletes, sets up clear power imbalance between athlete and coach, gives scope for separation of athlete from peers in time and space, and involves mixed sexes and ages sharing room on away trips. Concerning the structure: involves a hierarchical status system, gives rewards based on performance, links rewards to compliance with the authority system, has no formal procedures for screening, hiring and monitoring staff, and where technical/task demands legitimate touch (Brackenridge, 2001).

Perpetrators

Many of the articles on GSHA have concentrated on the coach as the perpetrator. This is important, but we also need to focus on the environment that surrounds the athletes, including the teammates and spectators. In the study from Kenya, for example, the major perpetuators were spectators (Rintaugu et al., 2014).

In the earlier studies in Norway and Czech Republic, no significant differences in the experiences of SHA from authority figures compared with SHA from peer athletes were found (Fasting et al., 2000). Later studies indicate, however, that peer athletes, not the coaches, are the major source of SHA, though the percentages vary according to the form of harassing behavior. Among those who had been sexually harassed in the United Kingdom study 66% mentioned that teammates had been involved, compared only to 21% who listed coaches. Among those who had been sexually abused (which was 3%) the equivalent figures were 88% from teammates and 8% from coaches (Alexander, Stafford, & Lewis, 2011). These results are in accordance with the results from a study in Nigeria. Elendu and Umeakuka (2011) found in a study among 1214 university male and female athletes that the perpetrators of gender harassment, sexual harassment, and sexual abuse first of all were fellow athletes, and not the coaches.

Apart from some information from media (Brackenridge, Bishopp, Moussalli, & Tapp, 2008), court reports (Fasting, Brackenridge, & Kjølberg, 2013), and interviews with athletes (Fasting & Brackenridge, 2009), we have little direct knowledge of the psychological profile of the abusive or harassing coach. However, analyses of accounts of sexual exploitation in sport indicate that perpetrators' feelings of power and control arise from feelings of confidence and superiority (Brackenridge, 1997; Cense, 1997; Kirby & Greaves, 1996). According to these studies, sexually abusive coaches have good social skills, high visibility, popularity, and a high level of sexual confidence. Popular media representations of harassing and abusive coaches also suggest that not only do they have a reputation for success; they also often are regarded as "very nice people."

Nielsen (2004, unpublished PhD thesis) analyzed cases in Denmark, in which the perpetrators had been found guilty and sentenced. These files yielded 160 cases that had occurred in the context of sport, during the period from 1980 to 2002. The average age of the perpetrators' first offence was 35 years, and average age of the sexually abused athletes was 12 years old. In nine out of ten cases, the perpetrator had used rewards to entice the victim to cooperate. In other cases, the perpetrator had played on the victim's feelings of guilt and shame.

A few years later, a study of Norwegian court reports of cases in which perpetrators also had been sentenced for sexual abuse in sport found that in 11 of 15 cases the perpetrators had been coaching their victims (Fasting et al., 2013). Further, all perpetrators were men, the youngest 19 years old and the oldest 58 years. The civil status of the perpetrators varied; none was a full-time coach. The author concluded that no clear profile of a perpetrator could be drawn.

Most perpetrators of sexual abuse and sexual harassment in sport never face the criminal justice system because of victims' fears of reprisals, "de-selection" (being barred from further training or advancement in their sport), or not being taken seriously. However, we might learn more about these perpetrators by listening to those whom they have harassed. From interviews with Norwegian elite female athletes who had been sexually harassed by their coaches, three main types of offending sports coaches emerged:

- The behavior of the Flirting-Charming Coach was characterized by constant flirting, joking, trying to touch, and so on.
- The behavior of the Seductive Coach was characterized by more extreme behavior and trying to "hit on" everyone.
- The Authoritarian Coach, in addition to displaying and using their power, often had a degrading and negative view of women in general. (Fasting & Brackenridge, 2009)

This study, however, concluded that rather than being one type only (ie, conforming to a single pattern), sexually harassing coaches may select from a repertoire of several harassment scripts that vary according to the situation.

In most cases, sexual harassment and sexual abuse are expressions of abuse of power. Examples of power relations in sports include the power that people in the support network always have in relation to athletes: This especially applies to the coach, who can help young athletes achieve their sporting goals. This type of trust and power relationship is often called an "expert" or "power of position" relationship, which can be exploited and lead to SHA. Coaches should, therefore, be aware of this power difference between themselves and their athletes, realize that the athletes are dependent on, see them as, the experts, and usually have complete trust in them. If misunderstood, this power imbalance can lead to exploitative sexual relationships with athletes. The same proposition is argued in a Canadian study that found coaches' power contributes to athletes' risk of abuse (Stirling & Kerr, 2009). This may also be related to the coaching style. In the European study of sport students, we found that the prevalence of sexual harassment was significantly higher among female athletes who had experienced an authoritarian type of coaching than those who had not (Sand et al., 2011).

Leahy, Pretty, and Tenenbaum (2004) found two dimensions of perpetrator methodology in a qualitative study of Australian athletes. These were: "The creation of a powerless victim and the creation of an omnipotent perpetrator" (Leahy et al., 2004, p. 531), both of which appear to confirm Brackenridge's (2001) earlier findings about coach/perpetrator risk factors, extracted from the analysis of interviews with abused athletes. The following quote is from the Czech study mentioned earlier and illustrates this:

> ... as time went on he started to act like I was his property ... Also I heard from him that I should take off some weight and what I should eat or shouldn't eat. And then off course he tried to seduce me as he tried to seduce many other women. He was married and I didn't want to have any relationship with him. (Fasting & Knorre, 2005, p. 41)

PREVENTION

In the mid-1990s, only a few sport organizations in the United Kingdom (National Coaching Foundation, 1995), Canada (Canadian Association for the Advancement of Women and Sport, 1994), and Australia (Active Australia, 1998) acknowledged or addressed child abuse and protection, but for a long time sport organizations did not recognize that SHA occurred in sport. They were in denial. Nevertheless, media attentions, sexual abuse scandals, and research have led to a rapid growth in interest in the issue internationally, particularly in relation to the protection of children and youth. Major organizations and institutions like Council of Europe (2000, 2015), European Union (Deutsche Sportjugend im Deutschen Olympischen Sportbund, 2012; European Commission, 2014), UNICEF (Brackenridge, Fasting, Kirby, Leahy, Parent, & Sand, 2010; UNICEF, 2014) and IOC (2015) have initiated projects. Different agencies adopt different foci, dependent on their overall mission. They can be divided into sport-specific (focusing on abuse prevention in sport), children's rights organizations (focusing on child protection around sports events) and humanitarian organizations (focusing on child development and protection through sport) (Brackenridge & Rhind, 2014).

The common labels for concern are child protection, children's welfare, and safeguarding. Child safeguarding can be defined as the set of actions, measures, and procedures taken to ensure that all children are kept safe from harm, abuse, neglect, or exploitation while in care (Council of Europe, 2015). An International Safeguarding Children in Sport Founders Group has worked with more than 50 organizations and developed safeguards for children in sport. These safeguards set out the actions that all organizations working in sport should have in place to ensure children are safe from harm. The safeguards are: "1) Developing your policy, 2) Procedure for responding to safeguarding concerns, 3) Advice and support, 4) Minimizing risks to children, 5) Guidelines for behaviour, 6) Recruiting, training and communicating, 7) Working with partners, and 8) monitoring and evaluating" (Mountjoy, Rhind, Tiivas, & Leglise, 2015, p. 3).

Much of the research has led to policy statements; actions plans; codes of practice for coaches, parents, and officials; coach education workshops; ethical guidelines for everyone involved in sport; rules for being alone with or even touching young athletes; and criminal checks of people working with children in sports. As an example, I will show you the following guidelines that shall apply to all Norwegian sports, to prevent GSHA:

1. *Treat everyone with respect, and refrain from all forms of communication, action or behaviour that may be perceived as offensive.*
2. *Avoid body contact that may be perceived as unwanted.*
3. *Avoid all types of verbal intimacy that may be perceived as sexually charged.*
4. *Avoid expressions, jokes and opinions that relate to the athlete's gender or sexual orientation in a negative way.*
5. *Seek to have both sexes represented in the support network.*
6. *Avoid contact with the athletes in private spaces unless there are several persons present or in agreement with parents/guardians or the sports management.*
7. *Show respect for the athlete's, coach's and leader's private life.*
8. *Avoid dual relationships. If a reciprocal relationship is established, the situation should be raised and clarified openly in the milieu.*
9. *Do not offer any form of reward with the purpose of demanding or antici-pating sexual services in return.*
10. *Take action and give notice if a breach of these rules is experienced.* (Norwegian Olympic and Paralympic Committee and Confederation of Sports, 2011, p. 4)

Though different preventive actions have been taken in many countries and sport organizations, in an international perspective, policies, including codes of conducts and reporting system, are often not in place. This is one reason why the European Commission last year in their *Strategic Action for Gender Equal-ity in Sport* devoted a chapter to the "Fight against gender based violence in and through sport" (European Commission, 2014). In the report, it is stated "The overall aim of preventing gender based violence in sport is to reduce its occur-rence and to contribute to the reduction of gender based violence in society" (p. 27). By 2020, the following objectives should be in place:

1. *A specific national strategy, including a policy and legal framework and action plan, grounded in evidence based data, is in place in all EU Member States.*
2. *Preventive tools and supporting services for victims developed in all EU Member States.*
3. *Human resource policies on volunteers and professionals are operational, including European cooperation regarding screening systems for all ap-plicants for coaching staff and volunteer positions to avoid cross border activities of perpetrators.*
4. *Evidence based programmes in sport are developed and disseminated in order to empower athletes against possible harassment and abuse in sport and society. Provide education and training to coaches to prevent them be-ing involved in gender based violence and to act in the right way preventing violence between peers or others.* (European Commission, 2014, p. 27)

For each of these objectives, three or four actions are suggested. Following are some examples from each of the objectives:

- "All sport federations/associations should develop and implement mandatory procedures when SHA occur, including complaint procedures" (objective 1, p. 29).
- "Member States and sport governing bodies should support the development of education and training programmes for different groups on GSHA and make training programs to prevent GSHA mandatory in all coach education" (objective 2, p. 30).
- "Member states and sport governing bodies should develop a registration system for sexual offenders in sport and distribute this to European and international sport governing bodies" (objective 3, p. 31).
- "Develop evidence based programmes for coaches, which should be made mandatory in all coach education to act and intervene in the right way preventing gender based violence between peers or others" (objective 4, p. 32).

In spite of the fact that many protection policies have existed for a while, we do not know very much about their impact, that is, very few of them seem to have been monitored and/or evaluated. Two articles have, however, been published in recent years in this area, one by Donnelly, Kerr, Heron, and DiCarlo (2014) and one by Kerr, Stirling, and MacPherson (2014). The first one was an examination of the requirements that Sport Canada mandated 17 years ago, stating that funding to the national sport organizations was contingent upon each national sport organization (NSO) having a harassment policy and trained harassment officers who would address complaints. The purpose of the study was to examine the current status of these policies. The results revealed that 86% of the national and 71% of the provincial sport organizations had accessible harassment policies. However, critical information, such as a detailed complaint process was missing, and only 10% and 14%, respectively, had harassment officers. Though these facts are probably much better than in most countries, the authors concluded that "Canada is falling short of the requirements initially stipulated by Sport Canada for athlete protection" (Donnelly et al., 2014, p. 1). They suggest the need for a centralized pool of trained officers to reduce the burden on individual sport organizations. The article concludes with recommending that an approach to athlete protection should be grounded in an ethic of care, because "such an approach would shift the focus from addressing problematic behaviors to methods of enhancing the holistic health and well-being of athletes" (Donnelly et al., 2014, p. 15). In the second article, seven child protection in sport initiatives were examined in terms of the extent to which they originated from research, had a content that was consistent with scholarly work, and were evaluated empirically (Kerr et al., 2014). The protection initiatives that were examined were: "Play by the Rules" from Australia; "Speak out" and "Respect in Sport" from Canada; "Safe4Athletes" and "Safe to Compete" from the United States; and the "Child Protection in Sport Unit" and "Children First" from the United Kingdom. The results indicated that these initiatives were not empirically nor derived theoretically for the most part, and were not evaluated. Lack of attention to the notion of power and other contextual information were missing, which according to the authors are central to the understanding of critical relationships and maltreatment. There is, however, some policy work that has been totally based on research, such as that of IOC. In 2007, based on the information from a meeting among international experts in the field, IOC adopted a consensus statement on SHA. This resulted in an interactive online video on the athlete's right to safe sport, which was published in 2012. The consensus statement from 2007 ended with the following recommendations to all sport organizations:

1. *Develop policies and procedures for the prevention of sexual harassment and abuse;*
2. *Monitor the implementation of these policies and procedures;*
3. *Evaluate the impact of these policies in identifying and reducing sexual harassment and abuse;*
4. *Develop an education and training program on sexual harassment and abuse in their sport(s);*
5. *Promote and exemplify equitable, respectful and ethical leadership*
6. *Foster strong partnerships with parents/carers in the prevention of sexual harassment and abuse; and*
7. *Promote and support scientific research on these issues.* (IOC, 2007, p. 5)

IMPLICATIONS FOR SPORT PSYCHOLOGISTS

Based on the knowledge that one has today, what should the implications for sport psychologists and sport psychology consultants be? Whatever the valid prevalence numbers are, statistically, sport psychologists are highly likely to be working with athletes who have been or are harassed or abused. Some may have treated victims or survivors, but some may also never have learned about their athletes' harassing and abusive experiences, though they may have had their suspicions. If knowledge about harassment and abuse never were in their training when becoming a sport psychologist or sport psychology consultants, they may not be able to see the signs, simply because they never did learn about it. In searching the literature, surprisingly few articles have written about the role of sport psychologists in preventing and treating harassed and abused athletes. Some of the few are from Trisha Leahy (2010a,b, 2011) from Hong Kong and from Ashley Stirling and Gretchen Kerr (2010) from Canada. In the following I draw heavily upon their work. All authors stress that the sport psychologists, because of their close involvement with a team, are often the first point of contact for athletes in distress, and thus need to be aware of the relevant social policy and procedures for reporting and referring. As gatekeepers for athletes' safety in identifying, intervening, and acting to prevent the sexual abuse of athletes in sport systems, the sport psychologists have a key safeguarding role (Leahy, 2010a). Leahy writes that "Implications for sport psychology practice involve individual assessment and intervention as well as, more generally, training and supervision programs for sport psychologists" (Leahy, 2011, p. 260), and that the implications for psychology practice may be understood as operating at both an individual and systemic level.

Concerning the individual level, assessment and treatment of athlete survivors of childhood sexual abuse implies that training programs for sport psychologists need to include comprehensive education in the assessment and treatment of childhood abuse and traumagenic symptomatology. Leahy (2011) also stresses that the sport psychology profession should become a more socially engaged discipline. This is embedded in the systemic issues when she refers to the necessity to be aware of the sociocultural context of organized competitive sport, which in some countries has been criticized for normalizing psychologically abusive coaching practice, particularly in relation to children and youth (Brackenridge, 2001; Leahy et al., 2004). The implications of this is the necessity of changing these accepted coaching styles, which masks sexual offender behaviors that rely on psychological abuse and emotional manipulation as primary strategies. A hierarchical power structure has also been found to be associated with the bystander effect, in which observing adults feel unable to intervene in high-risk or suspicious circumstances. The bystander effect may be a result of such an environment, and to overcome this, comprehensive and ongoing sexual abuse awareness education is imperative for all those involved in organized sport, not only the psychologist, but also athletes, parents, and other people, among the support personnel. Leahy (2011, p. 255) also writes that:

Before sport psychologists can step up to the role of gatekeeper, effectively acting to protect the rights of young people in sport, we must first insist on our own rights to be educated and provided with clear ethical guidelines and core competencies embedded in a support system that empowers us to act on behalf of young athletes at risk.

She stresses, however, that sport psychology training programs that primarily teach mental skills as performance enhancement techniques at the expense of training in related systemic policy, advocacy, and ethical systems will not "equip entrants to the profession with the necessary competencies to enable effective engagement with a biopsychosocial discourse and praxis" (Leahy, 2010a, p. 319).

Stirling and Kerr (2010) did a study with the purpose of assessing the experiences and perceived knowledge base for sport psychology consultants with respect to issue of child protection. Questions of interest included: "Are sport psychology consultants exposed to cases of child maltreatment in sport?," "Do sport psychology consultants believe they have the requisite knowledge and training to identify the various forms of relational maltreatment?," and "How might sport psychology consultants be better enabled to act as agents of child protection in sport?" (Stirling & Kerr, 2010, pp. 306–307). They used a mixed method research design where 75 sport psychology consultants completed a questionnaire. In addition, they did eight expert interviews.

The sport psychology consultants were also asked to rank their current knowledge of child protection policies in sport; about half reported "moderate" understanding, and 22% low understanding. Almost all also felt that they were aware of their duty to report incidences of child abuse, including both when and where they should report. The importance of knowledge, training, and competence about children, and of understanding warning signs, symptoms, and specific behaviors associated with child abuse were highlighted by many of the participants. One of them expressed it this way: "We need to know the legal and ethical ramifications and the potential psychological signs and not just be bystanders if at all possible" (Stirling & Kerr, 2010, p. 311). The majority of the participants also suggested supplemental education on athlete/child protection. Many proposed that information on child protection should be provided along with education on other ethical issues faced in the sport environment. The sport psychology consultants also talked about the need for child protection guidelines along with sport-specific examples of maltreatment and best practice in sport, accreditation in counseling ethics as a component of the SPC certification process, and the facilitation of discussion groups where case studies could be discussed with other professionals. The authors summarize the results concerning the recommendations in the following way:

> Regardless of the perceived prevalence of abusive or neglectful incidences in sport reported by the SPC's, the vast majority of the respondents reported that issues of child protection must be addressed by the community of sport psychology professionals. One expert SPC explained, "I don't think we do enough in terms of thinking outside of psychology skills. We need to think about the bigger picture of how we can protect children from a number of different types of abuse." (Stirling & Kerr, 2010, p. 312)

The analysis also revealed an inconsistency between the participants' reports of exposure to specific examples of abusive behaviors in sport and their reported exposure to the various forms of maltreatments. The authors therefore conclude that although the majority of consultants believe they are able to detect abusive and neglectful behaviors, this may not be the case and therefore indicated the need for further education about maltreatment and the behavioral constituents of each form of abuse.

The role and the work of sport psychologists and sport psychology consultants vary internationally. I will end this chapter by telling you a case story of how psychologists can work at a major sports event to both prevent and solve problematic issues that may occur. This is from the 2nd African Youth Games that were held in Gabarone, Botswana, in May 2014. The games had 2500 participants of both genders from all of the 54 African countries. The organizing committee of the games and the Norwegian Olympic and Paralympic Committee and Confederation of Sports (NIF) initiated a partnership to provide safety planning and establish precedence for the hosting of the games under a "safe games" theme (Huffman, 2014). Sport safety planning was defined as being aware, prepared, and active in promoting a Safe Games environment for players, coaches, officials, volunteers, and spectators. Many different actions were taken, but for this chapter I will only present the psychological services that were provided. In reading this, you should have in mind that it is not common in most African countries that psychologists are working with sport teams. In this case, contact was taken with the University of Botswana's Counselling Services Department. Together with The Botswana Association of Psychologists, and Childline, they developed a support and reporting system for the Games. Elements included were, for example, "Safe Games Reporting Box" in different locations throughout the athlete's village, a direct toll-free emergency call number, direct reporting to the psychologists at the place or the clinic, and participation by the psychologists at the daily chef du mission meetings where challenges were brought forward. The University of Botswana provided the venue and the staff for securing a confidential and professional service to the Games' participants. The group, which consisted of 38 people mostly psychologists and a few sociologists, called themselves "Safe Games Psychological First Aiders." There was a lot of aggression and violence going on and as an example of one of the things that the psychologist did was that they briefed the full medical team on abuse and child/youth safeguarding—recognizing signs of stress and abuse. The psychological First Aiders were assigned to different areas throughout the Games' 24 h, including competition venues, the athletes' village and residences. There were always three members of the team at the counseling clinic, and counseling services were provided for everyone. One person was assigned to roam all areas and carried a radio linked to the medical unit and police. The psychological team members were on alert all the time, and if they observed an abusive or potentially abusive situation, they would identify themselves and be available to calm a difficult situation before it became a major problem. They also had sessions with a whole team based on the reaction of coaches and athletes during the competitions on request from a team leader to assist with the levels of stress and anxiety. The main problems identified were related to stress and anger due to pressure to perform, but there were a high number of reports of abuse, particularly verbal abuse, to staff and volunteers, incidents that were managed by the Safe Games' Psychological First Aiders. They provided a number of interventions during the games for different individuals and teams including interviews; relaxation exercises; motivational workshops as requested by coaches, team leaders, or team attachés; counseling sessions; calming techniques; conflict resolution; and anger management. According to Diane Huffman from NIF who reported on the safe guarding of the Games, "an important result was the understanding by all parties of the value and need of such services at major Games where anxiety and stress levels are high" (Huffman, 2014, p. 2). She also writes that based on the experiences from these Games, The Botswana Association of Psychologists and the Botswana National Sports Council are now considering a proposal to work together and provide awareness problems and support systems to the sport associations of Botswana on an ongoing basis.

Based on the few publications presented in this last section, it is clear that the sport psychologists are in a unique position to protect, discover, hinder, and treat athletes from sexually harassing and abusive behaviors. But some prerequisites are necessary. First of all, the sport psychologist must have the necessary knowledge about what constitutes the different forms of harassment and abuse. Second, he or she should work in an environment that has policies for protecting not only the athletes, but also the people who are accused of GSHA, which theoretically could be a sport psychologist. Until a case has been researched and solved either by the sport organization itself or in a criminal court, it is important to have a system in place that take care of both parts. There is no research or statistics in sport about false accusations, and research outside sport is also very scarce. But it is of great importance that ethical guidelines are developed for everyone involved in sport. Such guidelines should also include guidelines for reporting and how cases should be taken care of. If policies and guidelines do not exist, the sport psychologists, if part of the athletes' entourage, should push for and see to that the sport club or association get it. By not being a bystander, but taking action when they observe or have suspicions about the occurrence of harassment and abuse, sport psychologists can and should play an important role in creating a safer sport environment for everyone involved in sport.

Both ISSP and FEPSAC have position statements related to violence in sport. ISSP (n.d.) is the oldest. It is titled "Aggression and Violence in Sport." It seems to have been written many years ago, and concerns primarily aggression as indicated in the title. It barely touches upon the problems described in this chapter. As previously mentioned, the role of the sport psychologists is important, and ISSP should therefore develop and decide upon a position statement in which the problems related to SHA in sport are much better addressed. FEPSAC (2002), on the other hand, has a position statement (# 6) on sexual exploitation in sport. With respect to what has been presented in this chapter, every paragraph is still relevant, but it could be somewhat broadened and updated based on the research that has taken place since it was written. This concerns different types of harassment and abuse, including neglect and hazing; a clearer separation between the child and adult athlete; a stronger focus on peer harassment and abuse; and the role of the sport psychologists in the prevention of the occurrence of such behavior. FEPSAC (2011) also decided upon a position statement (# 9) about ethical principles of the European Sport Psychology Federation. These are very relevant both for research on and treatment of athletes who have experienced SHA. A referral to this position statement could also be done in position statement (# 6) as previously mentioned. Together, if these positions are put into practice, that is, followed by the members of FEPSAC, the organization may be an important contributor in making sport a safer place for everyone.

REFERENCES

Active Australia (1998). Harassment free sport: guides for sports administrators, coaches, athletes and sport and recreation organizations. Canberra: Australian Sports Commission.

Alexander, K., Stafford, A., & Lewis, R. (2011). *The experience of children participation in organized sport.* Edinburgh: The University of Edinburgh.

Auweele, Y. V., Opdenacker, J., Vertommen, T., Boen, F., van Niekerk, L., Martelaer, K. D., & Cuyper, B. D. (2008). Unwanted sexual experiences in sport: perceptions and reported prevalence among Flemish female student-athletes. *International Journal of Sport and Exercise Psychology, 6,* 354–365.

Barak, A. (1997). Cross-cultural perspectives on sexual harassment. In W. T. O'Donohue (Ed.), *Sexual harassment: theory, research and treatment* (pp. 263–300). Boston: Allyn & Bacon.

Brackenridge, C. (1997). He owned me basically: women's experience of sexual abuse in sport. *International Review for the Sociology of Sport, 32,* 115–130.

Brackenridge, C. (2001). *Spoilsports: understanding and preventing sexual exploitation in sport.* London: Routledge.

Brackenridge, C. H., & Rhind, D. (2014). Child protection in sport: reflections on thirty years of science and activism. *Social Sciences, 3,* 323–340.

Brackenridge, C. H., Bishopp, D., Moussalli, S., & Tapp, J. (2008). The characteristics of sexual abuse in sport: a multidimentional scaling analysis of events described in media reports. *International Journal of Sport and Exercise Psychology, 6*(4), 385–406.

Brackenridge, C., Fasting, K., Kirby, S., Leahy, T., Parent, S., & Sand, T. S. (2010). *The place of sport in the UN study on violence against children.* Florence: UNICEF Innocenti Research Centre.

Bringer, J., Brackenridge, C., & Johnston, L. (2001). The name of the game: a review of sexual exploitation of females in sport. *Current Women's Health Reports, 1,* 225–231.

Canadian Association for the Advancement of Women and Sport (1994). *Harassment in sport: a guide to policies, procedures and resources.* Ottawa: Canadian Association for the Advancement of Women and Sport.

Cense, M. (1997). *Red card or carte blanche: risk factors for sexual harassment and sexual abuse in sport: summary, conclusions and recommendations.* Arnhem: NOC and NSF.

Cense, M., & Brackenridge, C. (2001). Temporal and developmental risk factors for sexual harassment and abuse in sport. *European Physical Education Review, 7,* 61–79.

Chroni, S., & Fasting, K. (2009). Prevalence of male sexual harassment among female sports participants in Greece. *Inquiries in Sport & Physical Education, 7,* 288–296.

Council of Europe (2000). Resolution on the prevention of sexual harassment and abuse of women, young people and children in sport (03/2000). Available from: http://www.coe.int/t/dg4/sport/resources/texts/spres00.3_en.asp.

Council of Europe (2015). Pro safe sport. Available from: http://pjp-eu.coe.int/en/web/pss.

Crooks, C., & Wolfe, D. (2007). Child abuse and neglect. In E. J. Mash, & R. A. Barkley (Eds.), *Assessment of childhood disorders* (4th ed., pp. 639–684). New York: Guilford Press.

Dansky, B., & Kilpatrick, D. (1997). Effects of sexual harassment. In W. O'Donohue (Ed.), *Sexual harassment: theory, research, and treatment* (pp. 152–174). Boston: Allyn & Bacon.

Deutsche Sportjugend im Deutschen Olympischen Sportbund. (Ed.) 2012. Prevention of sexual and gender harassment and abuse in sports: Initiatives in Europe and beyond. Available from: http://www.iss-ffm.de/m_88_dl.

Donnelly, P., Kerr, G., Heron, A., & DiCarlo, D. (2014). Protecting youth in sport: an examination of harassment policies. *International Journal of Sport Policy, 8*(1), 33–50.

Duffy, J., Wareham, S., & Walsh, M. (2004). Psychological consequences for high school students of having been sexually harassed. *Sex Roles, 50*, 811–821.

Elendu, I., & Umeakuka, O. A. (2011). Perpetrators of sexual harassment experienced by athletes in southern Nigerian universities. *South African Journal for Research in Sport Physical Education & Recreation, 33*, 53–64.

European Commission (2014). *Gender equality in sport: proposal for strategic actions 2014–2020*. Brussels: European Commission.

Fasting, K., & Brackenridge, C. (2009). Coaches, sexual harassment and education. *Sport, Education and Society, 14*(1), 21–35.

Fasting, K., & Knorre, N. (2005). *Women in sport in the Czech Republic: the experiences of female athletes*. Prague: Norwegian School of Sport Sciences and Czech Olympic Committee.

Fasting, K., Brackenridge, C., & Sundgot-Borgen, J. (2000). *Women, elite-sport and sexual harassment*. Oslo: The Norwegian Olympic and Paralympic Committee and Confederation of Sports.

Fasting, K., Brackenridge, C. H., & Walseth, K. (2002). Consequences of sexual harassment in sport for female athletes. *The Journal of Sexual Aggression, 8*, 37–48.

Fasting, K., Brackenridge, C., & Sundgot-Borgen, J. (2003). Experiences of sexual harassment and abuse among Norwegian elite female athletes and nonathletes. *Research Quarterly for Exercise and Sport, 74*, 84–97.

Fasting, K., Brackenridge, C., & Sundgot-Borgen, J. (2004). Prevalence of sexual harassment among Norwegian female elite athletes in relation to sport type. *International Review for the Sociology of Sport, 39*, 373–386.

Fasting, K., Brackenridge, C., & Walseth, K. (2007). Women athletes' personal responses to sexual harassment in sport. *Journal of Applied Sport Psychology, 19*, 419–433.

Fasting, K., Brackenridge, C., & Knorre, N. (2010). Performance level and sexual harassment prevalence among female athletes in the Czech Republic. *Women in Sport & Physical Activity Journal, 19*, 26–32.

Fasting, K., Chroni, S., Hervik, S., & Knorre, N. (2011). Sexual harassment in sport toward females in three European countries. *International Review for the Sociology of Sport, 46*, 76–89.

Fasting, K., Brackenridge, C. H., & Kjølberg, G. (2013). Using court reports to enhance knowledge of sexual abuse in sport: a Norwegian case study. *Scandinavian Sport Studies Forum, 4*, 49–67.

Fasting, K., Chroni, S., & Knorre, N. (2014). The experiences of sexual harassment in sport and education among European female sports science students. *Sport, Education and Society, 19*, 115–130.

Fejgin, N., & Hanegby, R. (2001). Gender and cultural bias in perceptions of sexual harassment in sport. *International Review for the Sociology of Sport, 36*, 459–478.

FEPSAC. 2002. Position statement #6: sexual exploitation in sport. Available from: http://www.fepsac.com/activities/position_statements/.

FEPSAC. 2011 Position statement #11: ethical principles of the European Sport Psychology Federation. Available from: http://www.fepsac.com/activities/position_statements/.

Gelfand, M. J., Fitzgerald, L. F., & Drasgow, F. (1995). The structure of sexual harassment: a confirmatory analysis across cultures and settings. *Journal of Vocational Behavior, 47*, 164–177.

Gruber, J., & Fineran, S. (2008). Comparing the impact of bullying and sexual harassment victimization on the mental and physical health of adolescents. *Sex Roles, 59*, 1–13.

Hartill, M. (2005). Sport and the sexually abused male child. *Sport, Education and Society, 10*(3), 287–304.

Hartill, M. (2009). The sexual abuse of boys in organized male sports. *Men and Masculinities, 12*, 225–249.

Holland, K. J., & Cortina, L. M. (2015). Sexual harassment: undermining the well-being of working women. In M. L. Connerly, & J. Wu (Eds.), *Handbook of well-being of working women* (pp. 83–102). London: Springer.

Huffman, D. (2014). *Gaborone 2014 2nd African youth games May 22–31: "safe games" report.* Oslo: The Norwegian Olympic and Paralympic Committee and Confederation of Sports.

Hunt, C. M., Davidson, M. J., Fielden, S. L., & Hoel, H. (2010). Reviewing sexual harassment in the workplace: an intervention model. *Personnel Review, 39*, 655–673.

International Olympic Committee (2007). *IOC adopts consensus statement on "sexual harassment and abuse in sport".* Lausanne: International Olympic Committee.

International Olympic Committee (2015). Sexual harassment and abuse in sport. Available from: http://www.olympic.org/sha.

ISSP. (n.d.). Aggression and violence in sport. An ISSP position stand. Available from: http://www.issponline.org/p_positionstands.asp?ms=3&sms=2.

Jolly, A., & Decamps, G. (2006). Les agressions sexuelles en milieu sportif: une enquête exploratoire. *Science & Motricité, 57*, 105–121.

Kerr, G., Stirling, A., & MacPherson, E. (2014). A critical examination of child protection initiatives in sport contexts. *Social Sciences, 3*, 742–757.

Kirby, S., & Greaves, L. (1996). Foul play: sexual harassment in sport. Paper presented at the Pre-Olympic Scientific Congress (pp. 11–15), Dallas.

Kirby, S. L., Greaves, L., & Hankivsky, O. (2000). *The dome of silence: sexual harassment and abuse in sport.* Halifax: Fernwood.

Koss, M. P. (1992). The underdetection of rape: a critical assessment of incidence data. *Journal of Social Issues, 48*, 61–75.

Koss, M. P. (1993). Detecting the scope of rape: a review of prevalence research methods. *Journal of Interpersonal Violence, 8*, 198–222.

Krauchek, V., & Ranson, G. (1999). Playing by the rules of the game: women's experiences and perceptions of sexual harassment in sport. *Canadian Review of Sociology & Anthropology, 36*, 585–600.

Krug, E. G., Dahlberg, L. L., Mercy, J. A., Zwi, A. B., & Lozano, R. (Eds.). (2002). *World report on violence and health.* Geneva: World Health Organization.

Leahy, T. (2010a). Sexual abuse in sport: implications for the sport psychology profession. In T. V. Ryba, R. J. Schinke, & G. Tenenbaum (Eds.), *The cultural turn in sport psychology* (pp. 315–334). Morgantown: Fitness Information Technology.

Leahy, T. (2010b). Working with adult athlete survivors of sexual abuse. In S. Hanrahan, & M. Andersen (Eds.), *Routledge handbook of applied sport psychology: A comprehensive guide for students and practitioners* (pp. 303–312). London: Routledge.

Leahy, T. (2011). Safeguarding child athletes from abuse in elite sport systems: the role of the sport psychologist. In D. Gilbourne, & M. Andersen (Eds.), *Critical essays in applied sport psychology* (pp. 251–266). Champaign: Human Kinetics.

Leahy, T., & Fasting, K. (2014). Sexual harassment and abuse in sport: Implications for health care providers. In M. Mountjoy (Ed.), *Handbook of sports medicine and science: the female athlete* (pp. 103–109). Hoboken: Wiley-Blackwell.

Leahy, T., Pretty, G., & Tenenbaum, G. (2002). Prevalence of sexual abuse in organised competitive sport in Australia. *Journal of Sexual Aggression, 8*, 16–36.

Leahy, T., Pretty, G., & Tenenbaum, G. (2004). Perpetrator methodology as a predictor of traumatic symptomatology in adult survivors of childhood sexual abuse. *Journal of Interpersonal Violence, 19*, 521–540.

Madzivire, D., Mkumbuzi, V., Nyaundi, A., Benza, R., & Mupaso, F. (2006). *Experiences of sexual harassment and abuse against Zimbabwean female athletes and non-athletes*. Harare: For Zimbabwe Olumpic committee.

Mountjoy, M., Rhind, D. J. A., Tiivas, A., & Leglise, M. (2015). Safeguarding the child athlete in sport: a review, a framework and recommendations for the IOC youth athlete development model. *British Journal of Sports Medicine*, *49*, 883–886.

Muchena, P., & Mapfuno, J. (2010). Sexual harassment among Zimbabwe elite sportswomen: a study at the Zimbabwe Tertiary Institutions Sports Union (ZITISU) Games 2012. *American Based Research Journal*, *2*(7), 95–104.

National Coaching Foundation (1995). *Code of ethics and conduct for sports coaches*. Leeds: NCF Coachwise.

Nielsen, J. T. (2001). The forbidden zone: Intimacy, sexual relations and misconduct in the relationship between coaches and athletes. *International Review for the Sociology of Sport*, *36*, 165–182.

Parent, S., & Bannon, J. (2012). Sexual harassment in sport: what about boys? *Children and Youth Services Review*, *34*, 354–359.

Parent, S., Lavoie, F., Thibodeau, M.-E., Hebert, M., & Blais, M. (2015). Sexual violence experienced in the sport context by a representative sample of Quebec adolescents. *Journal of Interpersonal Violence*, *2015*, 1–21.

Rintaugu, E. G., Kamau, J., Amusa, L. O., & Toriola, A. L. (2014). The forbidden acts: prevalence of sexual harassment among university female athletes. *African Journal for Physical Health Education, Recreation and Dance*, *20*, 974–990.

Sand, T., Fasting, K., Chroni, S., & Knorre, N. (2011). Coaching behavior: any consequences for the prevalence of sexual harassment? *International Journal of Sports Science & Coaching*, *6*, 229–242.

Shire, J., Brackenridge, C., & Fuller, M. (2000). Changing positions: the sexual politics of a women's field hockey team 1986–1996. *Women in Sport & Physical Activity Journal*, *9*, 35–64.

Stirling, A., & Kerr, G. (2009). Abused athletes' perceptions of the coach-athlete relationship. *Sport in Society*, *12*, 227–239.

Stirling, A., & Kerr, G. (2010). Sport psychology consultants as agents of child protection. *Journal of Applied Sport Psychology*, *22*, 305–319.

Timmerman, G. (2003). Sexual harassment of adolescents perpetrated by teachers and peers: an exploration of the dynamics of power, culture, and gender in secondary schools. *Sex Roles*, *48*, 231–244.

Tomlinson, A., & Yorganci, I. (1997). Male coach/female athlete relations: Gender and power relations in competitive sport. *Journal of Sport & Social Issues*, *21*, 134–155.

UNICEF. (2014). Child protection in football: what every coach needs to know. Available from: http://www.unicef.org/easterncaribbean/ECAO_Child_Protection_in_Football.pdf.

United Nations (2006). Ending violence against women: from words to action. Available from: http://www.un.org/womenwatch/daw/public/VAW_Study/VAWstudyE.pdf.

van Niekerk, R. L., & Rzygula, R. (2010). The perceptions and occurrence of sexual harassment among male student athletes with male coaches. *African Journal for Physical, Health Education, Recreation & Dance*, *16*, 49–63 (Supplement).

Volkwein, K. E., Schnell, F. I., Sherwood, D., & Livezey, A. (1997). Sexual harassment in sport: perceptions and experiences of American female student-athletes. *International Review for the Sociology of Sport*, *32*, 283–295.

Welsh, A. (2009). Sex and violence in the slasher horror film: a content analysis of gender differences in the depiction of violence. *Journal of Criminal Justice and Popular Culture*, *16*, 1–25.

Chapter 16

Theory-Based Team Diagnostics and Interventions

Jeannine Ohlert*, Christian Zepp**

*The German Research Centre for Elite Sport and Institute of Psychology, German Sport University, Cologne, Germany; **Department of Health and Social Psychology, Institute of Psychology, German Sport University, Cologne, Germany

Especially in team sports, many clubs with (semi-)professional teams spend at least one week during the preparation period for the next season with team-building interventions like constructing canoes for a team race or abandoning team members in a forest with the task to find their way back to civilization. Afterwards, everyone assures that it had had positive effects on the team, but after a few weeks of the season, the team goes back to normal, and besides some new friendships, nothing has changed.

This little example illustrates the typical way team building is done in many sports teams. One big intervention is undertaken, and the focus is "to do team building" without really thinking about what should be changed within the team. In many cases, the result is only a short-term effect on team processes (if any), and it wears out as soon as the season is in progress. In order to generate long-term effects of team-building interventions (and to save money), we argue that it is necessary to use a more systematic way of team-building interventions. We will describe a possible approach within this chapter.

In their metaanalysis on team-building interventions, Martin, Carron, and Burke (2009) examine different studies evaluating team-building interventions regarding their effectiveness. They find that not every intervention is equally successful in changing team processes, but that some interventions do not show any significant effects. For example, interventions targeting interpersonal relationships did not produce any significant results, and neither did interventions with interactive sport teams or interventions lasting less than 2 weeks. Keeping in mind these results, in order to be effective, a team intervention should meet several criteria: at first, as team functioning in general does *not* relate to one process within the team only, but to several different aspects of group dynamics, the "problem" or issue to be addressed within the team should be specified in

Sport and Exercise Psychology Research. http://dx.doi.org/10.1016/B978-0-12-803634-1.00016-9

advance as precisely as possible so that any activities can be tailored specifically to this issue. Second, as not all issues within a team are linked to team performance or team functioning, an intervention should be based on theoretical and empirical findings, which can explain why and how an intervention will generate a perceptible impact. And third, it should be kept in mind that, in most cases, it will not be possible to change group processes within a day or a week, thus the focus should be on long-term interventions that can be embedded into daily training (Martin et al., 2009).

In order to meet these criteria, we propose the following methodology when planning a team-building intervention: (1) get an overview of those group processes or team factors with theoretical and empirical relevance for team performance; (2) select valid instruments for a team diagnostics; (3) conduct the team diagnostic to detect factors that are in need of improvement; (4) based on the results of the diagnostics, select intervention methods that show empirical evidence regarding a specific effect on the respective factors, and that can easily be implemented into daily training; (5) conduct the intervention with a duration of several weeks; and (6) evaluate the effects of the intervention. In the following, we will discuss the different steps in detail.

TEAM FACTORS POSSESSING THEORETICAL AND EMPIRICAL RELEVANCE FOR TEAM PERFORMANCE

When it comes to theoretical approaches toward group processes in sport, the approach that is mostly named is the *conceptual framework for the study of sport teams* by Carron, Hausenblas, and Eys (2005). The model describes *input variables* that have an impact on *process variables*, which in turn influence the *output variables*. Input variables are the attributes of the different group members, but also the context and environment of the group, whereas group products (eg, group performance) and individual products are considered as output variables. Of greatest importance for team interventions are those aspects that according to this framework are called process variables. Carron et al. (2005) propose that the input variables first have an impact on the *group structure*. The group structure influences the *cohesion of the group* as central aspect within the process variables, and group cohesion in turn affects the *group processes*, which are directly linked to the output variables. Group structure are factors like team roles, status, or leadership structure, whereas, for example, communication, cooperation, and collective efficacy are considered as group process variables (Carron et al., 2005).

The following team factors are relevant for the performance of a sport team according to this theoretical model and supported by empirical evidence (see also, Kleinert et al., 2012): (1) motivational climate, (2) leadership structure within the team, (3) team roles, (4) team identification, (5) team identity, (6) group cohesion, (7) team communication, (8) collective efficacy, and (9) team trust.

Motivational Climate

The construct of motivational climate is based on the achievement goal theory (Ames, 1992) and is the social situation created by the coach and/or the other athletes with regard to achievement goal orientations (Duda & Balaguer, 2007). These goal orientations can be divided into two different factors, a mastery climate (also task oriented motivational climate), and/or an ego-oriented motivational climate. Within a mastery climate, the task to be performed is the goal for the athletes, so the focus is on exerting effort and improving personally in a specific task. High values of an ego climate would indicate that the focus is mostly on demonstrating superior performance compared to other athletes (Duda & Balaguer, 2007). Creating a mastery climate within a group has positive effects on performance (Balaguer, Duda, Atienza, & Mayo, 2002), but also on other group processes like peer relationships (Ommundsen, Roberts, Lemyre, & Miller, 2005).

Leadership Structure

A team always contains formal and informal team leaders (Fransen, Vanbeselaere, Cuyper, Vande Broek, & Boen (2014b); Loughead, Hardy, & Eys, 2006), thus the leadership structure of a team cannot easily be derived from the sport-specific abilities of the different athletes. Formal team leaders are often selected by the coach or by the team, whereas informal leadership develops throughout the interaction within a team (Fransen et al., 2014b). According to Fransen et al. (2014a,b), four types of informal leaders can be identified within a team: (1) the task leader is the person who takes care about the goals and the tactics of the team, (2) the motivational leader is the one who pushes the other players to give their best, (3) the social leader is responsible for good mood and positive relationships between the other players, and (4) the external leader takes care about contacts with the club, the media, and other persons or institutions outside the team.

The quality of leadership within a team affects the effectiveness of a team and helps reaching shared goals (Fransen, 2014; Glenn & Horn, 1993). Furthermore, effective leadership within a team is linked to group cohesion and motivation (Glenn & Horn, 1993).

Team Roles

Several aspects of team roles have been investigated within sport (Eys, Beauchamp, & Bray, 2006), however, role ambiguity is the aspect that is mainly considered when it comes to effects on performance. Role ambiguity describes the lack of information an athlete would need to perform his or her designated role within a team to his own satisfaction (Beauchamp, Bray, Eys, & Carron, 2002). It can constrain athletes and teams in their performance (Cunningham & Eys, 2007). Other aspects of team roles have not been proved to be directly linked to team performance, but it is widely accepted that different role aspects are important when it comes to group processes and team performance (Kleinert et al., 2012).

Team Identification

According to Tajfel (1978), relevant processes for team identification take place on a cognitive, an affective, and an evaluative level. Cognitive processes of identification relate to the perception of and comparison with a certain identity, whereas affective processes describe the emotional bonding toward a group. On the evaluative level, the relevance of belonging to a certain group is assessed. The process of team identification is always related to (1) the identification as a group, (2) the distinction from other (similar) groups, (3) the identification as an individual within the group, and (4) the personal meaning of belonging to a group. Group members who identify strongly with their team will show higher willingness to perform than members whose identification is weaker (Fielding & Hogg, 2000).

Identity

According to social identity theory (Hogg, 2006), people categorize themselves into different social categories to build their own social identity. Thus, groups like sport teams are more or less part of this identity. The underlying social categories are built from prototypical attributes of other group members. Attributes can be norms, rules, and values, but also perceptions, feelings, and behaviors (Zepp, Kleinert, & Liebscher, 2013). According to the social identity theory, it could be expected that a group identity within a sport team, which is shared by the majority of the members, will have positive influence on the team's performance, but also on other team-related constructs. Until today, no scientific studies exist in sport that aim to link team identity to team performance. Still, team identity was shown to have positive correlations with group cohesion (Carron, Colman, Wheeler, & Stevens, 2002) and effective team leading (Cremer, van Dijke, & Mayer, 2010).

Group Cohesion

Group cohesion is the central variable within the conceptual model by Carron and colleagues, and also the most investigated construct of groups (Carron et al., 2005). It is defined as "a dynamic process which is reflected in the tendency for a group to stick together and remain united in the pursuit of its instrumental objectives and/or for the satisfaction of member affective needs" (Carron, Brawley, & Widmeyer, 1998, p. 213). Even though the centrality of the construct has been challenged by other researchers (for a summary, see Birrer & Seiler, 2008), the influence of cohesion on performance in sport teams has been approved in several studies and summarized in the metaanalysis of Carron et al.

(2002b). Independent of the type of sport, the authors found a medium-sized effect on performance. Another metaanalysis by Castaño, Watts, & Tekleab (2013) comprising also studies outside sports even showed that the cohesion performance relationship is not influenced by any mediators; however, the effect sizes were lower than those found by Carron et al. Furthermore, a high level of group cohesion is associated with almost all other team factors (for a summary, see eg, Carron & Eys, 2012).

Team Communication

The communication within a team is widely accepted as an important factor for the capability of a group or team (Sullivan & Short, 2011). It has a positive influence on team performance and efficiency when team members talk openly about team-related aspects (eg, roles, tactics, relationships; Sullivan, 1993). Studies show correlations of communication with several other variables of the group structure or group processes, for example, motivational climate (Duda & Balaguer, 2007) or collective efficacy (Fransen et al., 2012). Thus, team communication can be seen as one of the central variables in sport teams.

Collective Efficacy

The shared belief in a team's ability to reach its goals despite of barriers and difficulties is called collective efficacy (Feltz & Lirgg, 2001). It is based on Bandura's concept of self-efficacy and the theory of social learning (Bandura, 1977). The influence of collective efficacy on the performance of a group was confirmed within several studies (for a meta–analysis, see Gully, Incalcaterra, Joshi, & Beubien, 2002). For example, Feltz and Lirgg (1998) found that the collective efficacy of hockey teams was able to predict team performance even better than the combined scores of self-efficacy beliefs of the individual players. Furthermore, collective efficacy correlates with other group processes, for example, group cohesion (Spink, 1990).

Team Trust

Team trust refers to the ability of the team and the single team members as well as to the meaning of the task to solve (Kleinert & Wippich, 2012), and is part of the VIST model by Hertel (2002). The VIST model was created to map motivational processes in work teams and consists of the four factors: *valence of the team goal, perceived instrumentality, perceived self-efficacy,* and *team trust.* For team performance, mainly trust between the single team members is important. Furthermore, team trust also correlates with a higher emotional bonding of team members, which subsequently reduces dropouts (Colquitt, Scott, & LePine, 2007).

SELECTING VALID INSTRUMENTS FOR TEAM DIAGNOSTICS

As outlined before, several team processes can be affected when things are not working within a team. Thus, before starting any team intervention, practitioners should know which factors are in need of improvement to be able to work with specified intervention methods. Therefore, it is useful to conduct a team diagnostics to determine factors with room for improvement. However, when selecting instruments for the diagnostics, as it is recommended to use only instruments that are carefully developed and validated. Doing diagnostics with an invalid instrument may cause more difficulties than doing no diagnostics as correct interpretation of the results are not warranted, and furthermore athletes may not acknowledge the outcomes (Kleinert et al., 2012). If no validated instrument exists for a certain area, we would rather recommend doing a diagnostic interviewing approach where the practitioner generates questions by him-/herself. In this manner, it is still possible to assess the area of interest in some way and use the sport psychologist's experience to evaluate the status quo.

However, even though the area of group dynamics is still a developing field, several validated instruments exist for the different relevant constructs. In the following, these instruments and approaches from our working experience are presented.

Motivational Climate Diagnostics

To assess a coach-created motivational climate in sport teams, two different validated methodologies exist. The commonly used instrument is a questionnaire, the PMCSQ-2 (Newton, Duda, & Yin, 2000). It is based on the achievement goal theory and consists of six first-order factors that can be summarized to two second-order factors: *ego-involving climate* and *task-involving climate*. Both factors possess good internal consistency ($\alpha = 0.87$ and 0.86, respectively), and the concurrent validity of the factors was verified as well. Still, a second, less used instrument exists for motivational climate: the observational assessment for motivational climate (BEST) by Morgan et al. (Morgan, Sproule, Weigand, & Carpenter, 2005). Its factors are based on the TARGET model by Epstein (1989; see also Harwood, "Theoretical Developments in Career Transition Research: Contributions of European Sport Psychology" in this book) and thus consists of the six categories—*task, autonomy, recognition, grouping, evaluation,* and *time,* which are components of the intervention program developed for physical education teachers (Ames, 1990). Within these categories, the observer rates the coach's behavior in different situations as ego-oriented or task-oriented. For the categories *autonomy, grouping,* and *time,* the duration of the behavior is also assessed. The system shows satisfying reliabilities, and for trained observers an inter-observer agreement of above 0.80 (Morgan et al., 2005). A validation of the BEST system for sport does not exist yet, but it shows a sufficient correlation with the factors of the PMCSQ-2 (Zepp, Ohlert, & Kleinert, 2014a).

Leadership Structure Diagnostics

Assessing the leadership structure within a team is a relatively new area of research within group dynamics. As it is rather difficult to measure leadership structure with a quantitative methodological approach, a qualitative way is mostly used to assess *who* is seen as the leader(s) by the team. The approach of Fransen et al. (2014b) uses this qualitative approach and is based on their model of leadership structure within a team (as reported earlier): The athletes first have to read the description of the four types of leaders. Afterwards, they are asked which person in the team (name of the person) has this role. It is also possible to note that no one has this role. Finally, the participants have to assess the degree of role fulfilment of the respective person on a single item. These four measures are combined by the authors to the factor *leadership quality* (Fransen et al., 2014a), which can be mapped with a CFA.

Team Roles Diagnostics

In the area of team roles, role clarity/role ambiguity is the factor that is linked to team performance. The Role Ambiguity Scale (RAS; Beauchamp et al., 2002) is the available questionnaire for this phenomenon. It consists of two parts: the offensive role and the defensive role. Within both parts of the questionnaire, the same 19 items have to be answered. They can be summarized to the four factors—*ambiguity related to the scope of responsibilities, role behavior ambiguity, role evaluation ambiguity*, and *role consequences ambiguity*. All factors provide good Cronbach alpha values from 0.79 to 0.90. A German version is also available (Zepp, Ohlert, & Kleinert, 2014b).

Based on the RAS, we also developed several interviewing questions for our team diagnostics (Zepp et al., 2014a): Within three questions, the general role clarity within the whole team, the role acceptance within the whole team, and the role fulfilment of the whole team are assessed. Two further questions are related to the role of the coach, and for youth teams also to the role of the parents. This way of measurement can be used to evaluate team roles from the perspective of the team members (each member evaluates the team as a whole, not only the own role), and thus creates a possibility to combine the different methodologies in order to get a better picture of this group aspect (see also part 3).

Team Identification Diagnostics

For the assessment of team identification, a scale was developed by Zepp and Kleinert (2015). Since identification can be divided into cognitive, affective, and evaluative categories (Tajfel, 1978), three distinct subscales were developed. Two items were used to assess *cognitive* (eg, "I see this group as part of who I am") and *evaluative* components of identification (eg, "Personally, it is very important to me to be part of this group"), respectively. To assess the *affective* category, three items were applied (eg, "I like being with my fellow team members"). In addition, two items are used as control items (eg, "Based on your feelings, how much do you identify with the other group members?"). The three factors show good Cronbach alpha values from .75 to .91.

Identity Diagnostics

Team identity can be measured via assessing the prototype of a team. The PWT ("Prototypenwahrnehmung in Teams" = perception of prototypes in teams) by Zepp et al. (2013) is a German language questionnaire that consists of 64 characteristics for the description of a team (eg, ambition, experience). The characteristics can be summarized into the five subscales—*performance, enjoyment, intelligence, distinctiveness*, and *creativity*. Cronbach alpha values for the subscales range from 0.61 for *distinctiveness* to 0.96 (the low value for *distinctiveness* can be explained from the heterogeneity of the items used in this particular factor, eg, uniqueness, dedication). The authors are currently working on an English version of the questionnaire and validating the German questionnaire.

Group Cohesion Diagnostics

The Group Environment Questionnaire (GEQ; Carron, Brawley, & Widmeyer, 2002) is the oldest and most often used questionnaire in the area of group dynamics. The questionnaire is based on the theoretical model of group cohesion by Carron et al. (1998) and assesses group cohesion via 18 items on the four factors: *individual attraction to the group–task, individual attraction to the group–social, group integration–task*, and *group integration–social*. Translations of the GEQ to other languages (Heuzé & Fontayne, 2002; Ohlert, 2012; Ohlert, Kleinknecht, & Kleinert, 2015), and adaptations to other contexts, for example, youth sport (Eys, Loughead, Bray, & Carron, 2009), children's sport (Martin, Carron, Eys, & Loughead, 2012), and older adult physical activity groups (Estabrooks & Carron, 2000; Kleinknecht, Kleinert, & Ohlert, 2014) are also available and commonly used.

Communication Diagnostics

The "Scale of Effective Communication in Team Sports 2" (SECTS-2; Sullivan & Short, 2011) is the instrument at hand when it comes to estimate team communication. The questionnaire consists of the four factors: *acceptance, positive conflict, negative conflict*, and *distinctiveness*, which show acceptable reliabilities from 0.77 to 0.81. Within two studies, the construct validity and predictive validity of the questionnaire were verified (Sullivan & Short, 2011).

Within our team diagnostics (Zepp et al., 2014a), we also created an interviewing approach as well as an observation tool targeting communication to avoid using only questionnaires for diagnostics. For the interviewing guide, the four factors from the SECTS-2 were transformed into 10 interviewing questions (eg, "Are there examples for respectful and appreciative contact between the athletes?" from the factor *acceptance*). Furthermore, five questions were added regarding a general estimation of the communication within the team (eg, "How do you estimate the communication within your team?"), and communication and handling of emotions within the team (eg, "How are emotions in your team generally expressed?").

The category system for the observation of effective communication was divided into the three factors: *verbal communication, nonverbal communication,* and *proximity.* Within the first two factors, categories were positive, negative, or neutral. Within *proximity,* we differentiated between distance and closeness. All categories had to be rated regarding their frequency during a predefined practice session or competition. Experiences from our first diagnostics showed good interrelations between the results of the two ways of measuring team communication (Zepp et al., 2014a).

Collective Efficacy Diagnostics

The Collective Efficacy Questionnaire for Sports (CEQS; Short, Sullivan, & Feltz, 2005) consists of 20 items on the five factors: *ability, unity, persistence, preparation,* and *effort.* The factors show good Cronbach alpha values from 0.81 to 0.91; construct validity has been verified (Short et al., 2005). A German version of this questionnaire, the KoWiS (Zepp, Boss, Wolf, & Kleinert, 2011) exists as well.

Team Trust Diagnostics

Team trust is being measured with a questionnaire based on the VIST-model (Hertel, 2002; Hertel, Konradt, & Orlikowski, 2004). The questionnaire consists of the three subscales: *trust in abilities, trust in integrity,* and *trust in the attitude of the coworkers.* It was constructed for the use in work teams, but can be transferred to sport teams by replacing the term "work" with "effort" (Zepp et al., 2014a). Reliability for the use in sport teams is good with Cronbach alpha values from 0.85 to 0.89.

CONDUCTING A TEAM DIAGNOSTICS

Conducting a team diagnostics is different from doing individual diagnostics in that there are several possibilities to analyze the gathered data (Dion, 2000): the most common way would be to simply aggregate the individual data from all team members and use the mean score as criterion. However, for most group constructs, theoretical models are not based on individual views but use group-level approaches, thus data analysis should also consider this different approach. Several methods of analysis are thinkable, from calculating an index of consensus (Carron et al., 2004) to using hierarchical linear modeling or conduction observations with the group as unit of observation (for an overview, see Dion, 2000).

Considering these different approaches, when doing team diagnostics, we would recommend using a triangulated design if possible. Triangulation means that different methods and viewpoints are integrated into one final result (Hackfort & Birkner, 2003). The advantage is that errors of single methods can be compensated by the different methodologies used, and different viewpoints can be integrated into one complete picture. Therefore, the repertoire should comprise sport psychological questionnaires, interviews with coaches and athletes, as well as systematic observations. These should be applied in training and competition to generate a view on all aspects influencing the team (Kleinert et al., 2012). Furthermore, various ways of analyzing the data should be used in order to meet the theoretical expectations of the referent construct. One example for a triangular approach is our "momentum TEAMdiagnostik" that has been set up for German sport teams (Zepp et al., 2014a) and that consists of diagnostics for all relevant team processes named earlier.

Some practical aspects also have to be considered when conducting a team diagnostics: First of all, as a triangular approach requires comprehensive methodological knowledge, a team diagnostics should not be conducted by a coach or other laypersons. The diagnostics itself, the data handling and analyses, as well as the interpretation of the results are complex tasks that should be executed by a trained person with a (sport-)psychological background only.

Second, coaches and teams will only accept a diagnostics if it is not time consuming and does not disturb regular training. Within our team diagnostics, we have therefore cut down the time with the coaches and the team to a minimum even though we capture all relevant constructs: After an initial discussion with the coach about his or her requests regarding the team diagnostics, the conduction of the diagnostics can be divided into four different parts. About ten days ahead, all players receive a link for an online questionnaire covering the relevant constructs that can be captured via questionnaires. Then a regular training session is observed via two video cameras; the coach has to wear a small portable microphone so it is possible to analyze all his statements. The same procedure takes place at a regular competition of the team. Lastly, interviews of about 15 minutes with the coach, the assistant coach, the team captain, the social leader, as well as two randomly selected team members are conducted. The interviews will take place before or after a regular training session. In this manner, it is possible to gather data via three different methodological approaches, but coaches will still not feel disturbed in their routines—as they stated when asked for an evaluation (Zepp et al., 2014a).

The third aspect to be considered is the duration of the analyses until the results can be delivered. Because coaches will need to have the results within a short period of time to be useful for them, it is necessary to deliver the results as soon as possible. In our experience, a period of two weeks will be accepted, but longer periods of time may lead to reduced compliance from the coach. As transcribing the interviews and analyzing the observational data will need a great amount of time, the whole process should be planned as much in advance as possible. We use a standardized, half-automated way to analyze the questionnaire data and to create the presentation for the coach to save time for the more time-consuming analyses of the interviewing and observational data. Furthermore, the results should be delivered in person, even if a self-explanatory presentation is used. Because the scientific interpretation of psychological factors differs from the common sense regarding several aspects, this is important to reduce misunderstandings.

Furthermore, when interpreting the results, it should be kept in mind that teams pass through different stages of team development. According to Tuckman and Jensen (1977), teams pass through a forming, storming, norming, and performing (and adjourning) phase during their team life cycle, and that cycle may be restarted as soon as any changes appear in the team (for example, even an injury of a core player or one person joining the team). Results of a team diagnostic should always be interpreted against the background of the stage a team is currently passing. For example, in the storming phase, a high amount of conflict and low level of group cohesion may be usual and even necessary to pass this stage quickly and enter the norming and performing stages.

Lastly, everyone doing a team diagnostics should keep in mind that sometimes just taking care about something or diagnosing a process will already lead to changes within the team regarding this phenomenon (Kleinert et al., 2012). Doing the diagnostics will certainly lead to team members talking about the diagnostics, and in this manner they probably already start discussing things that are not working well.

SELECTING EFFECTIVE INTERVENTIONS

When choosing methods for a team-building intervention, the same caution as with the diagnostics is advised: Again, it should be considered beforehand, which of the varying methods for intervention are really related to the structure or the process that needs to be improved. As intervention methods might have been created from nonresearchers without any theoretical background, it is necessary to think about the underlying structures and processes and choose practical methods that trigger (a) specific aspect(s) within these processes. Unfortunately, to our knowledge no compendium of intervention methods exists that clearly relates the different intervention methods to the theoretical constructs previously described. Thus, the practitioner has to judge by him- or herself if the method to be used is clearly associated with the aspect to be changed within the team.

Ideally, practitioners should choose those intervention methods that were evaluated to be effectively, not just for any team outcome in general, but as a specific effect on the particular aspect that was addressed, for example an intervention on team communications should first of all significantly improve the communication within the team. Currently, more than 16,000 publications are related to teambuilding and on how to conduct teambuilding interventions (Paradis & Martin, 2012). However, most of these publications lack power because of small sample sizes, (non)experimental designs and uncontrolled conditions (Martin et al., 2009). Below, we will present those studies that evaluate intervention methods using *specific* effects for the relevant construct.

Motivational Climate Interventions

Interventions to improve coach-created motivational climate focus on workshops that are conducted for coaches. Within such workshops (75–180 minutes), coaches develop behavioral guidelines based on previous research on coaching behaviors and their potential effects on team members (Smith & Smoll, 2007; Smoll, Smith, & Cumming, 2007). Two strong emphases are put on the (1) a clear distinction between positive and aversive behavioral control, as well as on (2) the conception of success as giving maximum effort, rather than focusing on winning (Smoll et al., 2007). These interventions are predominantly based on the procedures presented by Ames (1992) to create a mastery climate in classrooms. The major focus of these workshops is on the creation of a mastery climate. Interventions have shown specific positive effects on motivational climate created by the coaches (via player ratings; Smoll & Smith, 1989), as well as on athletes' performance anxiety, on training adherence and collective efficacy beliefs as important structural and process factors in sport teams (Kao & Watson, 2014; Smith & Smoll, 2007).

Leadership Structure Interventions

Specific effects from interventions on leadership structure have been successfully proven in several studies (Gifford, Davies, Tourangeau, & Lefebre, 2011; Santos, Caetano, & Tavares, 2015). Within these interventions, formal team leaders are asked to develop an action plan that involves a vision statement and goals, as well as desirable leadership behaviors (Gifford et al., 2011). Desirable leadership behaviors can be relations-oriented (eg, "I will mentor my fellow team mates by…"), change-oriented (eg, "I will reinforce this vision/ goal statement by…"), and task-oriented (eg, "I will clarify roles and expectations to fellow team members by…"). In another study by Vella, Oades, & Crowe (2013) team leaders are educated in athlete outcomes in sport, aspects of transformational leadership, and goal setting. The results of these studies show that working with the leadership structure and behavior positively affects, for example, role modeling and thus is able to reduce role ambiguity, and positive developmental experiences for athletes, potentially leading to increased performance (Vella et al., 2013).

Team Roles Interventions

In order to improve role clarity within sports teams, it is necessary that coaches unambiguously interact with their athletes, and that athletes receive constructive feedback from team members with similar roles (Mellalien & Juniper, 2006).

Moreover, role ambiguity can be reduced through interventions that give the athlete the opportunity to create an understanding about their own role from a different perspective, for example, by occupying the role of his or her opponent, as has been described as cross-training by Marks, Sabella, Burke, & Zaccaro (2002). Furthermore, communication is a strong tool that can be used to improve role clarity within sport teams. Through communication, athletes have the chance to gain more information about what is needed to successfully perform their role (Eys, Carron, Beauchamp, & Bray, 2005).

Group Cohesion Interventions

Interestingly, Carron and Spink (1993) state that group cohesion increases as soon as the group perceives itself as distinct from other groups (thus, its identity becomes clear), role clarity increases within the team, as well as interaction and communication are facilitated. Hence, high group cohesion might result from effective interventions in several other social-psychological subdomains, as has been demonstrated in a recent study by Shipherd, Basevitch, Renner, and Siwatu (2014). Nevertheless, coach-induced interaction between group members during different situations in training can be used to foster communication between participants in order to enhance group socialization, and to set distinct team goals for specific trainings. Thus, team goal-setting appears as a powerful intervention to enhance group cohesion within sport teams (Senécal, Loughead, & Bloom, 2008). Thus, it seems that there is almost no team-building activity that is able to improve group cohesion, that does not focus on other intragroup structures and processes.

Communication Interventions

Results show that sharing information and conducting open discussions of team functioning has positive effects on communication among team members on and off the pitch (Pain & Harwood, 2009). Within such interventions, athletes can be invited to share their thoughts and questions they have about the team, its structure, processes, and aims. In addition, communication can be improved by simple positive comments, mutual sharing of information, and most importantly by including all team members into the discussion. Consequently, communication improves not only among team members but also between athletes and the coach (Pain & Harwood, 2009). Deriving from other contexts, the facilitation of a regular briefing, debriefing, and problem-solving routine is also able to improve communication within groups (Christodoulidis, Papaioannou, & Digelidis, 2001). Moreover, interventions using personal-disclosure mutual-sharing (PDMS) approaches have been shown to positively influence interpersonal interaction and communication in various ways (Barker, Evans, Coffee, Slater, & McCarthy, 2014). As open communication within teams is also intensively connected to perceived trust among team members (Yukelson, 1993), it appears necessary to develop trust and communication at the same time.

Collective Efficacy Interventions

To improve collective efficacy within sport teams, imagery interventions that focused on the team can be applied (Munroe-Chandler & Hall, 2005; Shearer, Holmes, & Mellalieu, 2009). After practicing imagination for four to 13 weeks, group workshops and evaluations were conducted. They resulted in higher collective efficacy scores in athletes for both training and competition, proving that such interventions are applicable within sport teams in order to enhance collective efficacy beliefs. Furthermore, PDMS interventions focusing on athletes' best performances, building on vicarious experience information and verbal persuasion information are much likely to positively improve collective efficacy in teams (Barker et al., 2014). In addition, even interventions that strive to enhance mastery climates within sport teams positively impact on the perceived collective efficacy (Kao & Watson, 2014). Results show that athletes with higher collective efficacy beliefs are more motivated to work for the groups' goals, persist on difficulties, and are more confident in the teams' abilities (Yukelson, 1997).

Identity Interventions

One study has been identified that used PDMS interventions to affect the groups' social identity and its content (Barker et al., 2014). Within this intervention, the authors strived to enhance social identity and individual understanding and empathy in the teams' athletes by conducting workshops. The workshops consisted of speeches athletes had to hold in front of the team and a concluding reflection led by a sport psychologist. Results of this intervention program show an increase of social identity and social identity content in the team (Barker et al., 2014).

For team identification and trust among team members, no studies have been identified that specifically measured the effectiveness of an intervention on the desired construct. In one study, Pain and Harwood (2009) conducted a longitudinal intervention with a soccer team and were able to show changes in trust, cohesion, and communication on the pitch within the team. Still, they do only describe the three-step protocol of every workshop, but do not describe the explicit interventions delivered during the season, and the intervention was not focused on one single construct.

As can be summarized from the review of studies addressing the effectiveness of team-building interventions, three common flaws in research are evident: the first flaw is the absence of a clear focus of the intervention, so the aims are not stringent in a theoretical way. The second flaw is that interventions are not thoroughly described within the study, so it is impossible for practitioners to apply them. The second flaw is the use of unspecific and/or invalid outcomes as criteria, for example, not conducting quantitative analyses (Dunn & Holt, 2004) or using only general team constructs such as group cohesion as dependant variables, although the interventions focus is on specific constructs such as communication, team goals, role behavior, or social interaction (Stevens & Bloom, 2003).

Summarizing the results from the evaluation studies, it can be noted that only very few studies exist that are able to prove *specific* effects of particular interventions, and some of them are even conducted with work teams, not sport teams (Santos et al., 2015). Most studies focus on improving a team's cohesiveness by addressing variables such as communication, leadership, role ambiguity, or goal setting. Thus, theory-based research on interventions is still relatively scarce, as researchers in general focus more on fundamental research (because it is easier to produce scientifically relevant effects), whereas practitioners simply use those methods they generally use without thinking about any scientific evaluations. Thus, in cases of no existing evaluations for a construct, our recommendation would be to at least conduct a personal evaluation of the different methods and then to select the ones that will be most specific with regard to the intended effects.

CONDUCTING A TEAM INTERVENTION

Team interventions can be conducted either as one occasion for the team—for example, building a raft or finding the way through wilderness—or as a serial of small interventions during regular practice sessions. Both ways have their advantages and disadvantages. For some teams, it might be necessary to do a massive team intervention at one time to eliminate dynamics that have led to great conflicts within the team. After certain aspects are adjusted, the whole team gets back to performing. Also for a newly formed team in the norming stage, this kind of team intervention might be useful to find and stabilize roles in the team. The disadvantage of this method is that one big team event with going to some fancy place and introducing new and eventful tasks as an intervention is not helpful to ensure long-term improvement of any group dynamics. It would be against most theories of learning if one big event that is even using a task not related to daily life would result in long-term changes of group processes.

The advantage of incorporating short interventions within the regular sessions is that it will be easier for the athletes to transfer the effects from the intervention to their daily training and competitions as the tasks to complete will be more similar to the ones they are generally used to. Furthermore, in this manner, it is easier to repeat the same or similar exercises after some time to stabilize and automate the underlying processes. Thus, in the case that a team interventions is designed to optimize team dynamics in order to improve team performance, we would rather recommend providing only small units that take place before, during, or after regular training sessions, but over a longer period of time (Martin et al., 2009).

Another positive aspect of small intervention units is that they will surely not be as expensive as one big event where also travel and accommodation of the whole team have to be paid. And the last reason for integrating the optimization of group processes into daily training is that within a team, the dynamics will change repeatedly throughout a season. Besides the results and performances from the weekly competitions that will have an effect on the team, also, for example, injuries from important players or the crisis of a leader within the team are events that can completely change the roles within a team, the leadership structure, but of cause also processes like collective efficacy, group cohesion, or team trust. Thus, a long-term intervention is able to adapt to these changes and to ensure that established positive processes are being kept. Therefore, we would recommend a one-shot intervention only in the very special occasions named earlier.

Another aspect of team interventions that has to be noted is that it has been demonstrated that interventions in sport teams are more effective if only a *specific set of behaviors* is targeted, instead of focusing on broad sets of variables. For example, interventions targeting only goal setting have been found to be effective, whereas studies using a combination of interventions did not produce a significant impact (Martin et al., 2009). Thus, it should be noted that not only the method used, but also the way of introducing and leading an intervention influences the effectiveness and the thematic focus of an intervention method. Some methods may have several possible focuses and are thus suitable for several constructs. Nevertheless, it is inherently necessary to put the focus on specific behaviors and target variables to achieve more positive outcomes from interventions. Thus, it is very helpful for the practitioner to plan the introduction and guiding in detail in advance to make sure that the intended specific effect of an intervention can be assured.

When doing team interventions, it is also important to keep in mind that the reflection of the completed tasks directly after an intervention is also a part of the intervention, perhaps even the most important one. The effect of an intervention can be undermined if the participants fail to transfer the effect to daily training and competition. Of course, this transfer might also happen on an implicit way of learning, but the effect will be strengthened when the participants cognitively comprehended what the important processes and structures within the interventions were. Therefore, it is very important (1) to plan the contents and purpose of the reflection in advance, and also (2) to allow for sufficient time for the reflection so all participants have the chance to do the transfer to daily life by themselves. Lastly, if possible, an appropriate room or place for the reflection should be chosen in order to make sure that the participants can focus on the reflection and are not disturbed by other things happening around them.

EVALUATING THE INTERVENTION

In order to ensure that an intervention has been effective, it is recommended to also do an evaluation afterwards. An effect of an intervention can be evident on different levels. Kleinert and Brand (2011) use the analogy of an onion with different skins to describe the different levels of effect of an intervention: The inner skin, the *counseling level*, represents the effect of an intervention or counseling on trust and satisfaction of an athlete (or in our case: a team), this means that the primary effect of an intervention would be the satisfaction of the team with the intervention, and the trust of the team members in the practitioner. The secondary skin is the *skill level* and deals with new skills or techniques a person or team has learned during an intervention. And the third and outer skin, the *performance level*, would be the effect on well-being, processes, and performance of a team; this means the effect on important outcome variables. When evaluating an intervention, it should be kept in mind that the effect can be more or less evident on all three levels of evaluation with the inner skin being the groundwork for effects on higher levels: Only when effects on the *counseling level* are evident, changes in the *skill level* and subsequently the *performance level* are possible (Kleinert & Brand, 2011). Therefore, an evaluation ideally should include on all three levels of evaluation. A validated questionnaire that assesses the quality of sport psychological interventions based on the onion model by Kleinert and Brand (2011) is the German language QS17 (Kleinert & Ohlert, 2014), which consists of 17 items representing the three theoretical levels of the model. Every participant of an intervention is thus able to evaluate an intervention based on personal experience and opinion. However, it should be kept in mind that evaluation data is also group level data, so alternative methods of analysis should be considered (see the previous sections).

In addition to assessing the opinion of the participants, it is recommended to do a specific evaluation of the aspect(s) on focus of the intervention. This means that when an intervention was focused on team roles, an evaluation with the RAS (Beauchamp et al., 2002) would be the most useful way to make sure that role ambiguity was reduced or even eliminated within the team.

Regarding the use of objective performance results or other outcomes as evaluation of team interventions, some aspects should be kept in mind: According to the onion model of Kleinert and Brand (2011), *performance* is the outer skin of the onion and is therefore influenced not only by the things that are changing inside (like new skills or processes for the team), but also by other influencing factors from the outside, and is not as much under control of the practitioner as the two inner skins. Therefore, it might happen that despite of the best intervention, no effect on performance is visible because of changing environmental factors. And second, team processes are only one aspect among others that affect team performance, thus the objective effect may just be too small to be directly visible. Thus, in our view, objective measures can only be an optional addition for an evaluation, and a practitioner should never use these as an exclusive base for evaluation. In case of using outcome criteria, we would recommend to rather focus on improved processes and well-being than on results (Kleinert & Brand, 2011).

Besides these aspects, the question is also about the timing of the evaluation. The advantage of doing the evaluation immediately after finishing the intervention is that the effect on the counseling level and the skills level (especially on the subjective opinion of the participants regarding new skills) are probably stronger than when doing the evaluation later. On the other hand, a disadvantage might be that in general, the effect of an intervention regarding the performance factor of the onion model will only show after at least a few weeks of working with the new skills/processes, and also the skill or process itself might not be completely developed until after several weeks of practice within daily life. Thus, practitioners should be clear about the level of evaluation (counseling, skill, or performance) in focus before conducting an evaluation. In case of a long-term intervention, we would recommend doing an evaluation every three or four months, depending on the frequency of intervention units.

Last, practitioners should think about presenting the results of the evaluation to the coach and also to the team. Besides the fact that it might be an important feedback for the practitioner to discuss the results again and get additional information for improving later interventions, the feedback and discussing process might similarly be the next step of the intervention because it also has the potential to further change processes within the team.

LIMITATIONS AND PERSPECTIVES

Conducting team interventions is not a new area for practitioners; however, for researchers, theory-based team diagnostics and interventions is not a field of research with a long tradition because it is more difficult to assess and comprehend than individual processes and behavior. For this reason, limitations have to be kept in mind when working in this area. On the theoretical side, very few theories exist that assess group processes *within* teams (Hogg, 2006). Theories that are created for the field of sports are even more scarce. Thus, researchers are mostly working with adapted theories from other fields (Hertel, 2002) or with theoretical models (Carron et al., 2005) that still need to be verified completely. There is still a big need for theories on group processes, especially in sport (see McNeese, Cooke, Fedele, and Gray, Chapter 6).

Furthermore, instruments to measure different constructs, which also possess a theoretical groundwork, are only available for some group processes, thus there are still not many possibilities to generate more studies or evaluate interventions. Within the last years, more instruments were developed, but in some areas, besides some validation studies, only few findings exist. This also has an effect on evaluation studies, as it is necessary to have a theoretical foundation as well as validated instruments and theory-based intervention methods to generate evaluation studies that demonstrate specific effects. Furthermore, it appears necessary to conduct studies on the effectiveness of interventions with real sports teams, since the validity of findings from studies with (sport) teams will be higher compared to studies with students and spontaneously created groups.

Apart from that, it needs to be kept in mind that interventions may affect several team processes at once—even if focused on one process—so in addition to a specific effect there might also be more a general effect of people starting to think about group processes within their team, which in turn leads to other changes and makes controled studies very difficult. This might be one reason why many researchers stay with fundamental research and are not very willing to conduct controled, but also applied studies in the field.

Therefore, it is even more important to possess at least some basic knowledge about theories and empirical evidence in the area of group dynamics when working with teams. This chapter provides a first help for practitioners about what should be known. Especially the variety of constructs should be kept in mind and taken care of, as group dynamics are only too often reduced to just group cohesion (Birrer & Seiler, 2008). With this knowledge, practitioners should rethink their own choice of intervention methods, but also their instruction for the group beforehand and the postreflection or debriefing of the interventions, as all aspects are important when targeting a specific group construct.

Another aspect that should be considered by researchers as well as practitioners is the fact that group processes do not only happen within team in interactive sports, but also within training groups of individual and co-active sport athletes. Still, this area is rarely researched, and the focus for practitioners working in these sports is more on improvements on an individual level than on team interventions. Even if some constructs may have different emphases (like team roles or team trust), there is no reason why these processes should not play a role and be a relevant factor for performance in groups of co-acting athletes (Kleinert et al., 2012). Thus, this is still a neglected area that needs more research within the next decades.

To summarize, we propose that there is a need for theory-based team diagnostics and interventions, as the status quo is still in deficit, and effects could be increased considerably when specifying interventions and evaluating effects with validated instruments. The more value is placed on the aspects targeted here, the more it can be assured that doing team interventions is not just fun for the athletes, but also leads to long-term profit for the team.

REFERENCES

Ames, C. A. (1990). Motivation: what teachers need to know. *Teachers College Record, 91*(3), 409–421.

Ames, C. A. (1992). Achievement goals, motivational climate, and motivational processes. In: G. C. Roberts (Ed.), *Motivation in sport and exercise* (pp. 161–176). Champaign, IL: Human Kinetics.

Balaguer, I., Duda, J. L., Atienza, F. L., & Mayo, C. (2002). Situational and dispositional goals as predictors of perceptions on individual and team improvement, satisfaction and coach ratings among elite female handball teams. *Psychology of Sport and Exercise, 3*, 293–308.

Bandura, A. (1977). *Social learning theory*. New Jersey: Prentice Hall.

Barker, J. B., Evans, A. L., Coffee, P., Slater, M. J., & McCarthy, P. J. (2014). Consulting on tour: a dual-phase personal-disclosure mutual-sharing intervention and group functioning in elite youth cricket. *The Sport Psychologist, 28*(2), 186–197.

Beauchamp, M. R., Bray, S. R., Eys, M. A., & Carron, A. V. (2002). Role ambiguity, role efficacy, and role performance: multidimensional and mediational relationships within interdependent sport teams. *Group Dynamics: Theory, Research, and Practice, 6*(3), 229–242.

Birrer, D., & Seiler, R. (2008). Gruppendynamik und Teambuilding [Group dynamics and team building]. In: J. Beckmann, & M. Kellmann (Eds.), *Anwendungen der Sportpsychologie. Enzyklopaedie der Psychologie* (pp. 311–392). Goettingen: Hogrefe.

Carron, A. V., & Eys, M. A. (2012). *Group dynamics in sport* (4th ed.). Morgantown, WV: Fitness Information Technology.

Carron, A. V., & Spink, K. S. (1993). Team building in an exercise setting. *The Sport Psychologist, 7*, 8–18.

Carron, A. V., Brawley, L. R., & Widmeyer, W. N. (1998). The measurement of cohesiveness in sport groups. In: J. L. Duda (Ed.), *Advances in sport and exercise psychology measurement* (pp. 213–226). Morgantown, WV: Fitness Information Technology.

Carron, A. V., Brawley, L. R., & Widmeyer, N. W. (2002a). *The Group Environment Questionnaire: test manual.* Morgantown, WV: Fitness Information Technology.

Carron, A. V., Colman, M. M., Wheeler, J., & Stevens, D. (2002b). Cohesion and performance in sport: a meta analysis. *Journal of Sport & Exercise Psychology, 24*, 168–188.

Carron, A. V., Brawley, L. R., Bray, S. R., Eys, M. A., Dorsch, K. D., Estabrooks, P. A., . . . Terry, P. C. (2004). Using consensus as a criterion for groupness: implications for the cohesion-group success relationship. *Small Gr. Res., 35*(4), 466–491.

Carron, A. V., Hausenblas, H. A., & Eys, M. A. (2005). *Group dynamics in sport* (3rd ed.). Morgantown, WV: Fitness Information Technology.

Castaño, N., Watts, T., & Tekleab, A. G. (2013). A reexamination of the cohesion-performance relationship meta-analyses: a comprehensive approach. *Group Dynamics: Theory, Research, and Practice, 17*(4), 207–231.

Christodoulidis, T., Papaioannou, A., & Digelidis, N. (2001). Motivational climate and attitudes towards exercise in Greek senior high school: a year-long intervention. *European Journal of Sport Science, 1*(4), 228–241.

Colquitt, J. A., Scott, B. A., & LePine, J. A. (2007). Trust, trustworthiness, and trust propensity: a meta-analytic test of their unique relationships with risk taking and job performance. *Journal of Applied Psychology, 92*(4), 909–927.

Cremer, D. de, van Dijke, M., & Mayer, D. M. (2010). Cooperating when "you" and "I" are treated fairly: the moderating role of leader prototypicality. *Journal of Applied Psychology, 95*(6), 1121–1133.

Cunningham, I., & Eys, M. A. (2007). Role ambiguity and intra-team communication in interdependent sport teams. *Journal of Applied Social Psychology, 37*(10), 2220–2237.

Dion, K. R. (2000). Group cohesion: From "fields of forces" to a multidimensional construct. *Group Dynamics, 4*, 7–26.

Duda, J. L., & Balaguer, I. (2007). Coach-created motivational climate. In: S. Jowett, & D. Lavallee (Eds.), *Social psychology in sport* (pp. 117–130). Champaign, Ill.: Human Kinetics.

Dunn, J. G. H., & Holt, N. L. (2004). A qualitative investigation of a personal-disclosure mutual-sharing team building activity. *The Sport Psychologist, 18*, 363–380.

Epstein, J. (1989). Family structures and student motivation. In: C. A. Ames, & R. Ames (Eds.), *Research on motivation in education* (pp. 259–295). (Vol. 3). New York: Academic Press.

Estabrooks, P. A., & Carron, A. V. (2000). The Physical Activity Group Environment Questionnaire: an instrument for the assessment of cohesion in exercise classes. *Group Dynamics: Theory, Research, and Practice, 4*, 230–243.

Eys, M. A., Carron, A. V., Beauchamp, M. R., & Bray, S. R. (2005). Athletes' perceptions of the sources of role ambiguity. *Small Group Research*, *36*(4), 383–403.

Eys, M. A., Beauchamp, M. R., & Bray, S. R. (2006). A review of team roles in sport. In: S. Hanton, & S. D. Mellalieu (Eds.), *Literature reviews in sport psychology* (pp. 227–256). New York: Nova Science Publishers.

Eys, M. A., Loughead, T. M., Bray, S. R., & Carron, A. V. (2009). Development of a cohesion questionnaire for youth: the youth sport environment questionnaire. *Journal of Sport & Exercise Psychology*, *31*, 390–408.

Feltz, D. L., & Lirgg, C. D. (1998). Perceived team and player efficacy in hockey. *Journal of Applied Psychology*, *83*, 557–564.

Feltz, D. L., & Lirgg, C. D. (2001). Self-efficacy beliefs of athletes, teams, and coaches. In: R. N. Singer, H. A. Hausenblas, & C. M. Janelle (Eds.), *Handbook of sport psychology* (2nd ed., pp. 340–361). New York, NY: Wiley.

Fielding, K. S., & Hogg, M. A. (2000). Working hard to achieve self-defining group goals: a social identity analysis. *Zeitschrift für Sozialpsychologie*, *31*(4), 191–203.

Fransen, K. (2014). Athlete leaders as key figures for optimal team functioning. The mediating role of players' team confidence and their team confidence and their team identification (Dissertation). Doctoral School of Biomedical Sciences, Leuven.

Fransen, K., Vanbeselaere, N., Exadaktylos, V., Vande Broek, G., Cuyper, B. de, Berckmans, D., ... Boen, F. (2012). "Yes, we can!": perceptions of collective efficacy sources in volleyball. *J. Sport Sci., 30*, 641–649.

Fransen, K., Coffee, P., Vanbeselaere, N., Slater, M., Cuyper, B. de, & Boen, F. (2014a). The impact of athlete leaders on team members' team outcome confidence: a test of mediation by team identification and collective efficacy. *The Sport Psychologist*, *28*(4), 347–360.

Fransen, K., Vanbeselaere, N., Cuyper, B. de, Vande Broek, G., & Boen, F. (2014). The myth of the team captain as principal leader: extending the athlete leadership classification within sport teams. *Journal of Sports Sciences, 32*(14), 1389–1397.

Gifford, W., Davies, B., Tourangeau, A., & Lefebre, N. (2011). Developing team leadership to facilitate guideline utilization: planning and evaluating a 3-month intervention strategy. *Journal of Nursing Management*, *19*(1), 121–132.

Glenn, S. D., & Horn, T. S. (1993). Psychological and personal predictors of leadership behavior in female soccer athletes. *Journal of Applied Sport Psychology*, *5*(1), 17–34.

Gully, S. M., Incalcaterra, K. A., Joshi, A., & Beubien, J. M. (2002). A meta-analysis of team-efficacy, potency, and performance: interdependence and level of analysis as moderators of observed relationships. *Journal of Applied Psychology*, *87*, 819–832.

Hackfort, D., & Birkner, H.-A. (2003). Triangulation as a basis for diagnostic judgments. *International Journal of Sport and Exercise Psychology*, *1*(1), 82–94.

Hertel, G. (2002). Management virtueller Teams auf der Basis sozialpsychologischer Theorien: das VIST-Modell. [Managing virtual teams based on social psychological theories: the VIST model] In: F. Witte (Ed.), *Sozialpsychologie wirtschaftlicher prozesse [Social psychology of economic processes]* (pp. 172–202). Lengerich: Pabst.

Hertel, G., Konradt, U., & Orlikowski, B. (2004). Managing distance by interdependence: goal setting, task interdependence, and team-based rewards in virtual teams. *European Journal of Work and Organizational Psychology*, *13*(1), 1–28.

Heuzé, J.-P., & Fontayne, P. (2002). Questionnaire sur l'ambiance du groupe: a French-language instrument for measuring group cohesion. *Journal of Sport & Exercise Psychology*, *24*, 42–67.

Hogg, M. A. (2006). Social identity theory. In: P. Burke (Ed.), *Contemporary social psychology theories* (pp. 111–136). Stanford, CA: Stanford Social Sciences.

Kao, S.-F., & Watson, J. C. (2014). The multilevel effects of motivational climate on the collective effi- cacy in a cheerleading team. *International Journal of Sport Science and Coaching, 9*(4), 593–603.

Kleinert, J., & Brand, R. (2011). Qualitätsmanagement in der sportpsychologischen Betreuung im Leistungssport [Quality management for sport psychological counseling in elite sports]. *Zeitschrift für Sportpsychologie, 18*(2), 60–72.

Kleinert, J., & Ohlert, J. (2014). Ergebnisqualität in der sportpsychologischen Beratung und Betreuung: Konstruktion und erste Ergebnisse des Befragungsinventars QS17 [Result quality in sport psychologcial counseling and support: construction and first results of the inventory QS17]. *Zeitschrift für Sportpsychologie, 21*(1), 13–22.

Kleinert, J., & Wippich, S. (2012). Vertrauen als Merkmal von Beziehungsqualität: Modellentwick- lung und explorative Interviews im Kontext sportpsychologischer Betreuung [Trust as an aspect of relationship quality: development of a model and explorative interviews in the area of sport psychological support]. *Organisationsberatung, Supervision, Coaching, 19*, 425–441.

Kleinert, J., Ohlert, J., Carron, A. V., Eys, M. A., Feltz, D. L., Harwood, C. . . . Sulprizio, M. (2012). Group dynamics in sport: an overview and recommendations on diagnostic and intervention. *The Sport Psychologist, 26*, 412–434.

Kleinknecht, C., Kleinert, J., & Ohlert, J. (2014). Erfassung von "Kohäsion im Team von Freizeit- und Gesundheitssportgruppen" (KIT-FG) [Assessing of "Cohesion within teams of recreationary sport and health sport groups" (KIT-FG)]. *Zeitschrift für Gesundheitspsychologie, 22*(2), 68–78.

Loughead, T. M., Hardy, J., & Eys, M. A. (2006). The nature of athlete leadership. *Journal of Sport Behaviour, 29*, 142–158.

Marks, M. A., Sabella, M. J., Burke, C. S., & Zaccaro, S. J. (2002). The impact of cross-training on team effectiveness. *Journal of Applied Psychology, 87*(1), 3–13.

Martin, L. J., Carron, A. V., & Burke, S. M. (2009). Team building interventions in sport: a meta- analysis. *Sport and Exercise Psychology Review, 5*(2), 3–18.

Martin, L., Carron, A. V., Eys, M. A., & Loughead, T. M. (2012). Development of a cohesion in- ventory for children's sport teams. *Group Dynamics: Theory, Research & Practice, 16*, 68–79.

Mellalien, S. D., & Juniper, S. W. (2006). A qualitative investigation into experiences of the role episode in soccer. *The Sport Psychologist, 20*, 399–418.

Morgan, K., Sproule, J., Weigand, D., & Carpenter, P. J. (2005). A computer-based observational assessment of the teaching behaviours that influence motivational climate in physical educa- tion. *Physical Education & Sport Pedagogy, 10*(1), 83–105.

Munroe-Chandler, K. J., & Hall, C. R. (2005). Enhancing the collective efficacy of a soccer team through motivational general-mastery imagery. *Imagination, Cognition and Personality, 24*(1), 51–67.

Newton, M. L., Duda, J. L., & Yin, Z. (2000). Examination of the psychometric properties of the Perceived Motivational Climate in Sport Questionnaire-2 in a sample of female athletes. *Journal of Sports Sciences, 18*(4), 275–290.

Ohlert, J. (2012). "Kohäsionsfragebogen für Individual- und Teamsport – Leistungssport" (KIT-L) – a German-language instrument for measuring group cohesion in individual and team sports. *International Journal of Sport and Exercise Psychology, 10*(1), 39–51.

Ohlert, J., Kleinknecht, C., & Kleinert, J. (2015). Group cohesion reworded—measuring group cohesion feelings in sport. *Sportwissenschaft, 45*(3), 116–126.

Ommundsen, Y., Roberts, G. C., Lemyre, P.-N., & Miller, B. W. (2005). Peer relationships in ado- lescent competitive soccer: associations to perceived motivational climate, achievement goals and perfectionism. *Journal of Sports Science, 23*, 977–989.

Pain, M., & Harwood, C. (2009). Team building through mutual sharing and open discussion of team functioning. *The Sport Psychologist, 23*, 523–542.

Paradis, K. F., & Martin, L. J. (2012). Team building in sport: linking theory and research to practical application. *Journal of Sport Psychology in Action, 3*(3), 159–170.

Santos, J. P., Caetano, A., & Tavares, S. M. (2015). Is training leaders in functional leadership a useful tool for improving the performance of leadership functions and team effectiveness? *The Leadership Quarterly, 26*(3), 470–484.

Senécal, J., Loughead, T. M., & Bloom, G. A. (2008). A season-long team-building intervention: examining the effect of team goal setting on cohesion. *Journal of Sport and Excercise Psychology, 30*, 186–199.

Shearer, D. A., Holmes, P., & Mellalieu, S. D. (2009). Collective efficacy in sport: the future from a social neuroscience perspective. *International Review of Sport and Exercise Psychology, 2*(1), 38–53.

Shipherd, A. M., Basevitch, I., Renner, K. B., & Siwatu, K. O. (2014). Development and evaluation of a team building intervention with a US collegiate rugby team: a mixed methods approach. *Journal of Multidisciplinary Research, 6*(2), 31–48.

Short, S. E., Sullivan, P. J., & Feltz, D. L. (2005). Development and preliminary validation of the Collective Efficacy Questionnaire for Sports. *Measurement in Physical Education and Exercise Science, 9*(3), 181–202.

Smith, R. E., & Smoll, F. L. (2007). Effects of a motivational climate intervention for coaches on young athletes' sport performance anxiety. *Journal of Sport & Exercise Psychology, 29*, 39–59.

Smoll, F. L., & Smith, R. E. (1989). Leadership behaviors in sport: a theoretical model and research paradigm. *Journal of Applied Social Psycology, 19*, 1522–1551.

Smoll, F. L., Smith, R. E., & Cumming, S. P. (2007). Effects of a motivational climate intervention for coaches on changes in young athletes' achievement goal orientations. *Journal of Clinical Psychology, 1*, 23–46.

Spink, K. S. (1990). Group cohesion and collective efficacy of volleyball teams. *Journal of Sport & Exercise Psychology, 12*, 301–311.

Stevens, D. E., & Bloom, G. A. (2003). The effect of team building on cohesion. *Avante, 9*(2), 43–54.

Sullivan, P. A. (1993). Communication skills training for interactive sports. *The Sport Psychologist, 7*, 79–91.

Sullivan, P., & Short, S. (2011). Further operationalization of intra-team communication in sports: an updated version of the Scale of Effective Communication in Team Sports (SECTS2). *Journal of Applied Social Psychology, 41*(2), 471–487.

Tajfel, H. (1978). Social categorization, social identity and social comparison. In: H. Tajfel (Ed.), *European monographs in social psychology: Vol. 14. Differentiation between social groups* (pp. 61–76). London: Academic Press.

Tuckman, B. W., & Jensen, M. A. C. (1977). Stages of small-group development revisited. *Group & Organization Management, 2*(4), 419–427.

Vella, S., Oades, L., & Crowe, T. (2013). A pilot test of transformational leadership training for sports coaches: impact on the developmental experiences of adolescent athletes. *International Journal of Sports Science and Coaching, 8*(3), 513–530.

Yukelson, D. P. (1993). Communicating effectively. In: J. Williams (Ed.), *Applied sport psychology: personal growth to peak performance* (pp. 122–136). (Vol 2). Mountain View, CA: Mayfield Publishing.

Yukelson, D. P. (1997). Principles of effective team building interventions in sport: a direct services approach at Penn State University. *Journal of Applied Sport Psychology, 9*(1), 73–96.

Zepp, C., & Kleinert, J. (2015). Symmetric and complementary fit based on prototypical attributes of soccer teams. *Group Processes & Intergroup Relations, 18*, 557–572.

Zepp, C., Boss, M., Wolf, S. A., & Kleinert, J. (2011). KoWiS – Erfassung kollektiver Wirksamkeit im Sport [KoWiS – assessment of collective efficacy in sport]. In: J. Ohlert, & J. Kleinert (Eds.), *Sport vereinT. Psychologie und Bewegung in Gesellschaft [Sport unites. Psychology and exercise in the society]* (pp. 158). Hamburg: Feldhaus.

Zepp, C., Kleinert, J., & Liebscher, A. (2013). Inhalte und Strukturen prototypischer Merkmale in Fussballmannschaften [Contents and structures of prototypical aspects in football teams]. *Sportwissenschaft, 43*(4), 283–290.

Zepp, C., Ohlert, J., & Kleinert, J. (2014a). Wir brauchen gar keinen Kapitän…!" Entwicklung eines sportartübergreifenden Assessments zur sportpsychologischen Diagnostik von Sportmannschaften ["We do not need a team captain…!" Development of an assessment for the sport psychological diagnostics of sport teams independent of the type of sport]. *Leistungssport, 44*(2), 11–16.

Zepp, C., Ohlert, J., & Kleinert, J. (2014b). Übersetzung und Validierung der Role Ambiguity Scale (RAS) [Translation and validation of the Role Ambiguity Scale (RAS)]. In: R. Frank, I. Nixdorf, F. Ehrlenspiel, A. Geipel, A. Mornell, & J. Beckmann (Eds.), *Performing under pressure* (pp. 223). Hamburg: Feldhaus.

Section IV

Perspectives From Exercise Psychology

Chapter 17

Empowering and Disempowering Coaching Climates: Conceptualization, Measurement Considerations, and Intervention Implications

Joan L. Duda, Paul R. Appleton

School of Sport, Exercise and Rehabilitation Sciences, University of Birmingham, Birmingham, United Kingdom

An extensive body of research in sport psychology underscores the significance of coach behaviors to variability in athletes' sport experiences. In the case of youth sport participants specifically, the actions and attitudes of coaches are relevant to young athletes' emotional (eg, reported levels of enjoyment and anxiety), cognitive (eg, how confident they are) and behavioral (eg, likelihood of dropping out) responses and whether sport engagement holds positive or more negative implications for their health and well-being (Duda & Treasure, 2014).

Applied to the sporting context, theories of motivation [ie, achievement goal theory (AGT; Ames, 1992; Nicholls, 1989) and self-determination theory (SDT; Deci & Ryan, 1985, 2000)] have focused on the role of significant others, such as the coach, in engineering a psychological climate holding important implications for the athletes participating within this environment. This climate is understood to be comprised of what the coach does and says and how he/she structures the environment in training and competitions (Duda & Balaguer, 2007). The AGT and SDT literature identifies key dimensions of that coach-created environment (ie, which coach behaviors, perspectives, and emphases hold motivational significance) and also the motivational mechanisms via which of these dimensions of coach behavior impact upon how sport participants think, feel, and act.

In this chapter, we briefly review the major assumptions of AGT and SDT. Drawing from these two theoretical frameworks, we next present what are the

Sport and Exercise Psychology Research. http://dx.doi.org/10.1016/B978-0-12-803634-1.00017-0

373

features of the sporting environment that are deemed to be relevant to participants' motivation and functioning. A conceptualization of the coaching environment is subsequently described (Duda, 2013) which integrates both AGT- and SDT-based environmental dimensions and also incorporates the mechanisms by which the multidimensional motivational climate may impact athlete outcomes. This conceptualization particularly centers on the implications of more or less empowering and disempowering coach behaviors and communication style. In the next section, preliminary research focused on assessing empowering and disempowering motivational climates (and their interplay) in regard to athlete perceptions and objective ratings. We then turn to the evolution of and principles undergirding the *Empowering Coaching*™ training program, which aims to create healthy and adaptive motivational climates in sport via the promotion of more empowering and reduction in more disempowering coach behaviors. Finally, we highlight a coach education research trial (ie, the PAPA Project; www.projectpapa.org) involving the implementation and testing of *Empowering Coaching*™ in the case of grassroots football (soccer) across five European countries.

THE MOTIVATIONAL CLIMATE FROM AN ACHIEVEMENT GOAL THEORY PERSPECTIVE

Drawing from the major tenets of AGT (Ames, 1992; Nicholls, 1989), variability in the degree to which individuals tend to judge their competence and define success utilizing task- and/or ego-involved criteria is assumed to impact how they interpret and respond to achievement-related activities. With respect to task-involved criteria, emphasis is placed on exerting effort, experiencing improvement and/or witnessing mastery. An ego-involved conception of competence and subjective success is tied to the demonstration of superiority. In terms of the central features of the social environment, not surprisingly AGT points to the ramifications of motivational climates marked by more or less task- and/or ego-involving characteristics. Via interactions with athletes, a task-involving coach indicates that he/she places value on individuals working hard and working together to do their best (Newton, Duda, & Yin, 2000). In contrast, a strongly ego-involving coach-created climate is characterized by differential treatment of athletes based on levels of ability, and a focus on outperforming one's competitors (and perhaps even one's teammates) and punishment for mistakes (Newton et al., 2000).

There have been numerous AGT-based studies addressing the correlates of these two dimensions of the coach-created environment. Overall, the findings point to the benefits of participating in a task-involving climate for sport participants as perceptions of such an environment have corresponded with a variety of positive outcomes (eg, intrinsic motivation, positive emotions, beliefs about the value of trying hard, greater "sportsmanship" and reported use of problem-solving coping strategies; see Duda & Balaguer, 2007, for a review of earlier work). Recent studies have added to this compelling literature and have revealed perceptions of a task-involving coach-created climate to positively predict athlete engagement (Curran, Hill, Hall, & Jowett, 2015), enjoyment (Jaakkola, Ntoumanis, & Liukkonen, 2015), and team cohesion (García-Calvo et al., 2014).

Athletes' perceptions of an ego-involving atmosphere have been linked to negative or maladaptive responses (such as heightened anxiety, compromised moral functioning, and dropping out) (Duda & Balaguer, 2007). Research has revealed positive relationships between a coach-created ego-involving team environment and athletes' reporting of psychological difficulties and use of avoidance/withdrawal coping strategies (Kim, Duda, & Gano-Overway, 2011).

THE MOTIVATIONAL CLIMATE FROM A SELF-DETERMINATION THEORY PERSPECTIVE

Self-determination theory (SDT; Deci & Ryan, 1985, 2000) centers on the "why" of behavior, considering the determinants and consequences of more or less autonomous and controlled reasons for participation. A key concept within SDT is that of "basic psychological needs" (Ryan & Deci, 2000a,b; see also Ekkekakis & Zenko, Chapter 18); namely, the universal needs of competence (feeling one is effective in meeting environmental demands), autonomy (feeling authentic, acting with volition, having input), and relatedness (feeling connected with and cared for by significant others in the context at hand). SDT holds that greater need satisfaction will contribute to more autonomous striving (ie, participating in an activity because one enjoys it for it's own sake and/or personally values the benefits of the activity) and optimal functioning. Diminished or actively thwarted basic needs is linked to more controlled (eg, engaging in the activity for extrinsic rewards or out of feelings of guilt and pressure) reasons for engagement and the compromised welfare of those participants (Ryan & Deci, 2000a,b).

With respect to the prominent social contextual factors deemed relevant to need satisfaction/need thwarting, the motivation regulations underlying participation, and associated outcomes, SDT has considered the extent to which the environment created by significant others is more or less autonomy supportive and/or controlling. An autonomy supportive coach acknowledges athletes' preferences and tries to take their perspective, provides meaningful choice in training and competition and welcomes their input into decision making when and where possible (Mageau & Vallerand, 2003). A coach who is more controlling in his/her interpersonal style will tend to be pressuring, coercive, and intimidating when interacting with athletes (Bartholomew, Ntoumanis, & Thogersen-Ntoumani, 2010).

SDT also considers the impact of additional, albeit related, dimensions of the social environment, such as the level and quality of social support (or interpersonal involvement) exhibited and structure. A socially supportive coach would show he/she cares for and values each athlete, as an athlete and as a person (Mageau & Vallerand, 2003). According to Reeve and coworkers (Reeve, Jang, Carrell, Jeon, & Barch, 2004), structure is manifested when the coach clearly articulates what is expected of his or her athletes and provides clear, timely and informative feedback. It is assumed (Reeve, 2002) that structure can be provided in an autonomy supportive as well as controlling manner. Optimal engagement and more autonomous motivation in athletes would be expected in cases where a coach provides structure as well as supports their autonomy (Sierens, Vansteenkiste, Goossens, Soenens, & Dochy, 2009; Reeve, 2002).

A growing body of sport research has been supportive of the SDT assumed differential implications of autonomy supportive, controlling and socially supportive coach coaching style for athletes' need satisfaction, reasons for engagement, as well as their well-being and likelihood of continued participation (Duda & Balaguer, 2007; Ntoumanis, 2012). More autonomy and/or socially supportive coaching styles have been linked to greater need satisfaction, more autonomous motivation, enhanced interest and feelings of vitality, reduced intentions to drop out, and better sport performance (eg, Adie et al., 2012; Álvarez, Balaguer, Castillo, & Duda, 2009; Amorose & Anderson-Butcher, 2007; Gillet, Vallerand, Amoura, & Baldes, 2010; Reinboth, Duda, & Ntoumanis, 2004; Quested et al., 2013). Aligned with theoretical predictions (Reeve, 2002), recent research points to the positive implications of coach-provided structure on athletes' reported behavioral engagement and reduced disaffection in the case where such expectations and feedback are conveyed in an autonomy supportive manner (Curran, Hill, & Niemiec, 2013).

More and more studies have also begun to focus on the implications of controlling coaching for the reduced satisfaction and, indeed, active thwarting of athletes' needs to feel competent, a sense of autonomy, and respectful and caring connection within their sporting milieu (Balaguer et al., 2012; Bartholomew, Ntoumanis, Ryan, Bosch, & Thøgersen-Ntoumani, 2011; González, García-Merita, Castillo, & Balaguer, 2016). As predicted by SDT, controlling coaching have been found (either directly or via need thwarting) to correspond with negative outcomes such as burnout, negative affect, disordered eating, and lower feelings of self-worth (Balaguer et al., 2012 & Bartholomew et al., 2011).

THE CONCEPTUALIZATION OF EMPOWERING AND DISEMPOWERING COACH-CREATED CLIMATES

Recently, a conceptualization of the motivational climate integrating principles and concepts cutting across AGT and SDT was proposed by Duda (2013; see Fig. 17.1). This conceptualization holds that the motivational climate is multidimensional as well as hierarchical and could be considered more or less empowering and disempowering, depending on the most prominently emphasized psychological features. An "empowering" environment is one that is more task involving, autonomy supportive, and socially supportive. In contrast, a "disempowering" environment would be highly ego involving and controlling. As illustrated in Fig. 17.1, Duda's conceptualization also considers the mechanisms by which coaching climates can lead to differential responses in their athletes. It is assumed that more or less empowering and disempowering coach-created climates hold implications for the degree to which athletes' needs for competence,

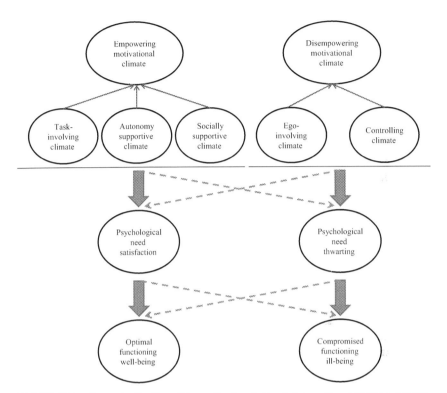

FIGURE 17.1   Conceptualization of the motivational climate integrating principles and concepts from AGT and SDT.

autonomy and relatedness are satisfied or thwarted. Pulling from Nicholls (1989) and tenets of AGT, the conception of competence embedded in this conceptualization is one that is based on task-involved criteria. When athletes' feelings of autonomy, relatedness, and task-involved competence are satisfied, positive outcomes are expected. In contrast, when the needs for autonomy, relatedness and a more mastery-grounded sense of competence are not satisfied, (or an ego-involved conception of competence is promoted) and/or especially thwarted, compromised functioning and ill-being should result.

ASSESSMENT OF EMPOWERING AND DISEMPOWERING CLIMATES

Conceptual models provide much needed guidance on what we should measure and how. It is also necessary to develop valid and reliable measurement tools to adequately test predictions emanating from our conceptual frameworks. A first challenge to furthering the application and evaluation of Duda's (2013) integrated framework, therefore, was to develop psychometrically robust (and hierarchically structured) measures of disempowering and disempowering coaching climates and their underlying dimensions. With this aim in mind, two assessments have been recently developed; one is a questionnaire assessing perceptions of the motivational climate and the other an observational tool that provides information on the objective features of the coach-created environment.

PERCEPTIONS OF EMPOWERING AND DISEMPOWERING FEATURES OF THE MOTIVATIONAL CLIMATE

Previous work that has measured the underlying dimensions of "empowering" and "disempowering" coach-created motivational climates in sport has employed multiitem questionnaires that are dispersed throughout the literature. Specifically, the 33-item Perceived Motivational Climate in Sport Questionnaire-2 (PMCSQ-2; Newton et al., 2000) or the 12-item Motivational Climate Scale in Youth Sport (MCSYS) (Smith, Cumming, & Smoll, 2008) have been used to measure task- and ego-involving dimensions, an adapted version of the 15-item or 6-item Health Care Climate Questionnaire (Williams, Grow, Freedman, Ryan, & Deci, 1996) has been employed to capture coaches' autonomy-support, the 15-item Controlling Coach Behaviors Scale (Bartholomew et al., 2010) as a measure of coaches' controlling behavior, and the 7-item Social Support Questionnaire (Sarason, Sarason, Shearin, & Pierce, 1987) has been utilized to capture coach-provided social support. In tapping all these different facets of the climate, athletes are required to respond to a lengthy list of statements that is time consuming and may be burdensome. Moreover, researchers generally use the individual climate scales (whether based on AGT and/or SDT) in combination with a battery of other instruments (eg, measuring the determinants, mediators, and potential consequences of the climate dimension), thus extending the overall length of the questionnaire. To overcome these issues as well as allowing researchers to more directly pull from Duda's (2013) model, a multidimensional scale that captures empowering and disempowering coach-created motivational climates, and that combines brevity with psychometric integrity, was clearly needed. In response, we (Appleton, Ntoumanis, Quested, Viladrich, & Duda, 2016) developed the 34-item Empowering and Disempowering Motivational Climate Questionnaire-Coach (EDMCQ-C). Using the data from 378 junior athletes, a series of confirmatory factor analyses (CFA) were initially employed to reduce the number of items required to measure the lower-order environment dimensions comprising empowering and disempowering climates from 67 to 34. A series of competing models were then tested using data from an additional 1917 junior athletes to determine the best representation of the questionnaire's factor structure. The findings revealed that bifactor exploratory structural equation modeling (ESEM) provided a better fit of the data to the hypothesized model than CFA solutions. While further work is needed to establish the psychometric properties of the EDMCQ-S, including its predictive and discriminant validity, initial evidence suggests this scale could be used to measure young athletes' perceptions of the degree to which their coach-created motivational climate is more or less empowering and disempowering.

OBSERVATIONAL ASSESSMENT OF EMPOWERING AND DISEMPOWERING FEATURES OF THE MOTIVATIONAL CLIMATE

The development of valid and reliable objective rating systems to assess motivationally relevant dimensions of coach-created environments has long been suggested as an important area for research (Duda & Balaguer, 2007). Objective data on the motivational climate created by coaches is especially important as it can be employed to address problems related to common method variance (De Meyer et al., 2014), provide information on the validity of self-reported data, and inform the development and evaluation of education programs aimed at modifying the motivational environment (Smith et al., 2015).

To date, there have been few observation systems informed by AGT or SDT to objectively capture features of the coach-created motivational climate. Research by Boyce, Gano-Overway, & Campbell (2009) represents a laudable step in assessing task- and ego-involving dimensions of the motivational climate in school sport athletes by using a novel observation checklist approach. Webster et al. (2013) developed the MPOWER observation system that specifically focuses on coaches' autonomy supportive behaviors. However, both the aforementioned systems focus on assessing the frequency of different coaching behaviors when providing a description of the degree to which the motivational climate is task and ego involving or autonomy supportive. They do not capture the quality or psychological potency of the motivational climate created by the coach, which is more in line with the perspective on the psychological environment held within AGT and SDT. Moreover, these systems do not simultaneously capture the broad range of climate dimensions proposed within Duda's (2013) hierarchical, multidimensional framework.

With these considerations in mind, Smith et al. (2015) developed the Multidimensional Motivational Climate Objective System (MMCOS). The MMCOS enables the opportunity to code and differentiate key empowering and disempowering coach-created styles. The observational rating system has a hierarchical structure whereby the coach-created motivational climate is coded according to the higher-order empowering and disempowering factors, seven lower-order dimensions (autonomy support, controlling, task involving, ego involving, relatedness support, relatedness thwarting, and structure), and 32 specific coach behavioral strategies identified within previous AGT- and SDT-based sport research (Smith et al., 2015). The MMCOS is a unique objective measure because it adopts a potency rating that captures the psychological meaning of the climate dimensions. That is, rather than simply rating the frequency of an observed coaching strategy strategy, the potency rating also considers the intensity or quality of the coach's delivery and how pervasive the environment was in terms of its motivational "meaning." After watching each clip of footage, a coder provides his/her potency rating for each of the environmental dimensions and higher-order factors on the following scale: 0 (*not at all*), 1 (*weak potency*), 2 (*moderate potency*), 3 (*strong potency*).

Initial psychometric evidence for the MMCOS provided by Smith et al. (2015) suggested coders' ratings (from three different countries; England, Greece, and France) were highly correlated and nonsignificantly different and coders' ratings reflected an adequate degree of reliability. The MMCOS (minus the ego-involving scale) demonstrated factorial validity, and predictive validity was established for a number of the lower-order environmental dimensions. Support for the MMCOS' concurrent validity has been demonstrated in research on grass-roots football coaches, revealing expected differences in the empowering and disempowering characteristics of the motivational climate manifested in training and matches (Smith, et al., in press). While more work is needed to further establish the psychometrics of this observational system and revise the tool as needed, the MMCOS provides a promising method to objectively capture the overarching empowering and disempowering features as well as the AGT- and SDT-based subdimensions (Duda, 2013) of the coach-created motivational climate.

INTERPLAY BETWEEN OBJECTIVE AND SUBJECTIVE ASSESSMENTS OF EMPOWERING AND DISEMPOWERING CLIMATES

Triangulating assessments of the motivational climate by collecting parallel data from coaches' and athletes', as well as independent observers, should provide a more comprehensive assessment of the environment (Duda, 2001a; Ntoumanis, 2012). Previous research has examined the associations between coaches', athletes', and observers' reports on discrete coaching behaviors. For example, Curtis, Smith, and Smoll (1979) used the Coaching Behavior Assessment System (CBAS; Smith, Smoll, & Hunt, 1977) and reported weak and nonsignificant relationships between coach, athlete, and observer ratings of coach behavior. An exception was for punitive dimensions of behavior where athletes', coaches', and observers' perspectives were significantly related. In another study, Boyce et al. (2009) found moderate correlations between coaches and athletes on task- and ego-involving dimensions of the environment. However, weaker relationships emerged between observers and coaches on the task-involving dimension, and observers and athletes on both the task- and ego-involving dimensions.

Smith et al. (2016) employed the MMCOS and EDMCQ-C to examine the associations between athletes', coaches', and observers' reports of empowering and disempowering climate features. With a sample of 74 grassroots football coaches and 926 athletes across 4 countries (ie, England, France, Greece, and Spain), results revealed nonsignificant associations between observed and athlete-perceived dimensions of the coach climate. In contrast, coaches' self-reported controlling behaviors were positively correlated with athletes' perceptions of their coach's controlling and ego-involving behaviors, and negatively associated with athletes' perceptions of the empowering climate dimensions.

In terms of coach and observer reports, observed autonomy support was positively correlated with coach-perceived autonomy support and relatedness support, and significantly and negatively related to coach self-reported disempowering climate dimensions. Conversely, observed disempowering features were significantly and positively correlated with coach-reported disempowering features and negatively correlated with coaches' perceptions of an empowering environment. Finally, the inclusion of the three measures of empowering and disempowering dimensions, in comparison to just an athlete self-report, provided a better fit to a model predicting athletes' autonomous motivation.

Overall, the findings reported by Smith and coworkers suggest some consistency in perceptions of empowering and disempowering features of the climate when measured from multiple sources. Importantly, the improvement in model fit when including the three sources of measurement indicates that when possible, researchers would benefit from assessing empowering and disempowering coaching climates from the perspective of athlete, coach and observer.

COACH EDUCATION TRAINING PROGRAMS DEVELOPED TO ENHANCE THE COACH-CREATED MOTIVATIONAL CLIMATE

Within the field of sport psychology, there have been continuous calls for more theory-based interventions. In the context of coach education specifically, the lack of theoretically grounded and evidence-based practice has been noted (Langan, Blake, & Lonsdale, 2013).

A number of coach education programs currently exist that pull from theory and aspire to modify the motivational climate operating in sport, and in particular youth sport. Each program has similar overarching purposes; namely, they aim to improve the sporting experience of children/adolescents and enhance their development and psychological well-being. Some intervention efforts (see Cecchini, Fernandez-Rio, Mendez-Gimenez, Cecchini, & Martins, 2014, for a recent example) have AGT as their conceptual foundation and have adopted Ames' (1992) advocation of Epstein's (1989) TARGET framework when developing strategies to promote a more task-involving sport environment. The TARGET framework considers modifying the task, authority, recognition, grouping, evaluation, and time-dependent facets of the motivational climate. Also with links to achievement goal theory is Smith and Smoll's "Mastery Approach to Coaching." The Mastery Approach to Coaching emerged from Smith and Smoll's earlier work on a cognitive-behavioral coach-based intervention entitled "Coaching Effectiveness Training" (CET) (Smith, Smoll, & Curtis, 1979). The aim of the Mastery Approach program is to help coaches promote healthy achievement in all areas of a child's life, including sports, by giving coaches specific behavioral guidelines on how they could create a more mastery-oriented climate in sport. Across a number of studies, Smith and Smoll have demonstrated the effectiveness of their intervention in fostering a task-involving sporting environment, as well as reducing children's anxiety in sport and increasing their task goal orientation (Smith, Smoll, & Cumming, 2007; Smoll, Smith, & Cumming, 2007a,b).

Specifically applied to football (soccer), Harwood (2008) designed the 5Cs (commitment, communication, concentration, control, and confidence) educational program (see Harwood, Chapter 11). This program also draws from AGT, and to a lesser extent SDT, as well as Smith and Smoll's CET. During a 5C's workshop, football coaches learn about eight coaching behavior directives, which are geared to shape their definition of success and failure, and thus potentially influence athletes' perceptions of the motivational climate. Harwood reported that, via changes in "commitment" and "communication," the 5C intervention should help coaches create a more task-involving climate that reflects a value on effort and cooperation, and was also socially supportive. In a study adopting a single-case multiple-baseline across individual designs, Harwood, Barker and Anderson (in press) delivered a training program to an academy soccer coach that sequentially focused on teaching principles relevant to each 'C'. Findings revealed that psychosocial responses of the five soccer players who were trained by this coach improved and their behaviors were more positive as self-rated and observed by the coach and their parents.

Langan, Blake, Toner, and Lonsdale (2015) determined the effect of an SDT-based coach intervention on motivation and reported burnout in the case of young athletes involved in Gaelic football. They found that the intervention delivery was both feasible and acceptable and it was possible to implement the training with fidelity. No significant effects were reported but the impacts of the training on player motivation and burnout were in the directions predicted by SDT. Cheon, Reeves, Lee, and Lee (2015) examined the longitudinal effect of an intervention designed to promote more autonomy supportive coaching (including providing structure in an autonomy supportive manner) as both coaches and their athletes prepared for a very pressure-packed and outcome-focused sporting event; namely, the 2012 Paralympic Games. In the control condition (in which the coaches did not receive the training), all the outcomes assessed were found to deteriorate over the assessment period while the levels of autonomous motivation, engagement more or less maintained. A significant effect on competitive performance was also observed as the athletes whose coaches received the training won more medals in these Olympic Games.

THE DEVELOPMENT AND PRINCIPLES OF *EMPOWERING COACHING*

The *Empowering Coaching*™ training program (see Duda, 2013, for a more detailed description) is a result of many years of research and applied work focused on the motivational climate. Initial workshop content was pulled extensively from achievement goal theory (eg, Duda, 1999, 2001b). However, as research interest began to center on connections between key constructs in AGT and SDT (eg, Duda, Chi, Newton, Walling, & Catley, 1995), the potential mediational role of psychological need satisfaction in the relationships between task- and ego-involving climates and targeted outcomes (eg, Álvarez, Balaguer, Castillo, & Duda, 2012; Reinboth & Duda, 2006; Sarrazin, Vallerand, Guillet, Pelletier,

& Cury, 2002), and the usefulness of considering both AGT and SDT-based dimensions of the environment (eg, Reinboth et al., 2004; Standage, Duda, & Ntoumanis, 2003), principles and constructs from SDT became embedded in the workshop as well. As it has evolved over time, the *Empowering Coaching*™ training programme is aligned with Duda's (2013) theoretically integrated conceptualization of the motivational climate and its effects.

Both interactive and self-reflective activities within *Empowering Coaching* training are geared toward facilitating coaches' understanding of optimal as well as more dysfunctional motivational processes and their impact on the degree to which their athletes are motivated in a quality way (ie, their sport engagement is more autonomously motivated). The workshop centers on enhancing awareness of the *what* and *why* of empowering (as well as disempowering) behaviors that they and/or other coaches exhibit. The content and embedded tasks (eg, as found in the workbook) comprising *Empowering Coaching*™ also aim to make it more likely that coaches will internalize the messages conveyed and feel more committed and competent about becoming more empowering coaches.

THE PAPA PROJECT: DELIVERING AND EVALUATING *EMPOWERING COACHING* IN YOUTH SPORT

The Promoting Adolescent Physical Activity (or PAPA Project) entailed the tailoring and delivery of the *Empowering Coaching*™ training program for grassroots football coaches. In essence, PAPA was a multiuniversity (8 in total), multi-country (namely, France, Greece, Norway, Spain, and England), multimethod (including questionnaires administered to players and coaches, observation, focus groups) and longitudinal (ie, across one season) research trial involving more than 7000 youth football players and their coaches (see Duda et al., 2013 for details on the aspects of the research protocol). Some of the coaches in this sample received the 6-hour, classroom-based version of *Empowering Coaching*™ and others did not.

Preliminary findings from the PAPA project point to the differential implications of empowering and disempowering coaching behaviors for players' emotional responses, desire to sustain their engagement, and overall health and levels of physical activity (eg, see Fenton et al., in press; Quested et al., 2013). The training program had a significant impact on the players' views regarding the motivational climate created by their coaches and their intentions to drop out (Quested et al., 2015). Four of the PAPA countries secured video footage of coach behaviors manifested in training sessions and analyzed these data with the MMCOS previously described (Smith et al., 2015). Objectively assessed empowering features of the motivational climate significantly improved from baseline (ie, at the start of the season and before the delivery of the training program in the case of the intervention coaches) through the end of the season in the case of the coaches who participated in the *Empowering Coaching*™ workshop when compared to those who did not (Tzioumakis et al., 2015).

OVERALL DISCUSSION

Coaches matter and it is important to optimize athletes' engagement in sport, to do all that we can to ensure that the environments created by coaches are as healthy and adaptive as possible. Within coach education, there is a pressing need for more theory-informed and evidence-based practice in general. Because of their significance to athletes' functioning, personal welfare and the likelihood that they will stay involved in sport, there is a particular necessity for theory-grounded training programs designed to enhance the motivational climates engineered by coaches. Over the past two decades, an impressive body of work has emerged that is grounded in contemporary theories of motivation and holds relevance for how coaches are trained and what should be the content of and approach adopted in that training. Within this chapter, we highlighted the evolution of and fundamental attributes of *Empowering Coaching*™, a training program that has at it's heart an amalgamation of tenets and constructs and research findings emanating from the achievement goal (Ames, 1992; Nicholls, 1989) and self-determination (Deci & Ryan, 1985, 2000; Ryan & Deci, 2000a,b) frameworks. Duda's (2013) theoretically integrated and hierarchical model of empowering and disempowering climates not only provides the conceptual backdrop to *Empowering Coaching*™ but it has also laid the bases for measurement development. The recently created objective and subjective assessments of the empowering and disempowering features of coaching behaviors and strategies will allow a more comprehensive examination of the motivational climates operating in different sports, at different competitive levels, and in different countries. They also will allow further implementations and refinements of *Empowering Coaching*™ to be tested, so we can see what works, what did not work as we had hoped for, and allow us to garner further evidence regarding what can be done to make the world of sport a better place.

ACKNOWLEDGMENT

The authors would like to express their gratitude to Professor Isabel Balaguer, University of Valencia, Spain, for her assistance in the preparation of this chapter.

REFERENCES

Adie, J. W., Duda, J. L., & Ntoumanis, N. (2008). Autonomy support, basic need satisfaction and the optimal functioning of adult male and female sport participants: a test of basic needs theory. *Motivation and Emotion, 32*, 189–199.

Adie, J., Duda, J. L., & Ntoumanis, N. (2012). Perceived coach autonomy support, basic need satisfaction and the well- and ill-being of elite youth soccer players: a longitudinal investigation. *Psychology of Sport and Exercise, 13*, 51–59.

Álvarez, M. S., Balaguer, I., Castillo, I., & Duda, J. L. (2009). Coach autonomy support and quality of sport engagement in young soccer players. *Spanish Journal of Psychology, 12*, 138–148.

Álvarez, M. S., Balaguer, I., Castillo, I., & Duda, J. L (2012). The coach-created motivational climate, young athletes' well-being and intentions to continue participation. *Journal of Clinical Sport Psychology, 6*, 166–179.

Ames, C. (1992). Achievement goals and adaptive motivational patterns: the role of the environment. In G. C. Roberts (Ed.), *Motivation in sport and exercise* (pp. 161–176). Champaign, IL: Human Kinetics.

Amorose, A. J., & Anderson-Butcher, D. (2007). Autonomy-supportive coaching and self-determined motivation in high school and colleague athletes: a test of self-determination theory. *Psychology of Sport and Exercise, 8*, 657–670.

Appleton, P. R., Ntoumanis, N., Quested, E., Viladrich, C., & Duda, J. L. (2016). Initial validation of the coach-created Empowering and Disempowering Motivational Climate Questionnaire (EDMCQ-C). *Psychology of Sport & Exercise, 22*, 53–65.

Balaguer, I., Gonzalez, L., Fabra, P., Castillo, I., Mercé, J., & Duda, J. L. (2012). Coaches' interpersonal style, basic psychological needs and the well- and ill-being of young soccer players: a longitudinal analysis. *Journal of Sports Sciences, 30*, 1–11.

Bartholomew, K. J., Ntoumanis, N., Ryan, R. M., Bosch, J. A., & Thøgersen-Ntoumani, C. (2011). Self-determination theory and diminished functioning: the role of interpersonal control and psychological need thwarting. *Personality and Social Psychology Bulletin, 37*, 1459–1503.

Bartholomew, K. J., Ntoumanis, N., & Thogersen-Ntoumani, C. (2010). The controlling interpersonal style in a coaching context: development and initial validation of a psychometric scale. *Journal of Sport & Exercise Psychology, 32*(2), 193–216.

Boyce, B. A., Gano-Overway, L. A., & Campbell, A. L. (2009). Perceived motivational climate's influence on goal orientations, perceived competence, and practice strategies across the athletic season. *Journal of Applied Sport Psychology, 21*, 381–394.

Cecchini, J. A., Fernandez-Rio, J., Mendez-Gimenez, A., Cecchini, C., & Martins, L. (2014). Epstein's TARGET framework and motivational climate in sport: effects of a field-based, long-term intervention program. *International Journal of Sports Science & Coaching, 9*(6).

Cheon, S. H., Reeves, J., Lee, J., & Lee, Y. (2015). Giving and receiving autonomy support in a high-stakes sport context: a field-based experiment during the 2012 London Paralympic Games. *Psychology of Sport and Exercise, 19*, 59–69.

Curran, T., Hill, A. P., Hall, H. K., & Jowett, G. E. (2015). Relationships between the coach-created motivational climate and athlete engagement in youth sport. *Journal of Sport and Exercise Psychology, 37*, 193–198.

Curran, T., Hill, A. P., & Niemiec, C. P. (2013). A conditional process model of children's behavioral engagement and behavioral disaffection in sport based on Self-Determination Theory. *Journal of Sport & Exercise Psychology, 35*, 30–43.

Curtis, B., Smith, R. E., & Smoll, F. L. (1979). Scrutinizing the skipper: a study of leadership behaviors in the dugout. *Journal of Applied Psychology, 64*, 391–400.

Deci, E. L., & Ryan, R. M. (1985). *Intrinsic motivation and self-determination in human behavior.* New York: Plenum Press.

Deci, E. L., & Ryan, R. M. (2000). The "what" and "why" of goal pursuits: human needs and the self-determination of behaviour. *Psychological Inquiry, 11*, 227–268.

De Meyer, J., Tallir, I. B., Soenens, B., Vansteenkiste, M., Aelterman, N., Van den Berghe, L., & Haerens, L. (2013). Does observed controlling teaching behavior relate to students' motivation in physical education? *Journal of Educational Psychology, 106*, 541–555.

Duda, J. L. (1999). The implications of the motivational climate in gymnastics: a review of recent research. In N. Marshall (Ed.), *The athlete wellness book*. Indianapolis, IN: USA Gymnastics Publications.

Duda, J. L. (2001a). Achievement goal research in sport: pushing the boundaries and clarifying some misunderstandings. In G. C. Roberts (Ed.), *Advances in motivation in sport and exercise*. Champaign, IL: Human Kinetics.

Duda, J. L. (2001b). The implications of the motivational climate in tennis (pp. 55–58). In M. Crespo, M. Reid, & D. Miley (Eds.), *Top tennis coaching*. London: ITF Ltd.

Duda, J. L. (2013). The conceptual and empirical foundations of Empowering Coaching™: setting the stage for the PAPA project. *International Journal of Sport and Exercise Psychology, 11*, 311–318.

Duda, J. L., & Balaguer, I. (2007). Coach-created motivational climate. In S. Jowett, & D. Lavallee (Eds.), *Social psychology in sport* (pp. 117–130). Champaign, IL: Human Kinetics.

Duda, J. L., Chi, L., Newton, M. L., Walling, M. D., & Catley, D. (1995). Task and ego orientation and intrinsic motivation in sport. *International Journal of Sport Psychology, 26*, 40–63.

Duda, J. L., Quested, E., Haug, E., Samdal, O., Wold, B., Balaguer, I., Castillo, I., Sarrazin, P., Papaioannou, A., Ronglan, L. T., Hall, H., & Cruz, J. (2013). Promoting adolescent health through an intervention aimed at improving the quality of their participation in physical activity ('PAPA'): background to the project and main trial protocol. *International Journal of Sport and Exercise Psychology, 11*(4), 319–327.

Duda, J. L., & Treasure, D. C. (2014). The motivational climate, athlete motivation, and implications for the quality of sport engagement. In J. M. Williams, & V. Krane (Eds.), *Applied sport psychology: personal growth to peak performance* (7th ed.). McGraw-Hill Higher Education.

Epstein, J. (1989). Family structures and students' motivation: a developmental perspective. In C. Ames, & R. Ames (Eds.), *Research on motivation in education Vol. 3 Goals and cognitions* (pp. 259–295). New York: Academic Press.

Fenton, S.A.M., Duda, J.L, Appleton, P.R., & Barrett, T.G. (in press). Empowering youth sport environments: implications for daily moderate-to-vigorous physical activity and adiposity. *Journal of Sport and Health Sciences*.

García-Calvo, T., Leo, F. M., Sanchez-Miguel, P. A., Gonzalez-Ponce, I., Mouratidis, A., & Ntoumanis, N. (2014). Multilevel analysis of perceived coach and peer motivational climate, cohesion, player satisfaction and role in semi-professional soccer teams. *Journal of Sport Sciences, 32*, 1738–1750.

Gillet, N., Vallerand, R. J., Amoura, S., & Baldes, B. (2010). Influence of coaches' autonomy support on athletes' motivation and sport performance: a test of the hierarchical model of intrinsic and extrinsic motivation. *Psychology of Sport and Exercise, 11*, 155–161.

González, L., García-Merita, M., Castillo, I., & Balaguer, I. (2016). Young athletes' perceptions of coach behaviors and their implications on their well- and ill-being over time. *Journal of Strength and Conditioning Research, 30*(4), 1147–1154.

Harwood, C. G. (2008). Developmental consulting in a professional soccer academy: the 5C's coaching efficacy program. *The Sport Psychologist, 22*, 109–133.

Harwood, C.G., Barker, J., & Anderson, R.J. (in press). Psychosocial development in youth soccer players: assessing the effectiveness of the 5C's intervention programme. *The Sport Psychologist*.

Jaakkola, T., Ntoumanis, N., & Liukkonen, J. (2015). Motivational climate, goal. orientation, perceived sport ability, and enjoyment within Finnish junior ice-hockey players. *Scandinavian Journal of Medicine and Science in Sports, 26*, 109–115.

Kim, M. S., Duda, J. L., & Gano-Overway, L. (2011). Predicting occurrence of and responses to psychological difficulties: the interplay between achievement goals, perceived ability, and motivational climates among Korean athletes. *International Journal of Sport and Exercise Psychology, 9*, 31–47.

Langan, E., Blake, C., & Lonsdale, C. (2013). Systematic review of the effectiveness of interpersonal coach education interventions on athlete outcomes. *Psychology of Sport and Exercise, 14*, 37–49.

Langan, E., Blake, C., Toner, J., & Lonsdale, C. (2015). Testing the effects of a self-determination theory-based intervention with youth Gaelic football coaches on athlete motivation and burnout. *The Sport Psychologist*, 29, 293–301.

Mageau, G. A., & Vallerand, R. J. (2003). The coach-athlete relationship: a motivational model. *Journal of Sports Sciences*, 21(11), 883–904.

Newton, M., Duda, J. L., & Yin, Z. N. (2000). Examination of the psychometric properties of the Perceived Motivational Climate in Sport Questionnaire-2 in a sample of female athletes. *Journal of Sports Sciences*, 18(4), 275–290.

Nicholls, J. G. (1989). *The competitive ethos and democratic education*. Cambridge, MA: Harvard University Press.

Ntoumanis, N. (2012). A self-determination theory perspective on motivation in sport and physical education: current trends and possible future research directions. In G. C. Roberts, & D. C. Treasure (Eds.), *Motivation in sport and exercise* (3rd ed., pp. 91–128). Champaign, IL: Human Kinetics.

Quested, E.J., Appleton, P.R., Wold, B., Balaguer. I., Sarrazin, P., Papaioannou, A., Hall, H.K., Ommundsen, Y., & Cruz, J. (2015). The impact of the Empowering Coaching training programme on the motivational climate and player responses. *14th FEPSAC congress*. Bern, Switzerland.

Quested, E., Duda, J. L., Ntoumanis, N., Viladrich, C., Haug, E., Ommundsen, Y., Van Hoye, A., Merce, J., Hall, H. L., & Zourbanos, N. (2013). Intentions to drop-out of youth soccer: a test of the basic needs theory amount European youth from five countries. *International Journal of Sport and Exercise Psychology*, 11, 395–407.

Reinboth, M., & Duda, J. L. (2006). Perceived motivational climate, need satisfaction and indices of well-being in team sports: a longitudinal perspective. *Psychology of Sport and Exercise*, 7(3), 269–286.

Reinboth, M., Duda, J. L., & Ntoumanis, N. (2004). Dimensions of coaching behavior, need satisfaction, and the psychological and physical welfare of young athletes. *Motivation and Emotion*, 28, 297–313.

Reeve, J. (2002). Self-determination theory applied to educational settings. In E. L. Deci, & R. M. Ryan's (Eds.), *Handbook of self-determination research* (pp. 183–202). Rochester, NY: Rochester University Press.

Reeve, J., Jang, H., Carrell, D., Jeon, S., & Barch, J. (2004). Enhancing high school students' engagement by increasing their teachers' autonomy support. *Motivation and Emotion*, 28, 147–169.

Ryan, R. M., & Deci, E. L. (2000a). Self-determination theory and the facilitation of intrinsic motivation, social development, and well-being. *American Psychologist*, 55, 68–78.

Ryan, R. M., & Deci, E. L. (2000b). The darker and brighter sides of human existence: basic psychological needs as a unifying concept. *Psychological Inquiry*, 11, 319–338.

Sarason, I. G., Sarason, B. R., Shearin, E. N., & Pierce, G. R. (1987). A brief measure of social support: practical and theoretical implications. *Journal of Social and Personal Relationships*, 4, 497–510.

Sarrazin, P., Vallerand, R., Guillet, E., Pelletier, L., & Cury, F. (2002). Motivation and dropout in female handballers: a 21-month prospective study. *European Journal of Social Psychology*, 32(3), 395–418.

Sierens, E., Vansteenkiste, M., Goossens, L., Soenens, B., & Dochy, F. (2009). The synergistic relationship of perceived autonomy support and structure in the prediction of self-regulated learning. *British Journal of Educational Psychology*, 79, 57–68.

Smith, N., Quested, E., Appleton, P., & Duda, J.L. (in press). Observing the coach-created motivational environment across training and competition in youth sport. *Journal of Sport Sciences*.

Smith, N., Tessier, D., Tzioumakis, Y., Fabra, P., Quested, E., Appleton, P. R., Sarrazin, P., Papaioannou, A., Balaguer, I., & Duda, J. L. (2016). The relationship between observed and perceived assessments of the coach- created motivational environment and links to athlete motivation. *Psychology of Sport and Exercise*, 23, 51–63.

Smith, N., Tessier, D., Tzioumakis, Y., Quested, E., Appleton, P., Sarrazin, P., Papaioannou, A., & Duda, J. L. (2015a). Development and validation of the Multidimensional Motivational Climate Observation System (MMCOS). *Journal of Sport and Exercise Psychology*, *37*, 4–22.

Smith, R. E., Cumming, S. P., & Smoll, F. L. (2008). Development and validation of the Motivational Climate Scale for Youth Sports. *Journal of Applied Sport Psychology*, *20*, 116–136.

Smith, R. E., Smoll, F. L., & Cumming, S. P. (2007). Effects of a motivational climate intervention for coaches on young athletes' sport performance anxiety. *Journal of Sport & Exercise Psychology*, *29*, 39–59.

Smith, R. E., Smoll, F. L., & Curtis, B. (1979). Coach effectiveness training: a cognitive behavioral approach to enhancing relationship skills in youth sport coaches. *Journal of Sport Psychology*, *1*, 59–75.

Smith, R. E., Smoll, F. L., & Hunt, E. (1977). System for behavioral-assessment of athletic coaches. *Research Quarterly*, *48*, 401–407.

Smoll, F. L., Smith, R. E., & Cumming, S. P. (2007a). Effects of coach and parent training on performance anxiety in young athletes: a systemic approach. *Journal of Youth Development*, *2*.

Smoll, F. L., Smith, R. E., & Cumming, S. P. (2007b). Effects of a motivational climate intervention for coaches on changes in young athletes' achievement goal orientations. *Journal of Clinical Sport Psychology*, *1*, 23–46.

Standage, M., Duda, J. L., & Ntoumanis, N. (2003). A model of contextual motivation in physical education: an integration of self-determination and goal perspective theories in predicting leisure-time exercise intentions. *Journal of Educational Psychology*, *95*, 97–110.

The PAPA Project (n.d.). Available from: http://www.projectpapa.org

Tzioumakis, Y., Smith, N., Tessier, D., Fabra, P., Balaguer, I., Papaioannou, A., Digelidis, N., Sarrazin, P., Quested, E., & Duda, J.L. (2015). Longitudinal effects of the *Empowering Coaching*™ programme on the observed coach behaviours in grassroots football across four European countries. *Annual Meeting of the International Society of Behavioural Nutrition and Physical Activity*, Edinburgh, Scotland (June 3–6, 2015).

Webster, C. A., Wellborn, B., Hunt, K., LaFleche, M., Cribbs, J., & Lineberger, B. (2013). MPOWER: an observation system for assessing coach autonomy support in high school varsity boys' soccer practices. *International Journal of Sports Science & Coaching*, *8*, 741–754.

Williams, G. C., Grow, V., Freedman, Z., Ryan, R. M., & Deci, E. L. (1996). Motivational predictors of weight loss and weight loss maintenance. *Journal of Personality and Social Psychology*, *70*(1), 115–126.

Chapter 18

Escape From Cognitivism: Exercise as Hedonic Experience

Panteleimon Ekkekakis, Zachary Zenko

Department of Kinesiology, Iowa State University, Ames, IA, United States

Several intriguing opinions on the psychology of exercise and physical activity can be found in the writings of the ancient Greeks (Ekkekakis, Hargreaves, & Parfitt, 2013) and other ancient texts. Reflections on human thoughts and feelings about exercise, some even remarkably detailed and insightful, also feature prominently in the writings of some of the fathers of modern psychology in the 19th century, including Alexander Bain, James Mark Baldwin, and William James (Ekkekakis, 2013). Occasional articles about a postulated role of exercise and physical activity in mental health, written by passionate physical educators and physicians, appeared during most of the 20th century, albeit basing rather bold claims on mere conjectures. Thus, by most accounts, the "dawn" of contemporary exercise psychology as a scientific field is conventionally demarcated by a series of preliminary investigations by William P. Morgan in the late 1960s, focusing on the relationships between exercise, physical fitness, and mental health (Dishman & O'Connor, 2005). This means that exercise psychology as a field of scientific inquiry is now approaching its first half-century mark. Although still very young, exercise psychology has seen rapid growth over these past decades (also see Chapter 3). This growth has been propelled by the widening recognition of the health benefits of physical activity and exercise and, at the same time, the intensifying need to increase the percentage of the population in Western countries who partake in these activities at levels sufficient to yield meaningful benefits. There are now several textbooks devoted exclusively to exercise psychology, some even in their third or fourth edition. Research articles related to exercise psychology are routinely published in a broad range of esteemed scientific journals, spanning the fields of clinical, preventive, and behavioral medicine, nursing, public health, gerontology, psychophysiology,

Sport and Exercise Psychology Research. http://dx.doi.org/10.1016/B978-0-12-803634-1.00018-2

and neuroscience. The publications of several highly successful researchers in exercise psychology have reached tens of thousands of citations. Some research teams manage multimillion-dollar grants. In several countries, young exercise psychologists beginning their academic careers in major research institutions are expected to procure extramural funding within a fiercely competitive environment, design and conduct large randomized controlled trials, and publish their findings in some of the most prestigious and selective journals in the world. Therefore, by conventional academic metrics, an appraisal of exercise psychology could lead to the conclusion that it is a dynamic, highly prolific, and rapidly growing field of scientific research. On the other hand, a skeptic could argue that an appraisal of the progress of the field should not be limited to academic metrics but must also encompass the crucial question of societal relevance and impact. Specifically, it would be reasonable to ask in what way exercise psychology research has improved the lives of people around the globe. This is not an unfair or unrealistic question. Other subdisciplines of exercise science (or "kinesiology"), despite having histories not much longer than that of exercise psychology, have already produced knowledge that has resulted in changes to practice norms on a global scale. For example, research from biomechanics has taught people to "bend their knees" when lifting heavy objects, thus reducing the rate of back strain injuries. Likewise, research in motor control has transformed several areas of clinical practice, ranging from stroke rehabilitation to the training of surgeons in eye-hand coordination. Research in exercise physiology has demonstrated that regular moderate-intensity exercise is not only safe but highly beneficial for individuals who have suffered a myocardial infarction (eg, exercise stimulates myocardial revascularization, improves contractility, enhances vasodilation, attenuates inflammation, and promotes fibrinolysis and thrombolysis). As a result, exercise-based cardiac rehabilitation has become the global standard of care for postinfarct patients.

One of the primary goals of exercise psychology is to initially understand and ultimately develop methods to influence the psychological processes involved in the decision to engage in, adhere to, and sustain long-term participation in physical activity or exercise. A second major goal is to evaluate and advance the application of physical activity and/or exercise in the promotion of mental health and well-being. A critical examination of practice norms at the societal level does not yield indications that research from exercise psychology has had a broad, meaningful influence. At schools, the practice of physical education still appears, by and large, unaltered and unaffected by developments in exercise psychology. At most schools in the United States, for example, children are still subjected to mandatory testing of their physical fitness (which is strongly influenced by genetics; eg, Maes et al., 1996), commonly resulting in deep-seated and lasting feelings of incompetence and embarrassment (eg, Hopple & Graham, 1995). Gymnasia and fitness facilities still feature wall-to-wall mirrors and typically employ staff members with exceptionally athletic bodies, thus exacerbating feelings of social physique anxiety among many of their clients. Although the managers of such facilities are greatly concerned about client retention, there is no indication that the fitness industry has considered the use of psychological interventions a worthwhile business investment. Despite evolving into highly sophisticated and laborious processes, the development of exercise prescription guidelines and physical activity recommendations still proceeds without direct input from exercise psychology theory and research. It seems reasonable to suggest that, after its first half century, establishing its societal relevance should be an important, if not urgent, goal for exercise psychology. This goal entails advancing basic research to the point that it can support translational research and, in turn, producing interventions of sufficiently demonstrated efficacy, effectiveness, and cost-effectiveness to support large-scale application.

SOCIETAL IMPACT: WHAT IS OUR TRACK RECORD?

Fig. 18.1 displays the results of an *ad hoc* meta-meta-analysis, synthesizing the pooled effect sizes from 18 meta-analyses from physical activity promotion trials. As can be seen, most pooled effects are "small," approximating one-fifth to one-fourth of a standard deviation. While this observation may be interpreted optimistically (ie, "better than nothing"), a more critical perspective suggests that these figures should be considered in the context of the following four caveats. First, the participants in all of the trials were volunteers, thus introducing a substantial self-selection bias. Second, in nearly all of the trials, physical activity was assessed by self-report rather than objective measures, thus introducing the possibility of expectancy bias inflating the reports of the intervention groups relative to the control groups. Third, few of the available trials involved truly randomized designs and most of the 18 meta-analyses included both experimental and preexperimental studies. Fourth, most assessments of methodological quality have concluded that the trials are characterized by "moderate" or "high" risk of bias. Each of these caveats likely led to an inflation of the reported effect sizes.

Given these research outcomes, it is unsurprising that participation rates at the population level remain low. What is perhaps surprising is *how low* these rates are. In the United States, the 2003–04 National Health and Nutrition Examination Survey found that, based on self-reports, 51% of the adult population accumulated 150 min per week of at least moderate-intensity physical activity in bouts of at least 10 min. At the same time, however, the figures based on objective measures (ie, accelerometers) were 3.5% for those 20–59 years of age and 2.4% for those 60 years or older (Troiano et al., 2008). When only activity performed in bouts of at least 10 min was considered, 93.5% of individuals were found to be inactive. More than half (56.1%) averaged approximately 0 min of moderate-to-vigorous activity per day. On 91.1% of days, participants averaged less than 1 min of vigorous-intensity activity. Fewer than 1% of adults registered 20 min of vigorous-intensity activity on at least 3 days per week

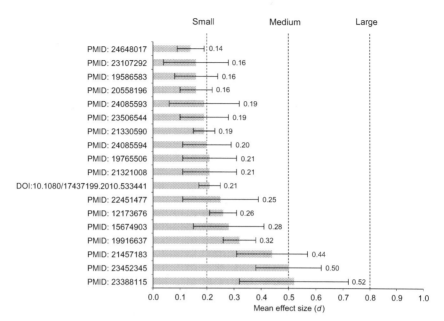

FIGURE 18.1   Summary of pooled effect sizes from 18 meta-analyses of intervention trials with physical activity as the outcome variable. Most effects are "small" and the overall average is $d = 0.26$, 95% CI 0.21–0.31. PMID is the record number of the respective meta-analysis in PubMed (http://www.pubmed.gov). DOI is the Digital Object Identifier (http://www.doi.org).

(Metzger et al., 2008). In Canada, based on self-reports collected in 2007, it was estimated that 65% of adults did at least the minimum recommended amount of activity (Bryan & Katzmarzyk, 2009). However, based on data collected with accelerometers between 2007 and 2009, it was found that 4.8% did at least 30 min of moderate-to-vigorous physical activity, accumulated in bouts of at least 10 min, on at least 5 days per week and 15.4% did at least 150 min per week of moderate-to-vigorous physical activity accumulated in bouts of at least 10 min (Colley et al., 2011). Similarly, according to the Health Survey for England, in 2008, based on self-reports, 39% of men and 29% of women aged 16 and over met the public-health recommendations for physical activity. At the same time, the percentages of those meeting the recommendation based on accelerometry data were only 6 and 4%, respectively (National Health Service Information Centre, Lifestyle Statistics, 2012).

The severity of the problem of physical inactivity is even more pronounced among medically vulnerable populations, such as adults with obesity, who could benefit greatly from higher levels of activity. Objective measurements in the United States show that fewer than 2% of adults with obesity are physically active at the level recommended for health promotion (Tudor-Locke, Brashear, Johnson, & Katzmarzyk, 2010). Women with obesity, in particular, show levels of noncompliance with the recommendations that are unmatched in the domain of public health. According to data from a nationally representative sample of 680 women with obesity from the 2005–2006 NHANES, fewer than 1.5% averaged 30 min of moderate-to-vigorous physical activity per day (Tudor-Locke et al., 2010). Based on the same data set, women with obesity performed, on average, only 13.8 min of moderate and 10.8 s of vigorous-intensity physical activity per day (Archer et al., 2013). Taken together, the data reviewed in this section suggest that the problem of physical inactivity remains poorly understood and resistant to intervention approaches that have been tried thus far.

WHY ARE WE FAILING? PERFECTING THE ART OF PEEKING AT THE UNIVERSE THROUGH A KEYHOLE

The main responses to criticisms about the slow rate of progress of the field of exercise psychology in delivering effective interventions are that (1) human behavior is complex and notoriously difficult to change, and (2) despite its importance, physical activity promotion has not received enough funding for research and implementation programs. While both arguments are valid, it should be pointed out that several of the "great public health achievements" recognized by the Centers for Disease Control and Prevention resulted from widespread changes in human behavior, some of them (such as the lowering of the rates of cigarette smoking and the increased use of condoms to prevent the spread of HIV) against considerable resistance (Koppaka, 2011). Moreover, while physical activity indeed receives less funding and fewer resources compared to certain other problematic health behaviors, there is no shortage of high-profile advocacy initiatives and social marketing campaigns (Kohl et al., 2012; Matheson et al., 2013; Trost, Blair, & Khan, 2014). So, why is the promotion of physical activity classified as one of the "catastrophic failures of public health" (Anonymous, 2004)?

This is a multifaceted and immensely complex problem. There can be little doubt, for example, that the layout of modern cities or the persistent unwillingness of traditionally trained medical professionals to recommend physical activity to their patients are partial contributors. Many such factors are outside the purview of exercise psychology. So, the emphasis here is on the theoretical frameworks that the field of exercise psychology has chosen to utilize and the intervention approaches it has developed and tested.

Even a cursory analysis of the research literature reveals that exercise psychology has been trying to understand and change physical activity and exercise behavior through a very small set of theories (see Fig. 18.2). As several theorists have pointed out over the years, these theories overlap to a great extent despite the use of different terms to describe the common constructs (Bandura, 2004; Maddux, 1993; Weinstein, 1993). Importantly, the constructs in question are all cognitive appraisals, thus typically sharing considerable common variance. What is my *perception* of threat? What is my *perceived* possible benefit from initiating the healthy behavior or the cost from neglecting it? What is the *perceived* confidence in my ability to carry out the recommended behavior? What are the *perceived*

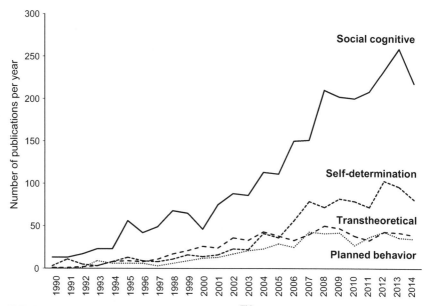

FIGURE 18.2   Number of entries in the PsycINFO™ database combining the terms "exercise" or "physical activity" with keywords associated with the Social Cognitive Theory, the Theory of Planned Behavior, the Transtheoretical Model, and Self-Determination Theory in the title or abstract (1990–2014).

expectations or likely support of important others? Recognizing that existing theories leave most behavioral variation unaccounted, researchers have recently proposed that, to advance the present understanding and possibly improve the quality of interventions, the best path forward would be the development of eclectic amalgamations of cognitive constructs (Hagger & Chatzisarantis, 2014).

What has been strikingly absent from the exercise psychology literature is any discourse at the level of metatheory. As a consequence, the field has not yet confronted the fact that all of its current theories are products of the same metatheoretical perspective, namely of the cognitivist paradigm that has dominated psychological thought since the middle of the twentieth century. Associated with the failure to confront this fact is the failure to consider and debate some of the fundamental assumptions underpinning the cognitivist perspective on human behavior. It is important, for example, to remember that cognitivist theories were inspired by the mind-as-computer analogy. As part of this legacy, cognitivist theories assume that the input is always information (such as the probability of future events), the workings of the mind can be modeled as computer algorithms that process this information, and, based on specific decision rules, produce behavioral decisions (Fig. 18.3). The theories also assume that, as in a computer software program, the algorithms that intervene between the data input and the behavioral output consist of logical and predictable cause-and-effect calculations, the goal of which is to select the option that optimally serves the self-interest of

Euclid's algorithm for the greatest common divisor of two numbers

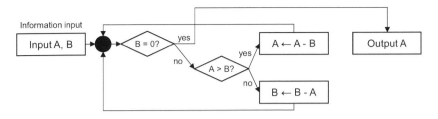

Bandura's algorithm for behavior

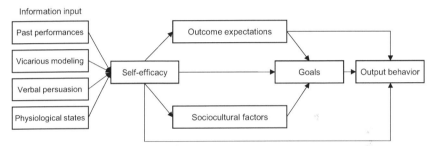

FIGURE 18.3   Illustration of the influence of computer analogies of the human mind on cognitivist models of behavior. Models are conceptualized as data-processing algorithms, with information as input, (rational) calculations within a central processing unit, and behavior as output.

the individual. These assumptions imply that human beings possess the capacity to collect and retain all pertinent information, that their behaviors result from the informational input in a rational and predictable manner, and that there is no alternative pathway that determines behavior besides the theorized (algorithmic and data-bound) cognitive processes. A further implication is that, if the behavioral output is undesirable (ie, suboptimal in promoting self-interest), this can be corrected by feeding the system with additional, more accurate, or more compelling data. In other words, the theories assume that, to change physical activity and/or exercise behavior (or any type of behavior for that matter), more information should be provided and subjected to rational cognitive evaluation.

Given that these assumptions form the conceptual foundation of all cognitivist theories presently in vogue within the field of exercise psychology, the fact that their soundness has yet to be debated is surprising. For example, within the *Theory of Reasoned Action* and the subsequent *Theory of Planned Behavior*, the reliance of behavior on the informational input and rational processing is explicit:

> *The totality of a person's beliefs serves as the informational base that ultimately determines his attitudes, intentions, and behaviors. Our approach thus views man as an essentially rational organism, who uses the information at his disposal*

to make judgments, to form evaluations, and arrive at decisions. (Fishbein &
Ajzen, 1975, p. 14, sexist language retained from the original)

Indeed, the assumption of rationality is one of the most fundamental assumptions of these theories. They are both based on the central premise that "people's behavioral intentions are assumed to follow reasonably from their beliefs about performing the behavior" (Ajzen & Fishbein, 2005, p. 193) and "human behavior can be described as reasoned" (p. 203). If the resultant behavior appears irrational, the theories attribute the apparent failure to the poor informational input, which led to the formation of "inaccurate, biased, or even irrational" beliefs (p. 193). Once beliefs have formed, they serve as "the cognitive foundation from which attitudes, perceived social norms, and perceptions of control—and ultimately intentions—are assumed to follow in a reasonable and consistent fashion" (pp. 193–194).

In *Social Learning Theory*, and its subsequent evolution into *Social Cognitive Theory*, people are conceptualized as constant information collectors and processors. Their thoughts and actions again follow rationally and deterministically from that information:

After people acquire cognitive skills and operations for processing information, they can formulate alternative solutions and evaluate the probable immediate and long range consequences of different courses of action. The result of weighing the effort required, the relative risks and benefits, and the subjective probabilities of gaining the desired outcomes influences which actions, from among the various alternatives, are chosen. (Bandura, 1977, p. 173)

Like other cognitivist theorists, Bandura anticipated the doubts about the occasional apparent irrationality of human behavior. He was, for example, well aware of the observation of Janis and Mann (1968) that "although a rational animal, man as a decision-maker can seldom claim to make purely rational judgments," with many judgments characterized instead by "oversimplifications, distortions, evasions, and gross omissions of relevant considerations" (p. 327). So, Bandura (1977) was quick, immediately after his description of a rational, information-based system for selecting behavioral options, to issue a caveat: "This is not to say that the decisions are necessarily good ones or that reason always prevails" (p. 173). However, like a true cognitivist, the only possible reason he noted for such failures was the unavailability of adequate or accurate information: "Decisions may be based on inadequate assessment of information and misjudgment of anticipated consequences" (p. 173). He further elaborated on this point in the description of his Social Cognitive Theory. In this iteration, seemingly irrational behavior can be attributed to (1) an immature (not fully developed) cognitive system, as in the case of children, (2) inadequate information, (3) incomplete consideration of available options, and (4) the misunderstanding or misinterpretation of information. In other words, in Social Cognitive Theory, adult humans, with fully developed cognitive faculties, if provided with adequate and complete information, which they have properly understood, are expected to behave rationally:

> *To say that people base many of their actions on thought does not necessarily mean they are always objectively rational. Rationality depends on reasoning skills which are not always well developed or used effectively. Even if people know how to reason logically, they make faulty judgments when they base their inferences on inadequate information or fail to consider the full consequences of different choices. Moreover, they often misread events in ways that give rise to faulty conceptions about themselves and the world around them. When they act on their misconceptions, which appear subjectively rational given their errant basis, such persons are viewed by others as behaving in an unreasoning, if not downright foolish, manner. (Bandura, 1986, p. 19)*

The *Transtheoretical Model*, despite incorporating some behaviorist concepts and methods (eg, counterconditioning, reinforcement management), is also, at its core, a cognitivist model. The main mechanism postulated to propel individuals across stages of change is a shift in their perceived "decisional balance," as conceptualized by Janis and Mann (1968). Specifically, action is predicted to occur after a critical "crossover" point, at which the anticipated pros of acting surpass the anticipated cons: "for most problem behaviors, people will decide that the pros of changing the behavior outweigh the cons before they take action to modify their behavior" (Prochaska et al., 1994, p. 44). With the main domain of application of the transtheoretical model being in smoking cessation, a quintessential example of a seemingly irrational behavior, Prochaska readily acknowledges that "behavioral change decision making is not as conscious or rational as traditional utility function theories would suggest" (Prochaska, 2008, p. 847). However, like other cognitivists, Prochaska attributes any irrationality to faulty information processing (ie, not being fully cognizant of the pros and cons), which the therapist is called upon to help correct. Then, with the proper decisional balance established, the individual should be ready to take appropriate action:

> *Smokers in the precontemplation stage, for example, are not aware that compared with their peers in other stages, they are underestimating the pros of quitting and overestimating the cons. Without expert help, patients can remain stuck in the precontemplation stage, if they are not particularly conscious that they are underestimating the pros of changing and overestimating the cons. (Prochaska, 2008, p. 847)*

Self-Determination Theory is commonly described as a "motivational" and "humanistic" theory, in contradistinction to "cognitive" theories. Deci and Ryan (1985) asserted that, while "cognitive" theories presume that behavior is the result of evaluating the likelihood and desirability of future outcomes and choosing among them, Self-Determination Theory considers the desire to satisfy certain basic needs as the "energy" that powers human motivation. Beyond this difference, however, Self-Determination Theory fully incorporates the cognitivist notions of symbolic representations and humans "striving to satisfy their needs by setting goals and choosing behavior that they believe will allow them to achieve these goals" (Deci, 1975, p. 16). It should be clear, therefore, that cognitive appraisals (eg, of autonomy, of competence, of relatedness) underpin the fundamental constructs of the theory. For example, Deci (1975), in describing the concept of intrinsic motivation, arguably the most central element within the theory, acknowledged that his approach focuses on "cognitive processes." The reasons for this, he wrote, are "simple": "not only do cognitions affect internal states such as attitudes and motives, but, as this work shows, individuals choose what behaviors to engage in on the basis of their cognitions about the outcomes of those and other behaviors" (Deci, 1975, p. vi). Thus, embedded within Self-Determination Theory are the assumptions that (1) "most behaviors are voluntary," (2) "people choose which behaviors to engage in," and (3) "these choices are made because people believe that the chosen behaviors will lead them to desired end states" (Deci, 1975, p. 20).

Most self-determination researchers openly endorse the assumption of rationality as the bedrock of their theorizing. For example, according to Helwig and McNeil (2011), "self-determination theory holds that people are *rational*, meaning-making agents who are self-governing (autonomous) and who exercise their autonomy and develop their competencies in relations with others" (p. 241, italics added). However, Deci and Ryan themselves have persistently avoided a direct endorsement of the assumption of rationality, presumably due to the association of the term with economic models of human behavior, which posit that humans act to maximize external (eg, monetary) rewards (eg, see Vansteenkiste, Ryan, & Deci, 2008).

Nevertheless, closer parsing of self-determination theory reveals its reliance on the assumption of rationality. In the framework of the theory, a dysfunctional motivational system is one in which there is a shift from intrinsic motivation (the optimal form of motivation) to amotivation. This is accompanied by a shift from behavior that is "self-determined" to behavior that is more "automatic." The distinguishing element between these two modes of behavior is the presence (versus absence) of conscious processing of information: "self-determined behaviors are chosen based on a conscious processing of information whereas automated behaviors are not" (Deci & Ryan, 1980, p. 34). Automatic behaviors are stimulus-bound impulses, such as smoking, nail-biting, and overeating, which will resist change as long as they remain outside conscious awareness. Thus, automatic behaviors are characterized as "mindless," whereas self-determined behaviors require "the higher cerebral functions" (p. 34). Ryan, Kuhl, & Deci (1997) invoked the ancient concept of "akrasia" (acting against one's better judgment) to describe the type of motivational failure in which behavior becomes mindless. In such cases, the goal of interventions is to strengthen the "capacity to be self-determining" (Deci & Ryan, 1985, p. 291) by (1) bringing problematic "mindless" behaviors into conscious awareness (Rigby, Schultz, & Ryan, 2014) and (2) providing information in the form of a "meaningful rationale" that focuses on the availability of choice and the controllability of motivational processes (Deci, Eghrari, Patrick, & Leone, 1994; Moller, Ryan, & Deci, 2006).

The cognitivist origins of contemporary theories used to understand exercise and physical activity behavior should be evident from the foregoing review. All these theories postulate that humans act on the basis of the rational analysis of information. Any instances of irrational behavior can be explained by a breakdown of the information-processing system, which can be corrected by supplying more or better information, raising the level of awareness, or correcting the evaluation or interpretation of the information. Not surprisingly, these essential postulates have fully permeated conceptual thinking and intervention approaches in the fields of health promotion and public health. What Weare (2002) calls the "rational educational" model forms the foundation of practice:

> *The world of health education in practice—in the school, the clinic, or the doctor's surgery—is still dominated by the commonsense view of "give the learner the facts (e.g. the helpful and informative leaflet, the lecture on the dangers of drugs by the policeman, or the chat on diet from the health professional) and they will surely then follow the advice and be healthy." This view is based on what is sometimes called the "rational educational" model, the fundamental assumption of which is that people are basically rational, and their behaviour driven by logically derived principles. (p. 107)*

Thus, at the core of the "rational educational" model, as the name implies, is the assumption that human beings act on the basis of rational information processing and its corollary, namely that the provision of information is the sole avenue for changing behavior. Whether explicitly stated or implied, these assumptions are ubiquitous in overviews of current theorizing. For example, "these theories are based on the notion that people are rational and that they typically engage in a process of weighing the pros and cons of engaging in any behaviours that affect their health" (Carmody, 2007, p. 106). Moreover, "it is further assumed that once in possession of the information, the clarified norms and values, and the decision-making skills, and with socio-cultural barriers removed, any rational person could not help but make the healthy choice" (Thorogood, 2002, p. 73).

In health promotion practice, the idea that "people need to be given factually correct information and then they will probably make a sensible decision" is increasingly deemed "far too naïve to be of much use to anyone" (Weare, 2002, p. 107). Within exercise psychology, however, although a rising number of investigators are willing to consider the role of nonconscious motivational processes (eg, Sheeran, Gollwitzer, & Bargh, 2013), the assumption of rationality (eg, Mogler et al., 2013; Shafir & LeBoeuf, 2002) remains unchallenged.

AFFECTIVE CONSTRUCTS? WHAT AFFECTIVE CONSTRUCTS?

Predictably, cognitivist theories have always had an uncomfortable attitude toward affective constructs. Moods, emotions, pleasures, and pains cannot be easily accommodated within conceptual frameworks that assume, as a fundamental premise, that decisions are based solely on the rational, deliberative analysis and evaluation of information. As a solution, some cognitivist models of behavior and decision making have simply ignored affective constructs altogether. As a case in point, a recent proposal for an integrative model of physical activity behavior (Hagger & Chatzisarantis, 2014) was criticized because it "may lack consideration of the affective domain in physical activity behavior over reasoned approaches to motivation" (Rhodes, 2014, p. 43). In actuality, the same is the case for all cognitivist models of exercise and physical activity behavior (Nigg, Borrelli, Maddock, & Dishman, 2008; Schwarzer, 2008; Spence & Lee, 2003). In other cases, affective constructs are considered either extraneous influences that bias the information-processing system or malleable "raw data," which are transformed into information meaningful to the individual only through cognitive appraisal (Baumeister, Vohs, DeWall, & Zhang, 2007; Carver & Scheier, 1990; Clore & Huntsinger, 2007; Forgas, 1995; Schwarz & Clore, 2003). According to one prominent such example, "the affect-as-information account posits that the *information* that affect provides is the key to such effects, *not* the affect itself" (Huntsinger, Isbell, & Clore, 2014, p. 602, italics in the original).

Similarly, although affective constructs appear in various degrees and forms in the main theories that have been used to understand and change physical activity and exercise behavior, their influence is persistently either devalued or considered subservient to cognitive processes. For example, in the *Theories of Reasoned Action and Planned Behavior*, affective constructs are described as "background factors" and, as such, their influence "is assumed to be indirect" (Ajzen & Fishbein, 2005, p. 203) in that they can merely color beliefs and evaluations: "people in a positive mood tend to evaluate events more favorably and to judge favorable events as more likely than people in a negative mood" (p. 203). This can "help explain why people sometimes seem to act irrationally" (p. 203). Ajzen has reiterated this point in response to criticisms that the theory of planned behavior overemphasizes rationality to the exclusion of other modes of behavioral decision making. He acknowledges that there may be instances of irrational beliefs and ensuant behavior. However, importantly, he maintains that this is not because the structure of the decision-making system inherently incorporates nonrational pathways but rather because the rational system is fed with faulty information: "Beliefs reflect the information people have in relation to the performance of a given behavior, but this information is often inaccurate and incomplete; it may rest on faulty or irrational premises, be biased by self-serving motives, by fear, anger and other emotions, or otherwise fail to reflect reality. Clearly, this is a far cry from a rational actor" (Ajzen, 2011, p. 1116). Thus, affective constructs are described as "biasing factors" (eg, people in a positive mood may tend to evaluate possible future consequences of a behavior more favorably or be more likely to recall positive events). Ajzen (2011) explicitly rejects the idea that "affect can influence behavior in a more direct fashion" (p. 1116).

In *Social Cognitive Theory*, affective constructs again enter the behavioral decision-making process as secondary and indirect influences. Affective states that generate "emotional arousal" are theorized to serve as information used in the formation of appraisals of efficacy. For example, during a stressful encounter, the emotional arousal associated with fear is *interpreted* as a sign of low efficacy, which in turns disrupts performance:

> Perceived self-efficacy and emotional arousal undoubtedly involve interactive (though asymmetrical) effects, with coping efficacy exercising the much greater sway. That is, perceived inefficaciousness in coping with potential threats leads people to approach such situations anxiously, and experiencing disruptive arousal may further lower their sense of efficacy that they will be able to perform skillfully. (Bandura, 1982, p. 140)

It is important to emphasize that the influence of affective constructs on behavior within the Social Cognitive Theory is *indirect* not only because they are theorized to operate through self-efficacy but also because they are thought to acquire meaning only through cognitive appraisal: "Information that is relevant for judging personal capabilities is not inherently enlightening. Rather, in the self-appraisal of efficacy these different sources of efficacy information must be cognitively processed, weighed, and integrated through self-reflective thought" (Bandura, 1989, p. 1179).

Many researchers within exercise psychology tend to think that *Self-Determination Theory* is different in that it assigns a central role to intrinsic motivation, a construct that is typically operationalized through assessments of the degree of enjoyment associated with various behavioral options. Closer reading of the theory, however, again reveals important nuances. As a fundamentally cognitivist theory, Self-Determination Theory assumes that affective constructs constitute *information* that is subjected to cognitive processing. For example, emotions are theorized to serve "as cues which provide information to the central information processing system to the effect that satisfaction can be experienced" (Deci, 1975, p. 97). What makes Self-Determination Theory different from other cognitivist theories is that it does recognize the possibility of affect having a direct influence on behavior, through the formation of associative bonds (eg, pleasant or unpleasant memories motivating the pursuit or avoidance of certain behavioral options). However, in the context of the theory, these inherent associations render the resultant behaviors non-self-determined. This is because the notion of the "self" is defined in terms of the involvement of "the higher cerebral functions" and, thus, by the mediation of conscious and deliberative cognitive processes:

> We suggest that when cues reintegrate affective experiences, the current affective experience is information that could lead to the formation of a motive and in turn to behavior. The behavior can be mediated by information processing and choice. This is in fact the critical point in self-determined versus non-self-determined,

affectively motivated behavior. If the behavior follows directly from an emotion,
because of associative bonds for example, the behavior is not self-determined.
(Deci & Ryan, 1985, p. 234)

With the reemergence of discussions on the Aristotelian distinction between hedonic and eudaimonic motives and well-being within positive psychology, Deci and Ryan have even added a moral dimension to the distinction between cognitively mediated (ie, "self-determined") and unmediated (non-"self-determined") affective motives. Thus, although the pursuit of pleasure and the avoidance of displeasure are considered possible motives, both their meaningfulness and their morality are evaluated as inferior to those that involve rationality and reflection:

The more directly one aims to maximize pleasure and avoid pain the more likely
one is to produce instead a life bereft of depth, meaning, and community. Pre-
scriptions based on maximizing pleasure are too often associated with dead-end
routes to wellness such as selfishness, materialism, objectified sexuality, and
ecological destructiveness, thus demonstrating how easily a map derived from
hedonic thinking can mislead. By contrast, specification of eudaimonic living
might not only be of value as a guide to a more complete and meaningful life; it
should also yield more stable and enduring hedonic happiness. (Ryan, Huta, &
Deci, 2008, pp. 141–142)

In summary, affective constructs have either been altogether omitted from the main theories used in the study of physical activity and exercise behavior or subjugated to an omnipotent cognitive apparatus. Consequently, the idea that affective constructs can serve as motivational forces has yet to enter mainstream thinking within the field of exercise psychology. Because the idea is incompatible with the current cognitivist paradigm, it is absent from most student textbooks and practitioner guidebooks. Most students graduating with doctoral degrees in exercise psychology remain uninformed about the essential theories of affect, mood, and emotion, thus perpetuating the narrowing of the conceptual perspective within the field (Ekkekakis & Dafermos, 2012).

DUAL-PROCESS CONCEPTUALIZATIONS OF HUMAN MOTIVATION AND DECISION MAKING

Given the failure to promote physical activity and exercise at the population level, it is reasonable to propose that a substantial expansion of the conceptual perspective may prove fruitful. It seems unlikely that exercise psychology research can produce the dramatic advances required to attain societal relevance by refining, expanding, or merging cognitivist models.

By most indications, postcognitivist theorizing will likely reflect a "dual-process" conceptualization. This approach suggests that two main classes of processes are involved in the decision-making process. These classes have been referred to by a variety of labels in the literature over the years. Evans (1984) used the terms *heuristic* and *analytic*. Heuristic processes were theorized to be "pre-attentive, rapid and indescribable by the person using them" (p. 452). Their function is "to select 'relevant' information for analytic processing" (p. 452). In contrast, "the function of analytic processes is to generate some form of inference or judgement from the information selected" (p. 451). Evans (1984) asserted that "arguments for rationality should center on the nature of analytic processes, but without an understanding of heuristic processes they are doomed to failure" (p. 452). Since then, authors have used a plethora of terms to describe pathways postulated to function analogously to heuristic and analytic processes, including *experiential* versus *rational* (Epstein, 1994), *associative* versus *rule-based* (Sloman, 1996), *affective* versus *analytical* (Peters & Slovic, 2000), *experiential* versus *analytic* (Slovic, Finucane, Peters, & MacGregor, 2002), *affective* versus *deliberative* (Figner, Mackinlay, Wilkening, & Weber, 2009), and *impulsive/reactive* versus *reasoned/reflective* (Alós-Ferrer & Strack, 2014; Strack & Deutsch, 2004).

In an effort to organize these proposals and help highlight their commonalities, Stanovich and West (2000) proposed the generic labels "System 1" to refer to heuristic processes and their analogues and "System 2" to refer to analytic processes and their analogues (for similar efforts at synthesis, see Evans, 2008; Sanfey & Chang, 2008). In an effort to provide further clarity, Evans and Stanovich (2013) suggested the adoption of the terms "Type 1" and "Type 2" to replace "System 1" and "System 2," respectively. Type 1 processes are intuitive, nonconscious, automatic, experience-based, and tend to rely on tacit knowledge and affective associations. On the other hand, Type 2 processes are slower, conscious, reflective, controlled, rule-based, require working memory, rely on explicit knowledge, and can involve inferential reasoning, mental simulation, and probabilistic predictions. Type 1 processes are theorized to be evolutionarily more primitive and to represent the default response mode unless overridden by the evolutionarily more recent Type 2 processes (Evans & Stanovich, 2013). However, because of the automaticity and effortlessness of Type 1 processes, Type 1 processes are thought capable of always modifying and biasing Type 2 processes. Further, the biases stemming from Type 1 processes may not always be apparent to the slower and more controlled Type 2 processes, thus potentially enhancing their biasing powers (Kahneman, 2011).

Type 1 processes are fast and efficient. They are assumed to be associated with the use of *heuristics* (Evans & Stanovich, 2013), namely simplified rules that help people make judgments and decisions efficiently, without the need for analysis of all possible alternative outcomes. In their seminal work on this subject, Tversky and Kahneman (1974) noted:

People rely on a limited number of heuristic principles which reduce the complex tasks of assessing probabilities and predicting values to simpler judgmental operations. In general, these heuristics are quite useful, but sometimes they lead to severe and systematic errors. (p. 1124)

Despite seemingly violating rationality and occasionally leading to "severe and systematic errors," heuristics and Type 1 processes have been preserved because they did offer advantages within the environment that shaped animal and hominid evolution (De Martino, Kumaran, Seymour, & Dolan, 2006; Evans & Stanovich, 2013; Kenrick et al., 2009; Santos & Rosati, 2015; Waksberg, Smith, & Burd, 2009). Theorists have argued that, within the modern, highly complex world, heuristics and Type 1 processes remain a necessity despite being nonoptimal. Such arguments follow from the notion of "bounded rationality" attributed to Simon (1978). According to Simon (1983), "human beings have neither the facts nor the consistent structure of values nor the reasoning power at their disposal" (p. 17). Thus, given their "bounded rationality," humans tend to "satisfice" rather than optimize. This notion gained acceptance within the fields of behavioral economics (Kahneman, 2011), psychology (Shafir & LeBoeuf, 2002), and medicine (Corrigan, Powell, & Michaels, 2015; Wegwarth, Gaissmaier, & Gigerenzer, 2009), in which authors increasingly recognize that real-world decisions are made under substantial, often insurmountable, constraints. Gigerenzer and Goldstein (1996) explain "satisficing" as follows:

> *Satisficing, a blend of sufficing and satisfying, is a word of Scottish origin, which Simon uses to characterize algorithms that successfully deal with conditions of limited time, knowledge, or computational capacities. His concept of satisficing postulates, for instance, that an organism would choose the first object (a mate, perhaps) that satisfies its aspiration level—instead of the intractable sequence of taking the time to survey all possible alternatives, estimating probabilities and utilities for the possible outcomes associated with each alternative, calculating expected utilities, and choosing the alternative that scores highest (p. 651).*

In summary, dual-process theories, which emerged from fields that operate (at least in part) outside of the confines of the cognitivist paradigm, acknowledge the role of nonrational, heuristic, automatic, and affective influences on decision making and behavior. This is in stark contrast to theories of physical activity and exercise behavior, which still focus on rational, deliberative, and controlled influences, as detailed in previous sections.

TOWARD A DUAL-PROCESS CONCEPTUALIZATION OF PHYSICAL ACTIVITY AND EXERCISE BEHAVIOR

A crucial step in the transition of exercise psychology to the postcognitivist era will be a broad agreement on the need to develop physical activity- and exercise-specific theoretical models, recognizing the unique features and challenges of these particular behaviors. This is a position also espoused by other authors, who have noted that "there is adequate, if not overwhelming, evidence to suggest that unique theories of [physical activity] should be pursued" (Rhodes & Nigg, 2011, p. 114). However, the arguments forwarded thus far, although correct (eg, exercise is an adoption rather than a cessation behavior, it is not necessary for immediate survival, it requires a significant time commitment, it is long-term), are incomplete. An important aspect of the "uniqueness" not addressed in previous accounts is the extent to which physical activity and exercise engage the affective system. Although Dishman (2003) had also made a related point, noting that "physical activity arguably offers more opportunities for pleasure than do most other health-related behaviors (compared to brushing, flossing, buckling up, and seeing the doctor, for example)" (p. 46), our view is different. From our perspective, at the core of the uniqueness lies a profound conflict between "Type 1" and "Type 2" processes, such that although most individuals recognize the health benefits of physical activity and exercise, they tend to regard them as unpleasant or inadequately pleasant to compete against other, more pleasant options vying for a portion of their discretionary time.

While knowledge and appreciation of the health benefits and rational, analytical, and deliberative reasons for exercising may influence behavior through Type 2 processes, automatic, affective processes can influence behavior through Type 1 processes. Unless these influences are congruent (ie, exercise is cognitively appraised as beneficial for health and well-being and is also experienced as pleasant), a conflict emerges. Because of the presumed default-nature of Type 1 processes, it is likely that a negative hedonic tone associated with exercise will prove to be a stronger determinant of behavior than the rational reasons for exercising (Loewenstein, Weber, Hsee, & Welch, 2001). Evidence indicates that time pressure and cognitive load, which enhance the salience or primacy of Type 1 processes, shift decision making in favor of hedonic options rather than "rational" or "cognitively favorable" options (Cabanac & Bonniot-Cabanac, 2007; Shiv & Fedorikhin, 1999). Exercise-specific dual-process theoretical models must account for the complex interplay between Type 1 and Type 2 processes (see Fig. 18.4).

The "affect heuristic" (Finucane, Alhakami, Slovic, & Johnson, 2000; Slovic et al., 2002) reflects the basic hedonistic premise that affect guides behavior, such that humans gravitate toward behavioral decisions likely to increase pleasure and

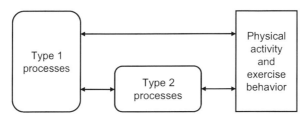

FIGURE 18.4   Dual-process models of physical activity and exercise will have to recognize the effect of noncognitive and nonrational processes on behavior. Moreover, physical activity and exercise will have to be conceptualized as stimuli that dynamically reshape Type 1 and Type 2 processes, rather than merely as the outcomes of information processing. Accordingly, the research agenda will have to encompass questions pertaining to (1) how physical activity and exercise can be modified to optimize both Type 1 and Type 2 processes and (2) how Type 1 and Type 2 processes can be modified to facilitate physical activity and exercise behavior.

tend to avoid those likely to decrease it (Ekkekakis & Dafermos, 2012). The affect heuristic has been called "probably the most important development in the study of judgment heuristics in the past few decades" (Kahneman, 2003, p. 710). In the conceptually similar risk-as-feelings model, both cognitive factors related to anticipated outcomes (eg, benefits and risks) and anticipatory affective responses felt at the time of decision making are theorized to influence behavior. These anticipatory affective responses are thought to (1) occur independently of Type 2 processes and (2) mediate the impact of Type 2 processes on behavior (Loewenstein et al., 2001). Applied to physical activity and exercise, the affect heuristic would suggest that automatically evoked (ie, cognitively unmediated) affective reactions at the moment of decision making, presumably stemming from a history of past experiences, would influence the behavioral decision. Given the presumed automatic evocation of such affective reactions, and the theorized "default" nature of the affect-centric Type 1 processes, negative past experiences could bias, override, or overpower a positive rational cost-benefit analysis under most circumstances.

This idea draws on a substantial body of research and theorizing over the past 30 years, albeit one that has been neglected within exercise psychology. The foundation was laid by Zajonc (1980, 1984), who questioned the assumption that "affect, such as that contained in preferences, is necessarily *postcognitive*" (Zajonc & Markus, 1982, p. 125, italics in the original). Further, he not only suggested that "affective responses, including preference judgments, may be fairly independent of cognition" but even went as far as to argue that "under some circumstances, affect or preference comes as the first experience, " whereas "the cognitions that have generally been taken to be the very basis of this preference can actually occur afterwards—perhaps as justification" (p. 125).

Zajonc also wrote of the formation of associations in memory linking ideas or past experiences with their attendant affective responses, as well as their associated "motor tendencies and other somatic manifestations" (Zajonc & Markus, 1982, p. 129). Thus, for example, whenever the idea of exercise is presented and a decision is made to engage in or refrain from exercise, the representation of exercise triggers the recollection of the associated affect, motor tendencies, and somatic manifestations. If positive (pleasure, eagerness, "endorphin high"), these recollections (presumed to be instantaneous and possibly intense) could precede and overpower any counteracting cognitive appraisals (eg, other commitments, such as work deadlines or social obligations). Conversely, if negative (displeasure, aversion, breathlessness), these recollections could again precede and overpower any counteracting cognitive appraisals (eg, awareness of health benefits). Zajonc postulated that the affective and somatic components may become independent of the associated cognitions, raising the possibility not only of substantial discrepancies but even of conflicts (eg, "I know exercise is good for me but I hate it"; see Bluemke, Brand, Schweizer, & Kahlert, 2010). In such cases, interventions are bound to face significant challenges. Those that exclusively target cognitions (eg, education campaigns, advice, counseling) are unlikely to be effective. Instead, a multipronged approach that seeks to change the affective experience and the associated action tendencies would be necessary:

> *While preferences have cognitive correlates, they may become functionally autonomous of these cognitive correlates and persist merely by virtue of the behavioral tendencies that have become their expressions. Once they are autonomous, behavioral tendencies that represent attitudes and preferences are hard to change, particularly if only cognitive means are to be employed. A simple communication is seldom sufficient to change a well-established behavioral habit. Methods are needed that can reach habitual behavior and motor output. (Zajonc & Markus, 1982, p. 129)*

If past affective experiences and established action tendencies are indeed as influential and as autonomous as Zajonc suggested, the implication for the promotion of physical activity and exercise is that interventions that merely seek to alter or strengthen cognitions (eg, of benefits, of efficacy, of social approval or support) have a limited possibility of success as long as these behaviors trigger memories of displeasure, embarrassment, pain, or exhaustion.

Although Zajonc's ideas, proposed at the height of the cognitivist revolution, were considered unorthodox and iconoclastic at the time, they are consistent with modern theorizing and clinical observations from the field of neurology (and subsequently endorsed by researchers in fields as diverse as addictions, eating behavior, and economic decisions). In a series of groundbreaking and compelling observations, Damasio (1996) described cases of patients with focused lesions in brain areas involved in linking stimuli to certain configurations of somatic state, namely the amygdala and the ventromedial prefrontal cortex. The amygdala is believed to be a critical neural substrate for activating somatic responses resulting from what Damasio labeled *primary inducers* (eg, seeing a snake, hearing a loud noise, experiencing dyspnea during exercise). In contrast, the ventromedial prefrontal cortex is believed to be critical in inducing somatic responses from *secondary inducers* (eg, watching the video of a mugging, hearing about a sick baby, thinking about exercising). Patients with lesions in these areas, despite exhibiting no cognitive deficits and being fully capable of enunciating the pros and cons of various behavioral options, manifest profound difficulties in making life decisions (eg, planning their day; choosing friends, partners, or activities). To explain this pattern of observations, Damasio (1996) proposed the somatic marker hypothesis: "The hypothesis attributes these patients' inability to make advantageous decisions in real life to a defect in an *emotional* mechanism that rapidly signals the prospective consequences of an action, and accordingly assists in the selection of an advantageous response option" (Bechara & Damasio, 2005, p. 339, italics added). The rationale for the function of this system incorporates the notions of "bounded rationality" and the "affect heuristic":

> *Deprived of this emotional signal, these patients rely on a reasoned cost-benefit analysis of numerous and often conflicting options involving both immediate and future consequences. The impairment degrades the speed of deliberation*

(e.g., choosing between two brands of cereal may take a patient a very long time because of endless reasoned analyses of the pros and cons of each brand), and also degrades the adequacy of the choice, i.e., patients may choose disadvantageously. (Bechara & Damasio, 2005, p. 339)

Damasio (1996) believes that, in decision making, different options may activate the "somatic marker" via one of two routes. In the so-called "body loop" scenario, there is an actual elicitation of a configuration of somatic state resembling that elicited during previous engagements in that option. For example, when asked whether one wants to ride a roller-coaster, one may get the same overall pattern of sympathetic activity elicited during previous rides (eg, racing heart, dilated pupils, clenched muscles), albeit perhaps a more faint version of it. All of these physiological responses are then relayed (looped) back to the brain (particularly the somatosensory and insular cortices) and are collectively felt as a particular affective cue (somatic marker) that sways the behavioral decision in one or the other direction, depending on whether the somatic marker is positively or negatively valenced. The alternative scenario is known as the "as-if body loop," as it does not involve the body proper. Instead, the relevant areas in the somatosensory and insular cortices are activated "as if" an actual configuration of somatic state was taking place, even though the body itself is bypassed.

CONCLUSIONS

Establishing its societal relevance should be a strategic target for exercise psychology. Progress toward this goal, however, has been slower than anyone in this field would have liked. In this chapter, we argued that, in part, the failure to deliver intervention methods that can reliably and meaningfully increase the level of physical activity may be due to an overly narrow metatheoretical perspective. We illustrated that all major theories in vogue within exercise psychology over the past decades are derivatives of the same (cognitivist) metatheoretical framework. As such, they all exhibit a crucial limitation, namely the relative disregard for the motivational properties of affective constructs, such as core affect, moods, and emotions.

Research over the past 15 years has demonstrated that the old adage of "exercise makes people feel better" is inaccurate. A description that is more in line with the empirical evidence is that the widely touted "feel-better" effect is conditional and relatively rare (ie, exercise *can* make *some* people feel better, given certain conditions). In actuality, many types and amounts of exercise make most people in western countries, who happen to be overweight and chronically sedentary, feel worse rather than better (Ekkekakis, Parfitt, & Petruzzello, 2011). In turn, a growing body of evidence indicates that affective responses to bouts of exercise are reliable correlates and predictors of the amount of physical activity people choose to do in their daily lives (Ekkekakis & Dafermos, 2012; Rhodes & Kates, 2015).

Thus, the central thrust of this chapter was to underscore the urgent need for the field of exercise psychology to transition to the postcognitivist era. This means acknowledging and testing dual-process models of behavioral decision making, which recognize and integrate nonrational and affective influences (Fig. 18.5). We especially highlighted the possibility that physical activity and exercise may be characterized by a profound conflict between "Type 1" (eg, prevalent nonpositive or even negative affective experiences) and "Type 2" processes (eg, awareness of significant health benefits). According

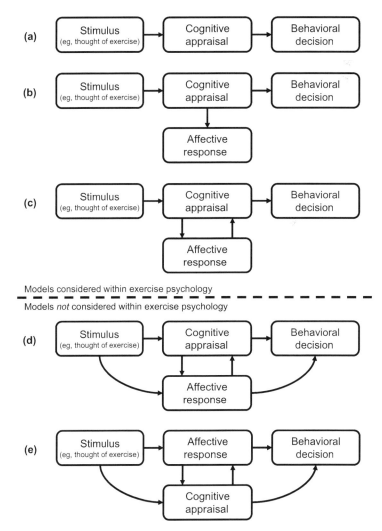

FIGURE 18.5   The role of affect within conceptual models of behavioral decision making that have been considered in the field of exercise psychology varies from (a) complete disregard, to (b) an inconsequential side-effect, to (c) an indirect influence entirely under the control of cognitive appraisal. Variations that have not been considered thus far include those suggested by dual-process models, namely (d) a direct influence parallel to a cognitive pathway but with cognition maintaining primacy, and (e) as a direct and primary influence, such as the versions proposed by Zajonc and Damasio.

to dual-process models, behavioral decisions in favor of physical activity or exercise should be considered unlikely unless the affective experiences are positive. The persistent failure to promote physical activity and exercise to larger segments of the population underscores the need for exercise psychology to reconceptualize its core phenomena of interest, namely physical activity and exercise, as hedonic experiences and, in turn, pursue a research agenda aimed at developing ways to enhance these experiences for the population at large, including individuals who are overweight and chronically sedentary.

REFERENCES

Ajzen, I. (2011). The theory of planned behaviour: reactions and reflections. *Psychology and Health*, *26*(9), 1113–1127.

Ajzen, I., & Fishbein, M. (2005). The influence of attitudes on behavior. In: D. Albarracín, B. T. Johnson, & M. P. Zanna (Eds.), *The handbook of attitudes* (pp. 173–221). Mahwah, NJ: Erlbaum.

Alós-Ferrer, C., & Strack, F. (2014). From dual processes to multiple selves: implications for economic behavior. *Journal of Economic Psychology*, *41*, 1–11.

Anonymous (2004). The catastrophic failures of public health. *Lancet*, *363*(9411), 745.

Archer, E., Hand, G. A., Hébert, J. R., Lau, E. Y., Wang, X., Shook, R. P., Blair, S. N. (2013). Validation of a novel protocol for calculating estimated energy requirements and average daily physical activity ratio for the US population: 2005–2006. Mayo Clinic Proceedings, *88*(12), 1398–1407.

Bandura, A. (1977). *Social learning theory*. Englewood Cliffs, NJ: Prentice-Hall.

Bandura, A. (1982). Self-efficacy mechanism in human agency. *American Psychologist*, *37*(2), 122–147.

Bandura, A. (1986). *Social foundations of thought and action: a social cognitive theory*. Englewood Cliffs, NJ: Prentice-Hall.

Bandura, A. (1989). Human agency in social cognitive theory. *American Psychologist*, *44*(9), 1175–1184.

Bandura, A. (2004). Health promotion by social cognitive means. *Health Education and Behavior*, *31*(2), 143–164.

Baumeister, R. F., Vohs, K. D., DeWall, C. N., & Zhang, L. (2007). How emotion shapes behavior: feedback, anticipation, and reflection, rather than direct causation. *Personality and Social Psychology Review*, *11*(2), 167–203.

Bechara, A., & Damasio, A. R. (2005). The somatic marker hypothesis: a neural theory of economic decision. *Games and Economic Behavior*, *52*(2), 336–372.

Bluemke, M., Brand, R., Schweizer, G., & Kahlert, D. (2010). Exercise might be good for me, but I don't feel good about it: do automatic associations predict exercise behavior? *Journal of Sport and Exercise Psychology*, *32*(2), 137–153.

Bryan, S. N., & Katzmarzyk, P. T. (2009). Are Canadians meeting the guidelines for moderate and vigorous leisure-time physical activity? *Applied Physiology, Nutrition, and Metabolism*, *34*(4), 707–715.

Cabanac, M., & Bonniot-Cabanac, M. C. (2007). Decision making: rational or hedonic? *Behavioral and Brain Functions*, *3*, 45.

Carmody, T. P. (2007). Health-related behaviours: common factors. In: S. Ayers, A. Baum, C. McManus, S. Newman, K. Wallston, J. Weinman, & R. West (Eds.), *Cambridge handbook of psychology, health and medicine* (2nd ed., pp. 102–109). New York: Cambridge University Press.

Carver, C. S., & Scheier, M. F. (1990). Origins and functions of positive and negative affect: a control-process view. *Psychological Review*, *97*(1), 19–35.

Clore, G. L., & Huntsinger, J. R. (2007). How emotions inform judgment and regulate thought. *Trends in Cognitive Sciences*, *11*(9), 393–399.

Colley, R. C., Garriguet, D., Janssen, I., Craig, C. L., Clarke, J., & Tremblay, M. S. (2011). Physical activity of Canadian adults: accelerometer results from the 2007 to 2009 Canadian Health Measures Survey. *Health Reports*, *22*(1), 1–8.

Corrigan, P. W., Powell, K. J., & Michaels, P. J. (2015). Beyond the rational patient: implications for health decisions and behaviors. In: P. W. Corrigan (Ed.), *Person-centered care for mental illness: the evolution of adherence and self-determination* (pp. 29–51). Washington, DC: American Psychological Association.

Damasio, A. R. (1996). The somatic marker hypothesis and the possible functions of the prefrontal cortex. *Philosophical Transactions of the Royal Society of London (Series B)*, *351*(1346), 1413–1420.

De Martino, B., Kumaran, D., Seymour, B., & Dolan, R. J. (2006). Frames, biases, and rational decision-making in the human brain. *Science*, *313*(5787), 684–687.

Deci, E. L. (1975). *Intrinsic motivation*. New York: Plenum.

Deci, E. L., & Ryan, R. M. (1980). Self-determination theory: when mind mediates behavior. *Journal of Mind and Behavior*, *1*(1), 33–43.

Deci, E. L., & Ryan, R. M. (1985). *Intrinsic motivation and self-determination in human behavior*. New York: Springer.

Deci, E. L., Eghrari, H., Patrick, B. C., & Leone, D. R. (1994). Facilitating internalization: the self-determination theory perspective. *Journal of Personality*, *62*(1), 119–142.

Dishman, R. K. (2003). The impact of behavior on quality of life. *Quality of Life Research*, *12*(Suppl. 1), 43–49.

Dishman, R. K., & O'Connor, P. J. (2005). Five decades of sport and exercise psychology: a festschrift for William P Morgan. *International Journal of Sport and Exercise Psychology*, *3*(4), 399–409.

Ekkekakis, P. (2013). Pleasure from the exercising body: two centuries of changing outlooks in psychological thought. In: P. Ekkekakis (Ed.), *Routledge handbook of physical activity and mental health* (pp. 35–56). New York: Routledge.

Ekkekakis, P., & Dafermos, M. (2012). Exercise is a many-splendored thing but for some it does not feel so splendid: staging a resurgence of hedonistic ideas in the quest to understand exercise behavior. In: E. O. Acevedo (Ed.), *The Oxford handbook of exercise psychology* (pp. 295–333). New York: Oxford University Press.

Ekkekakis, P., Parfitt, G., & Petruzzello, S. J. (2011). The pleasure and displeasure people feel when they exercise at different intensities: decennial update and progress towards a tripartite rationale for exercise intensity prescription. *Sports Medicine*, *41*(8), 641–671.

Ekkekakis, P., Hargreaves, E. A., & Parfitt, G. (2013). Envisioning the next fifty years of research on the exercise-affect relationship. *Psychology of Sport and Exercise*, *14*(5), 751–758.

Epstein, S. (1994). Integration of the cognitive and the psychodynamic unconscious. *American Psychologist*, *49*(8), 709–724.

Evans, J. S. B. T. (1984). Heuristic and analytic processes in reasoning. *British Journal of Psychology*, *75*(4), 451–468.

Evans, J. S. B. T. (2008). Dual-processing accounts of reasoning, judgment, and social cognition. *Annual Reviews of Psychology*, *59*, 255–278.

Evans, J. S. B. T., & Stanovich, K. E. (2013). Dual-process theories of higher cognition: advancing the debate. *Perspectives on Psychological Science*, *8*(3), 223–241.

Figner, B., Mackinlay, R. J., Wilkening, F., & Weber, E. U. (2009). Affective and deliberative processes in risky choice: age differences in risk taking in the Columbia Card Task. *Journal of Experimental Psychology: Learning, Memory, and Cognition*, *35*(3), 709–730.

Finucane, M. L., Alhakami, A., Slovic, P., & Johnson, S. M. (2000). The affect heuristic in judgments of risks and benefits. *Journal of Behavioral Decision Making*, *13*(1), 1–17.

Fishbein, M., & Ajzen, I. (1975). *Belief, attitude, intention and behavior: an introduction to theory and research*. Reading, MA: Addison-Wesley.

Forgas, J. P. (1995). Mood and judgment: the affect infusion model (AIM). *Psychological Bulletin*, *117*(1), 39–66.

Gigerenzer, G., & Goldstein, D. G. (1996). Reasoning the fast and frugal way: models of bounded rationality. *Psychological Review*, *103*(4), 650–669.

Hagger, M. S., & Chatzisarantis, N. L. D. (2014). An integrated behavior change model for physical activity. *Exercise and Sport Sciences Reviews*, *42*(2), 62–69.

Helwig, C. C., & McNeil, J. (2011). The development of conceptions of personal autonomy, rights, and democracy, and their relation to psychological well-being. In: V. I. Chirkov, R. M. Ryan, & K. M. Sheldon (Eds.), *Human autonomy in cross-cultural context: perspectives on the psychology of agency, freedom, and well-being* (pp. 241–256). New York: Springer.

Hopple, C., & Graham, G. (1995). What students think, feel, and know about physical fitness testing. *Journal of Teaching in Physical Education.*, *14*(4), 408–417.

Huntsinger, J. R., Isbell, L. M., & Clore, G. L. (2014). The affective control of thought: malleable, not fixed. *Psychological Review*, *121*(4), 600–618.

Janis, I. L., & Mann, L. (1968). A conflict-theory approach to attitude change and decision making. In: A. G. Greenwald, T. C. Brock, & T. M. Ostrom (Eds.), *Psychological foundations of attitudes* (pp. 327–360). New York: Academic.

Kahneman, D. (2003). A perspective on judgment and choice: mapping bounded rationality. *American Psychologist*, *58*(9), 697–720.

Kahneman, D. (2011). *Thinking, fast and slow*. New York: Farrar, Strauss and Giroux.

Kenrick, D. T., Griskevicius, V., Sundie, J. M., Li, N. P., Li, Y. J., & Neuberg, S. L. (2009). Deep rationality: the evolutionary economics of decision making. *Social Cognition*, *27*(5), 764–785.

Kohl, H. W. 3rd, Craig, C. L., Lambert, E. V., Inoue, S., Alkandari, J. R., Leetongin, G., & Kahlmeier, S. (2012). The pandemic of physical inactivity: global action for public health. *Lancet*, *380*(9838), 294–305.

Koppaka, R. (2011). Ten great public health achievements: worldwide, 2001–2010. *Morbidity and Mortality Weekly Report*, *60*(24), 814–818.

Loewenstein, G. F., Weber, E. U., Hsee, C. K., & Welch, N. (2001). Risk as feelings. *Psychological Bulletin*, *127*(2), 267–286.

Maddux, J. E. (1993). Social cognitive models of health and exercise behavior: an introduction and review of conceptual issues. *Journal of Applied Sport Psychology*, *5*(2), 116–140.

Maes, H. H., Beunen, G. P., Vlietinck, R. F., Neale, M. C., Thomis, M., Vanden Eynde, B., & Derom, R. (1996). Inheritance of physical fitness in 10-yr-old twins and their parents. *Medicine and Science in Sports and Exercise*, *28*(12), 1479–1491.

Matheson, G. O., Klügl, M., Engebretsen, L., Bendiksen, F., Blair, S. N., Börjesson, M., & Ljungqvist, A. (2013). Prevention and management of non-communicable disease: the IOC consensus statement, Lausanne. *Sports Medicine*, *43*(11), 1075–1088.

Metzger, J. S., Catellier, D. J., Evenson, K. R., Treuth, M. S., Rosamond, W. D., & Siega-Riz, A. M. (2008). Patterns of objectively measured physical activity in the United States. *Medicine and Science in Sports and Exercise*, *40*(4), 630–638.

Mogler, B. K., Shu, S. B., Fox, C. R., Goldstein, N. J., Victor, R. G., Escarce, J. J., & Shapiro, M. F. (2013). Using insights from behavioral economics and social psychology to help patients manage chronic diseases. *Journal of General Internal Medicine, 28*(5), 711–718.

Moller, A. C., Ryan, R. M., & Deci, E. L. (2006). Self-determination theory and public policy: improving the quality of consumer decisions without using coercion. *Journal of Public Policy and Marketing, 25*(1), 104–116.

National Health Service Information Centre, Lifestyle Statistics (2012). Statistics on obesity, physical activity and diet: England, 2012. Leeds: Author.

Nigg, C. R., Borrelli, B., Maddock, J., & Dishman, R. K. (2008). A theory of physical activity maintenance. *Applied Psychology, 57*(4), 544–560.

Peters, E., & Slovic, P. (2000). The springs of action: affective and analytical information processing in choice. *Personality and Social Psychology Bulletin, 26*(12), 1465–1475.

Prochaska, J. O. (2008). Decision making in the transtheoretical model of behavior change. *Medical Decision Making, 28*(6), 845–849.

Prochaska, J. O., Velicer, W. F., Rossi, J. S., Goldstein, M. G., Marcus, B. H., Rakowski, W., & Rossi, S. R. (1994). Stages of change and decisional balance for 12 problem behaviors. *Health Psychology, 13*(1), 39–46.

Rhodes, R. E. (2014). Adding depth to the next generation of physical activity models. *Exercise and Sport Sciences Reviews, 42*(2), 43–44.

Rhodes, R. E., & Kates, A. (2015). Can the affective response to exercise predict future motives and physical activity behavior? A systematic review of published evidence. *Annals of Behavioral Medicine, 49*(5), 715–731.

Rhodes, R. E., & Nigg, C. R. (2011). Advancing physical activity theory: a review and future directions. *Exercise and Sport Sciences Reviews, 39*(3), 113–119.

Rigby, C. S., Schultz, P. P., & Ryan, R. M. (2014). Mindfulness, interest-taking and self-regulation: a self-determination theory perspective on the role of awareness in optimal functioning. In: A. Ie, C. T. Ngnoumen, & E. J. Langer (Eds.), *Wiley Blackwell handbook of mindfulness* (pp. 216–235). Malden, MA: Wiley Blackwell.

Ryan, R. M., Kuhl, J., & Deci, E. L. (1997). Nature and autonomy: an organizational view of social and neurobiological aspects of self-regulation in behavior and development. *Development and Psychopathology, 9*(4), 701–728.

Ryan, R. M., Huta, V., & Deci, E. L. (2008). Living well: a self-determination theory perspective on eudaimonia. *Journal of Happiness Studies, 9*(1), 139–170.

Sanfey, A. G., & Chang, L. J. (2008). Multiple systems in decision making. *Annals of the New York Academy of Sciences, 1128*, 53–62.

Santos, L. R., & Rosati, A. G. (2015). The evolutionary roots of human decision making. *Annual Review of Psychology, 66*, 321–347.

Schwarz, N., & Clore, G. L. (2003). Mood as information: 20 years later. *Psychological Inquiry, 14*(3–4), 296–303.

Schwarzer, R. (2008). Modeling health behavior change: how to predict and modify the adoption and maintenance of health behaviors. *Applied Psychology, 57*(1), 1–29.

Shafir, E., & LeBoeuf, R. A. (2002). Rationality. *Annual Review of Psychology, 53*, 491–517.

Sheeran, P., Gollwitzer, P. M., & Bargh, J. A. (2013). Nonconscious processes and health. *Health Psychology, 32*(5), 460–473.

Shiv, B., & Fedorikhin, A. (1999). Heart and mind in conflict: the interplay of affect and cognition in consumer decision making. *Journal of Consumer Research, 26*(3), 278–292.

Simon, H. A. (1978). Rationality as process and as product of thought. *American Economic Review, 68*(2), 1–16.

Simon, H. A. (1983). *Reason in human affairs*. Stanford, CA: Stanford University Press.

Sloman, S. A. (1996). The empirical case for two systems of reasoning. *Psychological Bulletin, 119*(1), 3–22.

Slovic, P., Finucane, M., Peters, E., & MacGregor, D. G. (2002). Rational actors or rational fools? Implications of the affect heuristic for behavioral economics. *Journal of Socio-Economics, 31*(4), 329–342.

Spence, J. C., & Lee, R. E. (2003). Toward a comprehensive model of physical activity. *Psychology of Sport and Exercise, 4*(1), 7–24.

Stanovich, K. E., & West, R. F. (2000). Individual differences in reasoning: implications for the rationality debate? *Behavioral and Brain Sciences, 23*(5), 645–665.

Strack, F., & Deutsch, R. (2004). Reflective and impulsive determinants of social behavior. *Personality and Social Psychology Review, 8*(3), 220–247.

Thorogood, N. (2002). What is the relevance of sociology for health promotion? In: R. Bunton, & G. Macdonald (Eds.), *Health promotion: disciplines, diversity, and developments* (2nd ed., pp. 53–79). New York: Routledge.

Troiano, R. P., Berrigan, D., Dodd, K. W., Mâsse, L. C., Tilert, T., & McDowell, M. (2008). Physical activity in the United States measured by accelerometer. *Medicine and Science in Sports and Exercise, 40*(1), 181–188.

Trost, S. G., Blair, S. N., & Khan, K. M. (2014). Physical inactivity remains the greatest public health problem of the 21st century: evidence, improved methods and solutions using the '7 investments that work' as a framework. *British Journal of Sports Medicine, 48*(3), 169–170.

Tudor-Locke, C., Brashear, M. M., Johnson, W. D., & Katzmarzyk, P. T. (2010). Accelerometer profiles of physical activity and inactivity in normal weight, overweight, and obese U.S. men and women. *International Journal of Behavioral Nutrition and Physical Acticity, 7*, 60.

Tversky, A., & Kahneman, D. (1974). Judgment under uncertainty: heuristics and biases. *Science, 185*(4157), 1124–1131.

Vansteenkiste, M., Ryan, R. M., & Deci, E. L. (2008). Self-determination theory and the explanatory role of psychological needs in human well-being. In: L. Bruni, F. Comim, & M. Pugno (Eds.), *Capabilities and happiness* (pp. 187–223). New York: Oxford University Press.

Waksberg, A. J., Smith, A. B., & Burd, M. (2009). Can irrational behaviour maximise fitness? *Behavioral Ecology and Sociobiology, 63*(3), 461–471.

Weare, K. (2002). The contribution of education to health promotion. In: R. Bunton, & G. Macdonald (Eds.), *Health promotion: disciplines, diversity, and developments* (2nd ed., pp. 102–125). New York: Routledge.

Wegwarth, O., Gaissmaier, W., & Gigerenzer, G. (2009). Smart strategies for doctors and doctors-in-training: heuristics in medicine. *Medical Education, 43*(8), 721–728.

Weinstein, N. D. (1993). Testing four competing theories of health-protective behavior. *Health Psychology, 12*(4), 324–333.

Zajonc, R. B. (1980). Feeling and thinking: preferences need no inferences. *American Psychologist, 35*(2), 151–175.

Zajonc, R. B. (1984). On the primacy of affect. *American Psychologist, 39*(2), 117–123.

Zajonc, R. B., & Markus, H. (1982). Affective and cognitive factors in preferences. *Journal of Consumer Research, 9*(2), 123–131.

Chapter 19

Coach Behaviors and Goal Motives as Predictors of Attainment and Well-Being in Sport

Alison L. Smith

Department for Health, University of Bath, Bath, United Kingdom

Goal setting is a popular strategy endorsed and promoted by sport psychologists, coaches, trainers, and physiotherapists alike. Accordingly, the practice of setting and striving for goals is highly prevalent throughout all levels of sport. Within research, goal setting has also received considerable attention and gained support for the motivational and performance benefits. However, the topic of goal setting has not been without its controversies. Equivocal findings have prompted debate regarding the effectiveness of sports-based goals, with accompanying suggestions of a "goal effectiveness paradox" (Burton, Weinberg, Yukelson, & Weigand, 1998). While this discussion appears not to have deterred athletes from setting goals, the debate may have impeded the provision of clear recommendations. In response, this chapter presents a new avenue for enhancing goal setting by focusing upon the motives underlying athletes' goals.

THE ORIGINS OF GOAL SETTING

Advocacy for goal setting is rooted in organizational psychology and has developed almost solely from the work of Edwin Locke (1968). Responding to the absence of a work motivation framework, Locke and his colleagues engaged in a thorough and systematic examination of whether, and how, task performance may be regulated by goals. Locke broadly defined goals as "the object or aim of an action" (Locke, Shaw, Saari, & Latham, 1981, p. 126) and proposed that such goals are important antecedents of human behavior. Developing from his original work and drawing support from nearly 400 laboratory and field studies, including 88 tasks and over 40,000 participants, Locke and Latham

Sport and Exercise Psychology Research. http://dx.doi.org/10.1016/B978-0-12-803634-1.00019-4

415

(1990, 2002) refined goal-setting theory to include not only the benefits of goal setting, but also the characteristics of goals that enhance their efficacy as well as moderators and mediators of the relationship between goals and task performance. Specifically Locke and Latham advocated the motivating qualities of *specific* and *difficult* goals, described how such goals are moderated by individual ability, commitment, task complexity, performance barriers, and provision of feedback, and detailed their implications for task performance via focused attention, increased effort, strategic planning, and persistence.

GOAL SETTING IN SPORT

Buoyed by support for goal-setting theory in organizational settings, and acting upon a lack of goal-setting research in sport, Locke and Latham (1985) challenged researchers to test the theory in relation to sports-based tasks. Highlighting anecdotal support for sports goals and the comparable nature of organizational and sports-based tasks, Locke and Latham asserted that their theory should be generalizable across both contexts. Furthermore, it was proposed that goal effectiveness should be more evident in sport as performance is more measurable than in work settings.

Prompted by this challenge, and a concurrent interest in performance-enhancing strategies, an increase in goal-setting research was clearly evident throughout the 1980s and 1990s. Such work evidenced existing widespread use of goal setting (Weinberg, Burke, & Jackson, 1997; Weinberg, Burton, Yukelson, & Weigand, 1993) and provided initial support for the effectiveness of setting goals (see Burton & Weiss, 2008, for review). Furthermore, findings echoed Locke and Latham's (1990) endorsement of specific and difficult goals.

Early support for the effectiveness of goals fueled further promotion of goal setting as a fundamental strategy for sport (Hardy, Jones, & Gould, 1996). However, while the general outlook was positive, the findings were less convincing than expected. In their analysis of 36 studies, Kyllo and Landers (1995) reported an effect size of 0.34, notably lower than Locke and Latham (1990) and contradicting expectations that goal effectiveness should be more evident in sport. Furthermore, many researchers failed to provide evidence for the distinct benefits and optimal characteristics of sport-specific goals, with coaches similarly reporting difficulties with using goals effectively (Burton et al., 1998).

Unconvinced that these findings reflected poor applicability of goal-setting theory to sport, Locke (1991) contended that inconsistent results could be attributed to flaws in experimental methodology, including a lack of controls preventing participants from setting their own goals and failure to measure personal goals. While agreeing with the need for rigorous research, sports researchers were more hesitant to attribute findings to methodological problems alone. Instead, in their response to Locke, Weinberg and Weigand (1993) suggested that the highlighted causes of inconsistent findings (eg, spontaneous goal setting among participants) should be considered in terms of the difference between work and sport settings that they may reflect. Instead of preventing sports participants from setting their own goals, perhaps the tendency to set our own goals in sport should be examined in itself.

While the goal-setting debate may have hampered the provision of clear guidelines for sports-based goal setting, the debate may also have revealed a key factor in the pursuit of sports goals, namely the role of personal motivation. While Locke (1991) sought to control motivation through strict experimental conditions, Hall and Kerr (2001) argue that full understanding of sports goals requires consideration of the underlying motivation. This is due to a relevant difference between Locke's organizational settings and sport. In work settings, goal setting acts to ensure task completion in the absence of workers' own motivation. In contrast, sport is characterized by individuals who participate through their own volition. This inherent quantity of motivation can mask the distinct contribution of goals. Consequently, an understanding of sports-based goals requires an understanding of both the goals themselves and their underlying motives.

MOTIVATION FOR SPORT

Motivation has remained a consistent topic of interest in sport and exercise psychology, and has comprised numerous definitions and theories (see Roberts & Treasure, 2012, for review). Of these theories, self-determination theory (SDT; Deci & Ryan, 1985; see also Ekkekakis & Zenko, Chapter 18) has received considerable support in sport, as well as numerous other contexts. At its heart, the theory draws from humanistic and psychodynamic theories of personality (Maslow, 1955) and cognitive theories of development (Piaget, 1971) in recognizing the inherent tendency of humans to progress toward optimal functioning. However, the theory also recognizes contributions of operant behaviorist (Skinner, 1953) and social-cognitive (Bandura, 1986) interpretations of the conditioned and socially reactive human, respectively. The result is a comprehensive theory comprising the origins, nature, and implications of motivation.

SDT emphasizes the need to consider *quality* of motivation, in addition to *quantity*. Expanding upon previous notions of motivation as comprising intrinsic and extrinsic motivation (Deci, 1971), SDT proposes that multiple motives can be identified and organized along a continuum reflecting the extent to which they are self-determined (Deci & Ryan, 1985). At the least self-determined end of this continuum, *external motives* reflect externally controlled behavior prompted by rewards or punishments, such as the athlete motivated to avoid a coach's fitness punishment. Moving along the continuum, *introjected motives* include behaviors prompted by internal pressures of guilt, shame, or pride, for example, the athlete motivated to avoid the shame of defeat. *Identified motives* reflect more self-determined behavior mobilized by the identification of personal meaning or value, such as the athlete motivated by the value they identify in their training sessions. Finally, at the most self-determined end of the continuum, *intrinsic motives* underlie behaviors engaged in for their inherent interest or enjoyment. Consistent with SDT, research in sport has typically supported the benefits of more self-determined motives for improving task performance and psychological well-being (see Ntoumanis, 2012, for review). Accordingly, the basketball players engaging in training due to the enjoyment they experience (*intrinsic*) or because they identify value in the act of training (*identified*), will experience more positive outcomes than the players training due to guilt (*introjected*) or to avoid punishment (*external*).

SDT proposes that distinct motives are shaped by factors in the social environment (Deci & Ryan, 1985). Through the level of control emphasized and amount of information provided, social factors (eg, the coach) can either foster or undermine self-determined motivation (Deci & Ryan, 1980). Specifically, controlling environments that emphasize pressure (eg, continuous coach-driven pressure to perform) and minimize opportunities for choice undermine self-determined motivation and promote a move toward the less self-determined end of the continuum. In contrast, the provision of information (eg, task-relevant feedback) promotes self-determined motivation.

Vallerand and Losier (1999) proposed three social/environmental factors that can influence an athlete's self-determination; experiences of success versus failure, competition, and coach behaviors. Due to the possibilities for intervention, coach behaviors have received the greatest attention, with research primarily addressing this through the implications of *autonomy-supportive* versus *controlling* behaviors. Autonomy-support refers to behaviors that support the development of athlete autonomy through minimizing pressure, providing a rationale for actions, and providing opportunities for choice versus those that undermine autonomy and exert pressure. Research to date has typically supported the use of autonomy-supportive behaviors (Gagné, Ryan, & Bargmann, 2003). More recent findings have also highlighted the independent negative implications of controlling coach behaviors such as the use of controlling statements and the enforcement of punishments (Bartholomew, Ntoumanis, Ryan, & Thøgersen-Ntoumani, 2011; Duda & Appleton, Chapter 17).

In addition to expanding the concept of motivation and highlighting the role of social factors, SDT considers the link from these two elements to psychological health and well-being (Deci & Ryan, 1985). Specifically, SDT proposes three innate and universal psychological needs, the satisfaction of which is essential for optimal functioning. These needs include the need to experience oneself as the initiator of one's behavior (*autonomy*), the need to feel effective in one's actions (*competence*), and the need to feel connected to the social world (*relatedness*). These needs are not learned motives but reflect inherent requirements for psychological growth. Furthermore, these needs do not drive behavior but are supported or thwarted through our interaction with the social environment. Consistent with SDT, the link from need satisfaction to psychological well-being has consistently been evidenced in studies examining athlete groups (eg, Adie, Duda, & Ntoumanis, 2012; Reinboth, Duda, & Ntoumanis, 2004). In addition, these studies have emphasized the contribution of coach behaviors to the satisfaction of athletes' needs (see also Duda & Appleton, Chapter 17).

The expanded concept of motivation offered by SDT provides an opportunity to examine the inherent quantity of motivation to which inconsistencies in goal-setting research in sport have been attributed (Weinberg & Weigand, 1993). In contrast to minimizing the effect of such motivation as Locke (1991) recommends, SDT provides an approach through which the quality of motivation underlying goals can be explored in greater detail. The consideration of social factors also provides a mechanism through which practitioners (eg, coaches) can influence goal setting. Finally, the concept of psychological needs presents an area for further developing goal research to include the consequences for well-being.

Despite the apparent benefits of exploring goal setting through SDT, this approach has not been exploited in sports research until recently. However, such an approach was evident within wider psychology literature. In a refinement of SDT, Sheldon and Elliot (1999) proposed the self-concordance model to address the processes underlying goal striving and its effects upon psychological well-being. The model comprises two stages, namely *goal striving* and *goal outcomes*, which together reflect the entire sequence from goal selection to the consequences of goal attainment.

EXAMINING GOAL MOTIVES; THE SELF-CONCORDANCE MODEL

The self-concordance model is an application of the key principles of SDT to personal goal striving. Consistent with SDT, the model focuses on the quality of motives, in this case the motives underlying and driving goals, and proposes that goal motives can also be classified and placed on a continuum according to their level of self-determination. Furthermore, Sheldon and Elliot (1999) advocate the benefits of goals driven by motives at the more self-determined end of the continuum (*intrinsic* and *identified* motives) in comparison with less self-determined goals (*introjected* and *external* motives). The former, termed *autonomous* goal motives, are said to reflect the values and interests of the goal striver. In contrast, the latter, termed *controlled* goal motives, reflect goals driven by internal or external pressures of contingent rewards.

The first stage of the model focuses upon *goal striving*, encompassing the period from goal adoption to goal attainment. The model does not address the decisions underlying goal selection, focusing instead upon the implications of selected goals. In contrast to the work of Locke and Latham (1990) and their proposals for sports-based research (Locke & Latham, 1985), Sheldon and Elliot (1999) focused upon individuals' self-generated personal goals. Such goals may still originate from others, for example, when a student pursues a school grade expected by a parent or when an athlete pursues a goal assigned by a coach. However, the use of self-generated goals provides a more valid approach than researcher-assigned goals by examining personally relevant goals (Sheldon, 2002). Notably, such an approach also addresses the problem of spontaneous goal setting debated by Locke's (1991) and Weinberg and Weigand (1993), by making self-set personal goals the intentional focus of the research.

Due to their greater alignment with personal interests and values, *autonomous* goal motives are proposed to invoke their own motivational strength and, therefore, result in sustained goal-directed effort over time. In contrast, while *controlled* goal motives may prompt initial positive intentions and effort, the energy behind such goals quickly fades, particularly when an individual is presented with challenges (Sheldon & Elliot, 1998). As a result of sustained effort, autonomously motivated goals are more likely to be attained than goals driven by controlled motives. Importantly, Sheldon and Elliot (1999) emphasize that the benefits of autonomous goals cannot be solely attributed to the enjoyment experienced when pursuing such goals. Instead, the benefits are due to the sense of ownership individuals perceive in relation to their goals.

The second stage of the self-concordance model focuses upon the outcomes of goal striving. Drawing upon Carver and Scheier's (1990) model of self-regulation, which proposes the positive consequences of minimizing discrepancies between ideal and actual states, Sheldon and Elliot (1999) propose that goal attainment is associated with psychological well-being. However, in an exception to the positive outcomes, Sheldon and Elliot suggest that the link from attainment to well-being is dependent upon the motives underlying the goals. Specifically, when the goals are driven by autonomous motives, attainment results in increased well-being. In contrast, the goals driven by controlled motives will not increase well-being, regardless of attainment.

Providing the final link of the model, Sheldon and Elliot (1999) proposed that the benefits of autonomously motivated goals are enabled by satisfaction of the three psychological needs. Specifically, the attainment of goals that reflect personal interests and values satisfies innate needs for autonomy, competence, and relatedness. In turn, the satisfaction of these needs results in enhanced psychological well-being. In contrast, the attainment of goals prompted by internal pressures or external rewards do not satisfy these basic needs and, consequently, provide no benefit for well-being.

Research has consistently supported the benefits of autonomous goal striving (eg, Koestner, Lekes, Power, & Chicoine, 2002). This includes support across a variety of timeframes including short-term (eg, 2 weeks; Sheldon & Houser-Marko, 2001, Study 2) and medium-term goals (eg, semester long; Sheldon & Kasser, 1998), with persistent effects being found up to four years following the start of goal striving (Sheldon, 2008). Support for autonomous goal motives has also extended to a number of contexts with positive outcomes including increased job satisfaction (Judge, Bono, Erez, & Locke, 2005) and decreased psychopathology (Michalak, Klappheck, & Kosfelder, 2004). Finally, the benefits have been found to exist across cultures (Sheldon et al., 2004).

Encouraged by this support, the potential for applying the self-concordance model to sport-specific goal striving was explored through a series of related studies. The findings, including initial support and expansions of the model, provide a new avenue for exploring goal striving in sport.

GOAL MOTIVES IN SPORT

Guided by the self-concordance model (Sheldon & Elliot, 1999), the role of goal motives in sport was initially explored through two studies conducted with competitive athlete samples. In contrast to previous self-concordance research in which a *relative* motivation score was calculated (ie, autonomous minus controlled motives; eg, Sheldon & Elliot, 1999), the separate contributions of autonomous and controlled goals were explored to help identify unique contributions of each.

The first study tested the full self-concordance model using a cross-sectional approach to examine athletes' self-generated personal goals (Smith, Ntoumanis, & Duda, 2007). Consistent with the first stage of the model (ie, goal striving), sports goals driven by autonomous motives were associated with greater goal-directed effort, which, in turn, was linked with greater attainment. Additional analyses revealed that the benefits of autonomous motives were not reducible to goal characteristics such as goal difficulty, goal specificity, or the confidence athletes' felt in relation to their goals (goal efficacy) as previously promoted by Locke and Latham (1990). Supporting the second stage of the model (ie, goal outcomes), goal attainment predicted greater satisfaction of needs for autonomy, competence, and relatedness. In turn, need satisfaction was linked to greater psychological well-being. Notably, controlled goal motives did not predict goal-directed effort but were linked with decreased well-being.

Developing upon initial support, the focus was expanded to examine season-long goal striving (Smith, Ntoumanis, Duda, & Vansteenkiste, 2011). Supporting the model once again, autonomous goal motives at the start of the season were associated with goal-directed effort at mid-season, which, in turn, was linked to attainment at the end of the season. Goal attainment was associated with positive changes in need satisfaction during the season, which, in turn, predicted positive changes in psychological well-being. In addition, the relationship between goal attainment and need satisfaction was found to be stronger for athletes pursuing highly autonomous goals.

Findings from these initial studies support the self-concordance model as a framework for exploring goals in sport. In response to Hall and Kerr's (2001) recommendation, this framework goes beyond previous goal-setting research by examining the role of motivation. Furthermore, the focus upon self-set goals develops upon research designs proposed by Locke and Latham (1985) and does so without compromising the validity of the findings, satisfying Weinberg and Weigand's (1993) concerns regarding the control of self-set goals. These initial studies also support the model as a framework for exploring the consequences of sports-based goal striving. Developing upon these initial studies, this framework has been used to explore factors that could both influence, and be influenced by, athletes' goal motives. These factors provide further opportunities to explore athletes' goals, and how to support goal striving.

THE ROLE OF THE COACH DURING GOAL STRIVING

Coaches often adopt an active role in shaping athletes' goals (Weinberg, Butt, Knight, & Perritt, 2001). However, the impact of the coach upon the motivational quality of goals has received minimal attention. Drawing upon prior SDT research in sport, which has evidenced the impact of coach autonomy support versus controlling behaviors (Gagné et al., 2003), it was examined whether this impact extends to athletes' goal motives. Consistent with expectations, athletes' perceptions of coach autonomy support were found to be associated with both autonomous goal motives and satisfaction of basic needs for autonomy, competence, and relatedness (Smith et al., 2007, 2011). Furthermore, perceptions of controlling coach behaviors were associated with controlled goal motives (Smith, Ntoumanis, & Duda, 2010).

In addition to supporting the need for positive social influences in sport, these findings suggest that the impact of the coach may extend to the motives underlying athletes' goals and, in turn, both their level of attainment and resulting changes in psychological well-being. This is an important finding for coaches concerned with enhancing their athletes' use of goal setting. Such findings suggest that, in addition to promoting goal setting, coaches can positively influence goals by engaging in autonomy-supportive behaviors but must also avoid controlling behaviors that foster the internal and external pressures perceived in relation to goals (see also Duda & Appleton, Chapter 17).

MAKING PLANS; THE ROLE OF IMPLEMENTATION INTENTIONS

Implementation intentions are a cognitive strategy designed to aid goals by specifying when, where, and how goal striving will occur, in addition to creating "if–then" plans (Gollwitzer & Sheeran, 2006). The combination of autonomous goal motives and implementation intentions has been found to create an optimal situation for goal attainment outside of sport (Koestner et al., 2002). Autonomous goal motives have also been linked to higher levels of implementation planning (Carraro & Gaudreau, 2011). The research program outlined in this chapter extended this to demonstrate that intentions set by athletes may themselves be underpinned by autonomous or controlled motives (Smith et al., 2010). Specifically, athletes pursuing goals autonomously (ie, for enjoyment, interest, or identified value) may form similarly autonomous intentions. In contrast, athletes striving for goals due to internal or external pressures (ie, controlled goal motives) may develop pressured plans. Notably, the combination of a controlled goal with implementation intentions was also found to be linked with lower well-being, perhaps due to the additional pressures created by supplementing an already pressured goal, with pressured plans.

PERSISTENCE AND COPING WITH DIFFICULT GOALS

Goal striving in sport is rarely without its challenges. Due to internal conflicts (eg, conflicts over priorities) and external influences (eg, time limitations), goals can become increasingly difficult to achieve. Locke and Latham (1990) emphasized the need for sufficiently difficult goals to encourage personal investment and ensure goal attainment. Sheldon and Elliot (1999) also advocated the role of effort, but proposed that such investment is only sustained when goals are driven by autonomous motives. However, the self-concordance model does not detail *how* effort is maintained when an individual is faced with challenges.

The coping strategies employed by athletes are integral to persistence and performance (Lazarus, 2000), and have been associated with both goal attainment and athletes' general motivation for sport (Amiot, Gaudreau, & Blanchard, 2004; Gaudreau & Antl, 2008; Gaudreau, Carraro, & Miranda, 2012). Exploring this in relation to the athletes' goal striving revealed differing coping strategies used by athletes when pursuing their goals (Ntoumanis et al., 2013; Smith et al., 2011). Specifically, autonomous goal motives predicted the use of task-focused coping including planning and seeking instrumental support, which, in turn, have been linked to greater effort, attainment, and persistence when striving for increasingly difficult goals. In contrast, controlled goal motives have been associated with cognitive and behavioral disengagement from challenging goals and, consequently, with lower attainment and persistence. Furthermore, the differing associations of goal motives with coping strategies can be explained by differing appraisals of difficulties by athletes during goal striving (Ntoumanis et al., 2013). For athletes pursuing goals autonomously, difficulties are appraised as a challenge and an opportunity for personal mastery. In contrast, for those pursuing their goals with controlled motives, the same difficulties are appraised as threatening. In addition, controlled goals may be more mentally draining due to the internal and external pressures they reflect, leaving less energy to cope with difficult goals (Moller, Deci, & Ryan, 2006).

WHEN GOALS CANNOT BE ATTAINED

Regardless of the motives driving them, sports goals can progress beyond being difficult and become impossible to attain. Injury and illness, competing commitments, and external factors (eg, loss of funding) can all cause goals to become unattainable. The failure to attain a desired objective can be distressing for an athlete. However, despite the popularity of goal setting, relatively minimal focus has been directed toward unattainable goals and how to support athletes when this occurs.

Exploring wider life goals, Wrosch, Scheier, Carver, and Schultz (2003a) proposed that actively *disengaging* from an unattainable goal could prevent or, at least alleviate, the negative consequences of goal failure. Disengaging both effort and commitment prevents the accumulation of failure experiences, and frees personal resources for other activities. Furthermore, actively *reengaging* in alternative goals provides new opportunities for success. Importantly, these strategies function independently. Disengagement does not necessarily lead to reengaging in a new goal. Alternative goals may also be started without fully disengaging from the original goal. Each strategy also has its own unique benefits for well-being.

A growing body of evidence supports the use of such strategies when faced with unattainable goals in education (Boudrenghien, Frenay, & Bourgeois, 2012) and when attainment changes due to chronic health conditions (Arends, Bode, Taal, & Van de Laar, 2013). The benefits have also been extended to physical outcomes, including sleep quality and physical health (Wrosch, Miller, Scheier, & Brun de Pontet, 2007). Haase, Heckhausen, and Wrosch (2013) have also emphasized the value of these strategies for managing goals across the life span.

In sport, disengaging from a goal is often considered a sign of weakness. "Giving up" from goals conflicts with the wider cultural message of triumphing over adversity. Athletes are actively encouraged to pursue goals that push the limits of attainability. Consequently, disengaging from a goal may not be intuitively appealing. However, athletes and coaches also need to be strategic in how they utilize limited resources and energy, and when persistence is futile, disengagement and reengagement provide adaptive strategies for reallocating resources.

Although adaptive, individuals have been found to vary greatly in their ability to disengage from unattainable goals and reengage in new goals (Wrosch, Scheier, Miller, Schulz, & Carver, 2003b). More recent work has highlighted the role of goal motives in this process (Ntoumanis, Healy, Sedikides, Smith, & Duda, 2014; Smith & Ntoumanis, 2014). Suggesting a caveat to the benefits of autonomous goal motives, these motives have been linked with difficulties to disengage. Perhaps due to the greater personal investment of athletes in such goals and the potentially greater progress experienced up to the point of becoming unattainable, athletes striving for their goals autonomously appear to ruminate about the goal and find it more difficult to let go. Although this may enable athletes to fully explore the attainability of their goals, it may also expose them to lower well-being if attainment is not possible. However, such motives were also associated with intentions to identify, commit to, and begin alternative goals, particularly when the unattainability of the goal is realized early. In contrast, controlled goal motives were not linked to either strategy but were associated with shame and embarrassment experienced after realizing that a goal was unattainable.

RECOMMENDATIONS FOR PRACTICE

Goal setting is promoted as one of the primary psychological techniques for enhancing performance in sport, however, inconsistent findings have resulted in a lack of reliable advice for athletes and coaches. Examining goal motives provides a fresh perspective to the goal-setting problem. Importantly, it is not the intention of this work to disprove Locke and Latham's (1990) goal-setting theory. Prior research in sport supports the benefits of setting specific and difficult goals, combining short- and long-term goals, and adopting multiple goal types including outcome, process, and performance goals (see Burton & Weiss, 2008, for review). Consequently, each of these goal characteristics should be considered when setting goals. The intention of this chapter is to provide an additional framework for examining goals in terms of their motivational quality, and to provide an opportunity to further enhance goal striving.

Choosing the Right Goals

From the outset, more optimal goal striving can be achieved by selecting personally relevant goals. These goals will hold the motivational strength to be pursued through to completion, as well as benefiting psychological well-being. Sport psychologists and coaches are well placed to support athletes with identifying effective goals and often take responsibility for directing use of this performance strategy (Weinberg et al., 2001). Through such practices, practitioners should emphasize the importance of appropriate goal selection and facilitate athletes in selecting well. For coaches, the findings echo wider calls to be more proactive in the goal-setting process and, specifically, to "understand the reasons why players choose and action certain goals" (Maitland & Gervis, 2010, p. 340).

The ability to choose personally relevant goals, in itself, requires a sufficient level of self-awareness. Once again, practitioners can help by supporting athletes in developing an awareness of their own values and interests, and how they relate to their sport and their goals. Practitioners can also support by limiting the impression of their own values or interests upon athletes, at the expense of athletes developing their own.

Of course, decisions regarding goals may not always be the athlete's responsibility. Coaches often take the lead in deciding upon goals or communicating externally set goals. Although not self-selected, such goals can still be pursued autonomously if endorsed by the athlete and engaged in with a sense of choice or, at least, understanding of the rationale. This can be illustrated through the example of a gymnast setting the goal of learning specific techniques. In this example, the coach has selected the goal, perhaps based upon their knowledge of the gymnast's ability as well as consideration for the gymnast's safety. Although the gymnast has no choice in the content of her goal, the coach can enable the gymnast to identify value in striving for this goal by explaining the rationale. In doing so, the coach supports goal striving by fostering more autonomous goal motives.

Adopting Positive Coach Behaviors

In addition to facilitating goal setting, coaches can support the development of optimal goal motives through their use of autonomy-supportive behaviors, and through avoidance of controlling behaviors. Autonomy-supportive behaviors include adopting the athletes' perspective, providing relevant information and rationale (eg, communicating the purpose of a training session), providing opportunities for choice where possible, and minimizing pressure and demands. Controlling behaviors include the use of controlling statements (eg, you have to win this game) and punishments (eg, additional physical workout given when failing to win). Both types of behaviors are important for shaping athletes' goals, as they contribute independently to autonomous and controlled goal motives (Smith et al., 2010). Notably, coach behaviors have, in turn, been attributed to coaches' own sense of well-being, levels of job security, access to development opportunities, and work-life conflict, suggesting that support for athletes may begin with support for coaches themselves (Stebbings, Taylor, & Spray, 2015; Stebbings, Taylor, Spray, & Ntoumanis, 2012).

Setting the Right Intentions

Implementation intentions aid goal attainment by encouraging athletes to actively outline the details of goal striving (ie, when, where, and how striving will occur). For autonomously driven goals, the benefits of such motives are similarly expressed through these intentions and may further support goal pursuit and attainment. However, caution is needed when goals are pursued due to internal or external pressures. In this case, detailed planning may present a risk to well-being by amplifying these underlying pressures. While this does not prevent endorsement of implementation intentions, coaches and sport psychologists should be mindful of athletes' motives before engaging in such detailed planning. For example, consider the basketball player striving to achieve a given free-throw percentage to avoid punishments. In this example, detailing plans regarding when, where, and how this free-throw goal will be pursued may amplify external pressure experienced by the player and, consequently, risk greater detriments to the player's well-being.

Coping With Challenges During Goal Striving

Goals that are sufficiently difficult to prompt personal investment inherently bring challenges during striving. When faced with challenges, the coping strategies athletes adopt contribute significantly to goal attainment. Planning (eg, arranging additional training to address a technical weakness) and seeking instrumental support (eg, asking a coach for technical advice) have both been found to enhance goal attainment. In contrast, cognitively and behaviorally disengaging from a still attainable goal only serves to unnecessarily limit goal attainment. Sport psychologists and coaches are well situated to educate athletes about effective coping strategies for dealing with goal difficulties. In addition, effective coping can be promoted through positive coach behaviors, which indirectly impact upon coping by supporting autonomous goal striving.

Helping to Let Go and Move On

In addition to fostering persistence and coping, guidance may also be needed when athletes are faced with unattainable goals. Coaches are well placed to make reasoned judgments regarding the attainability of athletes' goals. When goals extend beyond being difficult and become unattainable, coaches should consider the strategic benefits of proactively disengaging from the current goal and reengaging in an alternative. Coaches can also support athletes to develop accurate assessments of goal difficulty by facilitating self-awareness of internal and external limits, and encouraging recognition of when attainability may be beyond the athlete's control (eg, due to injury). Finally, for autonomously driven goals, failure to attain may inevitably present challenges. Sport psychologists and coaches should be aware of this and ensure that support is provided (eg, information and social support), as well as helping to identify new goals. For example, in the case of an injured athlete striving to return to form for an upcoming competition, the coach can provide support by discussing the attainability of the goal. If such a goal is unattainable, the coach can support the athlete by helping to identify new competition targets and redirect goal striving.

The Use of Goal Setting by Other Practitioners in Sport

Recommendations for goal setting are not restricted to coaches and sport psychologists. Use and promotion of this tool is now widespread among sports practitioners including athletic trainers (Clement, Granquist, & Arvinen-Barrow, 2013), strength and conditioning coaches (Radcliffe, Comfort, & Fawcett, 2013), and physiotherapists (Wierike, van der Sluis, van den Akker-Scheek, Elferink-Gemser, & Visscher, 2015). In these disciplines, consideration of psychological approaches to enhance motivation reflects a holistic and interdisciplinary approach to athlete support. Consistent with recommendations for coaches and sport psychologists, these practitioners are also encouraged to consider the motivational quality of goals used by their athletes, as well as their impact upon the goal-striving process. Physiotherapists may also benefit from these findings in relation to unattainable goals, which often occur due to injury.

FUTURE DIRECTIONS

Examining goal motives provides a new direction for both research and applied work on goal setting. However, research into the motives underlying sports-based goals is still in its infancy, and there is considerable scope for further development. While a complete outline of future work is beyond the scope of this chapter, key areas are relevant for discussion.

The first topic for future work relates to how optimal goal motives can be developed and reinforced in applied settings. The research outlined in this chapter supports the benefits of autonomous goal motives and highlights the role of others (eg, the coach) in forming such motives. More recently, Ntoumanis et al. (2013) have evidenced that goal motives may also be primed by contextual factors such as videos and role models. Motivational primes prompt goal motives through the use of cues, which emphasize interest and enjoyment (autonomous) or internal and external pressures (controlled) in relation to the goal. The use of video priming is readily transferable to applied settings and has promise for widespread application; however, further research is warranted to establish reliable guidelines regarding specific cues and media.

A second, pertinent topic for further research is the athlete's simultaneous pursuit of multiple goals. Individuals frequently strive for multiple goals concurrently (Louro, Pieters, & Zeelenberg, 2007). Furthermore, dual pursuit of career and sporting goals is actively promoted to aid effective transitions postsporting career (European Commission, 2012). However, personal resources required to attain multiple goals are limited and competing goals can cause conflict. Further research is needed to explore the role of goal motives when athletes are faced with competing goals. Differing motives across goals may explain discrepancies in athletes' goal-related behaviors. Furthermore, goal motives may play a key role in the experience of goal conflict (Gorges, Esdar, & Wild, 2014). Such research may also reveal how those around the athlete can support the pursuit of multiple goals.

SUMMARY

Goal setting remains a consistently popular strategy in sport; however, prior research has been hindered by inconsistent findings, resulting in a lack of clear guidelines for athletes and coaches. The application of SDT and, specifically, the self-concordance model to goal striving in sport provides a new avenue for understanding and enhancing goal striving by examining the motivational quality of athletes' goals. Pursuing goals that reflect the values and interests of the athlete has been associated with goal-directed effort and persistence, positive coping strategies, higher levels of goal attainment, greater satisfaction of psychological needs, and enhanced psychological well-being. In contrast, goals driven by internal pressures (eg, guilt, shame, or pride) or by contingent rewards or punishments have been linked with more pressured planning, lower psychological well-being, and feelings of shame and embarrassment when goals cannot be achieved. Undoubtedly questions remain regarding athletes' and coaches' use of goal setting; however, it is hoped that these findings provide an impetus and framework for further developing our understanding of sports-based goals.

REFERENCES

Adie, J. W., Duda, J. L., & Ntoumanis, N. (2012). Perceived coach-autonomy support, basic need satisfaction and the well- and ill-being of elite youth soccer players: a longitudinal investigation. *Psychology of Sport and Exercise*, *13*, 51–59.

Amiot, C. E., Gaudreau, P., & Blanchard, C. M. (2004). Self-determination, coping, and goal attainment in sport. *Journal of Sport and Exercise Psychology*, *26*, 396–411.

Arends, R. Y., Bode, C., Taal, E., & Van de Laar, M. A. F. J. A. (2013). The role of goal management for successful adaptation to arthritis. *Patient Education and Counselling*, *93*, 130–138.

Bandura, A. (1986). *Social foundations of thought and action: a social cognitive view*. Englewood Cliffs, NJ: Prentice Hall.

Bartholomew, K. J., Ntoumanis, N., Ryan, R. M., & Thøgersen-Ntoumani, C. (2011). Psychological need thwarting in the sport context: assessing the darker side of athletic experience. *Journal of Sport and Exercise Psychology*, *33*, 75–102.

Boudrenghien, G., Frenay, N., & Bourgeois, E. (2012). Unattainable educational goals: disengagement, reengagement with alternative goals, and consequences for subjective well-being. *European Review of Applied Psychology*, *62*, 147–159.

Burton, D., Weinberg, R., Yukelson, D., & Weigand, D. (1998). The goal effectiveness paradox in sport: examining the goal practices of collegiate athletes. *The Sport Psychologist*, *12*, 404–418.

Burton, D., & Weiss, C. (2008). The fundamental goal concept: the path to process and performance success. In: T.S., Horn, (Ed.), *Advances in sport psychology*, (3rd ed., pp. 339–375). Champaign, IL: Human Kinetics.

Carraro, N., & Gaudreau, P. (2011). Implementation planning as a pathway between goal motivation and goal progress for academic and physical activity goals. *Journal of Applied Social Psychology*, *41*, 1835–1856.

Carver, C. S., & Scheier, M. F. (1990). Origins and function of positive and negative affect: a control-process view. *Psychological Review*, *97*, 19–35.

Clement, D., Granquist, M. D., & Arvinen-Barrow, M. M. (2013). Psychosocial aspects of athletics injuries as perceived by athletic trainers. *Journal of Athletic Training*, *48*(4), 512–521.

Deci, E. L. (1971). Effects of externally mediated rewards on intrinsic motivation. *Journal of Personality and Social Psychology*, *18*, 105–115.

Deci, E. L., & Ryan, R. M. (1980). The empirical exploration of intrinsic motivational processes. In: L. Berkowitz (Ed.), *Advances in experimental social psychology* (pp. 39–80). (Vol. 13). New York, NY: Academic Press.

Deci, E. L., & Ryan, R. M. (1985). *Intrinsic motivation and self-determination in human behavior*. New York, NY: Plenum Press.

EU Guidelines of Dual Careers of Athletes. (2012). *Recommended policy actions in support of dual careers in high-performance sport*. Brussels: Sport Unit of the Directorate-General for Education and Culture of the European Commission.

Gagné, M., Ryan, R. M., & Bargmann, K. (2003). Autonomy-support and need satisfaction in the motivation and well-being of gymnasts. *Journal of Applied Sport Psychology*, *15*, 372–390.

Gaudreau, P., & Antl, S. (2008). Athletes' broad dimensions of dispositional perfectionism: examining changes in life satisfaction and the mediating role of sport-related motivation and coping. *Journal of Sport and Exercise Psychology*, *30*, 356–382.

Gaudreau, P., Carraro, N., & Miranda, D. (2012). From goal motivation to goal progress: the mediating role of coping in the Self-Concordance Model. *Anxiety, Stress, and Coping*, *25*, 507–528.

Gollwitzer, P. M., & Sheeran, P. (2006). Implementation intentions and goal achievement: a meta-analysis of effects and processes. *Advances in Experimental Social Psychology*, *65*, 599–610.

Gorges, J., Esdar, W., & Wild, E. (2014). Linking goal self-concordance and affective reactions to goal conflict. *Motivation and Emotion*, *38*(4), 475–484.

Haase, C. M., Heckhausen, J., & Wrosch, C. (2013). Developmental regulation across the lifespan: toward a new synthesis. *Developmental Psychology*, *49*, 964–972.

Hall, H. K., & Kerr, A. W. (2001). Goal setting in sport and physical activity: tracing the empirical developments and establishing conceptual direction. In: G. C. Roberts (Ed.), *Advances in motivation in sport and exercise* (pp. 183–233). Champaign, IL: Human Kinetics.

Hardy, L., Jones, G., & Gould, D. (1996). *Understanding psychological preparation for sport: theory and practice for elite performers.* Chichester, UK: Wiley.

Judge, T. A., Bono, J. E., Erez, A., & Locke, E. A. (2005). Core self-evaluations and job and life satisfaction: the role of self-concordance and goal attainment. *Journal of Applied Psychology*, *90*, 257–268.

Koestner, R., Lekes, N., Power, T. A., & Chicoine, E. (2002). Attaining personal goals: self-concordance plus implementation intentions equals success. *Journal of Personality and Social Psychology*, *83*, 231–244.

Kyllo, L. B., & Landers, D. M. (1995). Goal setting in sport and exercise: a research synthesis to resolve the controversy. *Journal of Sport and Exercise Psychology*, *17*, 117–137.

Lazarus, R. S. (2000). How emotions influence performance in competitive sports. *The Sports Psychologist*, *14*, 229–252.

Locke, E. A. (1968). Toward a theory of task motivation and incentives. *Organizational Behavior and Human Performance*, *3*, 157–189.

Locke, E. A. (1991). Problems with goal setting research in sports—and their solution. *Journal of Sport and Exercise Psychology*, *16*, 212–215.

Locke, E. A., & Latham, G. P. (1985). The application of goal setting to sports. *Journal of Sport Psychology*, *7*, 205–222.

Locke, E. A., & Latham, G. P. (1990). *A theory of goal setting and task performance.* Englewood Cliffs, NJ: Prentice Hall.

Locke, E. A., & Latham, G. P. (2002). Building a practically useful theory of goal setting and task motivation: a 35-year odyssey. *American Psychologist*, *57*, 705–717.

Locke, E. A., Shaw, K. N., Saari, L. M., & Latham, G. P. (1981). Goal setting and task performance. *Psychological Bulletin*, *90*, 125–152.

Louro, M. J., Pieters, R., & Zeelenberg, M. (2007). Dynamics of multiple goal pursuit. *Journal of Personality and Social Psychology*, *93*, 174–193.

Maitland, A., & Gervis, M. (2010). Goal setting in youth football. Are coaches missing an opportunity? *Physical Education and Sport Pedagogy*, *15*(4), 323–343.

Maslow, A.H. (1955). Deficiency motivation and growth motivation. In: M.R. Jones (Eds.), *Nebraska symposium on motivation* (Vol. 3, pp. 1–30). Lincoln: University of Nebraska Press.

Michalak, J., Klappheck, M. A., & Kosfelder, J. (2004). Personal goals of psychotherapy patients: the intensity and the "why" of goal motivated behavior and their implications for the therapeutic process. *Psychotherapy Research*, *14*, 193–209.

Moller, A. C., Deci, E. L., & Ryan, R. M. (2006). Choice and ego-depletion: the moderating role of autonomy. *Personality and Social Psychology Bulletin*, *32*, 1024–1036.

Ntoumanis, N. (2012). A self-determination theory perspective on motivation in sport and physical education: current trends and possible future research directions. In: G. C. Roberts, & D. C. Treasure (Eds.), *Advances in motivation in sport and exercise* (pp. 91–128). Champaign, IL: Human Kinetics.

Ntoumanis, N., Healy, L. C., Sedikides, C., Duda, J., Stewart, B., Smith, A., & Bond, J. (2013). When the goal gets tough: the "why" of goal striving matters. *Journal of Personality*, *82*(3), 225–236.

Ntoumanis, N., Healy, L. C., Sedikides, C., Smith, A. L., & Duda, J. L. (2014). Self-regulatory responses to unattainable goals: the role of goal motives. *Self and Identity, 13*(5), 594–612.

Piaget, J. (1971). *Biology and knowledge*. Chicago: University of Chicago Press.

Radcliffe, J. N., Comfort, P., & Fawcett, T. (2013). The perception of psychology and the frequency of psychological strategies used by strength and conditioning practitioners. *Journal of Strength and Conditioning Research, 27*(4), 1136–1146.

Reinboth, M., Duda, J. L., & Ntoumanis, N. (2004). Dimensions of coaching behavior, need satisfaction, and the psychological and physical welfare of young athletes. *Motivation and Emotion, 28*, 297–313.

Roberts, G., & Treasure, D. (2012). *Advances in motivation in sport and exercise*. Champaign, IL: Human Kinetics.

Sheldon, K. M. (2002). The self-concordance model of healthy goal striving: when personal goals correctly represent the person. In: E. L. Deci, & R. M. Ryan (Eds.), *Handbook of self-determination research* (pp. 65–86). Rochester, NY: University of Rochester Press.

Sheldon, K. M. (2008). Assessing the sustainability of goal-based changes in adjustment over a four-year period. *Journal of Research in Personality, 42*, 223–229.

Sheldon, K. M., & Elliot, A. J. (1998). Not all personal goals are personal: comparing autonomous and controlled reasons for goals as predictors of effort and attainment. *Personality and Social Psychology Bulletin, 24*, 546–557.

Sheldon, K. M., & Elliot, A. J. (1999). Goal striving, need satisfaction, and longitudinal well-being: the self-concordance model. *Journal of Personality and Social Psychology, 76*, 482–497.

Sheldon, K. M., Elliot, A. J., Ryan, R. M., Chirkov, V., Kim, Y., Wu, C., Demir, M., & Sun, Z. (2004). Self-concordance and subjective well-being in four cultures. *Journal of Cross-Cultural Psychology, 35*, 209–223.

Sheldon, K. M., & Houser-Marko, L. (2001). Self-concordance, goal attainment, and the pursuit of happiness: can there be an upward spiral? *Journal of Personality and Social Psychology, 80*, 152–165.

Sheldon, K. M., & Kasser, T. (1998). Pursuing personal goals: skills enable progress, but not all progress in beneficial. *Personality and Social Psychology Bulletin, 24*, 1319–1331.

Skinner, B. F. (1953). *Science and human behavior*. New York: Macmillan.

Smith, A. L., & Ntoumanis, N. (2014). An examination of goal motives and athletes' self-regulatory responses to unattainable goals. *International Journal of Sport Psychology, 45*, 538–558.

Smith, A. L., Ntoumanis, N., & Duda, J. L. (2007). Goal striving, goal attainment, and well-being: adapting and testing the self-concordance model in sport. *Journal of Sport and Exercise Psychology, 29*, 763–782.

Smith, A. L., Ntoumanis, N., & Duda, J. L. (2010). An investigation of coach behaviors, goal motives, and implementation intentions as predictors of well-being in sport. *Journal of Applied Sport Psychology, 22*, 17–33.

Smith, A. L., Ntoumanis, N., Duda, J. L., & Vansteenkiste, M. (2011). Goal striving, coping, and well-being: a prospective investigation of the self-concordance model in sport. *Journal of Sport and Exercise Psychology, 33*, 124–145.

Stebbings, J., Taylor, I. M., & Spray, C. M. (2015). The relationship between psychological well- and ill-being, and perceived autonomy supportive and controlling interpersonal styles: a longitudinal study of sport coaches. *Psychology of Sport and Exercise, 19*, 42–49.

Stebbings, J., Taylor, I. M., Spray, C. M., & Ntoumanis, N. (2012). Antecedents of perceived coach interpersonal behaviors: the coaching environment and coach psychological well- and ill-being. *Journal of Sport and Exercise Psychology, 34*, 481–502.

Vallerand, R. J., & Losier, G. F. (1999). An integrative analysis of intrinsic and extrinsic motivation in sport. *Journal of Applied Sport Psychology, 11*, 142–169.

Weinberg, R. S., Burke, K. L., & Jackson, A. (1997). Coaches' and players' perceptions of goal setting in junior tennis: an exploratory investigation. *Sport Psychologist, 11*, 426–439.

Weinberg, R., Burton, D., Yukelson, D., & Weigand, D. (1993). Goal setting in competitive sport: an exploratory investigation of practices of collegiate athletes. *The Sport Psychologist, 7*, 275–289.

Weinberg, R., Butt, J., Knight, B., & Perritt, N. (2001). Collegiate coaches' perceptions of their goal setting practices: a qualitative investigation. *Journal of Applied Sport Psychology, 13*(4), 374–398.

Weinberg, R. S., & Weigand, D. (1993). Goal setting in sport and exercise: a reaction to Locke. *Journal of Sport and Exercise Psychology, 15*, 88–96.

Wierike, S. C. M., van der Sluis, A., van den Akker-Scheek, A., Elferink-Gemser, M. T., & Visscher, C. (2015). Psychosocial factors influence the recovery of athletes with anterior cruciate ligament injury: a systematic review. *Scandinavian Journal of Medicine and Science in Sports, 23*, 527–540.

Wrosch, C., Miller, G. E., Scheier, M. F., & Brun de Pontet, S. (2007). Giving up on unattainable goals: benefits for health? *Personality and Social Psychology Bulletin, 33*, 251–265.

Wrosch, C., Scheier, M. F., Carver, C. S., & Schulz, R. (2003a). The importance of goal disengagement in adaptive self-regulation: when giving up is beneficial. *Self and Identify, 2*, 1–20.

Wrosch, C., Scheier, M. F., Miller, G. E., Schulz, R., & Carver, C. S. (2003b). Adaptive self-regulation of unattainable goals: goal disengagement, goal reengagement, and subjective well-being. *Personality and Social Psychology Bulletin, 29*, 1494–1508.

Chapter 20

Health Assets and Active Lifestyles During Preadolescence and Adolescence: Highlights From the HBSC/WHO Health Survey and Implications for Health Promotion

Luis Calmeiro*, Margarida Gaspar de Matos**

*Department of Sport and Exercise Sciences, Abertay University, School of Social and Health Sciences, Dundee, Scotland; **Department of Education, Social Sciences and Humanities, University of Lisbon, Faculty of Human Movement, Lisbon, Spain

INTRODUCTION

In the last few decades, researchers have clearly shown the need for global community interventions that address family, school, and community contexts in which young people's health literacy and personal and social skills are developed. The family is fundamentally the first social environment that children experience; then, as children mature, they spend a vast proportion of their childhood and adolescence in schools. These two contexts have a critical role in promoting the health, well-being, and development of young people. As young people develop in a myriad of social contexts, it is also critical to establish networks and partnerships between family and school with local, regional, and national structures for the implementation of sustained and effective health promotion interventions.

Recently, studies have suggested the need "to give a voice to young people," to include them as active participants in all phases of school-based interventions, including problem identification, planning, implementation, and evaluation (see Matos, 2015, and Matos & Sampaio, 2009, for a review). How to create the conditions for such involvement and develop in youths the necessary sense of empowerment for participation is a challenge for practitioners. Nonetheless,

Sport and Exercise Psychology Research. http://dx.doi.org/10.1016/B978-0-12-803634-1.00020-0

433

to promote active and responsible citizens who have power over their own health and well-being, it is important to teach youngsters to develop their own strengths as human beings. Therefore, recent approaches to health promotion emphasize the importance of (1) focusing on positive and proactive aspects of individuals, (2) optimizing environmental factors and social support, and (3) encouraging individuals to participate by voicing their concerns and promoting their own health and well-being. In short, health promotion emphasizes "the potential of every individual for positive, healthy growth," which requires the development of "individuals and social contexts through strength-based policies and programs and through the empowerment of youth and families" (Theokas, Lerner, & Phelps, 2005, p. 27; see also Lerner & Benson, 2003). Our own work points in this same direction (Calmeiro & Matos, 2004; Matos, 2005, 2015; Matos et al., 2008; Matos & Equipa do Projecto Aventura Social e Saúde, 2011; Matos & Sampaio, 2009). In line with the previous frame of reference, in the present chapter we focus on the presentation of a model of health promotion, the assets model (Morgan & Ziglio, 2007), that emphasizes the strengths and opportunities that either are present or can be developed in individuals and communities.

ASSETS MODEL

According to the assets model (Morgan & Ziglio, 2007), individuals and communities hold a number of assets that allow them to identify their needs and actively engage in promotion of their health and well-being. The assets model integrates a number of concepts from positive psychology. Within this framework, a "health asset" is defined as "any factor (or resource) which maximizes the opportunities for individuals, local communities and populations to attain and maintain health and wellbeing" (Morgan & Ziglio, 2007, p. 18). Fergus and Zimmerman (2005) differentiated between *assets*, "positive factors that reside within the individuals," and *resources*, "positive factors that are external to the individuals" (p. 399). The identification of these health assets and resources allows policy makers and practitioners to deliver interventions that address these protective and promoting factors of individual and community health, empowering the communities as coproducers of health rather than treating them as passive consumers of already depleted healthcare services (Lerner & Benson, 2003).

The assets model is in contrast to the medical model, which focuses on the identification of health deficits and requires the use of high levels of professional resources and dependence on hospital and welfare services (Morgan & Ziglio, 2007). Ziglio and Morgan argued that while the medical model is concerned with the treatment of individuals' health problems and illnesses, the assets model is concerned with developing and optimizing individuals' or communities' capacities, strengths, and opportunities so that both individuals and communities can manage and savor their own health. In addition, focusing on promoting the "positive indicators" of health is preferable to focusing on the avoidance of the "negative indicators," as it provides guidance and a set of roles for what society delineates as desirable behaviors (Murphey, Lamonda, Carney, & Duncan, 2004). Thus, it can be argued that the assets model encompasses a broader understanding of the concept of health as an aptitude for developing and pursuing life goals and dreams (eg, holding future and educational expectations), individually and as a community, which has been shown to be associated with life satisfaction (Frasquilho, Matos, Gaspar, & Almeida, 2014). Evidence derived from the assets model "accentuates positive capability to jointly identify problems and activate solutions, which promotes the self-esteem of individuals and communities leading to less dependency on professional services" (Murphey et al., 2004, p. 18). One of the purposes of the assets approach is to empower individuals to be responsible contributors to their own health. Such empowerment demands the development of an awareness of what determines health. Thus, health promotion interventions focus in part on developing health-literate individuals, informed and demanding consumers who are aware of the protective and facilitative resources available in the community and make appropriate use of those resources to maintain health. Health promotion interventions encourage people to develop individual competences, such as interpersonal competences and self-regulation, or acquire and maintain appropriate social support. Such resources must be available at individual, group, and societal levels.

INDIVIDUAL, COMMUNITY, AND INSTITUTIONAL ASSETS

An assets approach starts by reflecting on what is working well in a group or community by asking, for example, "What external factors contribute to health and development?" "What opens us to more fully experience life?" "Which factors make us more resilient?" "What makes this a good place to be?" "What produces overall levels of well-being?" (Morgan & Ziglio, 2007, p. 19). Morgan and Ziglio operationalized an asset as any factor that constitutes a resource. Assets can take the form of social, financial, physical, environmental, or human resources and can be organized in three levels: *individual-level assets*, such as social competence, resilience, commitment to learning, positive values, self-esteem, and sense of purpose; *community-level assets*, for instance, a supportive family and friendship networks, intergenerational solidarity, community cohesion, and affinity groups; and *organizational-* or *institutional-level assets*, such as the environmental resources necessary for promoting physical, mental, and social health, employment, opportunities for volunteering, secure housing, political democracy and participation opportunities, social justice, and enhanced equity (Kawachi, 2010; Morgan & Ziglio, 2007; Search Institute, 2006).

The Search Institute (2006) described 40 internal (ie, resources within the individual) and external (ie, resources related to other people or within the community) assets that are thought to be associated with increased capacity to reinforce and maintain suitable and protective social contexts and the capacity to build one's own coping strategies and well-being (http://www.search-institute.org/research/developmental-assets). To effectively assess community capacity and address health inequalities, it is fundamental to list the presence and absence of particular assets, as research has shown that the more assets adolescents report experiencing, the more likely they are to report thriving behavior and the less likely they are to report risky behavior (Scales, 1999; Scales, Benson, Leffert, & Blyth, 2000; Theokas et al., 2005). Similarly, asset mapping involves the development of an inventory of the strengths of a community prior to intervention. Through such inventories, researchers, practitioners, and policy makers gather information concerning promotional and protective factors as well as the actions that need to be taken to create the necessary conditions for health. Producing valid and reliable asset maps requires the development of measures and assessment frameworks not only to properly assess the assets but also to determine the effectiveness of the proposed actions that derive from the process of assets mapping (Morgan & Ziglio, 2007).

To summarize, the assets model presented by Morgan (2007, 2010) proposes that attention should be shifted away from the problems and difficulties young people experience and toward their strengths and talents. Individuals have the potential to cope with the environmental and social risks they face in their lifetime, while valuing and protecting their health and well-being. Sometimes individuals may have to accept risks in their lives, and they need to understand just how far they should engage in this process.

CONCEPTS RELATED TO THE ASSETS MODEL

The assets model is not, in itself, a new perspective on health promotion. It is based on well-established concepts that have been associated with well-being. For example, this model brings together concepts such as salutogenesis, resilience, social competences, self-regulation, self-efficacy, social support, social cohesion, and social capital. Therefore, we now discuss how these concepts inform the assets model.

Salutogenesis

Health promotion is the process by which people increase their control over the determinants of their own health, thereby improving health and quality of life. In this context, quality of life refers to the perception that one is capable of managing one's health and life, that one's needs are being met, and that one is not being denied opportunities to achieve happiness and life satisfaction, regardless of eventual health, social, or economic limitations (World Health Organization, 1986). This perspective calls for a model of health promotion that emphasizes the development of empowerment and it is coherent with Aaron Antonovsky's concept of salutogenesis in which individuals are responsible, active, and participative (Eriksson & Lindström, 2006).

The theory of salutogenesis, or the salutogenic model (Antonovsky, 1996), represents a paradigm change in health promotion because it focuses on the factors that facilitate or optimize health rather than on the treatment or prevention of diseases (ie, the pathogenic model). Antonovsky suggested that health promotion has been overly concerned with risk factors rather than attempting to understand how people move in the direction of health. The salutogenic approach underlines the need for people to understand the factors that actively promote health instead of concentrating efforts and resources on negative outcomes. Hence, the assets model attempts to synthesize evidence based on the combination of factors that protect or promote health, well-being, and achievement (Morgan & Ziglio, 2007).

Antonovsky (1996) developed his salutogenic model during the Second World War, trying to determine what helps people maintain health under dramatic situations and how they recover from such situations. He suggested that those who have more favorable biological, psychosocial, and material resources, so-called general life resources (eg, money, social capital, cultural capital, intelligence), are more successful in dealing with life's challenges and recovering from life's problems than those who have fewer such resources (Rivera, Ramos, & Moreno, 2011).

Furthermore, Antonovsky (1996) referred to the importance of what he called the (internal) sense of coherence (SOC): a "generalized orientation towards the world, which perceives it, in a continuum, as comprehensible, manageable and meaningful" (p. 15). The SOC has three dimensions: the cognitive dimension or comprehensibility; the behavioral dimension or manageability, and the motivational dimension or meaningfulness. The SOC is thought to facilitate movement toward health because it provides the individual with the sense that the world and life events are understandable, ordered, and even predictable (ie, comprehensibility), the belief that one has the necessary resources to cope and manage events (ie, manageability), and the belief that life's challenges are worthy of investment of effort and resources (ie, meaningfulness; Rivera, Garcia-Moya, Moreno, & Ramos, 2013).

Research has supported the utility of the SOC in promoting health. Meta-analytic studies have demonstrated that the SOC is strongly associated with perceptions of health, optimism, and self-esteem and strengthens resilience, and it is negatively associated with anxiety and depression (Eriksson & Lindström, 2005, 2006). However, the relationship between the SOC and physical health is weaker (Flensborg-Madsen, Ventegodt, & Merrick, 2005). Therefore, the SOC can be considered an indicator of health and well-being, particularly when it is operationalized in terms of psychological health.

Resilience

The purpose of the assets model is to guide interventions and influence policies that focus on the development of individuals' resilience (Edwards,

Mumford, Shillingford, & Serra-Roldan, 2007) and on the promotion of positive youth development (PYD; Damon, 2004; Lerner, Phelps, Forman, & Bowers, 2009), and ultimately resilience (Catalano, Berglund, Ryan, Lonczak, & Hawkins, 2004). Resilience is "the process of adaptation in the context of adversity or risk" (Kobau et al., 2011, p. 3). Edwards et al. (2007) viewed resilience as the positive outcome of the interaction between the protective and promoting functions of assets and the exposure to risk. Rutter (1987) appeared to view resilience not as an outcome but as an antecedent of positive adjustment by defining it as the "protective factors which modify, ameliorate or alter a person's response to some environmental hazard that predisposes to a maladaptive outcome" (p. 316). Fergus and Zimmerman (2005) defined this concept as "the process of overcoming the negative effects of risk exposure, coping successfully with traumatic experiences, and avoiding the negative trajectories associated with risks" (p. 399).

Despite the inconsistency of the definitions of resilience (ie, antecedent, process, outcome), this concept is a key feature in the protection against risk-taking behavior and promotion of healthier outcomes (Kia-Keating, Dowdy, Morgan, & Noam, 2011). Resilience allows adolescents to cope with and respond adaptively to adversity and manage major problems in life, such as poverty, dysfunctional family environments, disadvantaged communities, and inadequate schooling (Edwards et al., 2007; Kobau et al., 2011). For example, Dumont and Provost (1999) demonstrated that resilient adolescents scored higher on self-esteem and problem-solving coping strategies and engaged less in antisocial and illegal activities compared to vulnerable adolescents.

The concepts of protection and promotion are integrated in Kia-Keating et al.'s (2011) theoretical framework that aims to explain healthy development through the presence of developmental assets, risk factors, and protective factors. Assets are factors that promote healthy development and are independent of the presence of risk. Risk factors increase the vulnerability to the onset or maintenance of a negative condition. Protective factors are safeguards that counteract the effect of risk and enhance the individual's capacity to resist stressful life events and promote adaptation and competence. These are distinguishable from assets in the sense that protective factors exist only in the presence of risks. Whereas assets influence PYD directly—the promoting pathway—risk and protective factors interact in developmental and socioecological contexts to explain healthy development—the protecting pathway. Hence, it is thought that the effects of "adversity upon individuals are not inherently determined by their exposure to negative stimuli, but rather that outcomes are negotiated by the individual" (White & Pulla, 2013, p. 128).

Indicators of assets, risk, and protection can be categorized in key domains: social, emotional, behavioral, moral, physiological, cognitive, educational, and structural (see Kia-Keating et al., 2011, for a review). These indicators, and the effects of their interactions, are likely to change throughout adolescence as a result of developmental and socioecological settings (eg, individual, family, school, community, culture). From a socioecological perspective (Bronfenbrenner, 1979), adolescents develop within multiple interacting systems, which implies that the development of resilience and PYD requires an understanding of the reciprocal interaction between individual and contextual characteristics (Kia-Keating et al., 2011).

Coping

Coping and resilience are often used interchangeably; however, these are distinct concepts (Fletcher & Sarkar, 2013). As an individual asset, resilience will influence coping efforts.

Fletcher and Sarkar (2013) pointed out that while resilience refers to the constellation of factors that promote assets and protect individuals from stressors, coping refers to the strategies individuals employ to deal with the stressors. According to the stress and coping literature, psychological well-being is more strongly influenced by the way individuals deal with stressful life events than by the mere presence of these events. Lazarus and Folkman (1984) defined coping as the "constantly changing cognitive and behavioural efforts to manage specific external and/or internal demands that are appraised as taxing or exceeding the resources of the person" (p. 141).

Therefore, cognitive appraisal processes are fundamental antecedents for the development of coping processes (Taylor & Stanton, 2007). Taylor and Stanton (2007) argued that the classification of coping strategies is usually based on the strategies' functions and is often discussed within a problem- and emotion-focused coping conceptualization (Lazarus & Folkman, 1984) or an approach-versus avoidance-oriented coping framework (Suls & Fletcher, 1985). Within Lazarus and Folkman's (1984) coping framework, problem-focused coping refers to attempts to change the characteristics of the stressful situation, whereas emotion-focused coping represents an attempt to regulate the emotions that arise as a result of the stressful situation without attempting to change. Within the approach- versus avoidance-oriented coping framework, individuals deal with stressful life events by approaching the conditions of the stressful situation or by tending to distance themselves from the source of stress. Whereas problem- and emotion-focused coping functions can coexist within a specific coping strategy, rather than being pitched against each other (Lazarus, 1999), approach- and avoidance-oriented coping seem to represent opposite functions.

It has been suggested that problem-focused and approach-oriented coping strategies are instrumental in helping adolescents reduce stress, depression, and health-compromising behaviors and are associated with better adjustment. Conversely, emotion-focused coping and mainly avoidance-oriented coping have been considered to be dysfunctional (Campos, Delgado, & Jiménez, 2012; Dumont & Provost, 1999). However, emotion-focused coping has been described as an effective coping strategy particularly when the individual has little control over the stressor (Lazarus, 1999). By the same token, avoidance-oriented coping may be an effective strategy to deal with severe stress in the short term only (Brodzinsky et al., 1992; Taylor & Stanton, 2007).

Brodzinsky et al., 1992 distinguished between cognitive avoidance and behavioral avoidance. Both types of avoidance strategies have been associated with internalizing and externalizing problems; Campos et al. (2012) found, however, that only cognitive avoidance protected adolescents who experienced many stressful life events from behavioral maladjustment. More active strategies (ie, approach strategies, such as seeking social support and problem solving) seem to be used more frequently than avoidance strategies throughout adolescence and stabilize during young adulthood; the opposite trend has been observed for avoidance strategies. Nevertheless, the bulk of research appears to indicate that beyond its association with impoverished physical and mental health and risk behaviors, avoidance-oriented coping obstructs the use of other more effective coping strategies (Taylor & Stanton, 2007).

Self-Regulation

All the definitions of self-regulation state that when individuals are self-regulatory, they adjust their behavior to pursue a goal or desired state (Carver & Scheier, 1998). Self-regulation refers to the processes by which individuals exercise control over their behavior, emotional states, and inner processes to achieve personally relevant goals or desired outcomes (Baumeister & Vohs, 2004). The importance of self-regulation has been one of the main topics of interest for researchers studying young people. Self-regulation has to do with the capacity to identify ecological risks and threats and develop adequate, relaxed, and competent coping strategies (Matos & Sampaio, 2009). It allows the relatively effortless management of emotions and desires that can lead to an alternative sense of well-being, competence, and self-fulfillment.

Self-regulation entails the use of strategies to attain desired outcomes or goals. These desired outcomes are, however, usually more positive in the long term than in the short term, which often means delaying gratification and resisting temptations (Vohs & Baumeister, 2004). However, the capacity to do so is difficult to develop. This is due to biological immaturity, which makes self-awareness challenging for children and adolescents, especially in real-life situations and very particularly in the presence of peers (Bjork et al., 2004; Bjork, Smith, Danube, & Hommer, 2007; Casey, Jones, & Hare, 2008; Casey, Jones, & Someville, 2011; Gardner & Steinberg, 2005; Oliva & Antolín, 2010; Steinberg, 2008).

Several studies have shown that the ability to regulate actions is developed progressively during childhood and adolescence. These periods require individuals to adjust to contexts and vice versa. This is a bidirectional regulation of the developmental process (Gestsdottir & Lerner, 2008). When applied to young children, the term "self-regulation" refers to various capacities, such as switching quickly between different tasks, focusing attention, or controlling emotions. Moreover, self-regulation measures adolescents' ability to monitor their activities, evaluate their performance, motivate themselves, and maintain their resilience while experiencing educational and social disappointments (Zimmerman, 2002).

The ability to identify, express, and manage (self-regulate) emotions is an important part of the successful development of adequate and competent coping strategies (Matos, 2005), making it possible for children to cope with and solve life threats, feel good about themselves, and promote wellness in others (Bryant & Veroff, 2007). Interventions should be designed to help individuals develop self-regulatory behaviors (Anderson, Winett, & Wojcik, 2007) and self-regulation cognitions and maximize the benefits of family and peer influences (Kalavana, Maes, & De Gucht, 2010). Furthermore, school curricula should also include a component that targets self-regulation and decision-making skills (Riggs, Sakuma, & Pentz, 2007).

Competence and Self-Efficacy

Perceptions of competence have been a central topic in human motivations. Deci and Ryan (2000) argued that the development of competence is a basic psychological need that influences people's cognitions, affect, and behaviors. Competence has multiple dimensions across five areas of youth functioning, including social, emotional, cognitive, behavioral, and moral competences (Catalano et al., 2004).

Social competence involves the use of interpersonal skills (eg, interpreting social cues, conflict resolution, making social decisions) to achieve specific social and interpersonal goals. Therefore, interventions in this dimension aim to enhance personal and interpersonal effectiveness and prosocial and health-enhancing values and beliefs and prevent maladaptive behavior. *Emotional competence* is "the ability to respond to feelings and emotional reactions in oneself and others" (Catalano et al., 2004, p. 104). It includes the ability to identify and manage the expression of emotions and show empathy. *Cognitive competence* involves, on the one hand, the ability to use cognitive skills, such as self-talk, self-awareness, problem solving, and decision making, and, on the other hand, the core capabilities for academic and intellectual achievement, such as logic, analytical thinking, and abstract reasoning. *Behavioral competence* denotes the effective use of verbal and nonverbal communication as well as the ability to take appropriate action. Finally, *moral competence* refers to the "ability to assess and respond to the ethical, affective, or social-justice dimensions of a situation" (Catalano et al., 2004, p. 105).

Competence is closely associated with self-efficacy. Self-efficacy refers to "beliefs in one's capabilities to organize and execute the courses of action required to produce given attainments" (Bandura, 1997, p. 3). Perceptions of self-efficacy are central to human behavior as they influence behavioral choices, the amount of effort put into behavioral pursuits, resilience in the face of adversity, and perseverance in the face of failure. Therefore, self-efficacy can be a powerful individual asset, for it holds the perceptions that one has the competence to exert control over one's own motivations, behavior, and social environment. Bandura's self-efficacy theory supports the use of cognitive interventions such as goal setting, self-talk, and observational learning to improve self-efficacy.

Competence and self-efficacy can be fundamental for the development of a sense of empowerment. Empowerment represents a perception of agency in as much as adolescents may develop a sense of ownership of their social environment. In this process, adolescents become aware that they have the capability to positively affect change in the environment and alter the manner in which they behave in it (Morton & Montgomery, 2011). Agency provides the motor for action. Awareness that the self is an active independent agent forms the basis of self-efficacy.

Self-Esteem

Self-esteem is a marker of psychosocial adjustment and represents a personal judgment of one's self-worth. Self-esteem is best understood in hierarchical models, as individuals can present a variety of levels of self-esteem, depending on the domain in which it is expressed (eg, academic, social, athletic) and the relevance individuals attribute to those domains (Guerra & Bradshaw, 2008). High self-esteem has been associated with high social support, resilience, life satisfaction (Dumont & Provost, 1999; Hoffman, Ushpiz, & Levy-Schiff, 1988), and long-term health and well-being (DuBois & Flay, 2004). Conversely, low self-esteem has been associated with a range of negative outcomes, such as depression and anxiety (Seifge-Krenk, 1995). Finally, self-esteem was the primary predictor of adolescent adjustment, indicating that positive personal perceptions about the self and one's own capabilities are important protective factors against stress and depression.

Social Connectedness

Social connectedness has been proposed as the primary determinant for youth adjustment (Guerra & Bradshaw, 2008). The need for relatedness is considered a basic human psychological need (Deci & Ryan, 2000) and adequate social support has been found to moderate the impact of stress on health (Dumont & Provost, 1999). Taylor and Stanton (2007) defined social support as "the perception or experience that one is loved and cared for by others, esteemed and valued, and part of a social network of mutual assistance and obligations" (p. 381). Adolescents' dissatisfaction with their social support has been associated with depression, anxiety, and poor sleep. In addition to feeling cared for, a sense of connectedness also involves caring about the social environment (Guerra & Bradshaw, 2008).

Social environments that provide adolescents with positive resources from significant others (eg, family, schools, communities) have been shown to facilitate more adaptive behavioral patterns characterized by fewer internalizing behaviors (eg, anxiety, depression), fewer externalizing behaviors (eg, hostility, isolation), and fewer academic problems, as well as more positive development opportunities, for example, with regard to social competence and self-esteem (Youngblade et al., 2007). The family context is fundamental in the development of well-adjusted, resilient adolescents. Family engagement, closeness, communication, and parental role-modeling were associated with adolescents' social competence, self-esteem, and health-promoting behavior (Youngblade et al., 2007). In addition, parental monitoring had a strong association with health behaviors (ie, dieting and physical activity) and a negative association with sedentary behaviors in youth with high risk of developing obesity (Lawman & Wilson, 2012).

Social support in the family context goes beyond the understanding of the traditional concept of family. Nowadays children live in diverse family structures. Researchers and practitioners need to consider the role of relationships with nonparental adults in adolescents' normative development (Sterret, Jones, McKee, & Kincaid, 2011). Sterret et al.'s review demonstrated that supportive nonparental adults (eg, extended family, teachers, community leaders, nonbiological care givers) have a positive impact on adolescents' academic functioning, self-esteem, and emotional and behavioral problems.

To develop connectedness, adolescents need to have social skills and opportunities to apply these skills; therefore, belonging to prosocial groups that model and encourage positive behaviors is psychologically rewarding (Guerra & Bradshaw, 2008). For example, adolescents who perceived their neighborhood as closely connected had greater social competence (Youngblade et al., 2007). Furthermore, participation in social activities has been correlated with self-esteem and perceptions of control (Dumont & Provost, 1999).

Social Capital

Social capital is a difficult concept to define because it encompasses a multiplicity of community-related characteristics that represent social determinants of health. Since the concept of community can be defined in a number of ways (eg, family, social groups, schools, neighborhood), social capital can be operationalized differently across social contexts. Vyncke et al. (2013) stated that "social capital refers to the idea that social networks are a potential resource for individuals, communities and society as a whole" (p. 3). Individuals establish a number of social networks, each one with its own specific characteristics and resources. These social networks represent the foundations of social capital. Social capital (Bourdieu, 1986; Putnam, 1993) includes strong ties among an exclusive group (eg, family), termed "bonding relationships," and more shallow relationships with a larger group (eg, friends and school colleagues) that are called "bridging relationships" (Morgan, Davies, & Ziglio, 2010; Morgan & Ziglio, 2007). Both bonding and bridging relationships are important for psychosocial development and well-being. Bonding relationships provide self-confidence, trust, and warmth, especially in the period before adolescence; bridging relationships provide company to explore the outside world, provide knowledge about cultures different from home, and are in a way the seed for human development. Bridging relationships pull together different perspectives and thus prevent the social stereotypes and xenophobic attitudes that arise from the "unknown." For example, "weak ties" with an enlarged social group (bridging relationships) encourage social progress and prevent xenophobic beliefs and attitudes. When individuals have the opportunity to engage in closer social contact with different kinds of cultures and ways of thinking, perceived interpersonal differences may be reinterpreted as beneficial to personal growth, lowering feelings of fear or mistrust (Granovetter, 1983).

A central issue in the construction and continuity of social capital is the feeling of "togetherness" or social cohesion in the family, school, and neighborhood (Kawachi, Kennedy, & Glass, 1999; Putnam, 1993). Social capital reinforces and is reinforced by feelings of trust, belonging, and social participation and engagement (Poortinga, 2006), both in school (or the workplace) and in the community. Extracurricular activities, volunteer activities, and leisure time out of school are important ways to strengthen young people's ties with their communities. This can help them develop their competence in leadership and decision making, increase their feeling of belonging, and get social support from adults (Brooks, 2006; Matos & Sampaio, 2009, 2015; Matos, Gaspar et al., 2012; Matos, Morgan, & Equipa do Projecto Aventura Social e Saúde, 2012).

Social capital can be operationalized in a number of ways depending on the context. For example, Morgan, Rivera, Moreno, and Haglund (2012) used measures of social capital and social support across a variety of social networks: family (eg, doing things together, allowing autonomy, monitoring), peers (eg, easy to talk to friends), neighborhood (eg, safety, friendliness, nice places to go), and school (eg, students are kind, helpful, and accepting; teachers are interested and encouraging). More recently, Garcia-Moya, Moreno, and Braun-Lewensohn (2013) found that SOC was negatively associated with neighborhood risks (ie, gang activity, social disorganization, and deprivation), and neighborhood assets (ie, resources associated with people, availability of recreational facilities, and neighborhood safety) were positively associated with SOC in a large sample of Spanish adolescents. Notably, while risks explained 4.1% of SOC variance, assets explained a further 6.5% of its variance, suggesting that social capital, mainly resources associated with significant people in the neighborhood, has the potential to play a protective role.

During adolescence, friends are an important source of social capital. Roth and Brooks-Gunn (2000) coined the acronym FRIEND to highlight a set of relevant aspects of peer relationships: *friendship, resisting* (peer pressure), *interests* (daily interests and commitments), *examples* (social role models), *numbers* (balance between risk and support), and *deviant* (association with deviant peers).

Even if during adolescence peers are a relevant factor, family remains a relevant factor, especially for long-lasting aspects of decision making. Letting young people participate in decision making in the family context helps them increase their sense of belonging, their responsibilities, and their expectations for the future (Werner & Smith, 2001). According to Frydenberg (2008), positive and supportive families have to be able to positively communicate with young people, provide support, optimize the expression of feelings and opinions, fully discuss problems, minimize conflicts, negotiate family plans, and develop cooperation and trust between parents and their children. Roth and Brooks-Gunn (2000) used the acronym TLC to summarize the characteristics of positive and supportive families: *time* (parents make time for their children), *limits* (they provide supervision, monitoring, and firm limits), and *connectedness* (they develop closeness and affective ties).

THE ASSETS MODEL AND A MORE ACTIVE AND HEALTHIER LIFESTYLE DURING PREADOLESCENCE AND ADOLESCENCE: HIGHLIGHTS FROM THE HEALTH BEHAVIOUR IN SCHOOL-AGED CHILDREN HEALTH SURVEY

The Health Behaviour in School-aged Children (HBSC) survey is a cross-European survey that aims at identifying, studying, and monitoring health and health behaviors of children and adolescents in their real social-life contexts (Currie, Hurrelmann, Settertobulte, Smith, & Todd, 2000; Currie et al., 2004, 2008, 2012). This large-scale international study includes children and adolescents from 11 to 16 years of age and uses gender-balanced national representative samples. The study began in the early 1980s and now includes 44 countries from Europe, the United States, Canada, and Israel (www.hbsc. org). The project involves researchers from various areas of health (eg, medical doctors, psychologists, sociologists, policy makers, public health experts, educators) and aims at influencing national public policies in the area of adolescent health.

The HBSC Portuguese research team has analyzed a variety of health-related behaviors [health-compromising or health-protective behaviors or social contexts, including physical activity, sedentary behaviors (mainly screen time), nutrition, body image, leisure, sports practice, violence, injuries, well-being, health symptoms, substance use, and sexual behavior], from a socioecological and assets model perspective. The Portuguese HBSC study has been conducted every 4 years, following the international protocol, since 1998. In 2014 the fifth wave was carried out. This repetition allowed the national team to monitor the lives and health of Portuguese adolescents in context. A few trends have been identified, but overall since 2002, the worst year for adolescent health in the country so far, Portuguese adolescents have become healthier and happier.

However, the most recent data from 2014 indicate an inversion in well-being and happiness perceptions following the recession period.

Besides identifying trends, researchers have conducted a systematic analysis of age- and gender-related differences in every wave, and results are rather consistent (Matos & Equipa do Projecto Aventura Social e Saúde, 2000, 2003, 2006, 2015). Younger children and boys reported doing more physical activity; older boys tended to attribute more importance to physical activity participation for their well-being; boys and younger children preferred to play team sports (ie, football, basketball), while girls did more gymnastics and swimming. In their leisure time, girls preferred sedentary activities, such as listening to music or hanging out with and talking to friends, while boys preferred to play video and computer games. Boys more often used the street, the school, and sports facilities in their leisure time, while girls preferred their own home or their friends' homes; school and own home were reported more frequently by younger children, while sports facilities and cafés were more frequently reported by older adolescents.

Physical activity can be seen as protective health behavior; however, this behavior often coexists with a variety of risk behaviors. For example, physical activity in boys was more frequently associated with reports of acts of violence, injuries, and withdrawal from school activities. These associations in behavioral patterns were not seen in girls, though (Matos, Calmeiro, Marques, & Loureiro, 2013). The reasons behind these associations are unclear and warrant further research, but similar results have been found with Greek adolescents (Papaioannou, Karastogiannidou, & Theodorakis, 2004) and North American high-school students (Demissie, Lowry, Eaton, Hertz, & Lee, 2014). Papaioannou et al. (2004) found a small positive relationship between sports involvement and sports violence and suggested the "winning-at-all-costs" sports culture as an explanatory mechanism. Demissie et al. (2014) found that engagement in physical fighting was associated with increased odds of daily physical activity and sports participation in boys particularly, suggesting a stronger role of peer context and tolerance to violence among boys compared to girls (Gardner, Roth, & Brooks-Gunn, 2009). Nevertheless, the association between health-enhancing and health-compromising behaviors warrants further research to clarify relevant mediating and moderating factors.

Physical Activity and Sedentary Behavior

The health benefits of physical activity are widely known and research that supports its usefulness as a health behavior is overwhelming (United States Department of Health & Human Services, 1996), leading to recommendations for adolescent physical activity that include 60 min of moderate-to-vigorous physical activity (MVPA) per day (Biddle & Mutrie, 2007). Nevertheless, studies have indicated that up to 80% of adolescents from countries around the world are not sufficiently active to comply with these recommendations (Hallal et al., 2012;

Kalman et al., 2015; Nader, Bradley, Houts, McRitchie, & O'Brien, 2008). Notably, Kalman et al. (2015) analyzed the trends in adolescents' physical activity from 2002 to 2010 in 32 countries included in the HBSC study and identified an increase of 1.6% in the proportion of 11- to 15-year-olds who met the recommendations of at least 60 min of MVPA daily. Changes in MVPA ranged from 11.9% and 5.7% for Finnish boys and girls, respectively, to 11.1% and 7.2% for Lithuanian boys and girls, respectively. These positive trends were verified for the 2002–06 period, with some reduction or at least maintenance during the period 2006–10. As expected, boys were not only more active than girls but also more likely to show a positive trend over the years. In addition, adolescents from higher socioeconomic backgrounds were more likely to be active than those from low socioeconomic backgrounds. Therefore, no evidence of a sharp decline in physical activity was observed, which can be seen as encouraging, considering the increasing opportunities for sedentary pursuits and less active forms of transportation.

The trend in Portugal was similar to the international trend with an increase in the percentage of boys (16–18.4%) and no change in the percentage of girls (8.4–8.5%) who met the recommended levels of MVPA (Kalman et al., 2015). Marques and Matos (2014) provided a more in-depth picture of these trends in Portugal. Because each cohort embodies a nationally representative sample of school children, comparisons between cohorts of different age groups were conducted to simulate a longitudinal design.

Results showed that there were no significant differences in the amount of physical activity performed by adolescents in the past 7 days during 2002, 2006, and 2010 within each age group (ie, 11–13 and 15–17), with the exception of 15- to 17-year-old boys. While the number of days per week of physical activity ranged from 4.2 to 4.4 in 11- to 13-year-old boys ($p = 0.243$), 15- to 17-year-old boys increased physical activity levels from 2002 to 2006, but then maintained this level in 2010 (respectively, 3.2, 3.9, and 3.8 days/week, $p = 0.019$). Concerning girls, the number of days per week of physical activity ranged from 3.3 to 3.5 in the 11- to 13-year-old group ($p = 0.456$) and from 2.7 to 2.9 in the 15- to 17-year-old group ($p = 0.056$). Moreover, there was a significant decline in physical activity among boys and girls when comparing the 2002–06 and 2006–10 cohorts (ie, 11- to 13-year-olds in 2002 vs 15- to 17-year-olds in 2006, and 11- to 13-year-olds in 2006 vs 15- to 17-year-olds in 2010). For both cohorts, the number of days per week of physical activity decreased in boys (4.2–3.9 days/week, $p = 0.001$ and 4.4–3.8 days/week, $p < 0.001$, respectively) and girls (3.5–2.7 days/week, $p < 0.001$ and 3.3–2.9 days/week, $p < 0.001$, respectively). These trends are troublesome as they suggest that efforts in the promotion of physical activity have been unsuccessful in reversing the tendency of adolescents to become less active as they age. Furthermore, the situation for teenage girls is particularly troublesome. For example, in three waves Portuguese girls were the least active of the participant countries in the HBSC (Currie et al., 2004, 2008, 2012; World Health Organization, 2009).

The physical and social characteristics of the neighborhoods in which adolescents live are important resources of social capital. Loureiro, Matos, Santos, Mota, and Diniz (2010b) evaluated the impact of the characteristics of the neighborhood on the physical activity of adolescents. Perceptions of the neighborhood as being unsafe were surprisingly associated with higher levels of children's outdoor practice and exercise. These results are likely to be a consequence of the search for more structure and supervised physical activities for children to engage in safely. In addition, the existence of places to spend time in the neighborhood and its aesthetic nature were associated with higher levels of physical activity in adolescents, as they have the necessary autonomy to walk or cycle to these places on their own.

Walking and cycling to and from school are opportunities to integrate physical activity into the adolescents' lifestyles. Loureiro and Matos (2014) recently analyzed the home–school transportation patterns in Portuguese adolescents and identified that 35% of the participants reported walking or cycling to school. Characteristics of the neighborhood influenced their decisions concerning active transportation; specifically, living in a residential area with good public services, aesthetically pleasant surroundings, and fewer nightlife entertainments were associated with active transportation. Conversely, unsafe and isolated areas were associated with less active transportation.

In a study with the 2010 cohort, Matos, Marques, Calmeiro, and Loureiro (2014) identified the behavioral profiles of adolescents and their association with physical activity, using both health behaviors (eg, physical activity, eating fruit) and risk behaviors (eg, engagement in violence, alcohol use). Cluster analysis resulted in the identification of four distinct profiles: The first profile consisted of adolescents who reported low engagement in both health and risk behavior (ie, low health and low risk behaviors); the second profile encompassed those who reported high frequency of health behaviors and low frequency of risk behavior (ie, high health and low risk behaviors); the third profile consisted of those who reported low frequency of health behaviors, high frequency of risk behaviors, and a positive perception of health (ie, low health, high risk behaviors with positive health perceptions); and the fourth profile was similar to Profile 3, except that participants reported low perceptions of health (ie, low health, high risk behaviors with negative health perceptions). Interestingly, adolescents who belonged to the clusters that featured high-risk behaviors reported higher levels of physical activity, which suggests that physical activity was not a protective factor against risk behavior. It would have been beneficial to differentiate the types of physical activities participants did, as some types may expose adolescents to a variety of risks that are typical of this developmental period. In fact, resilience develops in the face of risk and adversity (Kia-Keating et al., 2011). Although more active adolescents were more likely to report positive eating habits (ie, "eating fruit") and higher perceptions of life satisfaction and good health, physical activity was also associated with violent behavior, injuries, and alcohol abuse. Nevertheless, to promote physical activity, practitioners need to see beyond the beneficial and desirable health outcomes of participation and monitor and prevent associated risk behaviors (Matos et al., 2013).

Active lifestyles involve not only the promotion of physical activity but also the decrease of sedentary behaviors. Sedentary behavior has been defined by Pate, O'Neill, and Lobelo (2008) as "any activity that does not increase energy expenditure substantially and includes activities such as sleeping, sitting, lying down, and watching television and other forms of entertainment" (p. 173). These activities, often referred to as screen time, include watching TV, playing video games, and using computers, the Internet, and mobile phones, and recommendations suggest that children and adolescents should limit recreational screen time to less than 2 h per day (Tremblay et al., 2011a,b). Sedentary behavior affects health differently from physical activity (Hamilton, Healy, Dunstan, Zderic, & Owen, 2008). In a recent metaanalysis, Tremblay et al. (2011b) demonstrated that sedentary behavior was associated with reduced physical and psychosocial health in 5- to 17-year-olds. Specifically, TV viewing for more than 2 h per day was associated with poor body composition, low fitness levels, low self-esteem, fewer episodes of prosocial behavior, and decreased academic achievement.

Although screen-time behaviors appear to be at the low end of a physical activity continuum, recent evidence clearly suggests that physical activity and sedentary behavior are different behaviors with independent impact on health (Tremblay, Colley, Saunders, Healy, & Owen, 2010). For example, even among those individuals who have high levels of MVPA, those who spend more time watching TV are at a 1.5- to 2.0-fold increased risk of all-cause mortality (Matthews et al., 2012). In addition, time spent in sedentary screen-based activities was not associated with physical activity, suggesting that these behaviors can coexist (Biddle, Gorely, Marshall, Murdey, & Cameron, 2004; Beltrán-Carrillo, Beltrán-Carrillo, González-Cutre, Biddle, & Montero-Carretero, 2015). Therefore, the determinants of these two classes of behaviors should be studied carefully and interventions to increase physical activity and decrease sedentary behavior should be specifically designed.

International trends across HBSC countries indicate that leisure-time sedentary behavior tends to decrease from childhood to adolescence (World Health Organization, 2009). Prevalence data show that, in 2002, the proportion of adolescents who spent more than 4 h watching TV was approximately 24% on weekdays, with an increase to 43.3% on weekend days. In 2006, about two-thirds of the adolescents watched more than 2 h a day. Consistent with Beltrán-Carrillo et al.'s (2015) findings, boys reported watching more TV than girls (World Health Organization, 2009). Concerning computers, about one-third of the adolescents reported spending more than 2 h on weekdays playing games on a computer or game console. The use of computers to play games declined as children grew older, but it increased for Internet use and creative work (ie, writing, digital drawing). Boys reported more computer use than girls (49% vs 21% for 13-year-olds, and 46% vs 16% for 15-year-olds) on weekdays.

Portuguese HBSC data from 2010 (Matos & Equipa do Projecto Aventura Social e Saúde, 2011) and 2014 (Matos & Equipa do Projecto Aventura Social e Saúde, 2015) indicate some tendencies and gender differences in regard to sedentary behavior. The proportion of adolescents who reported spending between 1 and 3 h watching TV during the week decreased from 60.7% to 58.1% but during the weekend increased from 38.8% to 44.1%. Whereas in 2010 there were no gender differences, in 2014 girls reported more TV viewing during the weekend. Concerning the use of computers to play games, in 4 years there was a decrease from 41.8% to 38% on weekdays and from 43.2% to 39.5% on weekends. Boys reported playing computer games longer than girls. Finally, concerning the use of computers for activities such as browsing the Internet, chatting with friends, or doing homework, there was a decrease from 53.9% to 47.7% during the week and from 48.4% to 44.8% during the weekend. Interestingly, while in 2010 the boys reported more use of the computer for these activities, in 2014 there were no significant gender differences.

Loureiro, Matos, and Diniz (2010a) attempted to identify profiles of adolescents based on time spent watching TV and on time spent doing physical activity weekly (ie, active and TV viewers; nonactive and TV viewers; active and non-TV viewers, and nonactive and non-TV viewers). The main aim of this study was to explore the assumption that sedentary behaviors and physical activity coexist, and that individuals' behaviors can be described by two orthogonal axes, one active–nonactive and the other sedentary–nonsedentary. Nonactive TV viewers were more likely to be girls [odds ratio (OR) = 0.4] and adolescents with preobesity (OR = 2.7) or obesity (OR = 3.9) from a middle-class background (OR = 0.6). Active TV viewers were mostly boys (OR = 3.4) from a high economic background (OR = 1.7). Boys were more frequent in the active groups (ie, active TV viewers and active non-TV viewers) and girls were more frequent in the nonactive groups (ie, nonactive TV viewers and nonactive non-TV viewers). Older adolescents were more frequent in the group nonactive non-TV viewers, and younger adolescents were more frequent in the active non-TV viewers and active TV viewers. The results confirm that health promotion efforts should be directed at both increasing adolescents' activity and decreasing their sedentary behaviors.

Finally, Marques, Calmeiro, Loureiro, Frasquilho, and Matos (2015) studied the relation between screen-based behaviors, physical activity, and health complaints (ie, headaches, irritability, feeling nervous, and feeling low) and found that more screen time was positively associated with health complaints, with stronger effects on girls, and physical activity was negatively associated with these same health complaints, with stronger effects on boys. Further research needs to be conducted to explore how sedentary behavior and physical activity are associated with health assets to inform effective intervention strategies.

Life Satisfaction

The HBSC study identified a number of behaviors, self-perceptions, and environmental characteristics that are related to health and life satisfaction. Trends in self-rated health in Portugal followed the international trend for the HBSC countries overall: The proportion of adolescents who rated their health as "excellent" was significantly higher in 2006 and 2010 compared to 2002, but it remained unchanged when comparing 2006 and 2010. In addition, girls and older adolescents rated their health poorer than boys and younger adolescents. This pattern may be a consequence of the growing socioeconomic difficulties observed throughout Europe (Cavallo et al., 2015a).

Interestingly, the proportion of Portuguese adolescents who reported being satisfied with their lives remained similar from 2002 to 2006, but significant increases were observed when comparing 2002–06 and 2010. Again, girls and older adolescents reported lower life satisfaction than boys and younger adolescents (Cavallo et al., 2015b). Because life satisfaction may tap into emotional health, both life satisfaction and self-rated health provide an overall assessment of adolescents' health.

Nevertheless, a major concern in these trends is the impact of social inequalities in a variety of other indicators of health. For example, higher national income inequality resulted in less physical activity and life satisfaction and more psychological and physical symptoms (Elgar et al., 2015). These results reinforce the ecological nature of health behavior and adolescents' health and suggest the need for the development and implementation of political agendas that can tackle these health inequalities.

Calmeiro, Camacho, and Matos (2015) explored the influence of selected health assets in the prediction of life satisfaction in youth. Specifically, after controlling for gender and grade, sequential regression analysis showed that individual assets (persistence in learning, self-regulation, liking school, academic achievement, life objectives) explained 11.8% of adolescents' life satisfaction, while social assets (parental support, peer support, family relationship, parental monitoring, and school connectedness) explained a further 10.5% of the variance. Family relationships and school connectedness were the strongest predictors of life satisfaction, reinforcing the role of social interaction models in the promotion of PYD. The interaction between individual and social assets needs to be further understood for the development of effective interventions to improve quality of life.

IMPLICATIONS FOR HEALTH PROMOTION: MOVING FORWARD AND INFLUENCING PUBLIC HEALTH POLICIES

Steinberg (2008) claimed that young people lack the brain maturity needed to fully identify risks and cope with life threats, especially in real-life situations and in the presence of peers. He suggested that direct intervention programs are not efficient in reducing risk taking in young people. Young people may become better informed, but they do not change their behavior. Steinberg thus recommended changing national legislation to reduce their exposure to risk and make their involvement safer. Taking another approach, Matos and Sampaio (2009) proposed a model of intervention prescribing continued health promotional work directly with young people and their families and identifying the need to promote a safer environment and greater protection of adolescents (not only in the form of prohibitive measures, but also in the form of empowering interventions). This approach would make it possible to promote greater social cohesion, increase social capital, and develop social networks and social support (Morgan, 2007, 2010; Morgan & Ziglio, 2007; Morgan et al., 2010). In addition, it is strongly recommended that practitioners work directly with young people in real-life situations, helping them make decisions, identity threats and pitfalls, and become better informed about brain immaturity and resulting limitations; young people should be encouraged to develop additional ways of coping by promoting strategies of awareness, coping, and self-regulation and, if necessary, encouraging them to seek more information or help.

Yet health information is clearly insufficient. This is a fact that has been widely recognized and clearly documented, but it is just as ineffective to keep young people in a dependent situation, without autonomy, without a sense of responsibility, and overprotected by restrictive legislation, freeing them of personal responsibility and discouraging their social participation and civic commitment. Any solution that is put forward with the aim of discouraging risk taking in young people cannot involve overprotecting them until adulthood, giving them no autonomy, limited social participation and commitment, but also limited responsibility.

School and leisure time represent favorable contexts for social interaction and health promotion. Parents, schools, peer groups, neighbors, and the local community in general all must be jointly involved in a process of increasing social cohesion. There is clearly a need for a global community intervention in adolescent contexts (family, school, and community) to promote personal and social competence and increase social capital (Morgan, 2010; Morgan et al., 2010). The ultimate aim is the promotion of quality of life, well-being, competence, autonomy, and a personal sense of responsibility, which includes a sense of belonging and personal achievement, social participation, and commitment. A new approach to making people's lives more visible and better is the inclusion of target populations in all steps of health interventions: needs identification, defining objectives and priorities, defining and implementing strategies, evaluating and reformulating, making actions effective and sustainable (Matos, 2015).

In Portugal, after 20 years of studying adolescent health and health behaviors in the social contexts of their lives (Matos & Equipa do Projecto Aventura Social e Saúde, 2000, 2003, 2006, 2011, 2015), after designing, implementing, and evaluating promotional programs, mostly universal interventions in schools and in the communities (Gaspar, Morgan et al., 2012), and after a hard political advocacy for adolescents' health promotion (Working Group on Sexual Education, 2005, 2007; Matos et al., 2008), the next natural step was to create a youth-led participatory action research project. In this project, a nationwide group of young people was instructed to reflect on—and allowed to have a voice in—the public policies concerning their lives. This vision resulted in the Dream Teens project (http://www.dreamteens.aventurasocial.com, http://www.dreamteens2014-2015.blogspot.pt/ and http://dreamteensaventurasocial.blogs.sapo.pt/), started in May 2014, in which adolescents engaged in an enormous advocacy project over the course of 1 year. This work included two national meetings, several presentations and public debates at the regional level, and submission of a chart of recommendations to the Portuguese government (formally received by a high commissioner of the Ministry of Health and published on the Ministry of Health webpage). After the last meeting at the end of 2015, this group was formally organized as a youth association in order to achieve sustainability and support from the National Institute of Youth and Sports and the Choices Program of the High Commissioner of Migrations. The collaboration with the Dream Teens group resulted in the publication of a book in which the experience is described and the theoretical rationale is fully discussed (Matos, 2015).

CONCLUDING REMARKS

In this chapter, we emphasized the role of health assets as fundamental resources that allow individuals and communities to be active participants in health promotion. The basis of this approach lies in the assets model as a framework that focuses on the development of social and individual contexts that aim at optimizing personal and community resources. This approach guides the development of policies and programs through empowerment of youth and families within a health-enhancement perspective, in clear contrast to the prevailing medical model of disease management. Hence, the assets model uses concepts such as salutogenesis, self-regulation, resilience, and social capital as drivers of change.

The assets model is receiving increased attention from researchers and practitioners interested in public health from a variety of scientific areas. This is particularly visible in work on PYD that strongly relies on the ability of adolescents to realize their potential and manage risks. Health literacy is fundamental for adolescents to make reasonable, informed decisions concerning their health. With this in mind, the HBSC provides a plethora of crucial information for researchers, practitioners, and policy makers to develop a clearer understanding of the adolescents' view of the world. Attitudes, beliefs, life aspirations, social and physical environments, and behavioral patterns can form, or be influenced by, a number of resources that need to be identified, understood, and skillfully applied in intervention programs. Therefore, it is important to "give a voice" to adolescents, to listen to them and involve them in the decision-making process.

REFERENCES

Anderson, E. S., Winett, R. A., & Wojcik, J. R. (2007). Self-regulation, self-efficacy, outcome expectations, and social support: social cognitive theory and nutrition. *Annals of Behavioral Medicine, 34,* 304–312.

Antonovsky, A. (1996). The salutogenic model as a theory to guide health promotion. *Health Promotion International, 11,* 11–18.

Bandura, A. (1997). *Self-efficacy: the exercise of control.* New York, NY: Freeman.

Baumeister, R. F., & Vohs, K. D. (2004). Self-regulation. In: C. Perterson, & M. E. P. Seligman (Eds.), *Character strengths and virtues: a handbook and classification* (pp. 499–516). New York, NY: Oxford University Press.

Beltrán-Carrillo, V. J., Beltrán-Carrillo, J. I., González-Cutre, D., Biddle, S. J., Montero-Carretero, C. (2015). Are active video games associated with less screen media or conventional physical activity? *Games and Culture,* 1–17.

Biddle, S. J., & Mutrie, N. (2007). *Psychology of physical activity: determinants well-being and interventions* (2nd ed.). London, England: Routledge.

Biddle, S. J., Gorely, T., Marshall, S. J., Murdey, I., & Cameron, N. (2004). Physical activity and sedentary behaviours in youth: issues and controversies. *The Journal of the Royal Society for the Promotion of Health, 124,* 29–33.

Bjork, J., Knutson, B., Fong, G., Caggiano, D., Bennett, S., & Hommer, D. (2004). Incentive-elicited brain activation in adolescents: similarities and differences from young adults. *The Journal of Neuroscience, 24,* 1793–1802.

Bjork, J., Smith, A., Danube, C., & Hommer, D. (2007). Developmental differences in posterior mesofrontal cortex recruitment by risky rewards. *The Journal of Neuroscience, 27,* 4839–4849.

Bourdieu, P. (1986). The forms of capital. In: J. Richardson (Ed.), *Handbook of theory and research for the sociology of education* (pp. 241–258). New York, NY: Greenwood.

Brodzinsky, D. M., Elias, M. J., Steiger, C., Simon, J., Gill, M., & Hitt, J. C. (1992). Coping scale for children and youth: scale development and validation. *Journal of Applied Developmental Psychology, 13,* 195–214.

Bronfenbrenner, U. (1979). *The ecology of human development: experiments by nature and design.* Cambridge, MA: Harvard University Press.

Brooks, J. (2006). Strengthening resilience in children and youths: maximizing opportunities through the school. *Children & Schools, 28,* 69–76.

Bryant, F., & Veroff, J. (2007). *Savoring: a new model of positive experience.* Mahwah, NJ: Erlbaum.

Calmeiro, L., & Matos, M. G. (2004). *Psicologia da saude e do exercicio.* Lisbon, Portugal: Omniservicos.

Calmeiro, L., Camacho, I., Matos, M. G. (2015). Predicting life satisfaction in youth: the role of individual and social health assets. In: *Proceedings of the fifth ENSEC conference on social emotional learning and culture.* Lisbon, Portugal.

Campos, R. M. E., Delgado, A. O., & Jiménez, Á. P. (2012). Acontecimientos vitales estresantes, estilo de afrontamiento y ajuste adolescente: un análisis longitudinal de los efectos de moderación. *Revista Latinoamericana de Psicología, 44,* 39–53.

Carver, C. S., & Scheier, M. F. (1998). *On the self-regulation of behavior.* New York, NY: Cambridge University Press.

Casey, B. J., Jones, R., & Hare, T. (2008). The adolescent brain. *Annals of the New York Academy of Sciences, 1124,* 111–126.

Casey, B. J., Jones, R., & Somerville, L. (2011). Braking and accelerating the adolescent brain. *Journal of Research on Adolescence, 21,* 21–33.

Catalano, R. F., Berglund, M. L., Ryan, J. A., Lonczak, H. S., & Hawkins, J. D. (2004). Positive youth development in the United States: research findings on evaluations of positive youth development programs. *Annals of the American Academy of Political and Social Science, 591,* 98–124.

Cavallo, F., Dalmasso, P., Ottová-Jordan, V., Brooks, F., Mazur, J., Välimaa, R., & Raven-Sieberer, U. (2015a). Trends in self-rated health in European and North-American adolescents from 2002 to 2010 in 32 countries. *The European Journal of Public Health, 25*(Suppl. 2), 13–15.

Cavallo, F., Dalmasso, P., Ottová-Jordan, V., Brooks, F., Mazur, J., Välimaa, R., & Raven-Sieberer, U. (2015b). Trends in life satisfaction in European and North-American adolescents from 2002 to 2010 in over 30 countries. *The European Journal of Public Health, 25*(Suppl. 2), 80–82.

Currie, C., Hurrelmann, K., Settertobulte, W., Smith, R., Todd, J. (Eds.), (2000). *Health and health behaviour among young people.* Health Policy for Children and Adolescents, No. 1. Copenhagen, Denmark: World Health Organization.

Currie, C., Roberts, C., Morgan, A., Smith, R., Settertobulte, W., Samdal, O., Barnekow Rasmussen, V. (Eds.), (2004). Young people's health in context. *Health Behaviour in School-aged Children (HBSC) study: International report from the 2001/2002 survey.* Health Policy for Children and Adolescents, No. 4. Copenhagen, Denmark: World Health Organization.

Currie, C., Gabhainn, S., Godeau, E., Roberts, C., Smith, R., Currie, D., Barnekow, V. (Eds.), (2008). Inequalities in young people's health. *Health Behaviour in School-aged Children: International report from the 2005/2006 survey.* Health Policy for Children and Adolescents, No. 5. Copenhagen, Denmark: World Health Organization.

Currie C., Zanotti, C., Morgan, A., Currie, D., Looze, M., Roberts, C., Barnekow, V. (Eds.), (2012). Social determinants of health and well-being among young people. *Health Behaviour in School-aged Children (HBSC) study: International report from the 2009/2010 survey.* Health Policy for Children and Adolescents, No. 6.Copenhagen, Denmark: World Health Organization.

Damon, W. (2004). What is positive youth development? *Annals of the American Academy of Political and Social Science, 591,* 13–24.

Deci, E. L., & Ryan, R. M. (2000). The "what" and the "why" of goal pursuits: human needs and self-determination of behaviour. *Psychological Inquiry, 11,* 227–268.

Demissie, Z., Lowry, R., Eaton, D. K., Hertz, M. F., & Lee, S. M. (2014). Associations of school violence with physical activity among US high school students. *Journal of Physical Activity & Health, 11,* 705–711.

DuBois, D. L., & Flay, B. R. (2004). The healthy pursuit of self-esteem: comment on an alternative to the Crocker and Park 2004 formulation. *Psychological Bulletin, 130,* 415–420.

Dumont, M., & Provost, M. A. (1999). Resilience in adolescents: protective role of social support, coping strategies, self-esteem, and social activities on experience of stress and depression. *Journal of Youth and Adolescence, 28,* 343–363.

Edwards, O. W., Mumford, V. E., Shillingford, M. A., & Serra-Roldan, R. (2007). Developmental assets: a prevention framework for students considered at risk. *Children & Schools, 29,* 145–153.

Elgar, F. J., Pförtner, T. K., Moor, I., De Clercq, B., Stevens, G. W., & Currie, C. (2015). Socioeconomic inequalities in adolescent health 2002–2010: a time-series analysis of 34 countries participating in the Health Behaviour in School-aged Children study. *The Lancet, 385,* 2088–2095.

Eriksson, M., & Lindström, B. (2005). Validity of Antonovsky's sense of coherence scale: a systematic review. *Journal of Epidemiology and Community Health, 59,* 460–466.

Eriksson, M., & Lindström, B. (2006). Antonovsky's sense of coherence scale and the relation with health: a systematic review. *Journal of Epidemiology and Community Health, 60,* 376–381.

Fergus, S., & Zimmerman, M. A. (2005). Adolescent resilience: a framework for understanding healthy development in the face of risk. *Annual Review of Public Health, 26*, 399–419.

Flensborg-Madsen, T., Ventegodt, S., & Merrick, J. (2005). Sense of coherence and physical health. A review of previous findings. *The Scientific World Journal, 5*, 665–673.

Fletcher, D., & Sarkar, M. (2013). Psychological resilience: a review and critique of definitions, concepts, and theory. *European Psychologist, 18*, 12–23.

Frasquilho, D., Matos, M. G., Gaspar, T., & Almeida, J. M. C. (2014). Do adolescents' future expectations differ by parental employment situation? Highlights from the Portuguese HBSC/WHO survey. *International Journal of Development Research, 4*, 1981–1986.

Frydenberg, E. (2008). *Adolescent coping*. New York, NY: Psychology Press.

García-Moya, I., Moreno, C., & Braun-Lewensohn, O. (2013). Neighbourhood perceptions and sense of coherence in adolescence. *The Journal of Primary Prevention, 34*, 371–379.

Gardner, M., & Steinberg, L. (2005). Peer influences on risk taking, risk preferences and risky decisions making in adolescence and adulthood: an experimental study. *Development Psychology, 4*, 625–635.

Gardner, M., Roth, J., & Brooks-Gunn, J. (2009). Sports participation and juvenile delinquency: the role of the peer context among adolescent boys and girls with varied histories of problem behavior. *Developmental Psychology, 45*, 341–353.

Gestsdottir, S., & Lerner, R. M. (2008). Positive development in adolescence: the development and role of intentional self-regulation. *Human Development, 51*, 202–224.

Granovetter, M. (1983). The strength of weak ties: a network theory revisited. *Sociological Theory, 1*, 201–233.

Guerra, N. G., & Bradshaw, C. P. (2008). Linking the prevention of problem behaviors and positive youth development: core competencies for positive youth development and risk prevention. *New Directions for Child and Adolescent Development, 122*, 1–17.

Hallal, P. C., Andersen, L. B., Bull, F. C., Guthold, R., Haskell, W., & Ekelund, U. Lancet Physical Activity Series Working Group. (2012). Global physical activity levels: surveillance progress, pitfalls, and prospects. *The Lancet, 380*, 247–257.

Hamilton, M. T., Healy, G. N., Dunstan, D. W., Zderic, T. W., & Owen, N. (2008). Too little exercise and too much sitting: inactivity physiology and the need for new recommendations on sedentary behavior. *Current Cardiovascular Risk Reports, 2*, 292–298.

Hoffman, M. A., Ushpiz, V., & Levy-Schiff, R. (1988). Social support and self-esteem in adolescence. *Journal of Youth and Adolescence, 17*, 307–316.

Kalavana, T. V., Maes, S., & De Gucht, V. (2010). Interpersonal and self-regulation determinants of healthy and unhealthy eating behavior in adolescents. *Journal of Health Psychology, 15*, 44–52.

Kalman, M., Inchley, J., Sigmundova, D., Iannotti, R. J., Tynjälä, J. A., Hamrik, Z., & Bucksch, J. (2015). Secular trends in moderate-to-vigorous physical activity in 32 countries from 2002 to 2010: a cross-national perspective. *The European Journal of Public Health, 25*(Suppl. 2), 37–40.

Kawachi, I. (2010). The relationship between health assets social capital and cohesive communities. In: A. D. Morgan, M. Davies, & E. Ziglio (Eds.), *Health assets in a global context* (pp. 167–179). New York, NY: Springer.

Kawachi, I., Kennedy, B. P., & Glass, R. (1999). Social capital and self-rated health: a contextual analysis. *American Journal of Public Health, 89*, 1187–1193.

Kia-Keating, M., Dowdy, E., Morgan, M. L., & Noam, G. G. (2011). Protecting and promoting: an integrative conceptual model for healthy development of adolescents. *Journal of Adolescent Health, 48*, 220–228.

Kobau, R., Seligman, M. E., Peterson, C., Diener, E., Zack, M. M., Chapman, D., & Thompson, W. (2011). Mental health promotion in public health: perspectives and strategies from positive psychology. *American Journal of Public Health, 101*(8), e1–e9.

Lawman, H. G., & Wilson, D. K. (2012). A review of family and environmental correlates of health behaviors in high-risk youth. *Obesity, 20*, 1142–1157.

Lazarus, R. S. (1999). *Stress and emotion: a new synthesis*. New York, NY: Springer.

Lazarus, R. S., & Folkman, S. (1984). *Stress appraisal and coping*. New York, NY: Springer.

Lerner, R. M., & Benson, P. L. (2003). *Developmental assets and asset-building communities: implications for research policy and practice*. New York, NY: Kluwer Academic/Plenum Publishers.

Lerner, J. V., Phelps, E., Forman, Y. E., & Bowers, E. P. (2009). Positive youth development. In: R. M. Lerner, & L. Steinberg (Eds.), *Handbook of adolescent psychology, volume 1: Individual bases of adolescent development*. 3rd ed. (pp. 524–557). Hoboken, NJ: John Wiley & Sons.

Loureiro, N., & Matos, M. G. (2014). Why don't they walk or cycle? Reflections on active home–school transportation among Portuguese adolescents: the role of environmental perceptions. *Urban Planning and Transport Research, 2*, 265–273.

Loureiro, N., Matos, M. G., & Diniz, A. (2010a). Adolescentes activos e adolescents sedentarios: a realidade portuguesa. *Revista de Psicologia da Crianca e do Adolescente, 2*, 175–190.

Loureiro, N., Matos, M. G., Santos, M. M., Mota, J., & Diniz, J. A. (2010b). Neighborhood and physical activities of Portuguese adolescents. *International Journal of Behavioral Nutrition and Physical Activity, 7*, 33.

Marques, A., & Matos, M. G. (2014). Adolescents' physical activity trends over the years: a three-cohort study based on the Health Behaviour in School-aged Children (HBSC) Portuguese survey. *BMJ Open, 4*(10), e006012.

Marques, A., Calmeiro, L., Loureiro, N., Frasquilho, D., & de Matos, M. G. (2015). Health complaints among adolescents: associations with more screen-based behaviours and less physical activity. *Journal of Adolescence, 44*, 150–157.

Matos, M. G. (2005). *Comunicação gestão de conflitos e saúde na escola*. Lisbon, Portugal: FMH.

Matos, M. G. (2015). *Dream Teens: Adolescents in safe navigation through unknown waters*. Lisbon, Portugal: Coisas de Ler.

Matos, M. G., & Equipa do Projecto Aventura Social e Saúde. (2000). *A Saúde dos Adolescentes Portugueses* [*Portuguese adolescents' health*]. Lisbon, Portugal: Edições FMH. Available from www.aventurasocial.com

Matos, M. G., & Equipa do Projecto Aventura Social e Saúde. (2003). *A Saúde dos Adolescentes Portugueses (Quatro anos depois)* [*Portuguese adolescents' health: Four years later*]. Lisbon, Portugal: Edições FMH. Available from www.aventurasocial.com

Matos, M. G., & Equipa do Projecto Aventura Social e Saúde. (2006). *A Saúde dos Adolescentes Portugueses hoje e desde há 8 anos* [*Portuguese adolescents' health: Now and in the last 8 years*]. Available from www.aventurasocial.com

Matos, M. G., & Equipa do Projecto Aventura Social e Saúde. (2011). *A Saúde dos Adolescentes Portugueses nos últimos 12 anos* [*Portuguese adolescents' health in the last 12 years*]. Available from www.aventurasocial.com

Matos, M. G., & Equipa do Projecto Aventura Social e Saúde. (2015). *A Saúde dos Adolescentes Portugueses em tempos de recessão* [*Portuguese adolescents' health in times of recession*]. Available from www.aventurasocial.com

Matos, M. G., & Sampaio, D. (2009). *Jovens com saúde: Diálogos com uma geração*. Lisbon, Portugal: Texto Editores.

Matos, M. G., Baptista, M. I., Simões, C., Gaspar, T., Sampaio, D., Diniz, J. A., … Sardinha, L. (2008). Portugal: from research to practice-promoting positive health for adolescents in schools. In: *Social cohesion for mental well-being among adolescents*. WHO/HBSC FORUM 2007.

Matos, M. G., Gaspar, T., Ferreira, M., Tomé, G., Camacho, I., Reis, M., Melo, P., & Simões Equipa Aventura Social (2012a). Keeping a focus on self-regulation and competence: "Find your own style," a school based program targeting at risk adolescents. *Journal of Cognitive and Behavioral Psychotherapies*, *12*, 39–48.

Matos, M. G., Morgan, A., Equipa Aventura Social. (2012b). Roads to whatever or roads to a self-fulfilled future? Health assets and wellbeing in children and adolescents. In: F. C. Gulbenkian (Ed.), *Adolescence: roads to whatever*. Lisbon, Portugal: Gulbenkian.

Matos, M. G., Calmeiro, L., Marques, A., & Loureiro, N. (2013). Does physical activity promotion advantages need the identification of associated health compromising features such as injuries, alcohol use and interpersonal violence? Highlights from HBSC/WHO Portuguese Survey. *Journal of Child and Adolescent Behavior*, *1*, 1–6.

Matos, M. G., Marques, A., Calmeiro, L., & Loureiro, N. (2014). Differentes perfis comportamentais em adolescentes e associacao a pratica de actividade física [Different behavioral profiles in adolescents and their relationship with physical activity]. *Psicologia Saúde e Doenças*, *15*, 495–509.

Matthews, C. E., George, S. M., Moore, S. C., Bowles, H. R., Blair, A., Park, Y., & Schatzkin, A. (2012). Amount of time spent in sedentary behaviors and cause-specific mortality in US adults. *The American Journal of Clinical Nutrition*, *95*, 437–445.

Morgan, A. (2007). Frameworks for improving young people's mental well-being: assets and deficits models. *WHO/HBSC Forum: Social Cohesion and Mental Health, 2007*. Las Palmas, March 2007.

Morgan, A. (2010). Social capital as a health asset for young people's health and well-being. *Journal of Child and Adolescent Psychology*, *2*, 19–43.

Morgan, A., & Ziglio, E. (2007). Revitalising the evidence base for public health: an asset model. *Promotion and Education*, *14*(Suppl. 2), 17–22.

Morgan, A., Davies, M., & Ziglio, E. (2010). *Health assets in a global context: theory methods action*. New York, NY: Springer.

Morgan, A. R., Rivera, F., Moreno, C., & Haglund, B. J. (2012). Does social capital travel? Influences on the life satisfaction of young people living in England and Spain. *BMC Public Health*, *12*(1), 138.

Morton, M., & Montgomery, P. (2011). Youth empowerment programs for improving self-efficacy and self-esteem of adolescents. *Campbell Systematic Reviews*, 5. DOI: 10.4073/csr.2011.5

Murphey, D. A., Lamonda, K. H., Carney, J. K., & Duncan, P. (2004). Relationships of a brief measure of youth assets to health-promoting and risk behaviors. *Journal of Adolescent Health*, *34*, 184–191.

Nader, P. R., Bradley, R. H., Houts, R. M., McRitchie, S. L., & O'Brien, M. (2008). Moderate-to-vigorous physical activity from ages 9 to 15 years. *JAMA*, *300*, 295–305.

Oliva, A., & Antolín, L. (2010). Cambios en el cerebro adolescente y conductas agresivas y de asunción de riesgos. *Estudios de Psicología*, *31*, 53–66.

Papaioannou, A., Karastogiannidou, C., & Theodorakis, Y. (2004). Sport involvement, sport violence and health behaviours of Greek adolescents. *The European Journal of Public Health*, *14*, 168–172.

Pate, R. R., O'Neill, J. R., & Lobelo, F. (2008). The evolving definition of "sedentary". *Exercise Sport Sciences Reviews*, *36*, 173–178.

Poortinga, W. (2006). Social relations or social capital? Individual and community health effects of bonding social capital. *Social Science & Medicine*, *6*, 255–270.

Putnam, R. (1993). The prosperous community: social capital and community life. *American Prospect, 13*, 35–42.

Riggs, N. R., Sakuma, K. L. K., & Pentz, M. A. (2007). Preventing risk for obesity by promoting self-regulation and decision-making skills: pilot results from the PATHWAYS to Health Program (PATHWAYS). *Evaluation Review, 31*, 287–310.

Rivera, F., Ramos, P., & Moreno, C. (2011). Análisis del modelo salutogénico en España: aplicación en salud pública e implicaciones para el modelo de activos en salud. *Revista Española de Salud Pública, 85*, 137–147.

Rivera, F., García-Moya, I., Moreno, C., & Ramos, P. (2013). Developmental contexts and sense of coherence in adolescence: a systematic review. *Journal of Health Psychology, 18*, 800–812.

Roth, J., & Brooks-Gunn, J. (2000). What do adolescents need for healthy development? Implications for youth policy. *Social Policy Report, 14*, 3–19.

Rutter, M. (1987). Psychological resilience and protective mechanisms. *American Journal of Orthopsychiatry, 57*, 316–331.

Scales, P. C. (1999). Reducing risks and building developmental assets: essential actions for promoting adolescent health. *Journal of School Health, 69*, 113–119.

Scales, P. C., Benson, P. L., Leffert, N., & Blyth, D. A. (2000). Contribution of developmental assets to the prediction of thriving among adolescents. *Applied Developmental Science, 4*, 27–46.

Search Institute. (2006). *40 developmental assets for adolescents*. Available from http://www.search-institute.org/content/40-developmental-assets-adolescents-ages-12-18

Seifge-Krenk, I. (1995). *Stress, coping and relationships in adolescence*. Hillsdale, NJ: Erlbaum.

Steinberg, L. (2008). A social neuroscience perspective on adolescent risk taking. *Development Review, 28*, 78–106.

Sterrett, E. M., Jones, D. J., McKee, L. G., & Kincaid, C. (2011). Supportive non-parental adults and adolescent psychosocial functioning: using social support as a theoretical framework. *American Journal of Community Psychology, 48*, 284–295.

Suls, J., & Fletcher, B. (1985). The relative efficacy of avoidant and non-avoidant coping strategies: a meta-analysis. *Health Psychology, 4*, 249–288.

Taylor, S. E., & Stanton, A. L. (2007). Coping resources, coping processes, and mental health. *Annual Review of Clinical Psychology, 3*, 377–401.

Theokas, C., Lerner, R. M., & Phelps, E. (2005). Developmental assets and the promotion of positive development: findings from Search Institute data. *Focal Point, 19*, 27–30.

Tremblay, M. S., Colley, R. C., Saunders, T. J., Healy, G. N., & Owen, N. (2010). Physiological and health implications of a sedentary lifestyle. *Applied Physiology, Nutrition, and Metabolism, 35*, 725–740.

Tremblay, M. S., LeBlanc, A. G., Janssen, I., Kho, M. E., Hicks, A., Murumets, K., & Duggan, M. (2011a). Canadian sedentary behaviour guidelines for children and youth. *Applied Physiology Nutrition, and Metabolism, 36*, 59–64.

Tremblay, M. S., LeBlanc, A. G., Kho, M. E., Saunders, T. J., Larouche, R., Colley, R. C., & Gorber, S. C. (2011b). Systematic review of sedentary behaviour and health indicators in school-aged children and youth. *International Journal of Behavioral Nutrition and Physical Activity, 8*, 98.

United States Department of Health & Human Services. (1996). *Physical activity and health: a report of the Surgeon General*. Atlanta, GA: Center for Disease Control and Prevention.

Vohs, K. D., & Baumeister, R. F. (2004). Understanding self-regulation: an introduction. In: R. F. Baumeister, & K. D. Vohs (Eds.), *Handbook of self-regulation: research, theory, and applications* (pp. 1–9). New York, NY: Guilford Press.

Vyncke, V., De Clercq, B., Stevens, V., Costongs, C., Barbareschi, G., Jónsson, S. H., & Maes, L. (2013). Does neighbourhood social capital aid in levelling the social gradient in the health and well-being of children and adolescents? A literature review. *BMC Public Health, 13*(1), 65.

Werner, E., & Smith, R. (2001). *Journeys from childhood to midlife: Risk, resilience and recovery*. Ithaca, NY: Cornell University Press.

White, A., & Pulla, V. (2013). Strengthening the capacity for resilience in children. *Perspectives on Coping and Resilience, 1*, 121–159.

Working Group on Sexual Education. (2005). *Relatório preliminar do Grupo de Trabalho para a Educação Sexual, Ministério da Educação*. [*Preliminary report of the Working Group on Sexual Education, Ministry of Education*]. Available from http://www.dgidc.min-edu.pt/EducacaoSexual

Working Group on Sexual Education. (2007). *Relatório final do Grupo de Trabalho para a Educação Sexual, Ministério da Educação*. [*Preliminary report of the Working Group on Sexual Education, Ministry of Education*]. Available from http://www.dgidc.min-edu.pt/EducacaoSexual

World Health Organization. (1986). *Ottawa Charter for health promotion*. Geneva, Switzerland: World Health Organization.

World Health Organization. (2009). *A snapshot of the health of young people in Europe*. Copenhagen, Denmark: World Health Organization.

Youngblade, L. M., Theokas, C., Schulenberg, J., Curry, L., Huang, I. C., & Novak, M. (2007). Risk and promotive factors in families, schools, and communities: a contextual model of positive youth development in adolescence. *Pediatrics, 119*(Suppl. 1), S47–S53.

Zimmerman, J. (2002). Achieving academic excellence: a self-regulatory perspective. In: M. Ferrari (Ed.), *The pursuit of excellence through education* (pp. 85–110). Mahwah, NJ: Erlbaum.

Chapter 21

Emotional Experiences and Interpersonal Relations in Physical Activity as Health Prevention and Treatment—A Psychodynamic Group Approach

Kirsten Kaya Roessler

Department of Psychology, Faculty of Health Sciences, University of Southern Denmark, Odense, Denmark

INTRODUCTION

In general, exercise has been shown to improve self-experienced quality of life and health both for nonclinical and clinical populations (Pedersen & Saltin, 2006; Faulkner & Taylor, 2005). There is evidence that physical activity can lower blood pressure and reduce the risk of coronary heart disease and stroke (Cornellisen & Fagard, 2005; Lewington, Clarke, Oizilbash, Peto, & Collins, 2002), help people achieve weight loss and manage diabetes (Tuomilehto et al., 2001; Houmard et al., 2004), and reduce both pain (Nygaard Andersen et al., 2014; Zebis et al., 2011) and the risk of developing breast and colon cancer (Thune & Furberg, 2001).

With regard to mental health, physical exercise can relieve moderate depression (Babyak et al., 2000; Blumenthal et al., 1999), better the symptoms of dementia (Laurin, Verreault, & Lindsay, 2005), be an adjunct treatment for schizophrenia (Faulkner & Taylor, 2005), be a part of the treatment of alcohol and substance abuse (Brown et al., 2009a; Monti, Rohsenow, & Hutchison, 2000), and have an effect on social and motor deficiencies among autism disorder patients (Sowa & Meulenbroeck, 2012).

This chapter presents psychological aspects of physical exercise in the field of health promotion and treatment. Physical exercise can improve social skills, self-esteem, mood, and coping behavior and is in general associated with a person's psychological well-being. However, the initiation and maintenance of

Sport and Exercise Psychology Research. http://dx.doi.org/10.1016/B978-0-12-803634-1.00021-2
461

behavioral change with regard to exercise is extremely challenging and often characterized by failure. The aim of this chapter is therefore to draw attention to the relational and existential psychological aspects of exercise interventions.

THEORETICAL FRAMEWORK AND METHOD

The theoretical approach described in this chapter was developed at the Department of Psychology and the Department of Sport Sciences, University of Southern Denmark (Roessler, 2010, 2011). My colleagues and I use this approach to examine psychological aspects of group processes especially among patients with chronic somatic diseases. The approach focuses primarily on the significance of the interactional process, especially in supportive relationships (Roessler, Glintborg, Ravn, Birkebæk, & Andersen, 2012). Health-related interventions normally start with a specific context such as the organization (eg, hospital, community), the structure (eg, supervised, nonsupervised), the financing (eg, self-payment, paid), or the duration (eg, 12 weeks) of a project and use this to frame the examination of the outcomes of the intervention (eg, reduced weight, lower blood pressure, freedom from drug dependency, etc.).The processes that patients or participants experience and interpersonally create often remain in a "black box" (Fig. 21.1).

This chapter provides a closer analysis of the black box. Five relevant focus categories that influence the outcomes of an intervention are described: *feedback, cohesion, corrective emotional experience,* similarities in *suffering,* and group *climate* (Fig. 21.2). These five categories have their roots in the traditions of psychoanalysis and humanist psychology. In all the cases presented in this chapter, a psychodynamic approach (Alexander & French, 1946; Winnicott, 1965; Streeck, 2007; Egle, Hoffmann, Lehmann, & Nix, 2015) was chosen to look at the role of interpersonal relations in health interventions.

Our approach looks especially at the motivating role of learning (Yalom & Leszcz, 2005) that takes place in the interpersonal connection between participants, physiotherapists, general practitioners (GPs), and their environment. The term *corrective emotional experience* (Alexander & French, 1946) was introduced to describe learning and behavioral change during an intervention. Originally, it described the crucial process that takes place during psychotherapy, whereby the therapeutic setting is seen as a context in which patients are reexposed in a secure environment—created, for example, by the empathy and awareness of the therapist (Streeck, 2007; Streeck & Leichsenring, 2009)—to

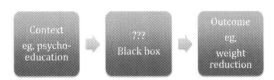

FIGURE 21.1   Context–black box–outcome.

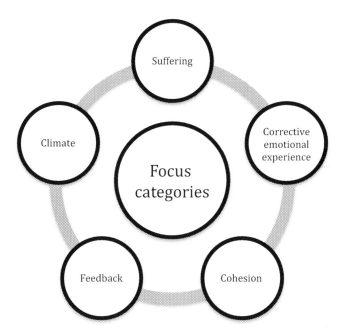

FIGURE 21.2   Five focus categories of a psychodynamic approach (Roessler, 2010, 2011; Roessler et al., 2012).

emotional situations that they could not handle in the past. To get better, the patient must undergo a corrective emotional experience that can repair the traumatic influence of previous experiences. For this purpose, the therapist adopts a "holding" attitude (Winnicott, 1964), which makes it possible for the patient first to undergo a therapeutic regression, then to have a corrective emotional experience, and afterwards to try out new behavior, initially in a secure environment and later in daily life. The corrective emotional experience in the context of an exercise program is understood as a *reeducation of emotions* that is linked to physical activity.

Using the five focus categories (Fig. 21.2), the aim is to understand how a change of behavior is brought about, or why a desired behavior is not achieved. The focus is on communication between people, and the aim is, on the one hand, to understand psychological and social processes and, on the other, to assist the analysis and evaluation of interventions. In any case, the black box of the classic model is extended by a description of the processes within a group.

Technique when Leading Group Sessions

During group counseling sessions, the group leader (psychologist, instructor, physiotherapist, etc.) uses a technique based on psychodynamic group therapy to create an empathic and safe atmosphere (Streeck & Leichsenring, 2009). The patients (or participants) react to a changing world of experience and have many opportunities to select or reject certain forms of behavior. The group leader tries to accept this individual reality rather than modify it. The patients' current experience of their disease provides a background for each session. The particular significance of the responding modus, here termed feedback, whereby the group leader reveals his or her own experience in a selective and purposeful way, is based on an interactional method that assumes that everyday challenges and problems of the participants will repeat themselves in a group situation and thus enable participants to change their behavior or attitude in a supportive environment (Leichsenring, Rabung, & Leibing, 2004).

Technique when Observing and Analyzing Group Sessions

When observing and analyzing group sessions, the observer has to answer several questions (Table 21.1). To establish the reliability of studies and to validate their findings, several steps are taken. Group counseling sessions are filmed, tape-recorded, and transcribed verbatim. Likewise, physical exercise sessions are videotaped, if possible, and the leaders write their observations and experiences down immediately after the session. The tapes and observations are coded and analyzed individually based on a question guide developed by Streeck and Leichsenring (2009; Table 21.1) and the five focus categories of the group approach (Roessler, 2010, 2011; Fig. 21.2). After the coding process, the main themes are described and analyzed with the focus on the five categories. The following section presents three Danish cases that describe attempts to change emotional experiences and behavior regarding physical activity.

TABLE 21.1 Question Guide for Analysis of the Group Sessions (Streeck & Leichsenring, 2009)

Questions
What are the participants talking about? (Theme of the session)
How can you describe the interaction? (Description of the situation)
Are there common rules or norms in the group?
Which emotions do the participants mention?
Which affects and emotions are visible?
Are there special relations between participants?
How can the participant differentiate between emotions? (Psychological functions)
What does the group leader do? (Interventions of the leader)

CASE 1: EXERCISE ON PRESCRIPTION—CHALLENGES OF A COMMUNITY-BASED PROGRAM

During the period 2004–07, Danish patients with lifestyle-related diseases received a prescription for exercise from their GPs. The program was based on primary health care and tried to help patients change their lifestyle by prescribing them physical training. To be included in the program, the patients had to have at least one of the following diagnoses: type 2 diabetes, above-normal cholesterol level (dyslipidemia), or above-normal blood pressure (hypertension). The patients received four months of supervised physical group training twice weekly, with the intention that they would continue to be physically active three times a week after that. After the four months of supervised training, the participants were expected to continue the training independently. The physical training supervised by physiotherapists used standardized exercises for strength and endurance. The health-related outcomes of the overall study ($N = 1156$; Roessler & Ibsen, 2009) showed an overall weight loss and improved fitness level from baseline to 12 months after start of the study. However, a second analysis of the results showed that some patients gained weight during the study, and the majority those patients were less likely to participate in the follow-up counseling after 12 months and had an increased tendency to drop out compared to the patients who lost weight. Therefore, we need a deeper understanding of the psychological processes supporting a lasting behavioral and emotional change with regard to physical activity.

For this reason, patients from five geographically different physiotherapy clinics in Copenhagen were included in an interview study to account for the different economic and social conditions of these quarters. Ninety semistructured interviews with 30 patients were conducted at baseline, four months after, and one year after having started their exercise by prescription. 22 women and eight men participated; the average age was 60 years. Several steps were taken to establish the reliability of the study and to validate its findings. First, the semistructured interview guides were designed using open questions to allow specific perspectives of the interviewees to be reflected. Second, an interview technique based on a psychodynamic approach was used (Streeck & Leichsenring, 2009), creating an empathic and safe atmosphere (see the previous description). Validation was given by the participants who were asked to confirm or refute the author's findings of the first interview at the beginning of the second and third interview.

A comparison of the participants interviewed and the total sample showed similarities with regard to sex, age, education, fitness level, and self-reported age. The participants were asked to provide information about their motivation, experience, and how they had changed their health and exercise behavior, including their expectations as well as self-assessment of their physical form, their experiences with mental motivational barriers, their attitudes toward physical activity and health in general, and reasons for changes in state of mind and

TABLE 21.2 Example of Interpretation of Quotes

Participant's spontaneous quote	Recurrent theme	Additional categories	Future questions
"I never expected to love the rowing machine. But I love it—I don't want to lose against her, I give everything" (male, 63 years old)	Enjoying being competitive	Motivating role of the training machines; machine as dialogue "partner"; gender aspect of competition	Role of *competition* and *control* in motivation

in relations—to the GP, partner, or family—during the period. The question of how the participant was affected by the fact that the training was organized in *groups* was given primary focus. The author talked with the participants individually, the first time at the physiotherapy clinic to create an atmosphere of trust, the second and third times at the participants' homes. These conversations were tape-recorded and subsequently transcribed verbatim. The transcripts were first broadly examined to identify recurrent themes among participants relating, for example, to motivation and expectation. Afterwards, the transcripts underwent closer analysis to refine emerging themes, focusing in more detail on the group aspects. The themes emerging from the first and second interviews were reported back to the participants at the beginning of the last interview. One example of the method of interpretation of the data is provided in Table 21.2. The participants' spontaneous responses were analyzed to identify recurrent themes and additional analytical categories. Three topics were central, namely, interpersonal relationships, existential emotions, and the experience of physical activity and their influence on individual behavior (Roessler, 2011).

Motives for and Barriers to Exercise Participation

The participants named seven motives for starting physical activity: to improve health, to lose weight, to reduce fear of dying, to improve well-being, to gain support, to be more physically active, and to enhance social interaction. These motives are often found in participants of interventions using physical activity as treatment (Biddle & Mutrie, 2005).

The most frequently named motives for participating in exercise were losing weight, getting psychological support, and fear of dying. Overweight characterized the majority of the participants interviewed, even though the three diagnoses identified as inclusion criteria—type 2 diabetes, hypertension, and dyslipidemia—are different, and both hypertension and diabetes can be developed without increasing weight. Participants identified the second motivation—getting psychological support—as the need for a psychological incentive, a "kick," to start a new way of living. This wish for a "kick" is interpreted as a wish for a *corrective emotional experience*. The third motive, fear of dying, was recognized in two ways. It was cited as a reason to engage in exercise as a response to a threat to life that had already been experienced, such as a thrombosis or a stroke. Here the motivation was to prevent another such event. The threat of heart failure after being physical active was also mentioned as a motive for *avoiding* exercise before starting physically the program.

Motives such as an interest in social interaction were mentioned occasionally but seldom appeared as a primary expectation. Some participants almost explicitly expressed anger at the assumption that they could participate for social reasons. In the first interviews seven participants mentioned that they were definitely *not* looking for any private networks or social contacts but were solely trying to improve their state of health.

The quantitative survey of the participants' expectations (Roessler & Ibsen, 2009) supported these findings, namely, that weight loss was the main motive while social aspects were of less interest. During the second and third interviews, immediately after the intervention and 1 year later, the weighting of these motives for participation, however, had changed. While weight loss continued as a main motive for participating, social motives increased. When they had finished the program, the majority of the participants reported that social aspects had motivated them. To know that the training group was waiting for them, to see how others struggled or succeeded with different exercises, and not feeling alone with being overweight were all reported as significant motivations.

The physiotherapists had a crucial role in maintaining physical activity in the groups. At the start of the intervention, the physiotherapist was seen as a person who gave "a kick" or extrinsic motivation, whereas later the role became that of an important other who gave care or attention. This is discussed next. The physiotherapist, the training group, and the family had a supportive role in the individual's motivation, but while the physiotherapist was central for the first four months, the group and especially the family were important for long-term motivation.

Characteristics of the Non-completers

The non-completers reported four reasons for dropping out or not maintaining a physical lifestyle—lack of weight loss, lack of time, lack of motivation, and lack of support. There may be more reasons. Some female participants claimed that exercise repetitions in the clinic were boring and annoying. However, the main reason for dropping out was disappointment about the lack of individual success. All of these participants put on weight; for them the result was a failure in relation to their main motives for participation. Compared to the adherent group, these participants had no episodes of weight loss at all that they could relate to increased physical activity.

Another frequent explanation for not exercising was the problem of "finding" time or support for exercise. Several participants reported that they felt that their family or partner was a barrier to exercising. The family or the partner can be an obstacle because of the demands they make or their lack of support. The participants had mentioned the expectation of an external "kick" or support as a motivating factor, while the family or the partner in some cases obviously could not fulfill this function and on the contrary acted as a barrier. For those participants who stopped exercising, fear of dying had lost its force as a primary motivation. Neither the experience of coronary thrombosis nor the recommendations of their GP could motivate them to exercise regularly.

The disappointment felt by the patients had two causes: either the training brought no measurable progress—for instance, weight loss—or the participants could not motivate themselves to exercise. One participant described the problem of motivating himself as "an appointment with your GP, but not with yourself." The lack of success seemed sometimes to be reduced to a question of personality. A 64-year-old male participant diagnosed himself and his family as "too lazy." For him, being overweight had been a lifelong condition. Almost all patients described their "failure" to exercise as a problem related to interaction, both intrapersonal and interpersonal. At the intrapersonal level, the formulation "I can't pull myself together" sets up an image of two people—one pulling the other. The motivated person cannot pull the lazy one, and it seems as if the lazy part wins over the motivated part. Another dimension was to feel broken, as not having control over their own existence, which was perceived as feeling fragmented. Regarding interpersonal interaction, the question of support or lack of support was crucial. Dropout participants described their family, partner, and GP as nonsupportive. Let us now have a comparative look at the participants who did complete the intervention.

Characteristics of the Completers

The participants who *were* able to complete the training and to change their exercise behavior reported three main reasons for this: the experience of feeling better during and after exercise, the supportive effect of structure, and the support of the group. Feeling better during and after exercise seemed to come as a surprise to the majority of the participants interviewed, who had often had negative experiences of exercise. Now, they improved their capacity for exercise and reported this to be both an indicator of health benefits and a correction of their self-image. The supportive function of the feedback on structured exercising was particularly highlighted by participants. Five of the eight male participants were thrilled by the possibility of being able to compete with the rowing machine. The "objective" information given by the machine, reporting distance, time, or just burned kilojoules, had the effect of external feedback. The physiotherapists were given the role of a "tough—but caring" parent, while the group members became encouraging siblings. "Most of us don't have the backbone

TABLE 21.3 Themes of Subgroups of Participants (Completers vs Non-completers)

	Subgroup	
Theme	**Non-completers**	**Completers**
Corrective emotional experience	Unpleasant feelings during exercise; no development through data points; confirmation of attitude; no readiness to change	Fun in competition with the machines; development through data points; lasting motivation from the machine data; experience that the group matters; structure and fixed patterns support change
Feedback	Feedback has no meaning	Machines give feedback; feedback supports motivation
Cohesion	No cohesion in the group	Building cohesion in the training group
Group climate	Lack of interest in the other group members	Teasing each other during the training sessions; taking the advice of the physiotherapist seriously
Control	Lack of control—the body and subconsciousness take over; the rigid structure is negative	Body control is life control; control by the rigid structure is positive
Social support	Lack of family support; family or partner remains inactive	Behavioral change of the patient is an integrated project of family or partner

to exercise on our own and we will stay home if it is raining. But knowing that four idiots will give you a telling-off if you didn't show up—well, that's enough to make me show up" (male, 61 years old). Overall the psychological effect of exercise was greater trust in one's ability to perform, reduced fatigue, and improved self-confidence (Table 21.3).

The idea behind the analysis of Case 1 was that an intervention that worked with a *holding attitude* of physiotherapists, the *feedback* of other group members, and a focus on *existential motives* such as fear of dying could counteract negative attitudes to exercise and provide a corrective emotional experience. It was assumed that this experience would support long-term change in health behavior. The analysis supported this with empirical material.

My goal in this chapter is to identify aspects of interpersonal learning in the context of health promotion with an exercise program. Research over recent decades has provided evidence that low social support and social isolation increase morbidity of cardiovascular disease (Kaplan et al., 1988) and that health behavior (such as exercise) has psychosocial dimensions (Williams, Vita, Manuck, Selwyn, & Kaplan, 1991).

Existential aspects such as fear of dying can motivate people and make them remain active. Many patients are in increased danger of a cardiac thrombosis or stroke. Near-death experiences or a warning from a concerned doctor seem to be good motivators to begin an exercise program. It is evident, however, that fear of death provides no lasting motivation for the majority of patients who would prefer to rely on pharmacological support rather than exercising. Many patients blame their lack of commitment on lack of time, lack of interest, or lack of knowledge. They ask for a superior and more rigid structure, that is, they want to leave responsibility to an external institution. In terms of psychology, this behavior can be seen as "regressive," as going back to an earlier stage of development (Balint, 1968). Patients who adhere successfully to a program see themselves at times as dependent on the physiotherapist. Once routines of exercising are established, participants can "grow" and take a more self-determined "adult" position.

A problem of this intervention was, however, that health professionals—such as the GPs and physiotherapists—were not trained in the interactional approach. A corrective emotional experience requires protected circumstances, empathy, and awareness from the therapist (Streeck, 2007). The health providers in this case study were young and obviously good at "kicking their participants," but they were not necessarily schooled to deploy the empathy or awareness that might be necessary to change long-term behavior. This can potentially change some participants' emotional response from therapeutic regression to a feeling of marginalization. Thus, the social arrangement of the training can work either as a barrier or as a motivation. For the completers in this study, the physiotherapist and the training group created a supportive environment. They became "siblings" with a common attitude toward exercise, sharing the feeling of all being in the same boat, and the opportunity to motivate each other. Their affective relations drawn from the primary family could explain the sense of cohesiveness created within the exercise group (Biddle & Mutrie, 2005). In this case, however, family and partners were mostly mentioned as demanding and nonsupportive, for example, because of unhelpful nutritional habits. This finding can be explained by the overrepresentation of lower socioeconomic status in diseases such as type 2 diabetes and dyslipidemia (Adler, Boyce, & Chesney, 1994). While Case 1 addressed a broad and heterogeneous population of participants with different lifestyle diseases, Case 2 concentrates on a specific group of clinical patients.

CASE 2: EXERCISE AND POLYCYSTIC OVARY SYNDROME—A CLINICAL INTERVENTION

Polycystic ovary syndrome (PCOS) is the most common endocrine disorder in women of reproductive age with a prevalence of 5–10% (Glintborg & Andersen, 2010). The disease is characterized by polycystic ovaries, menstrual dysfunction, and hyperandrogenism and is associated with many health risks including abdominal obesity, hypertension, hyperlipidemia, and insulin resistance (Dokras, 2008). More than 50% of the women with PCOS are overweight (Legro, Kunselman, Dodson, & Dunaif, 1999). In women with PCOS, changes in appearance, particularly obesity and unwanted hair growth (hirsutism), can reduce psychological well-being, while endocrine and metabolic parameters as well as menstrual irregularities and infertility seem to be less important (Hahn et al., 2005). Women with PCOS are significantly more prone to anxiety, depression, and low self-esteem (Barry, Kuczmierczyk, & Hardiman, 2011), and the challenges to feminine identity—such as hirsutism and menstrual problems—have an impact on mood, relationships, and psychological well-being (Teede, Deeks, & Moran, 2010). Low quality of life in women with PCOS may affect the patients' desire and ability to exercise and change their lifestyle (Glintborg & Andersen, 2010). Therefore, it is important to identify psychological and communicative aspects that are supportive for self-esteem and behavioral change.

Studies on the effect of exercise training on PCOS have shown positive effects on maximal oxygen uptake, weight, waist circumference (Brown et al., 2009b; Giallauria et al., 2009), and depression (Thomsen et al., 2010). Exercise has in general shown improved self-experienced quality of life both for nonclinical and clinical populations (Gorczynski & Faulkner, 2010), and especially group interventions have often shown positive psychological effects (Biddle & Mutrie, 2005). Group treatments combining disorder-specific and transfer-oriented aspects have shown positive results, and an intervention starting with a focus on communication about disease might support the opportunity to express emotional distress and to develop positive relationship patterns, which can facilitate a long-term change of health behavior (Nickel, Ademmer, & Egle, 2010).

One qualitative study looked at the impact of physical activity in combination with group counseling (Roessler, Birkebaek, Ravn, Andersen, & Glintborg, 2013b). Designed as a crossover study, it tested the effect of a high-intensity training program on weight, waist circumference, and quality of life of PCOS patients. Among the clinical results, statistically significant decreases in waist circumference and body mass index (BMI) and an increase in aerobic capacity were found; weight loss tended to be highest in the group that started with group counseling (Roessler et al., 2012).

In the counseling sessions, a psychodynamic approach was used (Roessler, 2010, 2011) in order to concentrate on the role of interpersonal relations for commitment to behavioral change. The aim of the study was to improve the cardiorespiratory fitness and quality of life in overweight and obese women with PCOS. For this, an understanding of the psychological and communicative processes during the group-counseling period is needed. The hypothesis was that group psychological treatment would enhance health behavior by focusing on disorder-specific aspects as well as on interpersonal problems from earlier experiences in the patients' lives, and the research questions aimed at understanding the influence of emotional experiences during the group sessions on changes in health and exercise behavior.

Patients were recruited via the Department of Endocrinology and the Department of Gynaecology and Obstetrics, Odense University Hospital. Women who met the diagnostic criteria for PCOS and had a BMI of 25–40 were invited to participate in the study. Exclusion criteria included pregnancy, diabetes, eating disorders, and the use of metformin or oral contraceptive pills. Patients with a history of cardiac angina or other physical symptoms that would limit exercise performance were excluded. Twenty-four women attended an information meeting, and 17 women aged 19–46 years agreed to participate. They were moderately obese with a mean BMI of 36.3 and a mean waist girth of 115.2 cm. The weight of the women varied between 72 and 127 kg, with a mean of 101 kg. After a baseline assessment, the participants were randomized to eight weeks of high-intensity aerobic exercise and eight weeks of 90-min group counseling per week, in a crossover design. The women underwent testing at baseline (week 0), crossover (week 8), and postintervention (week 16). The exercise program (described and analyzed in Roessler et al., 2013b) was conducted three days per week with indoor cycling and running.

Analysis of the Group Counseling

Group counseling sessions took place once a week for eight weeks. Each session lasted 90 min and was led by a psychologist. The aim of the counseling sessions was to improve the psychological and communicative skills of the participants with the ambition to encourage a health-oriented lifestyle. Skills were understood as (1) the ability to perceive others with *empathy*, *acceptance*, and unconditional positive *regard* (Rogers, 1951); (2) the ability to give *feedback* to other group members with regard to their experiences, for example, health-related problems; and (3) the ability to express communicative and behavioral experiences that changed attitudes toward health behavior.

The program was intended to enable participants to express emotions and receive support by communicating with emotion-focused expressions. Albrecht, Burleson, and Sarason (1992) showed that supportive interactions and relationships have a major role in physical health, emotional well-being, and performance. Especially emotion-focused expressions play a positive role (Burleson & Mortenson, 2003). Combining communication research with a psychodynamic perspective is important to appreciate the patient's disturbed attachment and relationship patterns. The term "corrective emotional experience" is understood as the ability to be empathic and supportive. Therefore, the focus of attention was directed toward the ability to give support by responding to other group members (Roessler, 2011). The investigation looked specifically at the motivating role of learning taking place among the participants and their environment.

During the group counseling sessions, the psychologist used a technique based on psychodynamic group therapy (Streeck & Leichsenring, 2009) to create an empathic and safe atmosphere. The psychologist tried to accept the individual reality rather than modify it. The patients' current experiences of their disease provided the background for each session. Through feedback, the psychologist revealed his or her own experience in a selective and purposeful way. This is based on an interactional method that assumes that the everyday challenges and problems of the participants will repeat in a group situation and should enable the participants to change their behavior or attitude in a supportive environment (Leichsenring et al., 2004).

To establish the reliability of the study and to validate its findings, methods were applied as previously described. The observations were structured as eight questions that are used in psychodynamic interactional therapy to analyze the group process (Streeck & Leichsenring, 2009); 2 postgraduate students coded and analyzed the tapes and the observations individually based on the question guide (see above). To sustain the intercoder reliability, the researchers coded the tapes individually and separately. After the coding process, the main themes were described and analyzed with a focus on the ability to give feedback, express empathy and acceptance, and describe changes in emotional experiences.

Topics Mentioned by the Patients

The participants talked about several topics during the group sessions. The group sessions showed different interactions, ranging from café meetings full of laughter and confessions—"I ate two chocolate bars that weekend"—to therapeutic sessions with a focus on individual problems. However, three topics emerged as most important in the group counseling sessions, namely, the influence of PCOS on daily life, existential emotions such as shame, and the experience of difficulties in changing lifestyle (Table 21.4). Especially for newly diagnosed patients, the disease was full of mysteries. The most important concern was connected to their bodily appearance, especially how to hide the increased hair growth. The hair growth was connected with self-esteem—a lot of hair was associated with lack of self-esteem and a reduced quality of life. The age difference in the two counseling groups seemed not to influence the group climate.

Encouraging Relationships

Three subgroups emerged during the group sessions. Nine of the participants built three smaller groups, each with a group cohesion of their own. Three of the younger women developed a certain pattern of relationship during the last counseling group sessions, which can be called teasing. The "teasers" constantly mocked each other, especially in the form of comments about their overweight and eating behavior. In the physical training sessions following the group counseling, they continued this pattern, commenting on their indoor cycling and bodily appearance. The universality of their suffering was their being overweight, their low self-esteem, and the problem of finding a partner.

Three of the middle-aged females, in their 40s, built another group, the "sisters." They all had well-established lives with marriage, jobs, and children. They

TABLE 21.4 Example of an Analysis of the Communication During Group Sessions (Roessler et al., 2013b)

Content	Results
What are the participants talking about?	PCOS and symptoms, especially hirsutism (hair growth); psychological aspects: shame, anxiety regarding telling others about the diagnosis; problems concerning food control and being overweight; importance of social support; difficulties in changing lifestyle
How can you describe the interaction?	Café meeting: laughter, mocking; therapy session: concentration, empathy, grief
Are there common rules or norms?	Precise start of the sessions; openness to talking about private issues; change from focus on the group leader to focus on the participants
Which emotions do the participants mention?	Shame about the hirsutism; shyness about showing up in a swimming suit or in the gym; relief about others with same problems and experiences; anger about the prejudice of nonoverweight people
Which emotions are visible?	Empathy, compassion, grief
Are there special relations between participants?	"The sisters"; "the curious"; "the teasers"
How can the participant differentiate?	Group members often anticipate situations, reflect on how people will comment or think about their overweight
What does the group leader do?	Changing from taking responsibility for the structure of the group session in the start to handing responsibility over to the group members in the following sessions

PCOS, polycystic ovary syndrome

did not tease each other but had a certain relationship by supporting each other in their everyday problems. One of them got divorced, on which they spent a lot of communication. Compared to the younger participants in the project, their self-esteem and quality of life was not affected by their disease, especially because they had not experienced problems with fertility. They instead talked about their motivation and issues of maintaining healthy food-related behavior. For example, they were planning to train together for a 5-km race during summer. The "sisters" were creating a different dimension of group cohesion from that of the "teasers"—their solidarity being based on their commitment to their families rather than on individual fun. As one of them said, "*My duty towards my children is to stay healthy.*"

A third subgroup, the "curious," consisted of three younger and newly diagnosed patients. Their common theme was their disease. They were curious to know more about the disease and to share experiences and knowledge especially about their problems and concerns, for example, with fertility or hirsutism. Especially the youngest of them was anxious about not being able to get pregnant. At the beginning of the group counseling sessions, she had not yet told her boyfriend about PCOS, because she was ashamed about the unwanted hair growth. The "curious" worked as a research team; they shared information—for example, where to get laser therapy, how to get the financial support—and they supported each other. The "curious" were focused on the dimension of hope.

The three subgroups showed different approaches to dealing with their disease. The "teasers" had a self-ironical approach, responding to the other members in a humorous way. The irony allowed them to discuss serious themes—such as the difficulty of finding a partner—in a light and innocent way. The "curious" had a similar light way of responding but acted more as a common research team. Their approach functioned as encounter, where old and new information about the disease could be exchanged. The "sisters" in contrast were most personal and private. They considered substantial answers, trying to bear the others' pain and maintain the desirable change of behavior.

The categories feedback, group cohesion, suffering, and corrective emotional experiences were meaningful for the analyses of the project material. Especially the feedback given by the other group members was very helpful for the development of group cohesion. Similarities in suffering supported the group climate. The group sometimes functioned as a place for confession and absolution. The experiences of success or failure influenced the change of behavior. All members of the counseling group had experiences with failed diet and were relieved by the confessions of other group members. Maintenance of physical activity was especially supported in the group who started with counseling sessions before the physical intervention.

Avoiding Social Isolation by Cohesiveness

Case 2 describes an intervention designed to identify additional psychological and communicative skills of patients undergoing an exercise and group counseling intervention. The results underline how important it is to express emotional experiences, to support group members through feedback, and to engage in exchange with patients who have the same disease. Research over the past decades has provided evidence that low social support and social isolation increase morbidity (Kaplan et al., 1988). Psychosocial dynamics and health behavior are connected (Williams et al., 1991). The overall attendance rate of almost 70% in the presented case can be interpreted as a positive result, considering that the participants had to motivate themselves for up to three weekly meetings.

If groups train together and are supported by counseling, this enhances the group cohesion, the motivation to follow an exercise intervention, and in general the quality of life (Chachamovich et al., 2010). It was therefore important to find out if aerobic exercise in groups combined with group counseling sessions would exert the same beneficial effects as previously demonstrated in studies focusing on individual training of women with PCOS, or whether it could improve the results.

The results showed that communication in a health intervention can be supportive, indeed. Because of their overweight, many PCOS patients are at an increased risk of cardiac thrombosis. It is evident, however, that individual fear provides no lasting motivation for the majority of the patients who would prefer surgery rather than exercise. Often patients blame their lack of commitment on lack of time, lack of interest, or lack of knowledge, and these patients ask for a superior and more rigid structure that would help devolve a part of their personal responsibility to an external institution (Roessler, 2011). In this study, it became clear that patients who adhered successfully to the program saw themselves as being connected not to a rigid structure but to other patients. The communication of emotional experiences, as suggested earlier, required protected circumstances, empathy, and awareness from the therapist (Streeck & Leichsenring, 2009). Here the social group condition evidently delivered motivation. The group created a supportive environment. The patients became "siblings" with a common attitude toward their disease. Sharing the feeling of all being in the same boat gave the participants an opportunity to motivate each other. If there were affective relations drawn from the primary family, this would explain the sense of cohesiveness created within the exercise group (Biddle & Mutrie, 2005). Interestingly, the threatening infertility—usually the main complication of the disease—was less important than other issues for the quality of life of the patients (in accordance with Hahn et al., 2005).

The results of the study indicate a significant postintervention reduction in weight and BMI among those who started with group counseling. The findings may therefore suggest a beneficial effect of group counseling *before* exercise. Furthermore, the women who started with counseling may have enhanced their motivation to change lifestyle during the group counseling sessions, and they may have started changes on a cognitive and emotional level, which resulted in a larger weight loss. This could also help explain the significant reduction in waist girth after the group counseling sessions. If one combines training and counseling sessions from the beginning of an intervention, this might be the most effective strategy to improve and sustain results. Future research requires studies of a longer duration examining the effects of high-intensity aerobic exercise in groups and group counseling sessions on overweight and obese women with PCOS.

In both Case 1 and Case 2, the participants were populations in which the main focus was on somatic diseases. The last case targets a population with high incidence of psychological and psychiatric symptoms, namely, addicts.

CASE 3: EXERCISE AND SUBSTANCE USE DISORDER—THE DANGER OF RELAPSE

The misuse of alcohol and drugs is a central issue for public health. Alcohol and drug consumption affects overall disease, and compared to the people of other countries, the Danish population has a large intake of alcohol (Hansen et al., 2011). Evidence-based treatment of alcohol and drug dependence includes different psychological interventions and forms of pharmacological treatment. However, the outcomes are limited (Cutler & Fishbain, 2005; Miller & Willbourne, 2002). Therefore, we have a strong need for developing new interventions to increase the effectiveness of treatment.

Physical exercise related to substance abuse is a quite new but promising treatment option (Read & Brown, 2003; Moore & Werch, 2005; Roessler, 2010; Roessler et al., 2013a; Sari, Bilberg, Søgaard-Nielsen, Nielsen, & Roessler, 2013). It can be used both as early prevention and as part of a continuous treatment process (Collingwood, Sunderlin, Reynolds, & Kohl, 2000; Biddle & Mutrie, 2005). There are several benefits of exercise for alcohol abusers. For example, exercise, especially moderate exercise (Monti et al., 2000), can decrease the urge to take substances. In addition, exercise can offer positive alternatives by providing pleasurable states, for example, through dopaminergic reinforcement (Read & Brown, 2003). Most important for adherence is probably that exercise improves psychosocial outcomes, such as mood management (Lane & Lovejoy, 2001), and reduces depression and anxiety (Martinsen, 2004; Babyak et al., 2000; DiLorenzo et al., 1999). In addition, resilience factors such as individual and social resources are strengthened by regular physical activity, especially as group activity (Brown et al., 2009a; Read & Brown, 2003).

Case 3 describes the experiences and outcomes of two interventions that used physical exercise in ambulant group treatments of patients with drug addiction and alcohol-abuse patients. The intervention with drug-addicted patients was carried out as a collaboration between West Zealand County Council and the University of Southern Denmark. It explored whether physical exercise can change behavior through an increased bodily awareness and self-confidence (Roessler, 2010). The second intervention was an offer to alcohol-abuse patients in Odense to participate in physical activity on a voluntary basis (Roessler et al., 2013a).

The drug addicts took part in different exercise activities focusing both on maximum oxygen uptake and social activity, such as spinning, running, volleyball, and badminton. The alcohol patients participated in a weekly running session.

The patients with drug addiction were selected through the Slagelse Addiction Centre or through social-service agencies. Drug addiction included cannabis, opiates, medicine, amphetamines, cocaine, and heroin. The team of the day clinic decided who among the about 60 users had the resources to participate in the intervention. People whose physical condition was too poor to exercise were excluded. Participants who missed three training sessions unexcused, who had to serve a prison sentence during the course of the intervention, or who committed a criminal offense while it was under way were likewise excluded. The patients being treated for alcohol abuse were recruited through Odense's alcohol treatment center.

Thirty-eight people with drug addiction who attended the day clinic were included. Their average age was 35 years. Only a few participants had their own income, and half of them had an abuse lasting longer than 10 years. The patients being treated for alcohol abuse were included in a pilot study. They were either working or unemployed; their average age was older. The pilot study took place in the treatment center at Odense. The patients participated on a voluntary basis and the experiences were integrated in the design of a large study (Sari et al., 2013).

Overall the goal was to change addiction behavior through exercise treatment. After finishing the interventions, the participants reported a better sense of the body expressed both as increased awareness of physical markers such as pulse and breathing, but also as increased sensitivity to pain. Generally, the participants reported a changed bodily awareness and a higher energy level. The increased energy level contributed to the participants' ability to cope with other duties of everyday life. Participants also reported a new self-confidence, since sports had provided an experience of being able to do more than they were aware they could. Several participants being treated for addiction spoke of the physical "kick" they got out of sport, one describing it even as similar to taking drugs. After the training phase, they all expressed their sense of a new quality of life, and new dreams or ideas for a future life.

Many of the participants revealed that they had only had few social relations at the start of the intervention. Some talked about how they had difficulties participating in social contexts. But at the end of the intervention, several participants were prepared to enter into social environments. Regarding adherence, two factors—in addition to the instructor's role—were shown to be of high importance and had an impact on behavior change: *feedback* and *suffering*. Feedback was related to the climate in the group. The participants experienced the running situation as a social context. In the empathic and safe environment, the level of honesty in giving feedback to others was high. The participants reported that exercising had a positive influence on their social relations, and the feedback of the instructor and the other group members increased their commitment. In this project, the group size was dependent on the participants who attended the running sessions twice per week. Therefore, feedback among the participants and between the instructor and the participants influenced commitment.

The experience of alcohol and drug misuse was—though not discussed explicitly—the common experience that created an emotional context. One participant (36 years old) said, "I would never talk to a group led by a psychologist about my alcohol problem. But when running together, I can express myself and have a little talk about my life."

Challenges when Working with Drug- and Alcohol-Abuse Patients

When working in the field of substance abuse, dropping out, lack of adherence, and relapse are a major problem (Cutler & Fishbain, 2005; Pedersen &

Hesse, 2009). A first barrier must be overcome by involving participants in lifestyle change and by increasing compliance. In the studies reported in Case 3, the patients participated on a voluntary basis and had expressed high interest in advance, but quite a number dropped out nevertheless. Some patients got upset at the fitness test at baseline because of their poor results, while others dropped out due to lack of energy or could not attend the training because of time issues. Lack of energy and motivation or injuries are often mentioned as barriers for change of behavior (Biddle & Mutrie, 2005). International studies of treatment projects for substance abusers have stressed two aspects of treatment in particular—the social element and the physical sensation (Donaghy & Ussher, 2005).

Physically, substance abusers get into better shape through programs (Brown et al., 2014). Regular physical exercise leads to an improvement in maximal oxygen intake, which finds expression in their fitness levels. In itself, it is not surprising that fitness levels improve, since this nearly always happens when a person is trained over a period of time. But the qualitative results of the substance-abuse treatment support the hypothesis that better fitness reduces the suffering associated with abstinence, a finding that has been supported by research about withdrawal symptoms of nicotine abuse and physical activity (Taylor & Ussher, 2005). The reduced intake could also be interpreted as a reinforcement (Smith, Schmidt, Iordanou, & Mustorph, 2008). Another central issue was that participants reported they could "feel" their body in a way that was different from before.

Socially, addicts may be especially vulnerable due to their lack of self-control and higher level of depression (Martinsen, 2004). International research studies have stressed in particular the social element and physical fitness (Donaghy & Ussher, 2005). There is a powerful link between the establishment of secondary networks and freedom from substance abuse after the end of treatment. Many of the participants had a tendency to be socially isolated and saw only a limited number of people in their daily lives. But this changed after treatment, with all of them reporting that they were now more open to the idea of becoming a part of new social contexts.

Also Case 3 shows the importance of social relationships and interpersonal learning in treatment. The organized and time-scheduled training and the engagement of the instructor helped the participants to exercise, and the training group gave space for interpersonal learning and positive feedback. Another social aspect might be the establishment of a secondary network. Peer group influence is central for maintenance of motivation; the same is true for the relationship to a trustworthy instructor.

Exercise alone can surely not change a lifelong addiction problem; it has to be an add-on to usual treatment, such as medical treatment and counseling. However, exercise can help patients become more independent and healthier. Exercise can distract thoughts, can become a "self-care" strategy (Collingwood et al., 2000), and can provide a possibility for self-control through body control.

GENERAL DISCUSSION

Health interventions using exercise to change lifestyle might end in failure because of high dropout rates or low adherence of vulnerable patient populations. Therefore, future studies should focus more on the central role of the instructor and group, as well as on the social network of the patients—partner, friends—to maintain compliance. Highly important is also the question of how to integrate a new behavior into the daily environment of the participants.

Improving Self-Image and Control Through Bodily Learning

For most of the involved patients and participants, the overall motivation was *getting a grip* on their own life. They expected changes of habits through bodily learning. Physical activity can act as a "self-care" strategy (Drumm, McBride, Metsch, Neufeld, & Sawatsky, 2005), particularly by improving people's self-image. Exercise provides the opportunity to distract oneself from the urge to take substances or food. Usually, physical pain is understood as a negative result, but here, it can be connected with an increased awareness of the body. All the participants in these three cases had a better sense of their body and, therefore, of pain and other physical problems than before they participated in a program. Participants felt their body whether they were out of breath or in pain. Through physical activity and an increased focus not only on physical markers such as pulse and exhaustion, but also on experiences like enjoyment and the feeling of having bodily control during activities, participants become more conscious of their bodies. Exercise treatment cannot change lifelong attitudes over a period of a few months, but it can offer a feeling of being in control. The challenge for practitioners is to focus on these bodily and interpersonal dimensions to identify further aspects and to strengthen compliance with exercise treatments in health science.

Group Dynamics

The case observations showed that it was very important to create a motivational environment around the group interventions and exercise sessions. It was of high importance that the instructor be receptive to the participants' questions, problems, and stories. Within the group interventions, different group dynamics developed. Two group processes in interventions with a focus on changing behavior were especially important: *feedback* and the universality of *suffering*. The participants experienced the movement environments as a social context, where the atmosphere encouraged them to react to others in a light way. The participants reported that the encouraging responses of instructor or group members increased their commitment. The common experience of a certain health-related problem—addiction, hormonal problems, pain, or nutrition habits—also supported the participants' exchange and commitment.

Health-related interventions often include recommendations for enhancing intrinsic motivation or self-determination (Ryan & Deci, 2000), but the specific theoretical point of view presented here suggests further recommendations. First, it is important to recognize that health interventions that focus on individual life threats may end in failure. Fear of death can provide a "kick-start" for motivating participation in exercise, but its impact decreases over the course of the intervention. The first recommendation, therefore, is to avoid threatening health campaigns, as they are unlikely to be successful. The second recommendation relates to feedback and support. If participants rely on personal feedback alone for confirmation, the chances of achieving high adherence levels are slight. However, when participants are exercising alone, focusing on more specific feedback information (eg, length of exercise, repetitions, training distance provided by heart rate monitors) can support the maintenance of a program. Highly motivated people with time-consuming jobs often want to exercise alone and in a self-organized way. They can relate to these monitors as external feedback. For people who lack inner structure, time-scheduled exercises in a stable group with continuous feedback from training machines can lead to a higher level of commitment because the structure of the exercise helps them relinquish responsibility. The time and exercise structures relieve the pressure on the participant and lead to a therapeutic regression, which supports a corrective emotional experience.

The third recommendation points to the need to strengthen interpersonal learning. Two central challenges were highlighted in these three cases. The first concerns the extent to which the existing social environment of the participants works as a barrier. Families and partners must become part of the project, helping the participants change their lifestyle. The second challenge concerns the training group as a place for interpersonal learning through corrective emotional experiences. In future research, greater attention should be devoted to group situations and group-oriented approaches.

These new insights demand an increased focus on the human resources of general practitioners and physiotherapists who handle the training. They should learn (1) about their supportive role for the participants, especially at the beginning of an intervention, (2) about the regressive urges of the participants, and (3) about the benefits of promoting group relations. The challenge is to focus on these interpersonal dimensions to identify further aspects of interaction in health science.

REFERENCES

Adler, N. E., Boyce, T., & Chesney, M. A. (1994). Socioeconomic status and health. The challenge of the gradient. *American Psychologist, 49*, 15–24.

Albrecht, T. L., Burleson, R., & Sarason, I. (1992). Meaning and method in the study of communication and social support: An introduction. *Communication Research, 19*, 149–153.

Alexander, F., & French, T. M. (1946). *Psychoanalytic therapy: Principles and application.* New York, NY: Ronald Press.

Babyak, M., Blumenthal, J. A., Herman, S., Khatri, P., Doraiswamy, M., Moore, K., … Krishnan, R. (2000). Exercise treatment for major depressions: maintenance of Therapeutic Benefit at 10 Months. *Psychosomatic Medicine, 62*, 633–638.

Balint, M. (1968). *The basic fault: Therapeutic aspects of regression*. London, England: Tavistock.

Barry, J. A., Kuczmierczyk, A. R., & Hardiman, P. J. (2011). Anxiety and depression in polycystic ovary syndrome: a systematic review and meta-analysis. *Human Reproduction, 26*, 2442–2451.

Biddle, S., & Mutrie, N. (2005). *Psychology of physical activity. Determinants, well-being and interventions*. London, England: Routledge.

Blumenthal, J. A., Babyak, M., Moore, K. A., Craighead, W. E., Herman, S., Khatri, P., ... Krishnan, R. (1999). Effects of exercise training on older patients with major depressions. *Archives of Internal Medicine, 159*, 2349–2356.

Brown, R. A., Abrantes, A. M., Read, J. P., Marcus, B. H., Jakicic, J., Strong, D. R., ... Gordon, A. A. (2009). Aerobic exercise for alcohol recovery: rationale, program description, and preliminary findings. *Behavior Modification, 33*, 220–249.

Brown, R. A., Abrantes, A. M., Minami, H., Read, J. P., Marcus, B. H., Jakicic, J. M., ... Stuart, G. L. (2014). A preliminary, randomized trial of aerobic exercise for alcohol dependence. *Journal of Substance Abuse Treatment, 47*, 1–9.

Brown, A. J., Setji, T. L., Sanders, L. L., Lowry, K. P., Otvos, J. D., Kraus, W. E., & Svetkey, P. L. (2009b). Effects of exercise on lipoprotein particles in women with polycystic ovary syndrome. *Medicine & Science in Sports & Exercise, 41*, 497–504.

Burleson, B. B., & Mortenson, S. R. (2003). Explaining cultural differences in evaluations of emotional support behaviors. Exploring the mediating influences of value systems and interaction goals. *Communication Research, 30*, 113–146.

Chachamovich, J. R., Chachamovich, E., Ezer, H., Fleck, M. P., Knauth, D., & Passos, E. P. (2010). Investigating quality of life and health-related quality of life in infertility: a systematic review. *Journal of Psychosomatic Obstetrics & Gynecology, 31*, 101–110.

Collingwood, T. R., Sunderlin, J., Reynolds, R., & Kohl, H. W. (2000). Physical training as a substance abuse prevention intervention for youth. *Journal of Drug Education, 30*, 435–451.

Cornellisen, V. A., & Fagard, R. H. (2005). Effects of endurance training on blood pressure, blood pressure-regulating mechanisms, and cardiovascular risk factors. *Hypertension, 46*, 667–675.

Cutler, R. B., & Fishbain, D. A. (2005). Are alcoholism treatments effective? The project MATCH data. *BMC Public Health, 5*, 75.

DiLorenzo, T. M., Bargman, E. P., Stucky-Ropp, R., Brassington, G. S., Frensch, P. A., & LaFontaine, T. (1999). Long-term effects of aerobic exercise on psychological outcomes. *Preventive Medicine, 28*, 75–85.

Dokras, A. (2008). Cardiovascular disease risk factors in polycystic ovary syndrome. *Seminars in Reproductive Medicine, 26*, 39–44.

Donaghy, M. E., & Ussher, M. H. (2005). Exercise interventions in drug and alcohol rehabilitation. In: G. E. J. Faulkner, & A. H. Taylor (Eds.), *Exercise, health and mental health* (pp. 48–69). New York, NY: Routledge.

Drumm, R. D., McBride, D., Metsch, L., Neufeld, M., & Sawatsky, A. (2005). "I'm a health nut"! Street drug users' accounts of self-care strategies. *Journal of Drug Issues, 35*, 607–629.

Egle, U. T., Hoffmann, S. O., Lehmann, K. A., & Nix, W. A. (2015). *Handbuch chronischer Schmerz. Grundlagen, Pathogenese, Klinik und Therapie aus bio-psycho-sozialer Sicht*. Stuttgart, Germany: Schattauer.

Faulkner, G. E. J., & Taylor, A. H. (Eds.). (2005). *Exercise, health and mental health: Emerging relationships*. London, England: Routledge.

Giallauria, F., Palomba, S., Vigorito, C., Tafuri, M. G., Colao, A., Lombardi, G., & Orio, F. (2009). Androgens in polycystic ovary syndrome: the role of exercise and diet. *Seminars in Reproductive Medicine, 27*, 306–315.

Glintborg, D., & Andersen, M. (2010). An update on the pathogenesis, inflammation, and metabolism in hirsutism and polycystic ovary syndrome. *Gynecological Endocrinology, 26*, 281–296.

Gorczynski, P., & Faulkner, G. (2010). Exercise therapy for schizophrenia. *Cochrane Database of Systematic Review, 12*(5), CD004412.

Hahn, S., Janssen, O. E., Tan, S., Pleger, K., Mann, K., Schedlowski, M., ... Elsenbruch, S. (2005). Clinical and psychological correlates of quality-of-life in polycystic ovary syndrome. *European Journal of Endocrinology, 153*, 853–860.

Hansen, A. B., Hvidtfeldt, U. A., Grønbæk, M., Becker, U., Nielsen, A. S., & Tolstrup, J. S. (2011). The number of persons with alcohol problems in the Danish population. *Scandinavian Journal of Public Health, 39*, 128–136.

Houmard, J. A., Tanner, C. J., Slentz, C. A., Duscha, B. D., McCartney, J. S., & Kraus, W. E. (2004). Effect of the volume and intensity of exercise training on insulin sensitivity. *Journal of Applied Physiology, 96*, 101–106.

Kaplan, J. R., Salonen, J. T., Cohen, R. D., Brand, R. J., Syme, S. L., & Puska, P. (1988). Social connections and mortality from all causes and cardiovascular disease: prospective evidence from eastern Finland. *American Journal of Epidemiology, 128*, 370–380.

Lane, A. M., & Lovejoy, D. J. (2001). The effects of exercise on mood changes: the moderating effect of depressed mood. *Journal of Sports Medicine and Physical Fitness, 41*, 539–548.

Laurin, D., Verreault, R., & Lindsay, J. (2005). Physical activity and dementia. In: G. E. J. Faulkner, & A. H. Taylor (Eds.), *Exercise, health and mental health: Emerging relationships* (pp. 11–26). London, England: Routledge.

Legro, R. S., Kunselman, A. R., Dodson, W. C., & Dunaif, A. (1999). Prevalence and predictors of risk for type 2 diabetes mellitus and impaired glucose tolerance in polycystic ovary syndrome: a prospective, controlled study in 254 affected women. *Journal of Clinical Endocrinology and Metabolism, 84*, 165–169.

Leichsenring, F., Rabung, S., & Leibing, E. (2004). The efficacy of Short-term Psychodynamic Psychotherapy in Specific Psychiatric Disorders: A Meta-Analysis. *Archives of General Psychiatry, 61*, 1208–1216.

Lewington, S., Clarke, R., Oizilbash, N., Peto, R., & Collins, R. (2002). Prospective studies collaboration. Age-specific relevance of usual blood pressure to vascular mortality: a meta-analysis of individual data for one million adults in 61 prospective studies. *Lancet, 360*, 1903–1913.

Martinsen, E. W. (2004). *Kropp og sinn. Fysisk aktivitet - psykisk helse - kognitiv terapi. [Body and mind. Physical activity—mental health—cognitive therapy].* Bergen, Norway: Fagbogforlaget.

Miller, W. R., & Willbourne, P. L. (2002). Mesa Grande: a methodological analysis of clinical trials of treatments for alcohol use disorders. *Addiction, 97*, 265–277.

Monti, P. M., Rohsenow, D. J., & Hutchison, K. E. (2000). Toward bridging the gap between biological, psychobiological and psychosocial models of alcohol craving. *Addiction, 95*, 229–236.

Moore, M. J., & Werch, C. E. C. (2005). Sport and physical activity participation and substance use among adolescents. *Journal of Adolescent Health, 36*, 486–493.

Nickel, R., Ademmer, K., & Egle, U. T. (2010). Manualized psychodynamic interactional group therapy for the treatment of somatoform pain disorders. *Bulletin Menninger Clinic, 74*, 219–237.

Nygaard Andersen, L., Kohberg, M., Juul-Kristensen, B., Gram Herborg, L., Søgaard, K., & Roessler, K. K. (2014). Psychosocial aspects of everyday life with chronic musculoskeletal pain: a systematic review. *Scandinavian Journal of Pain, 5*, 131–148.

Pedersen, M. U., & Hesse, M. A. (2009). A simple risk scoring system for prediction of relapse after inpatient alcohol treatment. *American Journal of Addiction, 18*, 488–493.

Pedersen, B. K., & Saltin, B. (2006). Evidence for prescribing exercise as therapy in chronic disease. *Scandinavian Journal of Medicine and Science in Sports*, *16*, 3–63.

Read, J. P., & Brown, R. A. (2003). The role of physical exercise in alcohol treatment and recovery. *Professional Psychology*, *34*, 49–56.

Roessler, K. K. (2010). The Odense group approach. *Conference abstract from Nordic Conference 2010 on interdisciplinary perspectives on health, participation and effects of sport and exercise*. Odense, Denmark.

Roessler, K. K. (2011). A corrective emotional experience—or just a bit of exercise? The relevance of interpersonal learning in exercise on prescription. *Scandinavian Journal of Psychology*, *52*, 354–360.

Roessler, K. K., Bilberg, R. M., Jensen, K., Kjærgaard, A. S., Dervisevic, A., & Nielsen, B. (2013a). Exercise as treatment for alcohol dependence: a pilot study. *Sport Science Review*, *12*, 205–216.

Roessler, K. K., Birkebaek, C., Ravn, P., Andersen, M., & Glintborg, D. (2013b). Effects of exercise and group counselling on body composition and VO2$_{max}$ in overweight women with polycystic ovary syndrome. *ACTA Obstreticia et Gynecological Scandinavia*, *92*, 272–277.

Roessler, K. K., Glintborg, D., Ravn, P., Birkebæk, C., & Andersen, M. (2012). Supportive relationships—psychological effects of group counselling in women with polycystic ovary syndrome (PCOS). *Communication & Medicine*, *9*, 125–131.

Roessler, K. K., & Ibsen, B. (2009). Promoting exercise on prescription: recruitment, motivation, barriers and adherence in a Danish community intervention study to reduce type 2 diabetes, dyslipidemia and hypertension. *Journal of Public Health*, *17*, 187–193.

Rogers, C. (1951). *Client-centred therapy*. London, England: Constable.

Ryan, R. M., & Deci, E. L. (2000). Self-determination theory and the facilitation of intrinsic motivation, social development, and well-being. *American Psychologist*, *55*, 68–78.

Sari, S., Bilberg, R., Søgaard-Nielsen, A., Nielsen, B., & Roessler, K. K. (2013). Physical exercise as a supplement to outpatient treatment of alcohol use disorder—a randomized controlled trial. *BMC Psychology*, *1*, 23.

Smith, M. A., Schmidt, K. T., Iordanou, J. C., & Mustroph, M. L. (2008). Aerobic exercise decreases the positive-reinforcing effects of cocaine. *Drug and Alcohol Dependence*, *98*, 129–135.

Sowa, M., & Meulenbroeck, R. (2012). Effects of physical exercise on autism spectrum disorders: a meta-analyses. *Research in Autism Spectrum Disorders*, *6*, 46–57.

Streeck, U. (2007). *Psychotherapie komplexer Persönlichkeitsstörungen.[Psychotherapy of complex personality disorders]*. Stuttgart, Germany: Klett-Cotta.

Streeck, U., & Leichsenring, F. (2009). *Handbuch psychoanalytisch-interaktionelle Therapie. Behandlung von Patienten mit strukturellen Störungen und schweren Persönlichkeitsstörungen. [Handbook of psychodynamic interactional therapy. Treatment of patients with severe personality disorders]*. Göttingen, Germany: Vandenhoeck & Ruprecht.

Taylor, A. H., & Ussher, M. H. (2005). Effects of exercise on smoking cessation and coping with withdrawal symptoms and nicotine cravings. In: G. E. J. Faulkner, & A. H. Taylor (Eds.), *Exercise, health and mental health: Emerging relationships* (pp. 135–158). New York, NY: Routledge.

Teede, H., Deeks, A., & Moran, L. (2010). Polycystic ovary syndrome: a complex condition with psychological, reproductive and metabolic manifestations that impacts on health across the lifespan. *BMC Medicine*, *8*, 41.

Thomsen, R. L., Buckley, J. D., Lim, S. S., Noakes, M., Clifton, P. M., Norman, R. J., & Brinkworth, G. D. (2010). Lifestyle management improves quality of life and depression in overweight and obese women with polycystic ovary syndrome. *Fertility and Sterility*, *94*, 1812–1816.

Thune, I., & Furberg, A. S. (2001). Physical activity and cancer risk: dose response and cancer, all sites and site-specific. *Medicine and Science in Sports & Exercise, 33*, 530–550.

Tuomilehto, J., Lindstrom, J., Eriksson, J. G., Valle, T. T., Hämäläinen, H., Ilanne-Parikka, P., … Uusitupa, M. (2001). Prevention of type 2 diabetes mellitus by changes in lifestyle among subjects with impaired glucose tolerance. *New England Journal of Medicine, 344*, 1343–1350.

Williams, J. K., Vita, J. A., Manuck, S. B., Selwyn, A. P., & Kaplan, J. R. (1991). Psychosocial factors impair vascular responses of coronary arteries. *Circulation, 84*, 2146–2153.

Winnicott, D. (1964). *Psychoanalytic explorations.* London, England: Karnac.

Winnicott, D. W. (1965). *The maturational processes and the facilitating environment.* London, England: Hogarth Press.

Yalom, I., & Leszcz, M. (2005). *The theory and practise of group therapy.* New York, NY: Basic Books.

Zebis, M. K., Andersen, L. L., Pedersen, M. T., Mortensen, P., Andersen, C. H., Pedersen, M. M., … Sjøgaard, G. (2011). Implementation of neck/shoulder exercises for pain relief among industrial workers: a randomized controlled trial. *BMC Musculoskeletal Disorders, 12*, 205.

Index

MMSE. *See* Mini Mental State Examination
(MMSE)
Modeling roles, 239
3×2×2 Model of goals, 232
Moderate-intensity exercise, 45, 389
Moderate-to-vigorous physical activity
(MVPA), 446–447, 449
Momentum TEAMdiagnostik, 356
Mood management, 477
Moods, 399
Moral behaviors, 212
Motivated agent, 293, 300
Motivating role of learning, 462, 472
Motivation, 202, 230, 237, 417. *See also*
Motivational climate
constraints, 229
quality, 425
for sport, 417
themes, 301
achievement, 301
commitment-investment, 302
desirability reward, 302
ease-effort, 302
getting ahead, 302
getting along, 302
learning and personal growth, 301
power, 301
Motivational climate, 221, 233, 349
from achievement goal theory
perspective, 374
ego-oriented, 349
empowering and disempowering features
interplay between objective and
subjective assessments, 380–381
observational assessment of, 379–380
perceptions of, 378
from a self-determination theory
perspective, 375–376
task oriented, 349
Motivational Climate Scale in Youth Sport
(MCSYS), 378
Motor action, 91, 96, 105
levels of action, 98
mental practice, 91
and mental representation development,
learning of, 99
physical practice, 91
system, 92, 112
Motor approach, 95
Motor control, 75, 389
accuracy, 205
and learning, 95
Motor-coordination training, 54

Motor cortex, 59
Motor imagery training, 91, 107
Motor learning, 31, 92, 94, 104
with competitive athletes, 31
with novices, 31
perceptual-cognitive approaches on, 95
perspectives on, 95
cognitive approaches, 95
ecological approaches, 95
processes, 43
Motor performance, 29, 43
Motor skill, 48
acquisition, 48
retention, 48
MPOWER observation system, 379
MRI. *See* Magnetic resonance imaging (MRI)
Multiculturalism, 217, 220, 222
Multicultural societies, 221
Multicultural understanding, 211
Multidimensional Motivational Climate
Objective System (MMCOS),
379, 380
Multiethnic societies, 218
Multilevel transitions, 269

N

Narcissism, 202
Narcissistic leadership literature, 175
Narrative identity, 293
National Institute of Sport, Expertise and
Performance (INSEP), 15
National Olympic Committees (NOCs), 18
National sport organization (NSO), 336
Negative-consequences coping, 256
NEO-FFI-3 serial winners' scores, 299
Neural level, functional changes on, 94
Neurological constraints, 237
Neurophysiology, 201
component, 204
processes, 202
theories, 205
Neuroticism, 205, 299
Ninth European Federation of Sport
Psychology (FEPSAC)
conference, 253
NOCs. *See* National Olympic Committees
(NOCs)
Noise, 201
Nomothetic research approaches, 295
Nonclinical and clinical populations,
health, 461
Noncompleters characteristics, 467–469

Printed in the United States
By Bookmasters